Epidemiologic Research

Epidemiologic Research

PRINCIPLES AND QUANTITATIVE METHODS

David G. Kleinbaum

Lawrence L. Kupper

Hal Morgenstern

JOHN WILEY & SONS, INC.

New York • Chichester • Weinheim • Brisbane • Singapore • Toronto

Library of Congress Cataloging-in-Publication Data:

Kleinbaum, David G.
   Epidemiology research.
   Includes bibliographies and index.
   1. Epidemiology—Research. 2. Epidemiology—Research—
Methodology. I. Kupper, Lawrence L. II. Morgenstern, Hal. III. Title
[DNLM: 1. Epidemiologic methods. 2. Models,
Theoretical. WA950 K64e]
RA652.4.K56   614.4.'072   82-79
ISBN: 0-471-28985-X

Printed in the United States of America

10

Contents

Table List

Preface

This text discusses the principles and methods involved in the planning, analysis, and interpretation of epidemiologic research studies. Our purpose in writing this book is to provide the applied researcher with a synthesis of current methodological thought and practice. In particular, we focus our discussion on quantitative (including statistical) issues that arise during the course of an epidemiologic investigation. Instead of restricting our focus just to statistical techniques and their various applications, we also address issues of study *design, measurement,* and *validity*. Where appropriate, we describe statistical considerations relevant to each such issue.

AIM

Throughout the text, we emphasize that validity should be the primary goal in an epidemiologic study, even if this means sacrificing generalizability. A study free of bias, even if restricted in scope, is preferred to a more general study with unresolvable validity problems. Sophisticated statistical analyses mean nothing if the data are unreliable. Or, to put it another way, "good statistical analyses do not salvage poor data."

For several of the topics we discuss (e.g., the treatment of confounding, the use of matching, multivariable analyses), there are differing points of view in the literature. Even when there is reasonable consensus, there are rarely clear-cut recommendations that can be made. Thus, rather than try to find the nonexistent "ideal" solution, we provide a quantitative framework through which such issues can be investigated. Whenever possible, we discuss both the advantages and disadvantages of various approaches to a given methodological problem.

PHILOSOPHY AND APPROACH

AUDIENCE AND PRE-REQUISITES

This book was written with several audiences in mind. Our primary audience includes epidemiologists and other health professionals, as well as graduate students in the health sciences. We assume that this audience has a good understanding of the basic principles of epidemiology. A second audience includes researchers or students in other human science disciplines. Finally, a third audience consists of statisticians and biostatisticians interested in the application of statistics to epidemiologic research.

The degree of mathematical sophistication required, particularly with regard to statistical prerequisites, will depend on the reader's learning objectives for each chapter. We have written primarily at the level of persons with a good understanding of basic statistical procedures of data analysis typically covered in a two-course sequence in applied biostatistics. It would also be advantageous—through not essential—for the reader to have a basic knowledge of the biostatistical methods used to analyze epidemiologic data. Because we do not draw heavily on statistical inference principles prior to Part III, the reader with minimal statistical knowledge will be able to follow the discussion of basic methodological principles given in Parts I and II.

OUTLINE OF TEXT

This book is divided into three parts, plus an introductory chapter (Chapter 1). This overview chapter provides a nonquantitative discussion of key methodological issues that are addressed in the remainder of the text.

Part I (Chapters 2–9) contains the epidemiologic foundation for the more quantitatively oriented (including statistical) treatment of methodological issues addressed in Parts II and III. Of the eight chapters in Part I, only Chapters 6, 7, and 8 contain material (including notation) that is absolutely prerequisite for Parts II and III.

Part II (Chapters 10–14) provides a quantitative, conceptual framework for evaluating validity. Part III (Chapters 15–24) provides a detailed quantitative discussion of procedures and strategies for the design and analysis of epidemiologic research studies.

We strongly recommend that the reader work the exercises provided at the end of the chapters. These exercises are intended to help the reader understand and apply the principles and methods presented in the text. Abbreviated answers to selected problems are provided in Appendix A. A detailed solutions manual for the exercises is available from the publisher.

ACKNOWL-EDGMENTS

We wish to acknowledge several people who contributed to the preparation of this text. The authors developed much of their interest in quantitative epidemiology from exposure to the pioneering and sometimes controversial research contributions of Olli Miettinen at Harvard University. They have also gained insight from the work of Norman Breslow and Nicholas Day, as well as from many others too numerous to list individually. We thank Beverly Cole for typing the many drafts and revisions of all chapters, for her assistance in helping us to communicate efficiently with our publisher, professional colleagues, and students, and for her patience and good cheer throughout this project. Dave and Larry thank Anna Kleinbaum and Cindy Kupper for once again providing much-needed emotional support during the writing of their second book. Hal thanks Cyndie Gareleck for her encouragement and friendship. We thank the many students and colleagues at UNC, Yale, and elsewhere for their helpful comments and interest. Finally, we thank our publisher, Alex Kugushev, for his highly valued enthusiasm, advice, and friendship.

Dave Kleinbaum
Larry Kupper
Hal Morgenstern

To our parents

Joslyn and Janet Kleinbaum

Louis and Sylvia Kupper

Joseph and Edith Morgenstern

SPECIAL ACKNOWLEDGMENT

We give special thanks to Sander Greenland of UCLA's School of Public Health for his many contributions: reviewing the manuscript, offering suggestions for improvement, and providing each of us with further insight into many aspects of the material in the text.

1

Key Issues in Epidemiologic Research: An Overview

CHAPTER OUTLINE

**1.0
PREVIEW**

As exemplified by John Snow's famous work on cholera (1936), the field of epidemiology was initially concerned with providing a methodological basis for the study and control of population epidemics. Currently, however, *epidemiology* has a much broader scope—namely, the study of health and illness in human populations. The range of topics now includes chronic and acute diseases, the quality of health care, and mental health problems. In fact, many health professionals believe that a variety of behavioral and biomedical factors affect the health status of an individual. This belief has enabled epidemiologic research to evolve as a synthesis of knowledge from several health-related disciplines.

As the focus of epidemiologic inquiry has broadened, so has the methodology. In recent history, we have seen a proliferation of new procedures and strategies, as well as new ideas and points of view, concerning methodology. Such developments call for efforts to bring the field of quantitative epidemiology up to date in a unified way; this is our motivation for writing this text.

Our purpose is to provide a synthesis of the current and most important methodological concepts, procedures, and strategies involved in epidemiologic inquiry about the etiology of disease. To promote a more complete perspective of methodological issues, we present this discussion in the chronology in which issues arise during the course of an epidemiologic investigation. In this chapter, we will provide some general perspective by highlighting three broad issues of concern, issues that will be treated in detail in subsequent chapters. In addition, certain terms and concepts will be mentioned in an introductory manner.

Our primary focus, here and throughout the text, will be on the assessment of a postulated association between a dichotomous study factor (i.e., *exposure*) variable (E) and a dichotomous *disease* variable (D). We will also discuss more general situations where the exposure variable can be polychotomous or continuous, and we will consider applications involving several exposure variables.

Issue 1.   In the assessment of an exposure-disease relationship, an important initial decision involves the *choice of the underlying measure of disease frequency* to be used and the corresponding measures of association dictated by this choice. This decision is not always straightforward; it depends on several study characteristics, including its purpose, the population under study, and the design strategy to be used.

Issue 2.   Regardless of the study design used, the investigator must be concerned about the extent to which the results obtained from a study may be distorted because of some biasing aspect in the study design and/or analysis. This issue concerns study *validity*.

Issue 3.   As a component of issue 2, there is the need to *take into account (control for) extraneous factors,* that is, factors other than the exposure and disease variables. This step is necessary to untangle the possible mixture of effects of such additional factors with the effect of the exposure variable on disease status.

We will now discuss each of the above three issues by using some realistic examples.

In a follow-up study of a human population, the fundamental concerns of the investigator are the measurement, the analysis, and the interpretation of an observed set of new events: incident cases of disease, deaths from one or more causes, or new occurrences of any health-related event. Two distinct indices may be employed to quantify the occurrence of such new (incident) events, namely, risk and rate.

1.1 MEASURING DISEASE FREQUENCY

Risk is the probability of an individual's developing a given disease or experiencing a health status change over a specified period (conditional on the individual's not dying from any cause during that period). Thus, risk can vary from zero to one, is dimensionless, and requires a specific period referent (e.g., the five-year risk of developing lung cancer). The most common way to estimate risk is to divide the number of newly detected cases that developed during follow-up by the number of disease-free subjects at the start of follow-up; we will adopt the term *cumulative incidence* (CI) for this proportion. In using this formula, we implicitly assume that the cohort is *fixed* in the sense that no entries into the cohort are allowed during the follow-up period. However, the size of the cohort is likely to be reduced during the follow-up period as a result of deaths or other sources of attrition; furthermore, the amount of the reduction will be directly proportional to the length of the follow-up period. This reduction presents a problem since we will not know whether a subject lost during follow-up developed the disease under study. Another difficulty is that subjects may be followed for different periods of time; the traditional estimate of risk will not make effective use of such information. A third problem arises if the population studied is regarded as a *dynamic population* rather than as a fixed cohort. The composition of a dynamic population is continually changing, allowing for the addition of new members during the follow-up period. As a result, new cases may emanate from those persons who entered this dynamic population after the beginning of the follow-up.

An alternative measure of incidence, designed to deal with the problems mentioned above, involves the concept of a rate. In general, a *rate* is an instantaneous potential for change in one quantity per unit change in another quantity; typically, this second quantity is time. A simple example of a rate is velocity, which may have the units miles per hour. Epidemiologists are particularly concerned with a "relative" type of incidence rate, defined as the instantaneous potential for change in disease status (i.e., the occurrence of new cases) per unit of time, *relative* to the size of the disease-free population at a given time.

An estimate of the incidence rate can be obtained by dividing the number of new cases of the disease by the amount of *population-time of follow-up* (e.g., person-years) of the disease-free population. This denominator can sometimes be obtained directly by summing the amount of disease-free time (e.g., in years) that each individual has been followed during the follow-up period. When the follow-up times are not available on an individual basis (e.g., when monitoring a large community for the detection of new cancer cases; see Cole et al., 1971), then the total population time of follow-up must be approximated (see Miettinen, 1976). We will refer to this ratio as the *average incidence density* (ID), as suggested by Miettinen (1976).

The choice of incidence measure (CI versus ID) depends on several conceptual and practical issues, which will be discussed in Chapter 6. Among these issues are the objective of the study, the type of disease condition under consideration, the nature of the population of interest, and the method of sampling.

EXAMPLE 1.1

As an example of a situation involving an average incidence density calculation, we present the following description of a hypothetical follow-up study of a midwestern urban population. The purpose of the study was to investigate the negative consequences of obesity among older women who, as a group, have not altered their weight-related behavior as much as have other age-sex groups in recent years. In particular, this investigation wished to evaluate the possible association between obesity and death from all causes among white women between the ages of 60 and 75.

The subjects for this hypothetical study were 450 white women between the ages of 53 and 74, all of whom could contribute one or more years of observation to the age interval 60–75 years. The follow-up period was the eight-year interval from 1960 through 1967, during which time 105 members of this female cohort died. For each fatality, the year of death was recorded. Obesity was measured (in 1960) by the Quetelet index, which is 100 times the ratio of weight (in pounds) to the square of height (in inches). For purposes of analysis, the top tercile (150 women) of the Quetelet index distribution was labeled "obese," and the remaining group of 300 was designated as "nonobese."

Despite the fact that this example is a follow-up study of a fixed cohort and there is no problem with competing causes of death (since the outcome variable involves *all* causes of death), an incidence density (ID) analysis is recommended, which will take into account the widely varying amounts of follow-up time contributed by the study subjects. Note, for example, that a 58-year-old woman in 1960 could potentially contribute up to five years of follow-up in the age interval 60–75, whereas a 72-year-old woman in 1960 would only have up to three years of potential follow-up time.

Analyses of these data are described in Chapter 15 (simple analysis) and Chapter 17 (stratified analysis). Average incidence density estimates

---

EXAMPLE 1.1 (*continued*)

for each group (obese or nonobese) are obtained by dividing the number of deaths in a given group by the number of person-years of follow-up computed for that group. The analyses include statistical tests for association and point and interval estimates of effect.

An important concern in any observational study is the possibility of an undetected flaw in either the research design or the analysis, which leads to spurious conclusions. In particular, the data may suggest a strong association between the study factor and the disease when, in fact, there is really no association at all. Or the data may indicate no association when, in reality, a strong association exists.

1.2 PROBLEMS OF VALIDITY

Difficulties of this sort are generally referred to as problems of *validity in estimation of effect*. A distortion that may result when estimating the association of interest is usually called a *bias*. As discussed in Chapters 10–14, sources of bias involve the selection of study subjects, incorrect information gathered on study subjects, and the failure to adjust for variables other than the study factor that are predictive of the disease. In many instances, particularly when the source of bias is subject selection, the information necessary to assess or correct for such bias is unavailable. However, even if an assessment of the magnitude of the bias is not possible, an assessment of the direction of the bias may be feasible (e.g., one may claim that an observed strong association is actually even stronger than the data indicate, or that a weak association is, if anything, even weaker than it appears). Problems of validity can become quite complex when many sources of bias have to be considered simultaneously in a given situation.

One of the lively controversies involving validity issues in epidemiology concerns the assessment of the putative (i.e., supposed) association between reserpine use and breast cancer. Several studies on this subject, carried out in the middle 1970s, yielded contradictory conclusions and considerable editorial comment in major epidemiological journals. We will consider one such study in the next example.

EXAMPLE 1.2

The Boston Collaborative Drug Surveillance Program's report on reserpine and breast cancer (1974) was one of the first to document a positive association. It has since been criticized on many grounds, most of which concern potential biases. This study of 24 Boston-area hospitals was de-

EXAMPLE 1.2 (*continued*)

signed to evaluate relationships involving a wide variety of drugs and diseases. Nurse monitors gathered information on some 25,000 patients admitted to medical and surgical wards. Patients who were too ill for interview or who were in the hospital less than 72 hours were excluded from the study. Subjects were interviewed shortly after admission, and information regarding the frequency and duration of drug use was recorded. The interviewers identified 350 women with breast cancer, but the study was restricted to the 159 newly diagnosed cases on whom full information regarding antihypertensive drug use was available. Two separate groups of women—one from surgical and the other from medical services—were chosen as controls. Each case was matched with four controls from each group, with matching on decade of age and hospital location. Excluded from the pool of about 6,500 potential surgical controls were 309 women whose first discharge diagnosis was any form of cancer and 180 women who used an "unknown" antihypertensive drug prior to admission to the hospital. Excluded from some 5,200 medical controls were 1,686 women whose first discharge diagnosis was any form of cancer or any form of cardiovascular disease and 171 women who used an "unknown" antihypertensive drug prior to admission.

A major criticism of the study concerned the exclusion from medical controls of the 1,686 women with any form of cardiovascular disease (CVD) and the exclusion from both control groups of the total of 351 women who used an unknown antihypertensive drug. The exclusion of CVD patients was criticized on the grounds that such patients would be expected to have a relatively high use of antihypertensive therapy, including reserpine use. Consequently, the proportion of controls with a history of reserpine use would be unfairly reduced relative to the corresponding proportion for cases; thus, the relationship between reserpine use and breast cancer would appear to be much stronger than it actually was. On the other hand, if *only* CVD patients (without breast cancer) had been designated as controls, the study could have been criticized as indicating a much weaker association than actually existed. As this discussion illustrates, a bias in the choice of control group can result from either the total inclusion or the total exclusion of a particular group of subjects. Unfortunately, in practice, the question of an appropriate control group rarely has a clear-cut answer. We will return to this issue of *selection bias* in Chapter 11. Finally, note that the exclusion from both surgical and medical controls of women with unknown antihypertensive drug use is yet another potential source of selection bias, since many of these might have been reserpine users.

Other potential sources of bias in this study are the sole use of hospital information and the failure to take into account certain other key variables. A bias resulting from a case-control study restricted to a hospital popula-

EXAMPLE 1.2 (*continued*)

tion is usually designated as "Berkson's bias," since Berkson (1946) was the first to publish a quantitative treatment of this aspect of selection bias. When only hospital patients are used, the selection of subjects for the study is influenced by these subjects' propensity for the utilization of hospital services. Different hospital utilization patterns among candidates for selection may make the hospital population sufficiently different from the community population to yield a biased estimate of effect.

For the Boston Collaborative study, the restriction to hospital data could have resulted in the case and control groups' differing markedly in socioeconomic status (SES), because high-SES women are generally more likely to seek diagnosis and treatment of breast cancer than are low-SES women. Moreover, hospital utilization rates for low-SES women are high for the disorders characterizing the control groups; hence, it is likely that the controls were mostly of low SES. Since SES is known to be positively related to both antihypertensive drug use and to breast cancer incidence, the strong association found in the study between reserpine and breast cancer may be attributable to the difference in the SES distributions in the case and control groups. If so, the variable SES would be called a *confounding variable,* since the effect of reserpine on breast cancer would be mixed up (i.e., confounded) with the effect of SES. Thus, the restriction to hospital patients in the Boston Collaborative study may have influenced subject selection so as to yield a spuriously high reserpine–breast cancer association because of the confounding effect of SES. A conceptual discussion of confounding is presented in Chapters 13 and 14. Various methods for adjusting an effect measure in order to control for confounding are summarized in Chapter 16 and are described in detail in subsequent chapters. Unfortunately, the SES variable was not recorded for the study subjects, so no such adjustment was possible.

The final source of bias to be introduced here is information bias, which will be discussed in Chapter 12. *Information bias* can result when the measurement of either the exposure variable or the disease variable (and possibly other variables) is systematically inaccurate. If the exposure and the disease variables are considered on a nominal scale, as they were in this reserpine–breast cancer example, information bias can result from errors in categorization of either variable; this special nominal scale case of information bias is called *misclassification bias*. In the Boston Collaborative study, misclassification errors are more likely to be attributable to the exposure variable (reserpine use) than to the disease variable (breast cancer status), since the histologic diagnosis of breast cancer is relatively reliable. The determination of exposure status was based on interview data only, and the report did not state that medical records were checked for validation purposes. Thus, there may have been undetected selective recall (e.g.,

---

EXAMPLE 1.2 (*continued*)

a patient in the hospital for a breast cancer biopsy may have more reliable recall of previous drug therapy than do other patients). Moreover, the investigators did not consider compliance with medication rules in their classification of reserpine use status, so that persons with poor compliance might have been classified as regular reserpine users. In Chapter 12, we will show how errors from misclassification can be corrected in certain situations. In the reserpine–breast cancer study, however, the information necessary for adjustment was not obtained.

1.3 PROBLEMS IN CONTROLLING FOR EXTRANEOUS FACTORS

From the discussion on validity, we see that the assessment of an exposure-disease relationship is invariably complicated by many potential sources of bias, including that concerned with the adjustment (or control) for extraneous factors not of primary interest to the investigator. Furthermore, the problems of interaction and confounding, in contrast to problems of selection and information bias, are associated with a wide variety of methods and strategies for their treatment. We will devote a considerable portion of this text to the discussion of such approaches, which can be implemented during the research design stage and/or during the analysis of the data.

A major source of difficulty in most studies is that several extraneous factors, as opposed to a single factor, need to be taken into account. And the decision about which of these variables to control requires consideration of the simultaneous, rather than the separate, effects of these variables. As the number of extraneous variables increases, more traditional methods of control (e.g., stratified analysis, to be discussed in Chapter 17) become unreliable and difficult to interpret because of small numbers. Consequently, some form of a mathematical-modeling approach is usually required. An additional complexity associated with the simultaneous control of several extraneous factors is the desire to obtain as much precision as possible in the estimate of effect without sacrificing validity. We will consider these issues in the next example.

EXAMPLE 1.3

As an example of an epidemiologic investigation involving the control of several variables, we will consider a follow-up study designed to examine the role psychosocial processes play in the etiology of chronic diseases. The objective was to assess the putative association of endogenous catecholamine (CAT) level in the blood with the subsequent incidence of coronary heart disease (CHD). There is, to date, a good deal of evidence from

EXAMPLE 1.3 (*continued*)

both animal and human studies that psychosocial factors influence the secretion of norepinephrine and/or epinephrine (two primary catecholamines) from the adrenal medulla. Furthermore, the acute cardiovascular effects of these catecholamines through the stimulation of the sympathetic nervous system are well known; these effects include constriction of the arteries, acceleration of the heart rate, and an increase in stroke volume, thereby elevating cardiac output. Nevertheless, little is known about the manner in which these biological mechanisms link a person's social environment to disease occurrence, nor is there much information about the role that other biological risk factors (e.g., cholesterol) play in this process.

The follow-up study data considered here derive from the 1960–1969 Evans County Heart Disease Study (Cassel, 1971); these data pertain to a cohort of 609 white males between the ages of 40 and 76, free of CHD and residing in Evans County, Georgia, in 1960. After seven years, the entire cohort was reexamined; at that time 71 new cases of CHD were identified. The level of circulating CATs, which is the exposure variable of interest, is the only factor whose values were artificially generated for the purpose of this discussion; all other variables were taken from the original Evans County study. CAT is a dichotomous variable that combines indicators of both norepinephrine and epinephrine levels into two categories: high (i.e., the top tercile) and low.

Other variables in this data set are described in Table 1.1. The measure of socioeconomic status (SES) is the McGuire-White index, which is a weighted sum of scores on three "prestige" scales: occupation, education, and source of income. All variables except CHD were measured in 1960.

As we mentioned previously, the primary goal of this study was to evaluate the putative association between CAT (as measured in 1960) and the subsequent seven-year incidence of CHD. As we will discuss in more detail later in the text, a simplified (or crude) analysis considers the CAT–CHD data in a 2×2 table of the following form:

		CAT	
		HI	*LO*
CHD	*Yes*	27	44
	No	95	443

EXAMPLE 1.3 (*continued*)

This crude data layout represents an initial approach for evaluating the nature and extent of the CAT–CHD association, but such a simple approach does not take into account the effects other known *risk factors* (see Chapter 13) have on the incidence of CHD. For example, AGE and cholesterol (CHL) may be distributed differently for high-CAT and low-CAT persons in the study. Consequently, the conclusions found from such a simple analysis might be altered drastically after adjusting for these potentially confounding variables.

Thus, the proper assessment of the CAT–CHD relationship requires the consideration of other risk factors for CHD. Which of the many variables listed in Table 1.1 need to be considered for control? What is gained or lost by controlling for too many or for too few extraneous variables?

Table 1.1   Code Book for Evans City Data

Variable Name	Variable Description	Variable Coding
CHD	Incidence of coronary heart disease	0 = noncase 1 = new case
CAT	Serum catecholamine level	0 = low 1 = high
SMK	Cigarette smoking	0 = never smoked 1 = smoker
ECG	Electrocardiogram abnormality	0 = normal ECG 1 = any abnormality
OCC	Type of occupation	0 = nonfarmer 1 = farmer
MAR	Marital status	0 = not married 1 = married
AGE	Age	Years
CHL	Serum cholesterol	mg/100 mL
SBP	Systolic blood pressure	mmHg
DBP	Diastolic blood pressure	mmHg
QTI	Quetelet index	$100[(\text{weight, in lb})/(\text{height, in in.})^2]$
HEM	Hematocrit	Percent
SES	Socioeconomic status	McGuire-White index
PLS	Pulse	Beats/min

EXAMPLE 1.3 (*continued*)

And, given a satisfactory strategy for determining the appropriate subset of variables to control, what different methodological approaches are available for carrying out the analysis, and how do these different approaches compare to one another?

We do not intend to provide a thorough discussion of the above questions in this overview chapter. We will comment, however, on some of the available approaches for dealing with such issues.

Regarding the design stage of this study, none of the potential control variables were manipulated prior to analysis; e.g., no matching was employed in the selection of exposed (high-CAT) and unexposed (low-CAT) subjects. Nevertheless, the variables requiring possible control should certainly be determined at the design stage; otherwise, they would not subsequently be measured. An alternative study design would restrict age to a narrow range for all subjects. If matching on age was used instead, only the nonexposed group would be restricted by design; e.g., each high-CAT person could be pair-matched at the start of the study with a low-CAT person of the same age. A systematic discussion of the advantages and disadvantages of matching will be given in Chapter 18. Methods for the analysis of matched data will be discussed there, as well as in Chapters 20, 21, and 24, which deal with mathematical-modeling approaches.

Regarding methods and strategies for taking into account extraneous variables at the analysis stage, the commonly used initial approach involves categorizing variables and then forming combinations of categories called *strata*. Stratum-specific associations and, where permissible, associations based on combining strata are then evaluated. This procedure is called *stratified analysis* and will be described in Chapter 17. Such an analysis for the Evans County data might involve, for example, categorization of the variables AGE (above 50, below 50), CHL (above 260, below 260), and DBP (above 90, below 90) and the formation of strata like the following:

Stratum A: AGE above 50, CHL above 260, DBP below 90.

Stratum B: AGE below 50, CHL above 260, DBP above 90.

Exactly which of the many variables to use and exactly how to categorize them for such an analysis are difficult to determine. In practice, such analyses are carried out for a wide variety of combinations of variables and categorization schemes. A valid criticism of stratified analysis is that information is lost by the process of categorization. Also, the larger the number of variables under consideration, the smaller is the amount of data expected in each stratum. Furthermore, the need to consider a variety of analyses for different subsets of variables (e.g., AGE alone, AGE and CHL,

EXAMPLE 1.3 (*continued*)

AGE–OCC–ECG, etc.) makes interpretation of results difficult. Consequently, although stratified analyses are very easy to carry out, they have sufficient drawbacks to warrant consideration of other approaches.

This is not to say that stratified analysis should be avoided; on the contrary, we recommend its use as an initial approach for control even when considering several extraneous variables. Moreover, the use of stratified analysis can provide important preliminary clues about the nature and extent of any interaction in the data. As an example, when stratifying on CHL for the Evans County data, the following two tables emerge:

<table>
<tr><td colspan="4" align="center">HIGH CHL</td><td colspan="4" align="center">LOW CHL</td></tr>
<tr><td></td><td></td><td>High CAT</td><td>Low CAT</td><td></td><td></td><td>High CAT</td><td>Low CAT</td></tr>
<tr><td></td><td>Yes</td><td>7</td><td>7</td><td></td><td>Yes</td><td>20</td><td>37</td></tr>
<tr><td>CHD</td><td></td><td></td><td></td><td>CHD</td><td></td><td></td><td></td></tr>
<tr><td></td><td>No</td><td>1</td><td>90</td><td></td><td>No</td><td>94</td><td>353</td></tr>
<tr><td></td><td></td><td>8</td><td>97</td><td></td><td></td><td>114</td><td>390</td></tr>
</table>

$$\text{risk ratio} = \frac{7/8}{7/97} = 12.13 \qquad \text{risk ratio} = \frac{20/114}{37/390} = 1.85$$

These data indicate that the risk ratios (i.e., relative risks) are extremely different for the high- and low-CHL groupings. This result, in turn, suggests that the interactive effects of CHL should be considered in any additional analyses involving risk ratios as measures of effect.

As previously indicated, the drawbacks to stratified analysis call for mathematical-modeling approaches to be used either in lieu of or in conjunction with stratification. Modeling, however, presents difficulties of its own, including those pertaining to the choice of model form, the variables to be included in the model, and the assumptions required for inference making. When the dependent variable is dichotomous (e.g., when it indicates the presence or absence of disease), a form of regression function popular with epidemiologists is the *logistic model*. A detailed treatment of logistic regression analysis will be presented in Chapters 20 and 21 (theory) and 22–24 (applications). Other modeling approaches, including the method of *confounder summarization*, will also be discussed in those chapters.

In this chapter, we have attempted to provide the reader with a nontechnical overview of the general subject of this text. The issues, concepts, and terminology introduced here will be described in detail, both quantitatively and qualitatively, in the remaining chapters.

**1.4
CONCLUD-
ING
REMARKS**

To provide the reader with a convenient reference to the variety of notation and symbols used in this text, we will present, at the conclusion of each chapter, when appropriate, a list of key *new* symbols introduced in that chapter. Each list will not necessarily contain all the new symbols appearing in the chapter but, rather, only those considered essential for a clear understanding of the material presented. The intended meaning of a symbol should, nevertheless, be obvious from its contextual use in each chapter.

NOTATION

   Because certain symbols and general notation are used throughout the text, we acquaint the reader with these now.

Mathematical Symbols

$\times$ or $\cdot$	Multiplication symbols.
Σ	Summation symbol (of a subscripted array of numbers).
Π	Product symbol (of a subscripted array of numbers).
ln	Natural logarithm (to the base e).
exp	Exponential function (e to some power).
$\mathbf{W}^{-1}$	Matrix inverse, where $\mathbf{W}$ is a square matrix.
$\mathbf{M}'$	Transpose of matrix $\mathbf{M}$.
$\mathbf{x}$	Column vector, say $(x_1, x_2, \ldots, x_n)'$.
$\mathbf{x}'$	Row vector, say $(x_1, x_2, \ldots, x_k)$.
C_j^n	Number of combinations of n things taken j at a time, equal to $n!/j!(n-j)!$, where ! denotes "factorial": $n! = n(n-1)\cdots 2\cdot 1$.
df/dx	Derivative of f with respect to x.
$\partial f/\partial x$	Partial derivative of f with respect to x.

Probability and Statistics Symbols

pr	Probability.
$pr(A\|B)$	Conditional probability statement (i.e., probability of event A given that event B has occurred), where | denotes "given."
$\mathscr{E}(X)$	Expected value of a variable X (e.g., population mean of X, say μ_X).

$\mathrm{Var}(X)$	Population variance of X (e.g., σ_X^2).
$\mathrm{Cov}(X, Y)$	Population covariance between the two variables X and Y.
$100(1 - \alpha)\%$	Confidence coefficient (e.g., 95% when $\alpha = .05$).
p	Proportion.
q	$1 - p$.
H_0	Null hypothesis.
H_A	Alternative hypothesis.
$\mathrm{Var}_0(X)$	Population variance of X under some null hypothesis H_0.
$\mathscr{E}_0(X)$	Expected value of X under some null hypothesis H_0.
Greek letters	Population parameters.
P	P-value.
χ^2	Chi-square statistic or distribution.
Z	Standard normal variable or distribution.
F	F statistic or distribution.
$\hat{\theta}$	An estimator of θ (the parameter θ being estimated appears underneath the "hat").
$\overline{X}$	Sample mean of a set of values of X.

The general 2×2 table format used throughout the text is as follows:

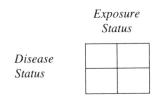

Tables for specific examples would appear as follows:

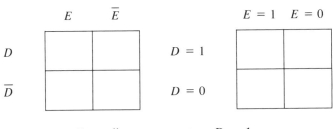

$$D \leftarrow \text{disease present} \rightarrow D = 1$$
$$\overline{D} \leftarrow \text{disease absent} \rightarrow D = 0$$

$$E \leftarrow \text{exposure present} \rightarrow E = 1$$
$$\overline{E} \leftarrow \text{exposure absent} \rightarrow E = 0$$

REFERENCES

BERKSON, J. 1946. Limitations of the application of fourfold table analysis to hospital data. *Biomet. Bull.* 2: 47–53.

Boston collaborative drug surveillance program's report on reserpine and breast cancer. 1974. *Lancet* 2: 669–671.

CASSEL, J. C. 1971. Summary of major findings of the Evans County heart disease study. *Arch. Intern. Med.* 128(8): 887–889.

COLE, P.; MONSON, R. R.; HANING, H.; and FRIEDELL, G. H. 1971. Smoking and cancer of the lower urinary tract. *N. Engl. J. Med.* 284: 129–134.

MIETTINEN, O. S. 1976. Estimability and estimation in case-referent studies. *Am. J. Epidemiol.* 103(2): 226–236.

SNOW, J. 1936. *Snow on cholera—A reprint of two papers.* New York: The Commonwealth Fund; pp. 1–175.

PART I

Objectives and Methods of Epidemiologic Research

2

Fundamentals of Epidemiologic Research

2.0
PREVIEW

The purpose of this chapter and the three that follow is to present an integrated discussion of the fundamental concepts and terms used in the planning of epidemiologic studies. In this chapter and the next, we develop a broad conceptual framework for defining epidemiologic research. In Chapters 4 and 5 we focus on the design of observational studies, which forms the foundation for the remainder of this book.

The generalized content of epidemiologic research is discussed in Section 2.1. In Section 2.2, we review causation and the basic strategy for conducting etiologic research. The intent of this chapter and the next is to present a broad perspective of epidemiologic research, thereby placing in context and laying the foundation for the chapters that follow.

2.1
EPIDEMIO-
LOGIC
RESEARCH

As an applied branch of science, *epidemiology* may be regarded simply as the study of disease and health in human populations. While this definition appears straightforward,* a few terms should be clarified before proceeding. "Disease" and "health" are not redundant; the former refers to pathological *processes,* and the latter refers to *states* of well-being. Health or a healthy state may not be equivalent to the absence of disease. Furthermore, each concept has at least three dimensions: biological or physical, perceptual or psychological, and social or behavioral. According to one elaboration of these dimensions (Susser, 1973, Chap. 1), we might say that a physician diagnoses the patient to be "diseased," the patient perceives himself to be "ill," and other persons or society label him as "sick." Although epidemiologists traditionally refer to health in the biological sense, the various dimensions are clearly related and sometimes cannot be easily distinguished in practice (Kasl and Cobb, 1966). For the purpose of presenting general concepts, principles, and methods of epidemiologic research, the term "disease" will be used to represent any dimension of either a pathological process or a state of well-being.

The use of populations distinguishes epidemiology from clinical medicine and other biomedical sciences, which typically involve a small number (often one) of individuals, tissues, or organs (Rose and Barker, 1978). Not that epidemiologists do not observe individuals, but, for the most part, their interpretations and conclusions are based on combining results from many subjects. Essentially, there are two reasons for the requirement of a population in epidemiologic research: (1) although our primary level of interest (biologically) is the individual, the ultimate goal of epidemiology and public health is to improve the health status of populations; (2) from a methodological standpoint, a population is required to make causal inferences about relationships between certain factors and disease. The latter reason will be discussed in more detail in Section 2.2. Throughout

---

*More elaborate definitions of epidemiology (e.g., MacMahon and Pugh, 1970; Susser, 1973; Lilienfeld and Lilienfeld, 1980) are not cited here because we believe that a scientific discipline should not be defined in terms of its methods or specific objectives.

the text, we will refer to the *study population* as the group of subjects for which we have observations and the *target population* as the larger group to which we would like to make inferences.

The following subsections deal with three broad aspects of epidemiologic research: aims and levels of investigation, theory and practice of epidemiology, and methods and procedures of empirical study.

The general aims of epidemiologic research are to (1) *describe* the health status of populations by enumerating the occurrence of diseases, obtaining the relative frequencies within groups, and discovering important trends; (2) *explain* the etiology of diseases by determining factors that "cause" specific diseases or trends and by discovering modes of transmission; (3) *predict* the number of disease occurrences and the distribution of health status within populations; and (4) *control* the distributions of diseases in the population by prevention of new occurrences, eradication of existing cases, prolongation of life with the disease, or otherwise improving the health status of afflicted persons.

2.1.1 Aims and Levels

Implied in the above list of aims are two different goals or levels at which epidemiologic research is conducted: understanding and intervention. Others have referred to this dichotomy as explanatory or scientific versus pragmatic or action-oriented (Schwartz and Lellouch, 1967). At the *understanding* level, we proceed from observations to inferences that lead to an accumulation of knowledge about disease occurrence and etiology (Shortell and Richardson, 1978). At the *intervention* level, we collect empirical information that can be used to make public health decisions. As illustrated in Figure 2.1, both levels may be conceived as a set of hypothetical connections among four types of occurrences relating to the natural history of a disease: (1) initiation of the etiologic process with the onset of the first cause; (2) initiation of the pathologic process with attainment of irreversibility (i.e., disease manifestation is inevitable); (3) detection of the disease through clinical signs and symptoms; and (4) outcome of the disease, including recovery, remission, change in severity, or death (Rothman, 1981).

The objective of research at the understanding level is to make scientific generalizations about the natural history of disease, which may be divided into three sequential processes: induction, promotion, and expression, each of which can be characterized by its duration (see Figure 2.1). Since the time at which a disease attains irreversibility is not generally known, in empirical research we usually regard induction and promotion as one process. In addition, the onset of the first cause for most diseases usually occurs at birth or before (Rothman, 1981). Consequently, epidemiologists have adopted the term *latency* to designate the period between the onset of any given cause and disease detection. With infectious diseases, this empirically estimable parameter is known as the *incubation period* (Fox et al., 1970). As a complement to latency, the period of ex-

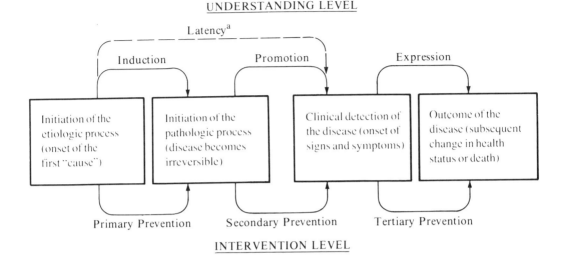

Observed duration from the onset of any *particular* cause to disease detection.

Figure 2.1 Levels of Epidemiological Research: A Conceptual Elaboration

pression between disease detection and disease termination (i.e., recovery or death) is typically called the *duration* of the disease (MacMahon and Pugh, 1970, Chap. 5).

On the basis of the distinction between latency and duration, we can define disease *chronicity* in two ways: as the period between initiation and detection or as the period between detection and termination. Thus, the concept of a chronic disease is two-dimensional. Table 2.1 lists some diseases that fit into a simple cross-classification of both dimensions. While the boundary between acute (i.e., short) and chronic (i.e., long) is arbitrary, the cutoff in Table 2.1 may be assumed to lie between 4 and 12 months.

The objective of research at the intervention level is to evaluate health practices, programs, and policies in order to prevent disease and promote good health. At this level, the three connections along the natural history sequence represent alternative strategies of prevention: primary, secondary, and tertiary (Caplan, 1967) (see Figure 2.1). These three strategies can best be defined by comparing the types and goals of the interventions involved in each strategy, as summarized in Table 2.2. Primary prevention is aimed at preventing or postponing first new occurrences of disease; secondary prevention is aimed at decreasing the duration of the disease or prolonging life; and tertiary prevention is aimed at making the disease outcome less severe (Ketterer et al., 1980).

The two levels of investigation involve fundamentally different interests, research strategies, and hypotheses. While an understanding of a dis-

Table 2.1   Disease Chronicity: Examples by Latency and Duration

	LATENCY	
Duration	Acute	Chronic
Acute	Influenza	Pancreatic cancer
	Botulism	Acute lymphatic leukemia
	Toxic shock syndrome	Acute schizophrenic episode
Chronic	Syphilis	Hypertension
	Tuberculosis	Osteoarthritis
	Spina bifida	Senile dementia

ease process may make an important contribution to our ability to control that disease, prevention does not require an extensive understanding. Conversely, an extensive understanding is not always sufficient for planning successful interventions (Renwick, 1973). In fact, there is often a conflict between persons who operate at different levels. Scientists tend to emphasize their doubts about the interpretation of empirical findings by questioning their assumptions. Policymakers or decision makers, on the other hand, advocate a position of action based on their perception of which results have practical implications and on their independently established priorities. Consequently, participants operating at different levels may respond to the same body of empirical evidence in very different ways (Lave and Seskin, 1979).

Table 2.2   Strategies of Prevention

Description	Type of Intervention	Goal of Intervention
Primary prevention	Modify the distribution of disease determinants in the population	Prevent or postpone first new occurrences of disease
Secondary prevention	Early detection of disease and subsequent treatment	Improve prognosis of cases—i.e., shorten duration of disease or prolong life
Tertiary prevention	Treatment and rehabilitation	Reduce or prevent residual defect and dysfunction or prolong life—i.e., make disease outcome less severe

**2.1.2
Theory and
Practice**

Currently, there is no unified theory of epidemiology that views the development of all diseases in populations through general etiologic principles. While few epidemiologists would argue the need for such a theory or even posit the existence of very general etiologic principles, there appears to have been a remarkable pattern of disease occurrence over long periods (Dubos, 1965, Chap. 9). The major causes of death in large populations have changed systematically, as if they formed a sequential series of overlapping secular epidemics. The widespread occurrence of chronic degenerative diseases (e.g., coronary heart disease and cancers) in post-industrial societies contrasts sharply with the predominance of infectious disease epidemics and malnutritional syndromes during the early period of industrialization, recurrent famines during primitive times, and chronic infections and parasitic infestations during the Stone Age (Hinkle, 1968).

Epidemiology, as a discipline, did not really flourish until after the *germ theory* had a firm basis in the late nineteenth century (Lilienfeld, 1973). However, the excitement generated by the discovery of the infectious model had some unfortunate consequences in the field of biomedical research. The new theory was so powerful that for decades researchers believed that knowledge of the appropriate microorganism was adequate to explain the relevant etiology of every disease (Cassel, 1964). A cogent argument can also be made that the germ theory continues to influence our thinking today about how and what phenomena should be studied, although few epidemiologists hold strictly to the specific correspondence between agent and disease (Cassel, 1964). We might claim, therefore, that the germ theory has guided much of the intellectual activity and achievement in epidemiology, at least until 1950.

Despite the current criticism of applying the underlying tenets of the germ theory for identifying etiologic factors (Cassel, 1964; Evans, 1978), it has not yet been replaced by any set of principles that is nearly as coherent or specific.* Nevertheless, the lack of a dominant theory does not indicate that epidemiology is atheoretical or merely common sense (Enterline, 1979), as suggested by many observers. Indeed, productive epidemiologic research borrows from and, to a certain extent, integrates the theories of several disciplines, including the biomedical sciences (pathology, physiology, microbiology, virology, immunology, and clinical medicine), the social sciences (psychology, sociology, anthropology, economics, and political sciences), and quantitative disciplines (mathematics, statistics, demography, and operations research).

Of course, all epidemiologists do not use each of the above disciplines to the same degree or in the same manner. In fact, we can distinguish three types of epidemiologic research, each of which is conducted by persons who are trained in very different ways and who use different methods (see

---

*The so-called multifactorial theory of disease does not specifically provide for the generation of refutable hypotheses (see Section 2.2.2). Thus, it is not a theory, as the term is used in this text.

the *International Journal of Epidemiology,* 1977). First, *laboratory research* applies the basic sciences to the technological development of procedures that enhance our ability to detect or control diseases and their determinants. For example, the laboratory researcher may be involved in the development of a vaccine or an assay procedure to identify certain antigens. Second, *epidemic investigation,* often called "shoe-leather epidemiology," deals with outbreaks of disease in specific populations. The objectives are to find the agent that caused the outbreak and its mode of transmission and to suggest appropriate control measures. Third, *population research* (or survey research) deals with the study of biological, environmental, and behavioral determinants of diseases and their prevention. Statistical techniques and other quantitative methods are used to make scientific generalizations that extend etiologic knowledge beyond observations. While this book deals almost exclusively with the third category of epidemiologic research, the basic principles and methods can also be applied to the other research activities.

Before proceeding to a more detailed discussion of research concepts, we will highlight some key methodological features of population research. First, population research is *empirical*—i.e., our pursuit of the aims discussed in Section 2.1.1 rests on the systematic collection of observations on the phenomena of interest in a defined population. While the notion of theoretical epidemiology has been put forth as a subdiscipline of epidemiology in which phenomena are studied in abstraction with mathematical models, advances in our knowledge of disease occurrence and etiology cannot accrue without a comparison of our observations with our deductions derived from the models (Lilienfeld and Lilienfeld, 1980, App. 2). Empirical research in epidemiology necessarily involves *quantification,* which is the numerical treatment of relevant factors (or theoretical constructs) by three related procedures: measurement of (random) variables, estimation of population parameters, and statistical testing of one or more hypotheses.

**2.1.3
Methods and
Procedures**

Measurement (in a broad sense) is the assignment of each unit of observation (e.g., subject) to a value or to a category of a set of values (variable) representing the factor of interest, according to an a priori rule. Thus, measurement of variables involves classification of persons into categories (e.g., case or noncase) as well as the positioning of persons along a continuum (e.g., age). For example, we might want to identify every new case of bladder cancer that occurred within a particular industrial population in 1975, which involves the assignment of every eligible person in the study population as either a case or noncase.

Estimation of population parameters involves the mathematical derivation of a summary value (i.e., estimator) for one or more quantities of interest. In epidemiology, estimation is used primarily to describe the frequency of disease in a population and to express the difference in frequency between two or more populations. For example, we might wish to estimate the incidence rate of bladder cancer in a particular industry in 1975 or the difference in the rates between two industries. Procedures for estimating common epidemiologic parameters will be presented in Chapters 6–9.

Statistical testing assesses the extent to which chance (or *sampling error*) may have accounted for our findings as represented by the estimates. A *test statistic* is computed from the data and compared to some theoretical distribution that characterizes the test statistic under the *null hypothesis* (i.e., no difference between groups). Results are generally expressed in terms of *statistical significance*, which concerns the probability of rejecting the null hypothesis if it is actually true. For example, we might wish to know whether the bladder cancer rate for one industry in 1975 is significantly different from the rate for all persons in the United States or from the rate for another industry. The basic procedure for statistical testing in epidemiology will be presented in Chapter 15.

Implied in the above paragraph is another fundamental aspect of epidemiologic methods: the *probabilistic nature* of the discipline—i.e., the use of statistical theory and applications in the analysis and interpretations of our data. While statistical theory allows epidemiology to be an empirical science, it also produces an inherent limitation to our predictive potential. For example, several thorough epidemiologic investigations of the etiology of bladder cancer in a particular industry will not allow us to predict with certainty (i.e., beyond reasonable doubt) *which* workers will develop the disease next year. However, we might be able to predict fairly well *how many* cases will develop during the year.

Lastly, most epidemiologic research (more specifically, studies not entirely limited to pure description) involves *comparisons* among groups, over time, or among studies. Typically, these comparisons are accomplished by testing and estimating the magnitude of an "association" between a putatively causal factor and its effect. In future discussions, we will refer to the putative cause as the *study factor* or *exposure* which may be personal (i.e., psychological, behavioral, biological, or genetic) or environmental (physical, chemical, social, or organizational). Other names commonly used for the study factor are characteristic, treatment, predictor, and independent variable. The hypothesized effect will be called the *disease,* otherwise known as the condition, health outcome, criterion, response, or dependent variable.

**2.2
ETIOLOGIC
RESEARCH**

Etiologic research is the search for the causes of a disease, their relationship to each other, and the relative magnitudes of their effects on the disease. Since etiology is a primary concern of most epidemiologists, we must clarify the meaning of "causality" before proceeding to options involved in designing a study.

Classically, the definition of *causality* is one of *pure determinism* in which a constant, unique, and perfectly predictable connection is postulated between two factors X and Y. X is a cause of Y if, in a completely stable system (i.e., all factors are initially fixed), any manipulation or change in *X alone* induces a subsequent change in Y (Blalock, 1964). More specifically, this definition of causation requires two criteria: *specificity of cause* and *specificity of effect*. The former indicates that X is the only cause of Y, and the latter indicates that Y is the only effect of X. The specificity-of-cause criterion implies that two other conditions must also be met: X is both a necessary and sufficient cause of Y. X is a *necessary cause* if all changes in Y must be preceded by changes in X; conversely, X is a *sufficient cause* if all changes in X inevitably induce changes in Y (Susser, 1973, Chap. 4). Both conditions can be quantitatively defined with respect to a possible causal factor (X) and a particular disease effect (Y) by reference to the hypothetical cross-classification in Table 2.3. If X is a sufficient cause of Y, cell C is always zero; if X is a necessary cause of Y, cell B is always zero. It should be noted that the two conditions are theoretically independent. That is, a factor may be a necessary but not sufficient cause, a sufficient but not necessary cause, both necessary and sufficient, or neither necessary nor sufficient. Moreover, neither specificity criterion necessarily implies the other.

The first major attempt in the health sciences to operationalize the criteria for pure determinism was made by Robert Koch nearly a hundred years ago (Evans, 1978). He proposed that three postulates be applied as tests to identify causative agents of disease: (1) the agent must be present in every case of the disease under appropriate circumstances (i.e., the necessary condition); (2) the agent should occur in no other disease as a fortuitous and nonpathogenic event (i.e., specificity of effect); and (3) the agent must be isolated from the body in pure culture and induce the disease

**2.2.1
Models of
Causality**

**Table 2.3   Hypothetical Cross-Classification of True Disease
Status (Y) by Category of a Possible Causal Factor (X)**

	X, POSSIBLE CAUSAL FACTOR	
Y, Possible Disease Effect	*Exposed*	*Unexposed*
Case	A	B
Noncase	C	D

Notes: 1. If X is a *sufficient* cause of Y, cell C is always zero.

2. If X is a *necessary* cause of Y, cell B is always zero.

3. If X is both a necessary and sufficient cause of Y, cells B and C are always zero.

anew in a susceptible animal (i.e., the sufficient condition). It is not clear whether Koch's omission of the specificity-of-cause criterion was an oversight or a deliberate decision. Possibly, he felt that this criterion was too stringent for demonstrating causality or that it could not be readily operationalized. In fact, Koch himself emphasized that the third postulate was not required to prove causation.

While many current biomedical researchers continue to apply Koch's postulates for demonstrating causality, this approach is often criticized and found to be inadequate for most diseases (Evans, 1978). The basic limitations of using the model of pure determinism to derive operational criteria for causation are summarized below.

1. *Multifactorial etiology.* There is an abundance of empirical evidence and substantial theoretical justification for accepting the widespread belief that diseases have more than one cause. Consequently, in any particular instance, we must challenge either the necessary or the sufficient condition for identifying a causal relationship. In the case of most infectious diseases, for example, we know that the presence of the microbial agent (which we *define* as a necessary condition) is not always accompanied by signs or symptoms characteristic of that disorder (Dubos, 1965). Thus, the agent is not sufficient to cause any pathological occurrence; rather, the effect may depend on several other factors, including nutritional deficiencies, toxic exposures, emotional stress, and the complex web of social networks. Regarding noninfectious chronic disease (not transmitted by genes at a single locus), there is no factor known to be present in every case. For example, smoking is not necessary for the development of lung cancer (of any a priori type), and no degree of coronary atherosclerosis is a necessary condition for myocardial infarction. Furthermore, if we recognize that certain causes of disease may not be physical agents, the classical model of causality does not enable us to consider causal chains of two or more factors that eventually result in disease. Thus, the agent may not be a necessary cause of the pathological occurrence.

2. *Multiplicity of effects.* Conversely, there is much evidence to support the contention that certain factors (though, perhaps not all) have more than one pathological effect. For example, smoking appears to be involved in the etiology of many diseases, including lung, bladder, esophageal, and oral cancers; coronary heart disease; emphysema; chronic bronchitis; perinatal mortality; and periodontal disease.

3. *Limited conceptualization of the putative causal factors.* Two aspects of the alleged cause make it difficult to generalize the criteria for pure determinism. First, we have maintained thus far that causation depends on a *change* in the causal factor. How do we then consider the roles of race, sex, genetic predispositions, and other fixed characteristics in disease etiology? While it is possible to maintain, in theory, that causality must involve the relationship between sequential changes, the investigator

may not always be able to observe, measure, or even identify the relevant changes. Second, the pure deterministic model does not allow a clear role for causal factors that are continuous, such as age, blood pressure, and obesity. For example, how high must blood pressure be in order to precipitate a cerebrovascular event? In this instance, we know there is no uniform cutoff value (or threshold) above which the effect occurs and below which no effect occurs.

4. *Imperfect knowledge*. Finally, we have an incomplete understanding of the disease and a limited ability to observe and measure the causal process. Thus, when studying the hypothesized effect of one factor, we can never be absolutely certain that the effects of other factors did not play a role in accounting for our findings. In addition, there is always some error in the measurement process, and we can never study every person whose experience bears on the causal issue.

Many current researchers have conceptualized a model of *modified determinism* to permit multiple causes of a single disease. Clusters of causal factors, rather than single factors, are treated as sufficient causes; and each sufficient cluster has an effect on that one disease, which is independent of the effects of factors in other clusters (Rothman, 1976). Within every sufficient cluster, the effect of each factor depends on the level of every other factor in that set. Thus, we could say that the factors forming a sufficient cause modify the effects of each other, yet they are independent of the effects of factors in other sufficient clusters. In this model, a cause need not involve an explicit change but may be an act, event, or a state of nature that initiates or permits the effect to occur. Any factor that occurs in at least one but not all sufficient clusters is called a *contributory cause* (Reigelman, 1979), and any factor that occurs in all sufficient clusters is a necessary cause, as in the previous model (Rothman, 1976).

Unfortunately, the modified model still does not meet our empirical needs because it does not consider the limited state of our knowledge regarding the causal process and how to observe it. In epidemiology, we use a probabilistic framework to assess evidence regarding causality—or, more properly, to make causal inferences. That is, we use probability theory and statistical techniques to test and estimate the magnitude of observed relationships that we hypothesize as causal. But a probabilistic viewpoint does not automatically negate our belief in a (modified) deterministic world (Blalock, 1964; Bunge, 1979). In other words, we need not regard the occurrence of disease as a random process; we employ probabilistic considerations to express our ignorance of the causal process and how to observe it.

Because of the lack of certainty in our results, epidemiologists generally use the term *risk factor* (instead of cause) to indicate a variable that is believed to be related to the probability of an individual's developing the disease, prior to the point of irreversibility (see Figure 2.1). Analogously, factors believed to be related to the time of disease detection, given sufficient etiology, are called *promoters,* if they are of etiologic importance, or *detection factors,* if they are not of etiologic importance. Thus, promoters speed up (or retard) the actual disease process; detection factors only alter the probability of cases being identified. Factors believed to be related to the probability of cases developing a certain outcome event are called *prognostic factors.*

Three general criteria must be met before we may suggest that a given factor is a risk factor for a particular disease (MacMahon and Pugh, 1970, Chap. 2; Nagel and Neef, 1979): (1) the factor must be observed to *covary* with the disease—i.e., the factor must be statistically associated with the development of the disease, or, equivalently, the frequency of disease must be observed to differ by category or value of the factor; (2) the presence of the risk factor (or a relevant change in the risk factor) must *precede* the occurrence of the disease—i.e., the factor and disease must not appear to be related simply because the value of the factor changed among diseased persons; and (3) the observed association must not be entirely due to any source of *error,* including chance or sampling error, the involvement of other (extraneous) risk factors, or other problems with the study design or data analysis. Evidence to support the understanding that a variable represents a certain risk factor accumulates from several epidemiologic studies in addition to the findings and theories of other scientists and clinicians. We will elaborate the operational criteria for identifying risk factors in Section 2.2.3.

A benefit derived from the probabilistic framework is that it permits the convenient treatment of continuous study factors (i.e., hypothesized risk factors). We can observe the frequency of disease for each category of the factor and fit the data to a mathematical model that treats disease frequency (or rate) as a function of the continuous factor. Thus, we may describe a *dose-response effect* in which various levels of the study factor are differentially related to the probability of developing the disease. An advantage of using mathematical models to describe dose-response relationships is that they provide a way of "smoothing" the data—i.e., reducing random fluctuations caused by sampling errors. Furthermore, the probabilistic model allows for the complex investigation of multiple effects of one or more factors since we may estimate the associations (not necessarily causal) among the diseases as well as between factors and diseases.

**2.2.2
Hypotheses and
Inference**

Epidemiologists, like other empirical scientists, must continue to bridge the gap between data and theory—what they observe versus what they believe. This ultimate quest rests fundamentally on the human process of reasoning or inference, which, in logic, means the claim that one statement (the conclusion) ought to be accepted because one or more other statements (the premises or evidence) are true. *Causal inference* in epidemiology is the logical development of a theory, based on observations and a series of arguments, that attributes the development of a disease to one or more risk factors. Essentially, there are two distinct types of arguments for making an inference: deduction and induction (Salmon, 1973).

A *deductive argument* is one in which the conclusion follows necessarily from the premises, such as a syllogism or the solution of an algebraic equation. Typically, the form of an argument can be recognized as deductive if it moves from general to specific statements (Salmon, 1973). If the conclusion must be true whenever the premises are true, we say the deductive argument is *valid*.

An *inductive argument* is one in which the conclusion does not necessarily follow from the premises and in which the conclusion contains information not present in the premises (Salmon, 1973). The premises in an inductive argument are usually called the *evidence*. Statements comprising the evidence are alleged to be facts from which the conclusion is induced. In contrast to deduction, induction moves from specific to general statements. The process of induction, therefore, is required to extend our knowledge of a phenomenon beyond our observation—i.e., to make scientific generalizations. The strength of an inductive argument is a matter of degree, rather than a dichotomy. Also, unlike a valid deductive argument, a logically correct inductive argument may have true premises and a false conclusion. All we can say from a logically correct inductive argument is that the conclusion is more *likely* to be true if the premises are true than if the premises are false.

The limited nature of inductive reasoning was discussed by the eighteenth-century philosopher David Hume (1946), who asserted that causality is a purely subjective concept, existing as an "idea" in one's mind. He maintained that the generalization of a necessary connection between cause and effect cannot be obtained strictly from experience but depends on two related ideas of "contiguity" and "succession," which are traceable to repeated observations. Without ever having defined the concept of induction, Hume recognized that causal inference depends on human insight, intuition, and imagination as links in the process connecting observations and theory.

Inferring that a given factor is a risk factor for a disease is a very complex process involving many uncertainties. There are several reasons for believing that causal inference depends on more than a single test of a hypothesis based on one set of observations. First, we cannot formulate the ideal or ultimate causal hypothesis, since this ability depends on our current state of knowledge and some degree of creative insight on the part of the investigator. Second, we cannot perfectly operationalize the causal hypothesis because of certain practical limitations—e.g., the limited availability and cooperativeness of the study population and restrictions in medical technology. Finally, we cannot draw a definitive conclusion from the results of one analytical test because of the inherent limitations of induction discussed above.

Acceptance of the above principles has guided several contemporary philosophers, including Karl Popper (1968), who maintains that scientific discovery is based solely on a hypothetico-deductive process and advances by disproof or refutations rather than by proof or confirmations. In fact, Popper maintains that the concept of induction is dispensable. He believes that the procedure of science is to generate a hypothesis with conjecture—creative leaps of the imagination—which is then refuted and used to generate new hypotheses. Each set of observations, or study, is an attempted refutation of a hunch, which leads to further hunches and tests. Thus, the major purpose of repeating (i.e., *replicating*) a study is to provide additional nonredundant refutations, enabling the investigators to refine their hypotheses and generalize their findings (Buck, 1975). For example, suppose we find that level of formal education is positively associated with blood pressure level among a large group of white urban males. Testing the association among black rural males might permit a better understanding of the role of education in the development of hypertension—i.e., what is deleterious about more or less education. A new hypothesis to explain the observations is advanced if it more adequately explains previous findings, unifies previously unconnected phenomena, or generates new predictions that can be tested.

While the value of Popper's philosophy for epidemiologists is hotly debated (Buck, 1975, 1976; Davies, 1975; Smith, 1975; Jacobsen, 1976; Peto, 1976), hypothesis formulation and refinement are widely regarded as central to all empirical research. Very often we find that otherwise sophisticated investigations suffer from at least one of several problems, including excessive replication without generating new explanations for our observations; reliance on advanced analytic techniques and computer technology as substitutes for new hypotheses; and hypotheses that are so broadly or specifically defined that they cannot be readily tested by using available epidemiologic methods (Buck, 1975). Indeed, good research depends as much on asking the right questions as it does on finding the solutions.

2.2.3
Causal
Inference in
Practice

The major objective of every investigator who tests an etiologic hypothesis is to eliminate alternative explanations for his or her findings—i.e., to convince others that the results of the study are internally valid. A *valid study* is one in which the observed association is not due either to the disease occurrence preceding the exposure or to various sources of error that might distort (bias) our results. But, as we suggested in the previous section, causal inference depends on synthesizing results from multiple studies, both epidemiologic and nonepidemiologic. To make matters even more complicated, conclusions drawn from this synthesis are often used to make decisions about medical practices, individual behaviors, and public policies.

Instigated by a federally sponsored effort to ascertain the hazards of smoking, researchers in the late 1950s and the early 1960s began to carefully define their operational criteria for making causal inferences. This effort focused on assessing the effects of exposures that cannot be randomly assigned (i.e., randomized) by the investigators. In 1964, the U.S. Department of Health, Education, and Welfare published a report that reviewed the research that dealt with the relationship between smoking and particular health outcomes (e.g., lung cancer). We will briefly examine the general criteria formalized by Bradford Hill (1971) and used in the 1964 document to assess the extent to which the available evidence supported a causal interpretation.

1. *Strength of the association.* The stronger the observed association, the less likely it is that the association is entirely due to various sources of error that might distort the results. Thus, in general, weaker associations do not lend as much support to a causal interpretation.

2. *Dose-response effect.* The observation that frequency of disease increases with the dose or level of exposure usually lends support to a causal interpretation. But in the absence of such an effect, the investigator may not be able to rule out certain alternative explanations, such as a threshold effect or a saturation effect (Rall, 1978; Falk, 1978; Lepkowski, 1978). In addition, an observed dose-response effect may be due entirely to a graduated distortion or bias (Weiss, 1981).

3. *Lack of temporal ambiguity.* It is very important for the researcher to establish that the hypothesized cause preceded the occurrence of the disease. In general, this task is more difficult when investigating diseases with long latent periods and study factors that change over time. As we will see in Chapter 4, the ability to establish the direction of the relationship largely depends on the study design.

The above criteria can be applied to the findings of a single study, and, thus, they may be regarded as internal validity issues. However, any of them may be satisfied in some studies and not in others that deal with the same hypothesis. The following criteria are not necessarily study-specific and depend, to a certain extent, on a priori knowledge.

4. *Consistency of the findings.* If all studies dealing with a given relationship produce similar results, a causal interpretation is enhanced. This criterion is particularly important if the studies involve different populations, methods, and/or study periods. Of course, there are bound to be some inconsistencies among studies, and we may have to give more subjective weight to those findings that we believe are more valid. Further complicating this inferential process is the possibility that inconsistencies are due to systematic changes in effect over time, not simply to methodological differences. Occasionally, inconsistencies can generate new hypotheses that lead to a better understanding of the disease (e.g., Morgenstern, 1980).

5. *Biological plausibility of the hypothesis.* If the hypothesized effect makes sense in the context of current biological knowledge, we are more likely to accept a causal interpretation. However, biological plausibility cannot be demanded of a hypothesis, since the current state of knowledge may be inadequate to explain our observations. In general, the less we know about the etiology of the disease and similar diseases, the less secure we are in rejecting a causal interpretation on the basis of this criterion.

6. *Coherence of the evidence.* If the findings do not seriously conflict with our understanding of the natural history of the disease or with other accepted facts about disease occurrence (e.g., secular trends), a causal interpretation is strengthened. In essence, this criterion combines aspects of consistency and biological plausibility and, therefore, is similarly delineated as described above.

7. *Specificity of the association.* If the study factor is found to be associated with only one disease, or if the disease is found to be associated with only one factor (after testing many possible associations), a causal interpretation is suggested. However, this criterion cannot be used to reject a causal hypothesis, because many factors have multiple effects and all (or most) diseases have multiple causes (see Section 2.2.1).

While the seven criteria listed above may help us to determine whether an exposure or characteristic is a risk factor for a disease, their application to a given hypothesis is never an uncomplicated or straightforward affair. None of the criteria are either necessary or sufficient for making a causal interpretation. In fact, strict adherence to any one of them without other considerations could result in incorrect conclusions (Hill, 1971).

**2.2.4
The Scientific
Method**

For more than a century, philosophers have attempted to characterize the scientific method by which observations and theories in all scientific disciplines are connected (Hershel, 1968; Pearson, 1911). Despite criticism of this concept and the belief by some that a single scientific method does not exist (Conant, 1951; Kaplan, 1964), certain basic elements of epidemiologic research are common to other empirical sciences and, therefore, can be generalized. It is, in fact, this potential for generalizing our methods that enables epidemiologists to investigate research questions in new areas and permits the development of a coherent framework by which new research is evaluated.

Figure 2.2 represents one idealized version of the scientific method that is particularly suited to epidemiology. Our knowledge of disease etiology is gradually modified and expanded by successive executions of several related processes in a continuous cycle, each of which is a transition between two "adjacent" content categories of empirical research. Given a certain understanding of a disease (refer to the top of Figure 2.2),

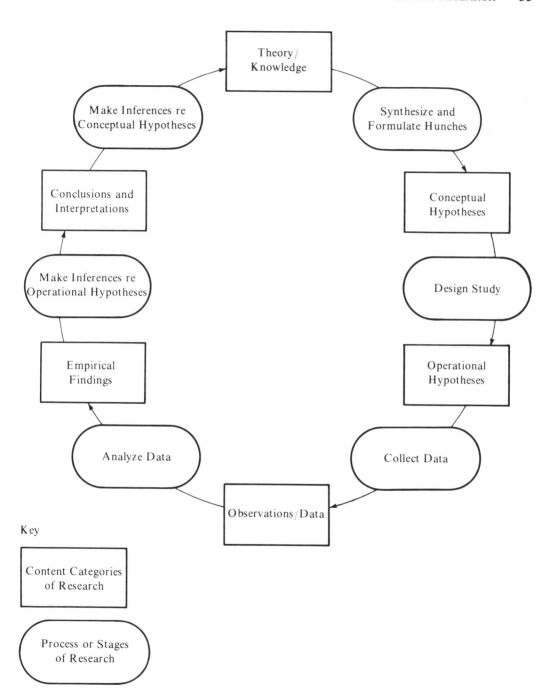

Figure 2.2 An Idealized Conceptualization of the Scientific Method

each researcher may formulate one or more conceptual hypotheses based on his or her insight and the hunches of others. The hypotheses are then operationalized by carefully defining the methods of research and collecting data according to a set protocol. The raw data are put into a usable format, summarized appropriately, and analyzed by testing the operational hypothesis. Using our results and the criteria discussed in the last section, we make causal inferences that allow us to modify existing theories and generate new hypotheses. Thus, the cycle continues with new findings generating new hypotheses, which, in turn, generate new empirical studies. Naturally, epidemiologic research does not always follow the exact order depicted in Figure 2.2. Nevertheless, the concept of a generalized approach to research is important for recognizing epidemiology as a scientific discipline as well as a part of public health practice.

A key stage of epidemiologic research is *study design*, the process of planning an empirical investigation, which will be our focus in the next three chapters. As shown in Figure 2.2, study design may be conceived as the link between one or more *conceptual hypotheses* (or simply hypotheses, as they are called by the philosophers) and the *operational hypotheses*, or testable conjectures. These two concepts are meant to emphasize the distinction between our ideas of nature and our empirical tests of these ideas. For example, suppose our conceptual hypothesis is that coffee consumption is a risk factor for CHD. The operational hypothesis might be that middle-age women who lived in a certain area in 1970 were more likely to have died during the next 10 years of ischemic heart disease if they reported an average consumption of two or more cups of coffee per day in a 1970 questionnaire than if they reported less consumption. What distinguishes the operational hypothesis from the conceptual hypothesis are the specifics of the study design, which enable the investigator to develop an idea into expected results.

Because the two types of hypotheses must be different, it follows that all study designs are potentially flawed, ignoring any inadequacies in the collection and analysis of data. There is no such thing as a perfect study design; therefore, it becomes most important to understand the specific limitations of each design. To achieve this understanding, we require a system for classifying types of epidemiologic research and an overall scheme for specifying the elements of a study design. *The central importance of study design to epidemiologic research cannot be overemphasized, because most serious problems or mistakes at this stage cannot be rectified in subsequent stages of the study. In particular, no type of sophisticated statistical analysis will salvage a poorly designed study.*

2.3 CONCLUDING REMARKS

Epidemiology is the study of health and disease in human populations. As applied scientists, contemporary epidemiologists are primarily concerned with the investigation of disease etiology—specifically, the possible effects of environmental, behavioral, and biological factors. Since we are relatively ignorant of the causal process and how to observe it, causal inference depends on a probabilistic approach to identify risk factors that purportedly influence the likelihood of disease occurrence. This complex process of scientific generalization involves modification of our theories on the basis of empirical findings from systematically collected data. Central to this linkage between our ideas and our observations in the conduct of research is study design—i.e., the planned specification of empirical methods for translating our conceptual hypotheses into testable predictions. In Chapter 3, we present a framework for classifying epidemiologic research. And in Chapters 4 and 5, we elaborate the options for and types of study design for the general category of research used most frequently by epidemiologists.

REFERENCES

BLALOCK, H. M., JR. 1964. *Causal inferences in nonexperimental research.* New York: Norton; Chap. 1.

BUCK, C. 1975. Popper's philosophy for epidemiologists. *Int. J. Epidemiol.* 4: 159–168.

———. 1976. Popper's philosophy for epidemiologists (letter to the editor re Buck's paper on Popper's philosophy). *Int. J. Epidemiol.* 5: 97–98.

BUNGE, M. 1979. *Causality and modern science.* 3rd rev. ed. New York: Dover; Chap. 1.

CAPLAN, G., and GRUNEBAUM, H. 1967. Perspectives on primary prevention: A review. *Arch. Gen. Psychiat.* 17: 331–346.

CASSEL, J. C. 1964. Social science theory as a source of hypotheses in epidemiological research. *Am. J. Public Health* 54: 1482–1488.

CONANT, J. B. 1951. *Science and common sense.* New Haven: Yale University Press; Chap. 3.

DAVIES, A. M. 1975. Epidemiological reasoning: Comments on "Popper's philosophy for epidemiologists" by Carol Buck (comment one). *Int. J. Epidemiol.* 4: 169–171.

DUBOS, R. 1965. *Man adapting.* New Haven: Yale University Press.

ENTERLINE, P. E. 1979. Epidemiology: "Nothing more than common sense"? *Occup. Health and Safety* 48: 45–48.

EVANS, A. S. 1978. Causation and disease: A chronological journey. *Am. J. Epidemiol.* 108: 249–258.

FALK, H. L. 1978. Biologic evidence for the existence of thresholds in chemical carcinogenesis. *Environ. Health Perspect.* 22: 167–170.

FOX, J. P.; HALL, C. E.; and ELVEBACK, L. R. 1970. *Epidemiology: Man and disease.* New York: Macmillan; Chap. 4.

HERSHEL, J. F. W. 1968. Scientific method. In *Science: Men, methods, goals,* edited by B. A. Brody and N. Capaldi, pp. 99–114. New York: W. A. Benjamin.

HILL, A. B. 1971. *Principles of medical statistics.* 9th ed. New York: Oxford University Press; Chap. 24, pp. 309–323.

HINKLE, L. E., JR. 1968. Relating biochemical, physiological, and psychological disorders to the social environment. *Arch. Environ. Health* 16: 77–82.

HUME, D. 1946. *A treatise of human nature.* Edited by L. A. Selby-Bigge. Oxford: Clarendon Press.

International Journal of Epidemiology. 1977. Epidemiology and health policy (editorial). 6: 99–100.

JACOBSEN, J. 1976. Against Popperized epidemiology. *Int. J. Epidemiol.* 5: 9–11.

KAPLAN, A. 1964. *The conduct of inquiry: Methodology for behavioral science.* Scranton, Pa.: Chandler.

KASL, S. V., and COBB, S. 1966. Health, behavior, illness behavior, and sick role behavior. *Arch. Environ. Health* 12: 246–266.

KETTERER, R. F.; BADER, B. C.; and LEVY, M. R. 1980. Strategies and skills for promoting mental health. In *Prevention in mental health,* vol. 1., edited by R. H. Price, R. F. Ketterer, B. C. Bader, and J. Monahan, Chap. 14, pp. 263–283.

LAVE, L. B., and SESKIN, E. P. 1979. Epidemiology, causality, and public policy. *Am. Scientist* 67: 178–186.

LEPKOWSKI, W. 1978. Extrapolation of carcinogenesis data. *Environ. Health Perspect.* 22: 173–181.

LILIENFELD, A. M. 1973. Epidemiology of infectious and non-infectious disease: Some comparisons. *Am. J. Epidemiol.* 97: 135–147.

LILIENFELD, A. M., and LILIENFELD, D. E. 1980. *Foundations of epidemiology.* 2nd ed. New York: Oxford University Press.

MACMAHON, B., and PUGH, T. F. 1970. *Epidemiology: Principles and methods.* Boston: Little, Brown.

MORGENSTERN, H. 1980. The changing association between social status and coronary heart disease in a rural population. *Social Sci. & Med.* 14A: 191–201.

NAGEL, S. S., and NEEF, M. 1979. *Policy analysis in social science research.* Beverly Hills, Calif.: Sage; App. 3.1.

PEARSON, K. 1911. *The grammar of science.* 3rd ed. London: A&C Black.

PETO, R. 1976. Cervical cancer and early sexual intercourse (letter to the editor). *Int. J. Epidemiol.* 5: 97.

POPPER, K. R. 1968. *The logic of scientific discovery.* New York: Harper & Row.

RALL, D. P. 1978. Thresholds? *Environ. Health Perspect.* 22: 163–165.

REIGELMAN, R. 1979. Contributory cause: Unnecessary and insufficient. *Postgrad. Med.* 66: 177–179.

RENWICK, J. H. 1973. Analysis of cause—Long cut to prevention? (editorial). *Nature* 246: 114–115.

ROSE, G., and BARKER, D. J. P. 1978. What is epidemiology? *Br. Med. J.* 2: 803–804.

ROTHMAN, K. J. 1976. Causes. *Am. J. Epidemiol.* 104(6): 587–592.

———. 1981. Induction and latent periods. *Am. J. Epidemiol.* 114(2): 253–259.

SALMON, W. C. 1973. *Logic.* 2nd ed. Englewood Cliffs, N.J.: Prentice-Hall.

SCHWARTZ, D., and LELLOUCH, J. 1967. Explanatory and pragmatic attitudes in therapeutical trials. *J. Chronic Dis.* 20: 637–648.

SHORTELL, S. M., and RICHARDSON, W. C. 1978. *Health program evaluation.* St. Louis: Mosby; Chap. 6.

SMITH, A. 1975. Epidemiological reasoning: Comments on "Popper's philosophy for epidemiologists" by Carol Buck (comment two). *Int. J. Epidemiol.* 4: 171–172.

SUSSER, M. 1973. *Causal thinking in the health sciences.* New York: Oxford University Press.

U.S. DEPARTMENT OF HEALTH, EDUCATION, AND WELFARE. 1964. *Smoking and Health.* PHS Publ. No. 1103. Washington, D.C.: Government Printing Office.

WEISS, N. S. 1981. Inferring causal relationships: Elaboration of the criterion of "dose-response." *Am. J. Epidemiol.* 113: 487–490.

3

Types of Epidemiologic Research

In this chapter we will employ two design criteria to create a basic typology **3.0** of epidemiologic research. The criteria are (1) whether the study factor is **PREVIEW** artificially *manipulated* by the investigators or others—i.e., whether dif-

Table 3.1   Types and Objectives of Epidemiologic Research

Type	Subtype	Objectives
Experimental (artificial manipulation of study factor with randomization)	Laboratory	Test etiologic hypotheses and estimate acute behavioral and biological effects
		Suggest efficacy of intervention to modify risk factors in a population
	Clinical trial	Test etiologic hypotheses and estimate long-term health effects
		Test efficacy of interventions to modify health status
		Suggest feasibility of population intervention
	Community intervention	Identify persons at "high risk"
		Test efficacy and effectiveness of clinical/societal interventions to modify health status within a particular population
		Suggest public health policies and programs
Quasi-experimental (artificial manipulation of the study factor without randomization)	Clinical/ laboratory	Same as clinical trial or laboratory experiment
	Program/policy	Evaluate extent to which public health goals are achieved
		Determine unanticipated problems or consequences of implementation and reasons for success or failure of the intervention
		Compare costs and benefits of intervention
		Suggest changes in current health policies or programs
Observational (no artificial manipulation of the study factor)	Descriptive	Estimate disease frequency and time trends and identify diseased individuals
		Generate etiologic hypotheses and suggest rationale for new studies
	Analytic (etiologic)	Test specific etiologic hypotheses and estimate chronic health effects
		Generate new etiologic hypotheses and suggest mechanisms of causation
		Generate preventive hypotheses and suggest potential for disease prevention

ferent categories of the study factor are allocated to subjects; and (2) if manipulated, whether categories of the study factor (i.e., treatments) are randomly allocated—i.e., *randomized*—to all subjects. Together, these two criteria delineate three mutually exclusive types of studies, as outlined in the following sections and summarized in Table 3.1.

3.1
EXPERI-
MENTS

Studies in which randomization is used to allocate subjects are called *experiments*. While many professionals in the health field believe that epidemiologists do not conduct "true" experiments, a well-defined tradition of experimental research has grown in epidemiology, largely in response to the need for testing the efficacy of new chemotherapies and vaccines (Harris and Fitzgerald, 1970; Comstock, 1978). More recently, population researchers have increased their use of experimental designs to examine the impact of other medical practices (Saracci, 1979; Wennberg et al., 1980) and behavioral programs intended to reduce morbidity and mortality in the community (Syme, 1978; Farquhar, 1978).

In the simplest type of experiment, one group of subjects is given an experimental *treatment* and another group (often called the *controls*) is given either no treatment, a sham treatment (e.g., a placebo drug), or, less preferably, the customary treatment under nonexperimental conditions (e.g., an available drug). After a period of follow-up, the change in the response variable (e.g., disease status) is measured for every subject, and the two groups are compared with respect to estimated summary values of the response. A difference in response between groups suggests an effect—beneficial or adverse—of the new treatment.

Experimental designs are specifically adapted to each study situation by modifying and/or restricting the randomization process. Most important among such features is the procedure of *double blinding,* in which neither the investigator nor the subjects know the treatments to which they have been allocated. In a clinical drug trial, double blinding is usually accomplished by having a third party assign groups and not informing either the examiners or the subjects about their treatments until after the trial. Double blinding is very important to experimental design because it helps to ensure that neither the investigator nor the subject influences the response in ways that promote bias. For more thorough discussions of experimental designs, see Harris and Fitzgerald (1970), Peto et al. (1976, 1977), and Weddell (1979).

3.1.1
Subtypes and
Objectives

We can define three subtypes of epidemiologic experiments; the classification depends on the approximate duration of the study and the selection of subjects.

The *laboratory experiment* has the shortest duration—usually, a matter of hours or days—and, therefore, is used to estimate acute biological or behavioral responses that are believed to be risk factors for the disease.

Typically, the study population is very highly restricted or self-selected so that it is seldom representative of the target population. For example, we might test whether a particular type of acute stressor (e.g., an unsolvable puzzle) increases catecholamine response among healthy subjects. A positive result would suggest a biological explanation for the well-known relationship between emotional stress and CHD.

The *clinical trial* has a longer duration, ranging from days to years, and usually is restricted to a highly selected population, such as a group of screened subjects, diagnosed cases, or other volunteers. This type of experiment has the longest tradition in epidemiology and has acquired a substantial literature describing all aspects of study planning, implementation, analysis, and interpretation (e.g., Harris and Fitzgerald, 1970; Peto et al., 1976, 1977; Weddell, 1979). The major objective of the clinical trial is to test the possible effect (i.e., efficacy) of a therapeutic or preventive intervention. For example, we may wish to assess to what extent, if at all, a new type of chemotherapy prolongs the life of children with acute lymphatic leukemia. Additionally, the clinical trial may be employed to examine specific etiologic relationships having no immediate therapeutic or preventive component, if such trials are ethically feasible.

Lastly, the more recently developed *community intervention* has a long duration (at least six months) and differs from the previous types in that it is conducted within a particular sociopolitical context of a naturally formed population (community). Thus, the objectives of the community intervention usually pertain to implementation and assessment of interventions aimed at primary prevention through risk factor modification in a well-defined population. Generally, we wish to determine the potential benefits of modifying certain individual behaviors, biological characteristics, or aspects of the environment.

In general, experiments afford the most control over the study situation because they best enable the investigator to isolate the observed effect of the treatment (i.e., study factor). With a large enough sample size, a well-designed experiment can be expected to control nearly all distorting effects from extraneous risk factors, including those that are unmeasured. The control is accomplished either by holding these extraneous factors fixed for all subjects or by randomization—so that all treatment groups have, on the average, the same distribution of the extraneous factors. However, even well-designed experiments are not free of all distorting influences since our procedures are subject to human errors and chance. Thus, the investigator may have to control for the potentially distorting influences of extraneous risk factors in the analysis of an experiment, in much the same way that control is accomplished in nonexperimental studies (Rothman, 1977) (to be discussed in Chapter 16). In fact, control of extraneous risk factors through randomization alone is made particularly difficult in the community setting, where it may be practically impossible to manipulate certain

**3.1.2
Advantages and
Limitations**

environmental or social factors (the treatment) while controlling for the effects of other risk factors. One way of handling this problem efficiently (in addition to analytic techniques) is to use a grouped design in which subjects are aggregated into relatively homogeneous groups before randomization. Thus, the experimental unit is actually the group, which may be any convenient aggregation, such as families, work groups, patient groups, or geographic areas (Sherwin, 1978; Cornfield, 1978).

One weakness of most experimental designs is related to their excessive control over the study situation—a weakness that, paradoxically, is also their strength. Because the experiment often takes place in an artificial setting among a selected sample, the study population may differ from the larger target population on several characteristics. If the true effect of the treatment depends on these characteristics, the observed effect in the study population could differ from the effect that exists in the target population. This difference may have important implications to public health activities, which are based on experimental findings.

The most often cited limitations of experiments are certain practical issues of implementing the design. Specifically, randomization may not be ethical if an arbitrary group of subjects must be denied an experimental treatment that is regarded as beneficial by clinicians or patients. In addition, the design may not be feasible, such as the artificial manipulation of a psychosocial attribute or the use of double blinding with a nonpharmacologic treatment. Solutions to these problems are sometimes offered by the use of special experimental options (e.g., Armitage, 1960; Zelen, 1979) or quasi-experimental designs.

3.2 QUASI EXPERI- MENTS

A study in which the study factor has been artificially manipulated but for which randomization has not been used is called a *quasi experiment*, a term borrowed from the social sciences (Campbell and Stanley, 1963) (see Table 3.1). These designs may involve one-group comparisons, multiple-group comparisons, or a combination of these.

With a *one-group* (or internal) *comparison*, each experimental unit serves as its own control by observing the response variable before and after one or more interventions. For example, we could observe the motor vehicle fatality rate in a state before and after the enforcement of a new speed limit. (Note that the experimental unit here is the state.)

With a simple *multiple-group* (or external) *comparison*, treatment or intervention groups are compared with each other, as they are in a simple experiment without randomization. In this design, treatment groups are formed from convenience (e.g., geographic areas) or according to the voluntary behavior of subjects (e.g., elective surgery). Using the previous illustration, we could compare the motor vehicle fatality rates in 1975 among several states, some of which had the new speed limit enforced in 1974 and some of which did not.

A mixed design combines elements of both internal and external comparisons, thereby enhancing the potential for making a causal inference. For example, we could observe the absolute changes between 1973 and 1975 in the motor vehicle fatality rates for states in which the new speed limit was first enforced in 1974 and compare these changes to comparable trends in states for which the new speed limit was not enforced.

As we suggested above, a quasi-experimental study can be conducted in a variety of ways. For a more thorough understanding of important principles and applications, see Nagel and Neef (1979), Campbell and Stanley (1963), Isaac and Michael, (1971), Alwin and Sullivan (1975), and Campbell and Cook (1979).

We may distinguish two subtypes of quasi experiments on the basis of how the manipulation or intervention has been done: (1) clinical or laboratory studies and (2) program or policy studies.

3.2.1 Subtypes and Objectives

In *clinical/laboratory studies,* the investigators or their colleagues execute the intervention themselves with a specific group of subjects. Essentially, the clinical/laboratory quasi experiment is a clinical trial or laboratory experiment without randomization and has objectives similar to those of its experimental counterparts (see Table 3.1). This type of quasi experiment is often done when an experiment would be too costly, infeasible, or unethical. For example, we might test the efficacy of treating mild hypertension with dietary modifications by comparing the periodic blood pressure levels of a voluntary test group of mild hypertensives who receive special instruction on diet with the levels of another group of mild hypertensives who do not receive the instruction.

In a *program/policy study,* the intervention typically is planned and implemented by others not involved in the immediate investigation, generally with the intent of alleviating a social problem (which need not be health-oriented). This subtype of quasi experiment is analogous to a community intervention (experiment) without randomization and is closely connected to the process of health planning. The major objectives of a program/policy study are to evaluate the effectiveness of a planned intervention and to suggest program or policy changes in response to this evaluation. An experimental design often cannot be used in this situation, because the intervention has already been initiated when the study begins. Moreover, even when the evaluation is planned prior to the onset of the new program or policy, it is not generally consistent with program/policy objectives to deprive a portion of the target population of the treatment. Thus, the program/policy study is not used primarily to test the efficacy of a therapeutic or preventive measure (which is often assumed); rather, it is used to evaluate the extent to which public health goals have been achieved (i.e., the effectiveness of the intervention).

Because a program/policy study usually is directed toward a large target population, the intervention may not involve the direct manipulation of the known or suspected risk factor of the outcome event. Sometimes, the strategy is to modify or regulate the sociopolitical or physical environment in such a way as to produce desired changes among targeted individuals, which will, in turn, have an impact on the health status of the population. For example, since we know that blood pressure level is an important determinant of cardiovascular disease, we might wish to evaluate a statewide program aimed at educating the populace about the etiology, effects, and treatment of hypertension.

3.2.2 Advantages and Limitations

As already implied, the chief advantage of the quasi experiment over the experiment is the smaller number of practical obstacles. Thus, in general, quasi experiments are likely to be more feasible and less expensive for conducting large studies—and, occasionally, they may be the only alternative.

On the other hand, the lack of randomization also means that the investigator has less control over the influence of extraneous risk factors. Actual control, however, can vary considerably among quasi-experimental designs. On one extreme, failure to randomize can introduce serious distortion in the results that cannot be corrected in the analysis. For example, a nonrandomized comparison of a new drug with traditional therapy for treating diagnosed cases might inadvertently favor the new drug if that test group consisted of cases with better prognoses. Conceivably, this distortion could result if a physician who advocates the new drug is the person who diagnoses the cases, allocates patients into groups, or measures the response.

Some *natural experiments* are quasi experiments,* and they may afford as much control as a true experiment. The design is called a natural experiment because the allocation process appears to be random, although no deliberate attempt was made to randomize. For example, consider the work done by John Snow in London during the middle of the nineteenth century (Snow, 1855). Snow believed that the cholera outbreaks of that period were due to contaminated water supplies, and he took advantage of a natural experiment to test his hypothesis. Shortly before the 1854 epidemic, one of the companies that supplied water to London residents changed its source of intake to the upper part of the Thames, where the water was noticeably cleaner. Fortunately, the houses supplied by that company were randomly distributed throughout London and were not set off from the other houses by divisions of economic status, factory affiliation, or other factors. In fact, very frequently, the residents did not know from which companies they got their water. Using the records of the water companies, census information, and the exact residential location of each new case fatality, Snow was able to compare the mortality rates for cholera

---

*Natural experiments may also be observational studies.

among consumers of the various companies. As predicted, he found a lower mortality rate within homes that received the cleaner water.

Epidemiologists most often use the *observational study,* in which there is no artificial manipulation of the study factor. While an observational study can take many forms, as we will see in Chapter 4, the simplest design closely resembles an experiment or quasi experiment. For example, we could identify a group of elderly hypertensives and a group of elderly normotensives from a baseline exam and follow both cohorts for several years. If the observed relative frequency of senile dementia is greater in the former group, we might infer that blood pressure is a risk factor for the disease. In addition, we could observe the association between blood pressure change or variability (without intervention) and the subsequent development of senile dementia.

Because observational studies are central to epidemiologic research, a more thorough presentation of these designs will be undertaken in Chapters 4 and 5. You may also wish to consult MacMahon and Pugh (1970), Susser (1973), Lilienfeld and Lilienfeld (1980), Cochran (1965), and McKinlay (1975).

Observational studies are commonly divided into two subtypes on the basis of the degree of a priori knowledge regarding the disease.

A *descriptive study* usually is conducted when little is known about the occurrence, the natural history, or the determinants of a disease. The objectives are to estimate the disease frequency or time trend in a particular population and to generate more specific etiologic hypotheses. For example, since we have limited knowledge of the mental health of the elderly, we might plan a community study to estimate the relative frequency of specific mental disorders. Suppose we found that a particular type of depression was very common in this age group, compared to the general population. We might initiate future investigations to explain the relative excess of this disorder and to discover other social and health implications.

An *analytic* (or etiologic) *study* is conducted when enough is known about the disease before the investigation so that specific a priori hypotheses can be tested. The objectives are to identify risk factors for the disease, estimate their effects on the disease, and suggest possible intervention strategies. An example of this subtype is the hypothetical senile dementia study mentioned above, for which high blood pressure was hypothesized to be a risk factor for the disease.

While descriptive and analytic studies are often treated as two mutually exclusive categories, they are, in fact, opposite ends of a continuum. At one end, we know very little about the disease and are searching for clues; at the other end, we know a great deal about the disease and are testing specific hypotheses. Very often, as our understanding of a disease increases, an investigation planned as a descriptive study will become more analytic after data collection begins.

**3.3.2
Advantages
and
Limitations**

Observational research is often the most practical or feasible to conduct because the study factor is not manipulated. However, for reasons that will be discussed in Chapter 4, these studies are not uniformly less expensive nor do they always take less time than other types of studies. Another potential advantage is that observational studies are often carried out in more natural settings, so that the study population is more representative of the target population. As we suggested in Section 3.1.2, this feature has important implications to health planners and policymakers who base their decisions partly on the results of epidemiologic investigations.

The major limitation of observational designs is that they afford the investigator the least control over the study situation; therefore, results are generally more susceptible to distorting influences. Consequently, a greater burden is placed on the investigator, particularly in the analysis stage, to deal with these potential sources of error that threaten the validity of his or her findings.

Because the investigator achieves relatively little control in the design stage, observational studies tend to be unique, making them very difficult to replicate and, therefore, making scientific generalizations less secure (Jamison, 1980). Yet epidemiologists can take advantage of this replication problem by using apparently inconsistent results to refine their hypotheses.

**3.4
CONCLUD-
ING
REMARKS**

In this chapter, we have briefly outlined three broad categories of empirical research: experiments, which involve randomization of study factor categories (or treatments) among all subjects; quasi experiments, which involve artificial manipulation of the study factor without randomization; and observational studies, which involve no artificial manipulation of the study factor. Since epidemiologists, overall, conduct more observational than nonobservational studies, the next two chapters will deal with the specific options and types of observational study designs. Throughout the remainder of this book, in fact, all principles and methods of epidemiologic research are presented in terms of observational studies. Nevertheless, most of the topics and discussions that follow, including validity considerations in Part II and analysis in Part III, apply also to nonobservational studies.

REFERENCES   ALWIN, D. R., and SULLIVAN, M. J. 1975. Issues of design and analysis in evaluation research. *Sociol. Meth. & Res.* 4: 77–100.

ARMITAGE, P. 1960. *Sequential medical trials*. Springfield, Ill.: Thomas.

CAMPBELL, D. T., and COOK, T. D. 1979. *Quasi-experimentation: Design and analysis for field settings*. Chicago: Rand McNally.

CAMPBELL, D. T., and STANLEY, J. C. 1963. *Experimental and quasi-experimental designs for research*. Chicago: Rand McNally.

COCHRAN, W. G. 1965. The planning of observational studies of human populations. *J. R. Stat. Soc. A* 138: 234–265.

COMSTOCK, G. W. 1978. Uncontrolled ruminations on modern controlled trials. *Am. J. Epidemiol.* 108: 81–84.

CORNFIELD, J. 1978. Randomization by group: A formal analysis. *Am. J. Epidemiol.* 108: 100–102.

FARQUHAR, J. W. 1978. The community-based model of life style intervention trials. *Am. J. Epidemiol.* 108: 103–111.

HARRIS, E. L., and FITZGERALD, J. D., eds. 1970. *The principles and practice of clinical trials*. Edinburgh: Livingstone.

ISAAC, S., and MICHAEL, W. B. 1971. *Handbook in research evaluation*. San Diego: EDITS.

JAMISON, J. R. 1980. The use of inferential statistics in health and disease: A warning. *South Afr. Med. J.* 57: 783–785.

KEMPTHORNE, O. 1978. Logical, epistemological and statistical aspects of nature-nurture data interpretation. *Biometrics* 34: 1–23.

LILIENFELD, A. M., and LILIENFELD, D. E. 1980. *Foundations of epidemiology*. 2nd ed. New York: Oxford University Press.

MCKINLAY, S. M. 1975. The design and analysis of the observational study—A review. *J. Am. Stat. Assoc.* 70: 503–523.

MACMAHON, B., and PUGH, T. F. 1970. *Epidemiology: Principles and methods*. Boston: Little, Brown.

NAGEL, S. S., and NEEF, M. 1979. *Policy analysis in social science research*. Beverly Hills, Calif.: Sage; App. 3.1.

PETO, R.; PIKE, M. C.; ARMITAGE, P.; BRESLOW, N. E.; COX, D. R.; HOWARD, S. V.; MANTEL, N.; MCPHERSON, K.; PETO, J.; and SMITH, P. G. 1976. Design and analysis of randomized clinical trials requiring prolonged observation of each patient. I: Introduction and design. *Br. J. Cancer* 34: 585–612.

———. 1977. Design and analysis of randomized clinical trials requiring prolonged observation of each patient. II: Analysis and examples. *Br. J. Cancer* 35: 1–38.

ROTHMAN, K. J. 1977. Epidemiologic methods in clinical trials. *Cancer* 39: 1771–1775.

SARACCI, R. 1979. Controlled studies. In *Health care and epidemiology,* edited by W. W. Holland and L. Karhausen, Chap. 13, pp. 194–207. Boston: Hall.

SHERWIN, R. 1978. Controlled trials of the diet-heart hypothesis: Some comments on the experimental unit. *Am. J. Epidemiol.* 108: 92–99.

SNOW, J. 1855. *On the mode of communication of cholera*. 2nd ed. London: Churchill.

SUSSER, M. 1973. *Causal thinking in the health sciences*. New York: Oxford University Press.

SYME, S. L. 1978. Life style intervention in clinic-based trials. *Am. J. Epidemiol.* 108: 87–91.

WEDDELL, J. 1979. Experimental studies. In *Health care and epidemiology,* edited by W. W. Holland and L. Karhausen, Chap. 14, pp. 208–225. Boston: Hall.

WENNBERG, J. E.; BUNKER, J. P.; and BARNES, B. 1980. The need for assessing the outcome of common medical practices. *Annu. Rev. Public Health* 1: 277–295.

ZELEN, M. 1979. A new design for randomized clinical trials. *N. Engl. J. Med.* 300: 1242–1245.

4

Design Options in Observational Studies

CHAPTER OUTLINE

**4.0
PREVIEW**

In this chapter, we outline the general options available to an investigator planning an observational study. The vast array of design options for conducting observational research may be divided into two broad categories: the selection of subjects and methods of observing subjects. Each category is elaborated in the following sections. Those familiar with non-observational methods will recognize that a few of the options discussed below also pertain to experimental and quasi-experimental research.

**4.1
SUBJECT
SELECTION**

Alternative procedures for selecting the subjects will be considered separately in the context of three methodological areas: (1) restricting the eligibility of potential subjects into the study population; (2) incorporating probability (i.e., random) sampling procedures in the selection process; and (3) stratifying (i.e., categorizing) the distribution of potential subjects prior to selection.

**4.1.1
Restriction**

Restriction refers to the process of narrowing the eligibility of potential subjects and is the major option available to the investigator for selecting a study population in observational research. We restrict eligibility by excluding potential subjects according to the categorization of one or more variables. Typically, each excluded category of a restricted variable is one of the following types: (1) a category of a known risk factor for the disease, such as age or race; (2) a particular medical procedure that influences the diagnosis of disease among persons who otherwise might not be detected, such as a screening procedure or treatment that enhances the degree of medical surveillance; (3) other diseases or conditions thought to be associated with the study factor, which may not be risk factors for the disease; (4) categories of other factors closely related to the convenience of sampling, such as area of residence or time of diagnosis; or (5) categories of the study factor itself.

In the first three cases, restriction is used to control for extraneous risk factors or selection procedures that otherwise might distort our results. By excluding designated persons from the study, we attempt to make our compared groups (e.g., exposed and unexposed, or cases and noncases) similar with respect to the restriction variables. For example, in comparing the development of hypertension in obese and nonobese women, we might restrict our study population to white women between the ages of 40 and 50, because age and race are risk factors for hypertension. Not only does restriction improve comparability between groups, thereby providing some control of distorting effects, but, for any given sample size, it may enhance the statistical efficiency of our tests. As we will see in Chapter 16, failure to deal with extraneous risk factors in the study design requires the investigator to deal with the distorting effects of these factors in the analysis.

The fourth type of restriction (on "convenience" variables) is used to reduce the cost or enhance the feasibility of selecting and observing subjects. For instance, an investigator might wish to limit his or her study population to residents of one state or to workers in a single factory.

While it is possible to restrict the variability of the study factor in the study population (the fifth type of restriction), this procedure is often counterproductive statistically if it sharply reduces the range of study factor values. On the other hand, careful restriction of the study factor can be advantageous. For example, we might limit the study population in an occupational investigation to workers with very intense exposures and workers with no exposure to a specific chemical (the study factor). If a monotonic relationship* exists, for any given sample size, this approach would improve our chance of demonstrating an association.

Methodologically, there are two basic types of restriction: complete and partial. *Complete restriction* establishes uniform eligibility requirements for all potential subjects in the study population, as in the previous examples. *Partial restriction,* also known as *matching,* limits the eligibility of potential subjects for one or more comparison groups, on the basis of observations of another independently selected index group. For example, a series of noncases (comparison group) is matched or selected to be similar to a series of cases (index group) with respect to the latter's age distribution (the matching variable). Thus, only the eligibility of potential comparison subjects is actually restricted by the matching procedure.

In practice, we match either by *pairing* one or more comparison subjects to each index subject with respect to the matching variables (i.e., *individual matching*) or by forcing the *distribution* of matching variables in the comparison groups to be similar to the distribution in the index group (i.e., *frequency matching*) (MacMahon and Pugh, 1970, Chap. 12). Individual matching may be further divided into artificial and natural procedures. *Artificial matching* indicates that the investigator does the matching from his or her knowledge of the matching variables in a larger pool of potential comparison subjects. This basic procedure is the one we alluded to in the previous paragraph. *Natural matching,* on the other hand, indicates that paired subjects (or matched sets) are formed without the aid of the investigator. For example, we could study twins or sibling pairs in which one member (index subject or proband) has a disease or trait and the other (comparison subject) does not. The key difference between artificial and natural matching is that while the matching variables are explicitly defined and measured in the former case, they are only implicitly defined in the latter. Thus, for example, twins may be similar on several genetic and environmental factors, any of which may be related to the disease of interest. The topics of matching and the analytic techniques that accompany matching will be presented in Chapter 18.

---

*A monotonic relationship is one in which the risk of disease increases with increasing exposure or in which the risk decreases with increasing exposure.

**4.1.2
Random
Sampling**

Random sampling refers to the selection of subjects in such a way as to give each potential subject in the target population a known probability of being included in the study (Hansen et al., 1953). The case in which all selection probabilities are equal is known as *simple random sampling*—i.e., in this design, each person has the same probability of being sampled. The cornerstone of survey research, random sampling ensures that the study population is *representative* (on the average) of the target population with respect to all factors relevant to the investigator, including the joint distribution of the disease and its determinants. Random sampling, therefore, allows the researcher to make statistical inferences regarding certain target population parameters from his or her estimates in the study population. Thus, the researcher may conclude, with a certain degree of confidence, that his or her findings are not due to errors of sampling.

Random sampling should be distinguished from the random allocation of treatments to all subjects in an experiment (i.e., randomization). As we discussed in Section 3.1, randomization attempts to distribute evenly the presence of extraneous risk factors among groups in order to ensure comparability. Unlike random sampling, which is aimed at achieving representativeness of the study population (on the average), randomization is aimed at achieving control over the study situation (on the average). Viewed another way, random sampling is a formal procedure for dealing with (random) sampling errors, and randomization is an analogous device primarily for dealing with potential (nonrandom) systematic errors. Thus, in general, random selection in observational studies cannot replace randomization in experiments.

**4.1.3
Stratified
Sampling**

Stratified sampling is the independent selection of subjects from mutually exclusive subpopulations, or *strata*, of the target population; that is, each stratum is sampled separately. Very frequently, random sampling is used within each stratum (i.e., stratified random sampling), so that members of different strata may have different probabilities of being selected. Strata are formed from categories of one or more variables of the following types: (1) known or suspected risk factors for the disease; (2) factors related to the convenience of sampling; (3) the study factor(s); or (4) the disease of primary interest.

We often use stratified sampling within categories of a strong risk factor in order to ensure adequate numbers of cases for a wide range of the risk factor. For example, in a study of coronary heart disease, we might oversample younger adults since the disease is less frequent earlier in life. Alternatively, if a major objective of the study were to compare the effect of the study factor on the disease for different racial or ethnic groups, we might select an equal number of blacks and whites despite unequal numbers in the target population. In both cases, we use stratified sampling to ensure a more statistically efficient test for any given sample size. Like restriction, stratified sampling also might facilitate the implementation of the study, such as sampling from separate hospitals (even if the disease rate does not vary by hospital).

Using the study factor to stratify in the selection of subjects may be convenient if certain categories or values of the study factor occur much less frequently than others. For example, in the comparison of vasecto-mized and nonvasectomized men, it may be advantageous to select the former group from the patients of a vasectomy clinic, since most men in the target population have not had this surgery. Equal numbers of the two compared groups also will ensure a more statistically efficient test for any given sample size.

The major reason we stratify on disease status before subject selection is to deal with an infrequent (or rare) disease—in much the same way that we stratify on the study factor to deal with a rare exposure. However, this strategy has other design implications, which will be discussed in Section 4.2.3. We may conclude that, in all other examples cited above, stratified sampling is used to make the analysis more efficient or the data collection more feasible. In this regard, it is less important to observational study design than are the options of restriction and random sampling.

Stratified sampling should be distinguished from two other forms of stratification: (1) stratification, or *blocking*, in the allocation of treatments in an experiment and (2) stratification in the analysis (of any study design). In an experiment with a blocked design, randomization is done separately within subgroups (i.e., blocks) of the study population. Generally, *blocks* are defined by the cross-classification of one or more variables (i.e., blocking variables) that either are believed to be associated with the outcome or are convenient for collecting data. Like stratified sampling, blocking ensures a more statistically efficient test of the null hypothesis.

In *stratified analysis*, all observations are categorized into separate strata after the data are collected, according to one or more extraneous variables. The analytic treatment of such data is presented in Chapter 17. Unlike the other forms of stratification, stratified analysis controls for extraneous risk factors that would otherwise distort our results.

The following subsections deal with six related options pertaining to methods of observing the study population. Together with the options presented in Section 4.1, they comprise a vast assortment of design choices available to planners of observational research.

**4.2
METHODS OF
OBSERVA-
TION**

The type of study population refers to the nature of the experience of subjects during the course of empirical investigation. Either the experience is *cross-sectional,* indicating single observations at one hypothetical point in time, or *longitudinal,* indicating at least two sets of observations or ongoing surveillance of the study population over a given follow-up

**4.2.1
Type of
Population**

period. Longitudinal studies may involve either a fixed cohort* or a dynamic population.

A *fixed cohort* is a group of subjects identified at a hypothetical point in time and followed for a given period for detection of new cases of disease. The cohort is "fixed" in the sense that no entries are permitted into the study after the onset of follow-up, though subsequent losses may occur as a result of nonparticipation, migration from the study area, death, or other forms of attrition. Generally, the average age of a fixed cohort increases as the duration of follow-up increases.

A *dynamic population* may gain and lose subjects over the course of the follow-up period. For example, we might follow the residents of a county or the employees of a work force between 1980 and 1985 for new cases of malignant melanoma. If the size and the age distributions of the dynamic population remain constant during the follow-up period, we refer to it as *stable*.[†] Thus, the average age of a stable, dynamic population remains fixed as the follow-up period progresses.

Sometimes we can view a dynamic population as a hypothetical fixed cohort if entry into the study corresponds to an event marking the onset of the relevant risk period (i.e., the period during which the subject is a candidate for developing the outcome event). For example, in an investigation of the relationship between smoking and subsequent coronary events among a group of coronary heart disease (CHD) cases, we might collect data on all first myocardial infarctions diagnosed in one hospital during a three-year period, obtain the patients' smoking histories, and follow those patients until a certain time for subsequent coronary events. Although the design involves a dynamic population, we may analyze it as a fixed cohort by defining the onset of the (hypothetical) collective follow-up period as the occurrence of the first myocardial infarction, regardless of the date on which it actually occurred. Of course, this approach almost always results in different lengths of follow-up for subjects.

4.2.2
Definition of
Disease Status

In epidemiologic research, the disease may be characterized as either a *state* of health or a *change* in health status over a follow-up period. In each case, the disease variable may be *continuous* (quantitative), such as blood pressure level or change in blood pressure, or *categorical* (qualitative), such as the presence of hyptertension or the development of hypertension (Kleinbaum and Kupper, 1978). The special case of a two-category variable is called a *dichotomy* and commonly is applied to most clinically defined entities (e.g., hypertensive versus normotensive). Despite the widespread appeal, conceptually and analytically, of measuring disease

---

*Defined in the most general terms, a cohort is a group of people who have something in common. For example, a birth cohort is a group of people who were born in the same year or period (see Section 7.3).

[†]Regarding a specific disease, a more restricted definition of a stable population states that the distributions of *all* risk factors (including age) remain fixed.

status as a dichotomy, our knowledge of many conditions and their clinical detection make this convention somewhat dubious and possibly misleading (Rose and Barker, 1978). For example, the diagnosis of adult-onset diabetes is made from several clinical signs and symptoms, including the results of a glucose tolerance test. Yet no level of glucose tolerance clearly differentiates cases from noncases, especially for persons over 65.

The dichotomous measurement of a disease state is called *prevalence* —i.e., prevalence is the presence of a disease at a hypothetical point in time (MacMahon and Pugh, 1970, Chap. 5). Thus, prevalent cases are existing cases for which the duration of the disease may remain unknown to the investigator. In any cross-sectional survey, the observed prevalent cases tend to exclude early fatalities, which are not available for selection, and tend to overrepresent cases who survive longer.

The dichotomous measurement of a change in disease status is called *incidence*—i.e., incidence is the development of the disease during a given period (MacMahon and Pugh, 1970, Chap. 5). Thus, incident cases are new occurrences—or, in practice, newly diagnosed events during the follow-up period. Depending on the disease and the objectives of the study, we may be interested in (1) first occurrences of the disease among subjects who never previously had the condition (i.e., first incidence), such as the development of an incurable chronic disease (e.g., coronary heart disease or diabetes); (2) all occurrences of one disease among subjects who may have multiple episodes (i.e., total incidence), such as the development of an infection (e.g., influenza) or a remittent disease (e.g., arthritis); or (3) death from one or more diseases either among the total study population (i.e., mortality) or among cases of the disease (i.e., fatality). Note that the part of the study population at risk of developing an incident event—i.e., the *candidate population*—differs by the type of event. For example, while subjects with a disease are not eligible to become new cases of that disease, they are eligible to develop subsequent occurrences and to die of the disease, if the disease is curable and if cases do not acquire lifelong immunity.

Directionality is a key dimension of observational study design, referring to the temporal relationship between our observation of study factor level and our observation of disease status (Miettinen, 1975). In a study with *forward* directionality, the investigator starts with observations of the study factor in the candidate population and follows that group for subsequent detection of incident cases or other changes in health status. Thus, in a forward design, the investigator proceeds from observations of the hypothesized risk factor to observations of the disease. In fact, all experiments and quasi experiments involve forward directionality; most observational studies do not.

In a *backward* design, the investigator begins with the classification of disease status (e.g., case versus noncase) and obtains information about individual histories of the study factor—i.e., previous exposures, events,

**4.2.3
Directionality**

or characteristics. Thus, the backward design proceeds from observations of the disease to observations of previous factors that are hypothesized as risk factors. Notice that, in both forward and backward designs involving incident cases, the investigator is able to ascertain, in theory, whether the study factor actually preceded the occurrence of the disease.

In a *nondirectional* design, the investigator observes simultaneously both the study factor and the disease, so that neither variable may be uniquely identified as occurring first. A nondirectional study may be cross-sectional, with selection of the sample from one target population. In this typical situation, disease status must be defined as prevalence at the time of observation. Alternatively, a nondirectional design may involve a follow-up period if changes in *both* the study factor and disease are observed concurrently. For example, suppose we test the association between individual change in blood pressure from 1960 to 1970 and the incidence of CHD during the same period. In either situation, we cannot ascertain from the study design whether the hypothesized cause actually preceded the occurrence of the disease.

Directionality is central to the interpretation of epidemiologic findings because it governs the researcher's ability to distinguish antecedent from consequent—a criterion for identifying risk factors (see Section 2.2). In addition, we will see in Chapters 10 and 11 that directionality is important in assessing the validity of our results.

4.2.4 Timing

Timing refers to the chronological relationship between the onset of the study (or, more specifically, the time of the most recent data gathering) and the occurrence of the primary phenomena under study (i.e., the study factor and the disease) (Miettinen, 1975). In a completely *prospective study,* the researcher observes directly both the study factor and the disease after the onset of the study so that observations can be recorded according to a study protocol. Thus, the directionality of a completely prospective study is forward or nondirectional, never backward.

In a completely *retrospective study*, both the study factor and the disease occur before the onset of the study. The researcher obtains information on the primary variables from records (e.g., censuses, insurance records, vital statistics) and/or from the recall of previous events by subjects, their relatives, or friends. A completely retrospective study may have any directionality, but it often involves a forward design; seldom does it involve a nondirectional design. As an example of a completely retrospective design with forward directionality, an investigator in 1980 might use company records to compare the lymphoma mortality rate between 1960 and 1979 for workers exposed to benzene during the 1950s with the rate for unexposed workers.

Many studies combine features of both prospective and retrospective designs. In such *ambispective designs*, either one primary variable is measured prospectively and the other retrospectively or one primary variable is measured in both ways. An example of the former type is a forward study of the possible effect of childhood development on the incidence of cancers later in life. We might identify a group of middle-age adults, question them about childhood experiences and social relationships (retrospective), and follow them into the future for subsequent detection of cancers (prospective). This example could also be made ambispective in the latter way by including previous occurrences of cancer before the onset of the study—that is, cancer incidence could be measured both retrospectively and prospectively.

Unlike directionality, timing does not directly influence our ability to distinguish between antecedent and consequent. Nevertheless, timing may have important implications for the quality of our data and thus for our ability to make inferences. In general, retrospective data, based on either records or recall, are more likely to involve measurement errors than are prospective data. We will see in Chapter 12 that this source of error is particularly important if subjects' recall of previous events or behaviors is itself influenced by current disease status.

The *unit of observation* for a particular variable is the level of human aggregation upon which a direct measurement is actually taken. It may be the individual or a collection of individuals, such as the family, community, or county. Because the level of primary biologic interest to epidemiologists is the individual, most epidemiologic data are based on the individual unit of observation.

**4.2.5
Units of
Observation
and Analysis**

The *unit of analysis* is the common level for which the data on all relevant variables is reduced and analyzed (Dogan and Rokkan, 1969). In epidemiology, the unit of analysis is generally the individual (*individual analysis*) or the group (*ecologic* or *aggregate analysis*), both of which may be done in forward or nondirectional studies. However, backward studies usually involve the analysis of individuals. The key difference between individual and ecologic analyses is that, in the latter, we do not know the joint distribution of the study factor and the disease within each group (unit of analysis), while in the former, we do know the joint distribution.

If the units of observation and analysis for a particular variable are identical, the variable is called *primary* (Dogan and Rokkan, 1969). For example, we might assess cardiovascular disease (CVD) mortality status and the average hardness of water consumed by every member in the study population. If we perform an individual analysis, both variables are primary. Alternatively, the unit of analysis for a primary variable may be the group if the variable is constructed without aggregating the experiences of individuals. For example, suppose we observed the ecologic association between average water hardness and CVD mortality among several contiguous regions, each with its own water supply. If we obtain water hardness levels from each region's water supply without aggregating individually assessed consumption levels, the study factor in this analysis is also primary.

If the units of observation and analysis are different, the variable is called *derived* (Dogan and Rokkan, 1969). Using the previous example, we could assign the water hardness value of the local water supply to every subject in that region in order to perform an individual analysis of the possible association between water hardness and CVD mortality. The study factor in this case is derived, because the unit of observation is the region and the unit of analysis is the individual. Alternatively, the study factor also would be derived in an ecologic analysis if we averaged individually measured water hardness levels for all subjects within each region in order to construct a regional index. In this last example, the disease variable also would be derived, because it is based on the aggregation of individual disease statuses to estimate the rate for each region.

Thus, we may classify each variable in a particular analysis into one of four categories: (1) primary variable, using individual analysis; (2) primary variable, using ecologic analysis; (3) derived variable, using individual analysis; (4) derived variable, using ecologic analysis. When you wish to make causal inferences about disease etiology, the first category generally is preferable for treating all relevant variables.

**4.2.6
Method of
Data Collection**

Data collection can be considered primary or secondary; the classification depends on the conditions under which observations were first recorded.

Primary data are those collected for purposes of the study, according to the study protocol. Such data may be prospective, retrospective, or ambispective and involve any type of directionality. The data are obtained through personal interviews, medical examinations and tests, questionnaires, or the direct observations of behavior.

Secondary data are those collected for purposes other than those of the study. Generally, secondary data must be abstracted and modified for the study. Secondary data are obtained from records of individuals (e.g., medical records, employment records, death certificates, disease registries) or from group records (e.g., the U.S. census, vital statistics, or national health examination surveys) (MacMahon and Pugh, 1970, Chap. 6). Thus, secondary data are usually retrospective, and they are frequently used to perform ecologic analyses, since study factor and disease information often is not available at the individual level in large populations.

While secondary data are generally much less expensive to collect than are primary data, the latter are typically more appropriate to the specific objectives of the study. Consequently, primary data are usually superior for testing a new hypothesis.

**4.3
CONCLUD-
ING
REMARKS**

We have divided the choices available in the design of observational research into options related to the selection of subjects and options related to the methods of observation. Regarding subject selection, the investigator must decide how to narrow the eligibility requirements of the study population by complete restriction or matching, how to make the study population representative of the target population by random sampling, and whether to stratify to make the study more feasible or to make the analysis more statistically efficient. Regarding methods of observation, the investigator must define the nature of the study population as cross-sectional, fixed cohort, or dynamic; select among measures of disease incidence, prevalence, or mortality; establish the directionality of the design as forward, backward, or nondirectional; specify the timing of variable measurement as prospective, retrospective, or ambispective; choose the units of observation and analysis as individual or ecologic; and decide between primary and secondary data sources. Although these choices define a large assortment of design combinations, sets of options are often used together—e.g., an ecologic study with secondary mortality data, or a prospective cohort study with forward directionality and primary incidence data. In the next chapter, we present types of observational studies corresponding to the most common groupings of these design options.

REFERENCES

DOGAN, M., and ROKKAN, S., eds. 1969. *Social ecology.* Cambridge, Mass.: MIT Press; Introduction, pp. 1–15.

HANSEN, M. H.; HURWITZ, W. N.; and MADOW, W. G. 1953. *Sample survey methods and theory.* Vol. II: *Theory.* New York: Wiley.

KLEINBAUM, D. G., and KUPPER, L. L. 1978. *Applied regression analysis and other multivariable methods.* Boston: Duxbury Press; Chap. 2.

MACMAHON, B., and PUGH, T. F. 1970. *Epidemiology: Principles and methods.* Boston: Little, Brown.

MIETTINEN, O. S. 1975. Principles of epidemiologic research. Unpublished manuscript. Cambridge, Mass.: Harvard University.

ROSE, G., and BARKER, D. J. P. 1978. What is a case? Dichotomy or continuum? *Br. Med. J.* 2: 873–874.

5

Typology of Observational Study Designs

CHAPTER OUTLINE

Because there are so many possible combinations of the design options, as we saw in Chapter 4, it is convenient to classify observational studies into a small number of types or study designs. The following subsections describe 15 such designs grouped into three broad categories: basic designs, hybrid designs, and incomplete designs. In practice, certain studies may be classified into more than one category, and the designs may be defined differently by various epidemiologists. Nevertheless, the following definitions and terms, in general, are those found in the current methodological literature.

5.0 PREVIEW

Each design is accompanied by a flow diagram that represents a simple illustration of that approach. These figures treat both the study factor and the disease as dichotomous variables and are created from a set of standard symbols. The following letters will be used in the flow diagrams to represent groups of individuals:

$$N = \text{target } population$$
$$C = prevalent \text{ cases}$$
$$D = incident \text{ cases or deaths}$$
$$\overline{C} \text{ or } \overline{D} = \text{noncases or survivors}$$
$$E = \text{subjects } with \text{ the } study \ factor \text{ (exposed)}$$
$$\overline{E} = \text{subjects } without \text{ the } study \ factor \text{ (unexposed)}$$
$$F = \text{subjects with another study factor}$$
$$\overline{F} = \text{subjects without another study factor}$$

A key to the graphic symbols used in the flow diagrams is shown below.

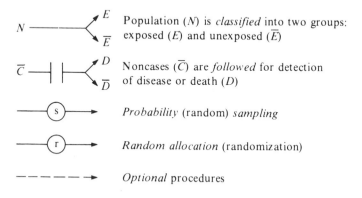

N ———— $\begin{cases} E \\ \overline{E} \end{cases}$ Population (N) is *classified* into two groups: exposed (E) and unexposed ($\overline{E}$)

$\overline{C}$ —||— $\begin{cases} D \\ \overline{D} \end{cases}$ Noncases ($\overline{C}$) are *followed* for detection of disease or death (D)

——(s)——➤ *Probability* (random) *sampling*

——(r)——➤ *Random allocation* (randomization)

– – – – ➤ *Optional* procedures

Basic designs consist of three principal types of studies (these types are usually given the most emphasis in epidemiologic texts): cohort studies, cross-sectional studies, and case-control studies (MacMahon and Pugh, 1970; Miettinen, 1975; Friedman, 1980). The objectives of the first two approaches may be descriptive or etiologic; the objectives of case-control studies are traditionally etiologic. All three types involve the individual as the unit of analysis.

5.1 BASIC DESIGNS

5.1.1
Cohort Study

The *cohort study* (Figure 5.1)—also called a follow-up, incidence, panel, or prospective study—involves a design in which information about the study factor (E and $\bar{E}$) is known for all subjects at the beginning of the follow-up period. The population at risk of developing the outcome event —either disease incidence or mortality—is followed for a given period through reexaminations or population surveillance, during or after which new cases or deaths (D) are identified. A cohort study involving incident cases of a chronic disease is concerned with first occurrence of the disease; thus, the candidate population is composed of all persons ($\bar{C}$) in the study population without the disease who are eligible to become cases.

EXAMPLE 5.1

Cohort designs often are used to study relatively frequent occurrences, such as coronary events, motor vehicle injuries, common infections, or deaths from all causes. For example, we might test the possible association between type A behavior pattern (Friedman and Rosenman, 1971) and CHD by comparing the frequency of incident cases for a group of type A subjects with the frequency of incident cases for a group of type B subjects. We exclude from the study population prevalent cases identified at the onset of the follow-up period (see Figure 5.1), and we follow both groups for the same duration. If a greater proportion of type A than type B subjects develop the disease, we may conclude that the study factor is statistically associated with disease incidence. Thus, assuming no distortion of our results, we may infer that behavior pattern is a risk factor for CHD.

A cohort study may be completely prospective, retrospective (using secondary data), or ambispective. Since a prospective cohort study is the type of observational design that most closely resembles an experiment, it is generally preferred for making causal inferences. Yet, a retrospective cohort study may be more feasible for studying a rare disease or a disease with a long latent period. The retrospective design, of course, depends on the availability of previous study factor information on a well-defined population that has been followed for detection of new cases or deaths. A potential problem in any type of cohort study, particularly those involving disease incidence and long follow-up periods, is the loss of subjects because of migration, lack of participation, and death. As we will see in Chapter 11, attrition of the study population over the follow-up period can lead to distortion of results, which cannot easily be corrected in the analysis.

The cohort study involves either a fixed cohort, which gets followed for a given period, or a dynamic population, for which the individual follow-up period of every subject is known (or assumed) by the investiga-

Figure 5.1 Cohort Study

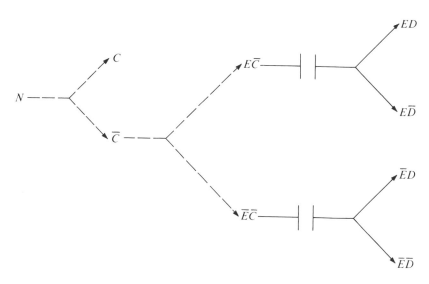

tor. As suggested in Figure 5.1, the compared groups—i.e., exposed (E) and unexposed ($\bar{E}$)—may be selected from separate populations; however, causal inference depends on the assumption that the populations are comparable with respect to factors other than the exposure of interest.

The major methodological advantage of the cohort design is that the study factor level on each subject is observed at the onset of the follow-up period—i.e., before the disease is detected. Consequently, the investigator can be reasonably sure that the hypothesized cause preceded the occurrence of the disease and that disease status did not differentially influence the selection of subjects by study factor level. In other words, cohort studies are relatively free of certain types of selection bias that can seriously limit other basic designs. It is this same design feature, however, that also accounts for the chief weaknesses of the cohort study. Because study factor information must be observed at the onset, a cohort study is not very good for generating new etiologic hypotheses regarding a certain disease after the follow-up period has begun. Furthermore, the cohort design is statistically and practically inefficient for studying rare diseases, because study factor information must be collected on a large number of subjects, of which only a small number will become cases.

5.1.2 Cross-sectional Study

A *cross-sectional study* (Figure 5.2)—also called a survey or prevalence study—involves a nondirectional or backward design of a study population that has been selected from a single target population. As indicated in Figure 5.2, this type of design involves disease prevalence (C), not incidence, and usually involves random sampling of the dynamic target population (N). After the selection process, all participating subjects are exam-

Figure 5.2 Cross-sectional Study

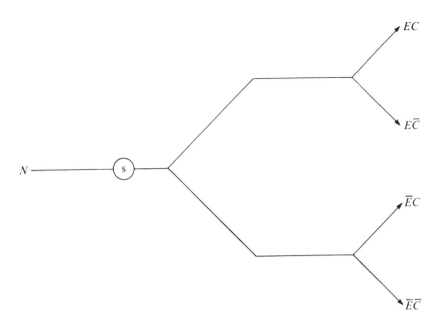

ined, observed, and/or questioned about their disease status, their current
or past study factor level, and other relevant variables.

EXAMPLE 5.2

Cross-sectional studies are particularly useful for studying conditions that
are quantitatively measured and that can vary over time (e.g., blood
pressure) or relatively frequent diseases that have long durations (e.g.,
chronic bronchitis). For example, we might draw a random sample of all
persons over the age of 20 in the state of Connecticut, question the
respondents about their smoking habits, and determine whether each
subject has chronic bronchitis by using a standard clinical examination.
We could then estimate the proportion of persons in the state who have the
disease (i.e., the prevalence rate) and compare such frequency measures
for different categories of smoking. If smokers are more likely than
nonsmokers to have chronic bronchitis, we may conclude that smoking is
statistically associated with disease prevalence. However, we cannot infer
that smoking is a risk factor for chronic bronchitis from these findings,
because we do not know how long the cases had the disease. That is, in
a cross-sectional study, we cannot distinguish empirically between risk

---

EXAMPLE 5.2 (*continued*)

factors and prognostic factors without additional information. In this example, therefore, smoking may not be related to the development of chronic bronchitis among disease-free individuals, but perhaps smoking is related to duration of survival among cases. Moreover, prevalence data cannot be used in the same way as incidence data to ascertain the direction of the relationship between study factor and disease, if an association is found. The investigator cannot determine from the study design alone whether the hypothesized cause was an antecedent or a consequent of the disease.

Sometimes cross-sectional studies do not use random (probability) sampling. But without random sampling, a cross-sectional study has limited value for describing the frequency of disease or other characteristics in a large population, and it has serious limitations for making causal inferences. As we will see in Chapter 11, not knowing the probability that an individual in the target population will be selected can lead to a distortion of our results if either disease status or study factor level inadvertently influences the probability of selection. On the other hand, carefully conducted probability sampling substantially increases the likelihood that the study population is *representative* of the target population. While this feature does not ensure the validity of our comparisons for making causal inferences, it does make cross-sectional studies particularly useful for describing characteristics of a target population (Feinstein, 1978). Thus, they are often used by administrators to plan health facilities, services, and programs.

Because the cross-sectional design does not involve a follow-up period, it is often used to generate new etiologic hypotheses regarding study factors and/or diseases. However, cross-sectional studies are not appropriate for studying rare diseases or diseases with short durations. In fact, this disadvantage is worse for cross-sectional studies than for cohort studies, because the latter design permits the regulation of the follow-up period, which governs the number of incident cases. In a cross-sectional study, however, rarity of the disease is defined by prevalence, which cannot be regulated by the design without introducing distortion.

5.1.3 Case-Control Study

The *case-control study* (Figure 5.3)—also known as a case-referent, case history, or retrospective study—involves a backward or nondirectional design that compares a group of cases (D) and one or more groups of noncases ($\overline{C}$) (i.e., controls) with respect to a current or a previous study factor level (E and $\overline{E}$). As indicated in Figure 5.3, the investigator selects these groups from separate populations of available cases and noncases; there-

Figure 5.3 Case-Control Study

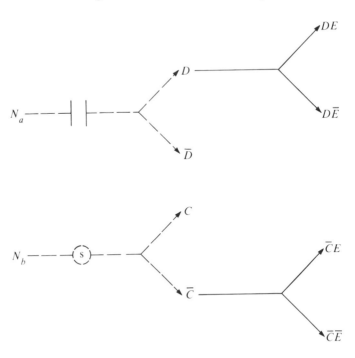

fore, this study differs from a cross-sectional design, which involves selection from a single target population. Another difference is that case-control studies, unlike cross-sectional studies, may involve incident cases of disease; i.e., cases and noncases may be identified over time, as is done in a cohort study. However, the occurrences of disease in a case-control study are not usually linked to a single, well-defined population. To make a causal inference, the investigator must assume that the comparison subjects ($\overline{C}$) are representative of the same candidate population (N_a) from which the cases (D) developed—i.e., N_a and N_b are equivalent. A case-control study may also be done with prevalent cases (C) identified from N_a.

EXAMPLE 5.3

Case-control studies are well suited to testing etiologic hypotheses for specific rare diseases. Since the ratio of cases to noncases can be fixed by the investigator, analyses are more statistically efficient than they are for other designs for a given sample size and study cost. For example, consider the investigation of the possible relationship between oral contraceptives and

EXAMPLE 5.3 (*continued*)

breast cancer. We might identify all newly diagnosed cases of the disease reported in a hospital during a given period and compare them to an equal number of noncancer patients from the same hospital, matched on age and race. Alternatively (or, perhaps, in addition), we might compare the cases to an equal number of healthy women selected from the region that the hospital serves. If cases and noncases have the same distribution of oral contraceptive use, we might (tentatively) infer no effect of the study factor on the disease. On the other hand, if cases are significantly more likely than noncases to have been prescribed oral contraceptives, or if they took the pill for longer periods of time or at higher estrogen dosages, we might infer a deleterious effect of the drug. Essentially, we are reasoning that, because cases are more likely than noncases to have used the pill, users are more likely to have developed breast cancer (Cornfield and Haenszel, 1960).

Although matching (i.e., partial restriction) is seldom used in cohort or cross-sectional studies, it is used often in case-control studies. We will see in Chapter 18 that the relatively frequent use of matching in case-control studies cannot be solely justified either by the greater need to control for the effect of extraneous risk factors (which must actually be controlled in the analysis after matching) or by the enhancement of statistical efficiency (which may be counterproductive in case-control studies). Rather, the widespread use of matching in case-control studies must also be explained by practical considerations, such as the convenience or cost of subject selection and, perhaps, by the intuitive appeal of the procedure for dealing with extraneous risk factors (instead of relying solely on complex statistical techniques).

The case-control design has been used by biomedical researchers for more than a century (Lilienfeld and Lilienfeld, 1979) and is probably the major contribution of epidemiologists and their predecessors to the general area of research methods. In recent years, the number of published case-control studies has increased dramatically (Cole, 1979), generating many insights into the etiology of chronic diseases, such as lung, cervical, and vaginal cancers, intravascular thrombosis, and congenital defects (Sartwell, 1974; Pearson, 1979). These past successes are largely the result of the practical advantages of conducting case-control studies when other basic designs would be much less feasible. Not only does the case-control design afford the opportunity to study diseases that occur very infrequently, but it also allows for the investigation of diseases with any latent period or duration of expression (see Figure 2.1). Furthermore, the convenient sampling strategy and the relatively short study period usually make case-control studies less time-consuming and less expensive than cohort or cross-sectional studies. Nevertheless, the use of the case-control design has generated a good deal of controversy among epidemiologists (Ibrahim, 1979; *British Medical Journal,* 1979; Mann et al., 1979) because it is most different, methodologically, from the classical experiment (Schneiderman and Levin, 1973).

The principal limitations of case-control studies derive from two key features of the study design: study factor information is obtained *after* the occurrence of the disease; and the compared groups of cases and noncases are selected from *two* separate populations. Consequently, it is difficult to ensure that cases and noncases in the study population are comparable with respect to extraneous risk factors and other sources of distortion. We will discuss in Chapter 11 how typical strategies for selecting the study groups can lead to certain types of bias that cannot readily be corrected in the analysis.

Aside from the above selection problems, case-control studies have other practical limitations. Of course, the disease must be measured as a categorical variable (e.g., case versus noncase), and it must be recognized as the one health outcome of interest before subjects are selected. Thus, the case-control design may not be appropriate for exploring the possible health effects of a certain study factor. Without additional information, this design is also not appropriate for estimating the frequency of the disease in a population. Furthermore, because case-control studies cannot have forward directionality, the ability of the investigator to distinguish antecedent from consequent depends on the retrospective ascertainment of study factor information. Either these data must be collected from records, which are often inadequate or incomplete, or they must be obtained from the recall of past events and habits, which is subject to substantial human errors. The use of subject recall is particularly problematic when respondents are aware of the association being tested or when the study factor involves a very subjective assessment. In these latter situations, self-reported study factor level is likely to be influenced by the disease status of the subject. Such "selective recall" would distort results, usually making the observed association between study factor and disease stronger than the actual association.

**5.2
HYBRID
DESIGNS**

Hybrid studies, as their name implies, are composite designs that (1) combine elements of two basic designs, (2) extend the strategy of one basic design through repetition, or (3) combine elements of a basic design with elements of a nonobservational design. In this section, we will describe the major type of hybrid design, the ambidirectional study, and we will briefly review several other hybrid studies that have not been well delineated in the literature. In fact, researchers commonly label hybrid studies as cohort, cross-sectional, or case-control studies by focusing on one design feature and ignoring others. We distinguish the hybrid designs here in order to emphasize the diversity of design options in observational research and to encourage a more careful classification of design types.

Figure 5.4 Ambidirectional Study

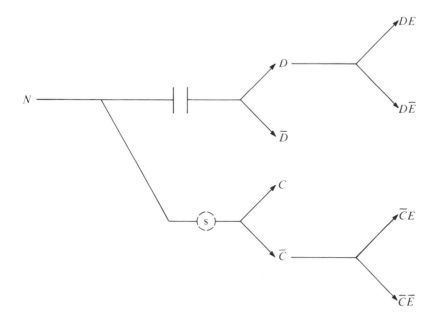

The *ambidirectional study* (Figure 5.4) (Miettinen, 1975)—also called a nested case-control study—combines elements of cohort and case-control designs. A single candidate population (N) is defined at the onset, without reference to study factor information, and is followed for a given period for detection of all new cases of a disease (D). The incident cases are then compared with a group of noncases ($\overline{C}$) sampled from the same population with respect to previous or current study factor levels (MacMahon and Pugh, 1970, Chap. 12; Miettinen, 1975, 1976; Kupper et al., 1975). Either the comparison subjects are sampled randomly from the candidate population or they are matched to incident cases. The candidate population may be fixed, as in a cohort study, or dynamic; but, in the latter case, the investigator need not observe the amount of follow-up time (at risk) contributed by each individual (Miettinen, 1976). As we will discuss in Chapter 6, the investigator can estimate the frequency of disease in the population by assuming that the candidate population is stable.

**5.2.1
Ambi-
directional
Study**

EXAMPLE 5.4

The ambidirectional study is the most important type of hybrid design, because it effectively combines a few of the major advantages of both

EXAMPLE 5.4 (*continued*)

cohort and case-control studies (Miettinen, 1976; Kupper et al., 1975). The most appropriate situation for an ambidirectional design is the etiologic study of one or more rare diseases, where the investigator can determine the time of diagnosis for each case. Frequently, an investigator will be able to identify most new cases of a disease in a large dynamic population by using existing information systems, such as employment or insurance records, a disease registry, or vital records.

Suppose we use the Connecticut Tumor Registry to identify all primary cases of bladder cancer in the state during a given period. We might then compare this group to a sample of noncases in the state who have been matched on age and time of diagnosis. We interview all subjects or their surviving relatives to collect information on saccharin consumption and other known risk factors for the disease. Since the prevalence of the disease is small, there will be very few existing cases in the comparison group; nevertheless, we usually must verify this classification with physical exams, a review of medical records, or medical histories. The design allows us to estimate the average bladder cancer rate during the study period as well as the strength of the association between saccharin consumption and bladder cancer (Miettinen, 1976).

Of course, this application of an ambidirectional design in a dynamic population depends on complete ascertainment of all (or most) new cases and may be limited by unknown rates of migration into or out of the population. Consequently, in practice, this design merges with the case-control design in which there is no direct link between observed noncases and the candidate population from which observed cases developed.

Sometimes an ambidirectional study is contained within a prospective cohort study (typically involving a fixed cohort), either when an etiologic hypothesis emerges after the beginning of follow-up (for a factor that was not measured) or when it is too expensive to measure the exposure level of every subject in the study population. Thus, as occurred in the previous application, exposure information is collected for only a fraction of the noncases. Since the follow-up mechanism in this design usually involves individual assessment (instead of population surveillance), we can be more confident than we were in the previous application that observed noncases are representative of the same candidate population from which the observed cases developed.

The major advantage of an ambidirectional design over a case-control design is that, in the former, cases and noncases are identified from the same well-defined candidate population. Thus, the ambidirectional design reduces, somewhat, the potential for certain types of selection bias in the estimation of effect and enables the investigator to estimate the frequency of disease in the population. The chief advantage of the ambidirectional design over the cohort design is the feasibility of studying rare diseases, since study factor information in ambidirectional studies is obtained on only a small fraction of the noncases in the candidate population. Of course, this latter advantage means that the hybrid study also has one potential limitation of the case-control study: the ability to distinguish antecedent from consequent depends on the ability to assess study factor levels retrospectively. And in Section 4.2.3, we argued that such a procedure may result in measurement errors or omissions, which can lead to distortion of the estimated effect.

5.2.2 Other Hybrid Studies

The following hybrid designs often get grouped or confused with the basic designs described in Section 5.1. In many situations, however, the distinctions we make here are important in order to understand the general limitations of such studies for making causal inferences. The labels defined below will not be found in other published works; we have chosen them to characterize the fundamental nature of each design, using terms already introduced.

A *follow-up prevalence study* (Figure 5.5) combines elements of cohort and cross-sectional designs, but neither basic design is preserved in its entirety. We begin, as we did in a prospective cohort study, by obtaining study factor information (E and $\bar{E}$) on a fixed cohort that is to be followed over time. However, disease status is not known at the onset and is not ascertained until a subsequent examination is conducted. Thus, the analysis involves prevalent cases (C) and is restricted to those members of the orig-

Figure 5.5 Follow-up Prevalence Study

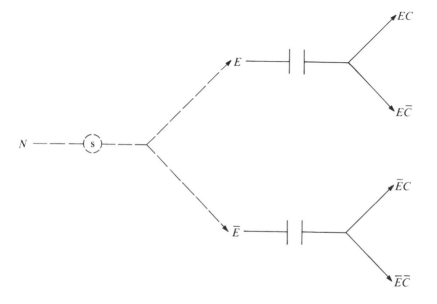

Figure 5.6 Selective Prevalence Study

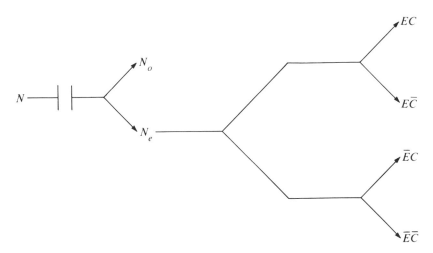

N_e = persons characterized by an event that designates eligibility for observing cases of the disease

N_o = persons who are not eligible to become cases in the study

inal cohort who were not lost to follow-up. This design is often used when, in the planning stage of a study, the investigator does not consider the particular disease as a possible consequent of the study factor.

A *selective prevalence study* (Figure 5.6) also combines elements of cohort and cross-sectional designs, but it does so differently from the follow-up prevalence design. A fixed or dynamic population (N) is followed over time for subsequent identification of events (N_e) (e.g., live births or visits to a health facility) that designate eligibility for observing cases of the disease. A cross-sectional study is then conducted within the group of "eligible" persons who are selected for study. Note that prevalence, not incidence measures, is estimated, because N_e does not represent the candidate population. Thus, a prevalence analysis is done for a selected group of subjects who have been isolated from the follow-up of a well-defined population. A selective prevalence design might be the best way of investigating the etiology of certain diseases (e.g., birth defects) for which the candidate population cannot readily be identified.

A *backward prevalence study* (Figure 5.7) is another hybrid derivative that combines elements of cohort and cross-sectional designs. Essentially, it is a cross-sectional study in which previous case occurrences (incident events) for a given period before selection are identified retrospectively. There is no follow-up period and, typically, the disease is an acute condition (e.g., a common infection). Since the study population does not represent the appropriate candidate population for the disease, only selected survivors, the frequency measure estimated in this study is prevalence, not incidence measures—even though case occurrences reflect incident events (refer to Chapter 7). Backward prevalence studies are used

Figure 5.7 Backward Prevalence Study

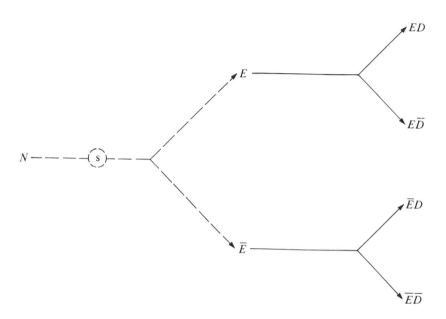

as relatively inexpensive, but inferior, substitutes for cohort studies involving acute diseases.

A *repeated survey* (Figure 5.8) is a sequence of two or more cross-sectional studies conducted within the same dynamic target population (N and N') and generally spaced at least a few years apart. For each probabil-

Figure 5.8 Repeated Survey

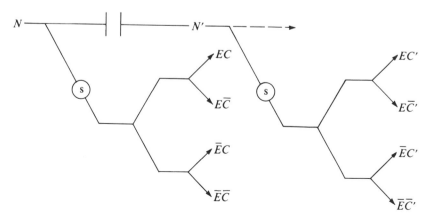

N and N' represent one dynamic population sampled at two or more successive times

ity sample, we obtain information about individual study factor levels (E/E' or $\overline{E}/\overline{E}'$) and disease prevalence (C/C' or $\overline{C}/\overline{C}'$). Yet, we do not actually follow individuals; we follow the population. In fact, it is unlikely that a single respondent will appear in more than one sample. Repeated surveys are used to assess overall health status changes in large populations and to determine to what extent these trends are due to differences or changes in the levels of one or more study factors.

A *survey follow-up study* (Figure 5.9) combines cross-sectional and cohort designs back to back. A cross-sectional study involving a random sample of a target population (N) is succeeded by a cohort study of that portion of the original study population still at risk of developing the disease. Thus, the investigator can estimate both prevalence and incidence rates of disease for the same target population.

A *repeated follow-up study* (Figure 5.10)—also called a repeated measures study—is a forward design with two or more contiguous follow-up periods. Essentially, this hybrid design is a fixed cohort study in which the total follow-up period is divided into two or more subperiods. Generally, the study is implemented by conducting three or more examinations and/or interviews, spaced several months or years apart, resulting in the collection of study factor and disease status information on all participating subjects at each exam. Incidence measures can then be estimated for different exposure groups for two or more subperiods, defined by the spacing of the periodic exams. Repeated follow-up studies are particularly useful to investigate the possible association between study factor change and disease occurrence, to investigate the etiology and natural history of a remittent disease, and to investigate the relationship between two diseases.

Figure 5.9 Survey Follow-up Study

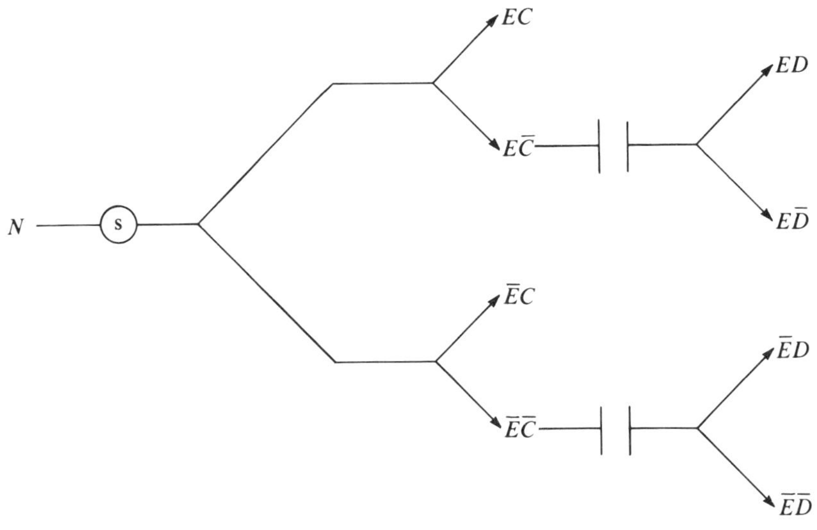

Figure 5.10 Repeated Follow-up Study

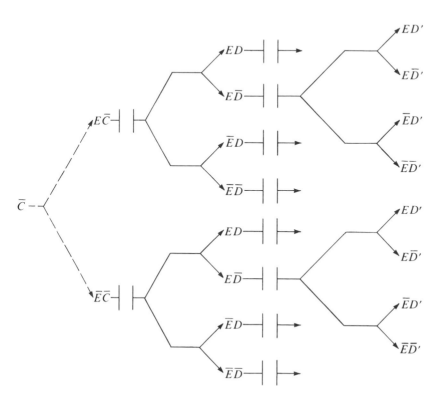

An *intervention follow-up study* (Figure 5.11) combines all or part of a nonobservational design (experiment or quasi experiment) with a cohort design, each having a different outcome event. We start with a fixed cohort, which may or may not be randomly allocated to study factor (or treatment) groups (E and $\bar{E}$), and we follow it for two successive periods. Typically, the first follow-up period is short (e.g., a few minutes to several days) and is intended to estimate an acute biological or behavioral effect (F and $\bar{F}$). The second period is usually longer (e.g., several months or years) and is intended to estimate a long-term or chronic effect (D and $\bar{D}$). By observing longitudinally the associations among three primary variables, we can examine the relationship between acute responses and chronic health effects. In intervention follow-up studies, therefore, we can test for short-term biological or behavioral mechanisms that act as *intervening variables* (F) (Susser, 1973) causally linking the study factor (E) with the disease (D).

Incomplete designs are studies in which information is missing on one or more relevant factors. In one sense, all empirical studies are incomplete, since we can never know whether *all* distorting influences of extraneous

**5.3
INCOMPLETE
DESIGNS**

Figure 5.11 Intervention Follow-up Study

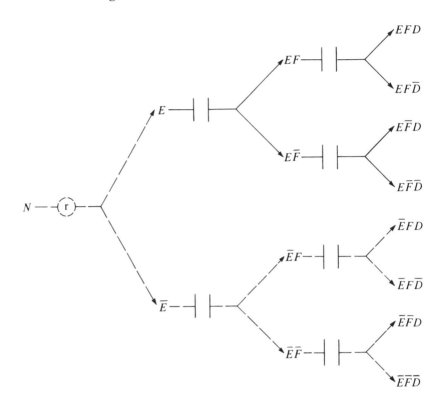

risk factors or selection procedures have been controlled. However, the four types presented in this section—ecologic, proportional, and two types of cluster studies—are limited to designs for which information is missing on either the study factor, the disease, or their joint distribution in the study population.

Incomplete designs, especially ecologic and proportional, are frequently used when data are not readily available for conducting another type of study. It is often relatively inexpensive or convenient to make use of secondary data sources to test or generate hypotheses with these designs before spending considerably more time and money on primary data collection.

Most of the incomplete study designs were developed and applied before the widespread use of the basic or hybrid designs. While the essential features of these incomplete designs are rather simple compared with other designs, they involve a few key methodological subtleties that may seriously limit causal inference.

**5.3.1
Ecologic Study**

An *ecologic study,* also called an aggregate or descriptive study, is one in which the unit of analysis is a group, most often defined geographically (see Section 4.2.5). Ecologic analysis may involve incidence, prevalence, or mortality data, but the latter is most common because of the widespread availability of such data. The primary analytic feature of an ecologic study is that we do not know the joint distribution of the study factor(s) and the disease *within* each group (unit of analysis). That is, we know the number of exposed persons and the number of cases within each group, but we do not know the number of exposed cases.

We may distinguish two types of ecologic studies: a simple comparison of frequency measures among k groups at one point in time or during one period (where k is usually large—e.g., $k \geq 10$), and an assessment of trends in one or more groups over time. In an *ecologic comparison study* (Figure 5.12), we estimate the frequencies of the exposure (E and $\overline{E}$) and the disease (D and $\overline{D}$) in each group. In an *ecologic trend* (or time series) *study* (Figure 5.13), we estimate the changes in both frequency measures during the study period. In addition, we may combine both types, estimating the change in average exposure level and the change in disease frequency for several groups.

EXAMPLE 5.5

Ecologic designs are most attractive when we must combine large data sources (e.g., the census and vital statistics) in order to obtain information on both the study factor(s) and disease for the same populations. For example, consider the work of the nineteenth-century sociologist Emil Durkheim (1951), who collected data on the frequency of suicides and the religious makeup of many contiguous provinces in Western Europe. He found that, on the average, provinces with greater proportions of Protestants had higher suicide rates and that provinces with greater proportions of Catholics had lower suicide rates. Durkheim concluded from these data that Protestants are more likely to commit suicide than are Catholics. While the conclusion may be true, the causal inference is not logically correct, because it may have been Catholics in predominantly Protestant provinces who were taking their own lives. This logical flaw, called the *ecological fallacy* (Selvin, 1958), results from making a causal inference about an individual phenomenon or process (e.g., suicide) on the basis of observations of groups. The problem occurs because the composition of each group is not homogeneous with respect to the study factor; e.g., most of the provinces in Durkheim's study included a substantial number of both Protestants and Catholics.

The ecological fallacy was first demonstrated mathematically, nearly a hundred years after Durkheim's study, by another sociologist, William Robinson (1950), who showed that the correlation between two ecologic variables is often markedly different from the corresponding individual correlation within the same populations. More recently, other social scien-

Figure 5.12 Ecologic Comparison Study

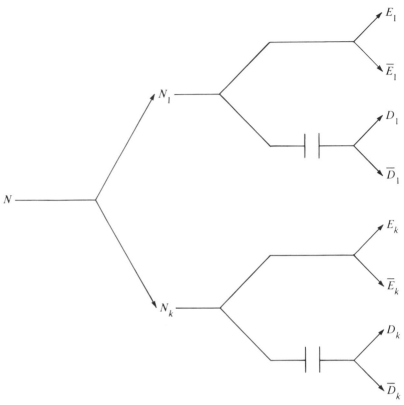

Figure 5.13 Ecologic Trend Study

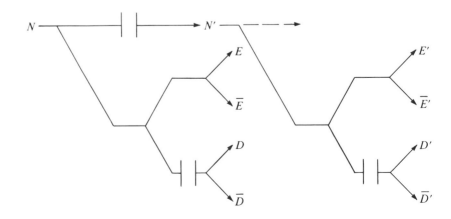

tists have specified the assumptions required to make causal inferences from ecologic data (Goodman, 1953, 1959; Valkonen, 1969; Langbein and Lichtman, 1978; Firebaugh, 1978), and health researchers have begun to incorporate these ideas in their studies of disease etiology (e.g., Kalimo and Bice, 1973; Stavraky, 1976; Oreglia and Duncan, 1977).

The ability to make a causal inference from ecologic data often can be enhanced by comparing time trends in disease frequency among several groups that have experienced different changes in average exposure level. Suppose that Durkheim had found that the suicide rate increased only in provinces where there was a net immigration of Protestants and decreased only in provinces where there was a net emigration of Protestants, regardless of the original religious composition. We then might be less willing to ascribe the results to an ecological fallacy—i.e., we are more likely to infer that Protestants have a greater probability of committing suicide than do Catholics.

Unfortunately, the magnitude of the association between two sociodemographic variables tends to be substantially higher in ecologic analyses than it is in individual analyses (Stavraky, 1976). This problem of *multicollinearity* makes it very difficult to separate the effects of two such variables in the analysis. For example, Durkheim probably would have had trouble isolating the independent effects of religion and income on suicide rate, because predominantly Protestant provinces had much higher average income levels than did Catholic provinces.

Despite their limitations for testing etiologic hypotheses, ecologic analyses are useful for evaluating the impact of intervention programs on the health status of target populations. Once the important modifiable determinants of a disease have been identified, the effectiveness of our public health initiatives to control that disease must be judged through ecologic assessment. In practice, however, we cannot completely distinguish between the testing of etiologic hypotheses and the evaluation of intervention strategies, because our knowledge of disease etiology is never perfect. Consequently, ecologic studies generally are used to understand natural phenomena at the same time they are used to test the application of our knowledge.

A *proportional* or *proportionate study* (Figure 5.14) is one that only includes observations on cases (D) without information about the candidate population at risk of developing the (index) disease(s) (MacMahon and Pugh, 1970, Chap. 5; Hill, 1971). The design may involve incident cases (proportional morbidity) or deaths (proportional mortality), though the latter is much more common because of the availability of mortality data. As indicated in Figure 5.14 the cases or deaths may be identified from the follow-up of a defined population (N); yet, study factor information is not known for noncases ($\overline{D}$), who were at risk of developing the index disease(s). Proportional studies may be regarded as either a special type of cross-sectional study (Hill, 1971; Kupper et al., 1978; Decouflé et al.,

5.3.2
Proportional
Study

Figure 5.14 Proportional Study

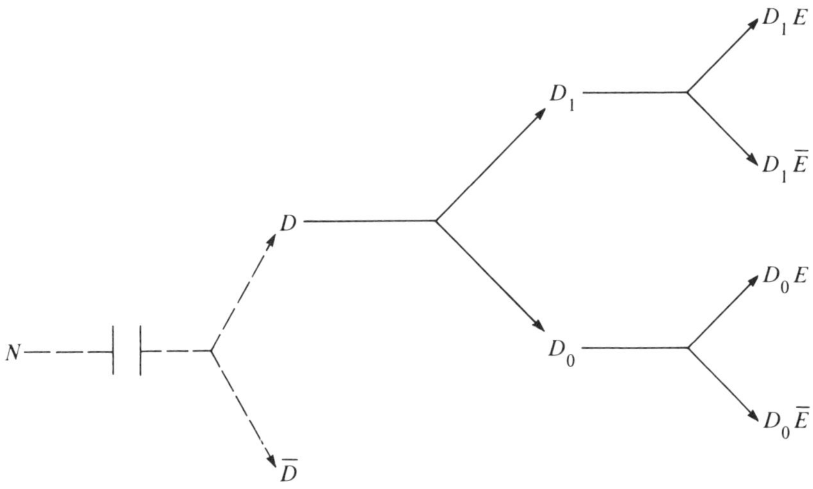

1980) or a special type of case-control study (Miettinen and Wang, 1981). According to the former conceptualization, we obtain study factor information on all deaths or a sample of deaths occurring in one population. We then compare the prevalence (i.e., proportion) of total deaths resulting from the index disease among categories or levels of the study factor. Treating the data as a case-control study, we would compare cases of one type (the index diseases, D_1) with cases of another type (e.g., one or more other causes of death, D_0) with respect to study factor level.

EXAMPLE 5.6

Since cause of death is often available for the deceased members of large residential or industrial populations, proportional studies are used to generate new hypotheses or to conduct preliminary tests of etiologic hypotheses without collecting much additional data. As an illustration, consider the Hanford study of nuclear power workers, designed to test the possible relationship between low levels of ionizing radiation and cancer (Mancuso et al., 1977). Among the 3,500 certified deaths that occurred among plant workers between 1944 and 1972, a significantly greater proportion of exposed workers (i.e., with one or more positive badge readings) than unexposed workers had died of reticuloendothelial system (RES) cancers. Stated another way, a greater proportion of RES cancer deaths than other deaths had been exposed to radiation at the plant. Because the data are incomplete, however, we cannot conclude that exposure

EXAMPLE 5.6 (*continued*)

was positively associated with RES cancer mortality among nuclear power workers. All that we can infer, assuming no distortion, is that the association between radiation exposure and RES cancer mortality is stronger than the association between radiation exposure and all other causes of death.

Thus, as shown in Example 5.6, if we assume there is no statistical association between the study factor and the comparison diseases, the results of a proportional study can be used to test the relationship of primary interest. This feature suggests an appropriate strategy for designing proportional studies (using the case-control formulation): select a comparison group that includes diseases believed to be unrelated to the study factor. Of course, even with this approach, proportional mortality studies are subject to many of the problems described for case-control and cross-sectional studies. In addition, most proportional mortality studies are based on death certificates, which have been shown to include a substantial proportion of misclassification errors (Percy et al., 1981).

As we will see in Chapter 17, the use of stratified analyses to control for extraneous risk factors typically requires information about the size of the candidate population (i.e., the denominator) within each stratum. Since this information is not available in proportional studies, the analytical control of distorting (confounding) effects must be based on "numerator" data. One group of researchers has found, however, that correction for such bias in the analysis of proportional studies appears to lie within acceptable limits for a variety of testing situations (Kupper et al., 1978).

5.3.3 Space/Time Cluster Studies

Space/time cluster studies (Figure 5.15) are a class of designs in which study factor levels are not observed directly; sometimes, a potential disease determinant is not even defined clearly by the investigator. In the absence of this information, we observe k allegedly nonrandom aggregations or clusters of disease (incidence, prevalence, or mortality), differentially distributed in space, over time, or together in space and time (where k is usually two or more) (MacMahon and Pugh, 1970, Chaps. 8–10). As indicated in Figure 5.15, the cases may be linked to a candidate population (N), but no study factor data need be collected.

Space clustering is a nonuniform distribution of cases over the total study area, relative to the distribution of the candidate population, and is often used by epidemiologists to suggest an environmental etiology of the disease. The simplest type of space clustering analysis is, essentially, an ecologic comparison of geopolitical areas without study factor data. For example, international comparisons of CHD prevalence, incidence, and mortality reveal large variations among industrial nations, with the United

Figure 5.15 Space/Time Cluster Study

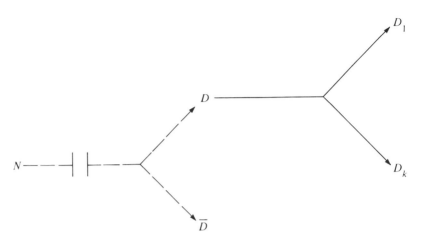

States having a frequency several times that of Japan (Keys, 1970). While such results are very provocative and often motivate new research efforts, they tell us very little about the etiology of CHD; in fact, the observed difference in CHD for these two countries may be explained predominantly by either genetic or environmental factors. One way to clarify the meaning of international comparisons is to study the disease among persons who migrate between the two countries and among their offspring. For example, a group of investigators found that, for men of Japanese ancestry, the frequency of CHD was lowest in Japan, intermediate in Hawaii, and highest in California (Marmot et al., 1975). Of course, this gradient could be due to several alternative explanations, including changes in dietary habits, smoking, physical activity, occupational stress, and/or social support. Additional studies must be conducted for tests of these specific hypotheses.

Time clustering is a nonuniform distribution of cases over the duration of the study for a given candidate population. The objective of studies designed to discover such clustering is (1) to identify long-term secular trends of disease frequency in large populations, (2) to identify and investigate local epidemics of a disease, or (3) to identify cyclic fluctuations in disease occurrence. Incomplete trend studies are merely crude ecologic analyses that lack study factor information (see Section 5.3.1). They alert health researchers and planners to major shifts in the general health status of a population and in the distribution of (unknown) disease determinants. In epidemic investigations, and, perhaps, in studies of cyclic variations, time clustering suggests that an infectious agent is involved in the disease etiology, though the agent or the nature of its transmission may remain unknown to the investigator. For example, a study of Down's syndrome in Israel revealed a fairly dominant six-month cycle, with disease frequency peaking for spring and fall births (Harlap, 1974). While many infectious diseases exhibit seasonal cycles, as observed for Down's syndrome, an infectious agent may not be involved in the etiology of the disease. Alternatively, deleterious intrauterine exposures may reflect different seasonal behavior patterns of pregnant women throughout the year.

One method for strengthening the inference of an infectious etiology is to observe the occurrence of cases in both space and time. *Space/time clustering* involves the interaction between place of onset and time of onset, such that cases that occur close in space also occur close in time. The major difficulty with this type of analysis is in determining that the observed clustering did not occur by chance. While statistical tests for cyclic variations are fairly straightforward (e.g., see Freedman, 1979), tests for space/time clustering involve more mathematical sophistication (e.g., see Pike and Smith, 1968).

Family cluster studies are another class of designs in which specific study factor levels are not observed directly; instead, patterns of disease occurrence (or trait distributions) are examined within families. The primary aim of such investigations is to elucidate and quantify the effect of genetic mechanisms in the pathogenic process. Since no disease is determined solely by either genetic or environmental factors (McMahon and Pugh, 1970, Chap. 14), the purpose of family cluster studies is *not* to dichotomize diseases into two types, genetic and nongenetic. Rather, the ultimate purpose is to identify specific gene-environment interactions that result in particular patterns of disease occurrence in populations. We know, for example, that the clinical manifestation (i.e., phenotype) of a disease that depends on a single gene locus (i.e., genotype), such as phenylketonuria, can still be attributable to environmental factors, particularly if the genotype is very common in the population. Most attempts to identify clustering of a disease within families can be classified into three design strategies: familial aggregation studies, twin studies, and pedigree studies.

5.3.4 Family Cluster Studies

A *familial aggregation study* (Figure 5.16) is a special type of cohort or cross-sectional design in which study factor information need not be collected but in which all subjects are stratified into k family units ($k \geq 10$) both before subject selection and in the analysis. This type of study may involve disease incidence (as in a cohort study) or prevalence (as in a cross-sectional study). Analytically, the objective is to compare variability of the disease (or trait) *within* families with the variability *between* families. The greater the between-family variance, relative to the within-family variance, the more extensive is the degree of familial aggregation—also known as *intraclass correlation* for continuous variables (Snedecor and Cochran, 1967). Yet, familial aggregation can result from genetically transmitted susceptibilities to the disease or from shared characteristics of the family environment. The fact that cases of schizophrenia tend to cluster in families, for example, does not necessarily reflect a genetic mechanism; it is quite possible that the environmental causes of this disorder are rooted in the family structure.

Figure 5.16 Familial Aggregation Study

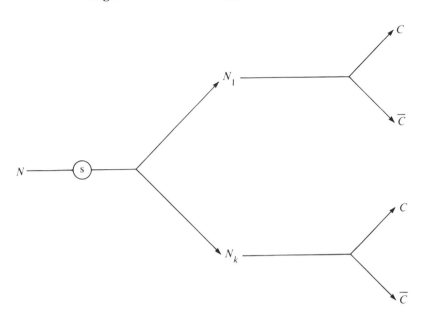

A more powerful method for identifying a genetic role in the etiology of a disease is the classical *twin study* (Figure 5.17). All twin pairs (N_p) are divided into monozygotic pairs (N_{mp}) and dizygotic pairs (N_{dp}), and all pairs are classified by disease status. Each pair may be concordant with respect to the disease (i.e., CC or $\overline{C}\overline{C}$) or discordant (i.e., $C\overline{C}$ or $\overline{C}C$). Since monozygotic pairs share all their genes and dizygotic pairs do not, greater similarity (or concordance) with respect to the disease between members of monozygotic pairs than between members of dizygotic pairs suggests a genetic component in the etiology of the disease (MacMahon and Pugh, 1970, Chap. 14). The principal estimated parameter in twin studies is the proportion of the total phenotypic variance that is due to genetic factors—i.e., heritability (Elston and Rao, 1978). For example, if a monozygotic schizophrenic is more likely to have a schizophrenic twin than is a dizygotic schizophrenic, we might infer a genetic mechanism in the etiology of schizophrenia. However, even with a significant difference in concordance between the two types of twins, one cannot entirely rule out an environmental explanation. It is certainly possible that monozygotic twins simply share more relevant environmental influences than do dizygotic twins—i.e., the estimated heritability may be distorted by environmental factors.

A *pedigree study* (Figure 5.18) is an investigation of a disease (or trait) in one or more large families, each of which is composed of at least three generations (Elston and Stewart, 1971). The purpose of such an investigation is to identify specific genetic mechanisms for certain diseases and to classify individuals according to their genotypes. Pedigree studies

Figure 5.17 Twin Study

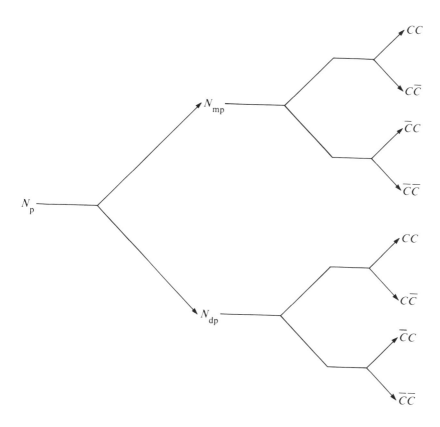

Figure 5.18 Pedigree Study

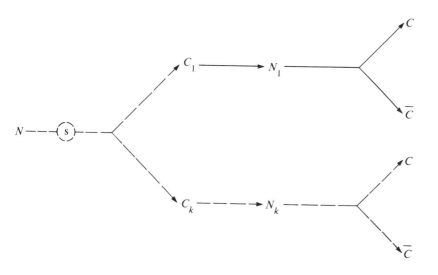

provide the most genetic information and are particularly useful for study-ing quantitative traits (e.g., blood pressure) or traits whose phenotype is influenced to a large degree by the environment (e.g., certain cancers and mental disorders) (Elston and Stewart, 1971). We conduct the study by (randomly) selecting k ($k \geq 1$) index cases (probands), constructing their family trees (i.e., pedigrees), and collecting data on as many relatives as possible. Each subject in every pedigree is then classified by disease status (i.e., phenotype). By assuming an underlying genetic model, we can de-rive the probability that a particular set of pedigree data will be observed. Therefore, not only can we estimate the heritability of a given phenotype within the population, but we can also describe its mode of inheritance (El-ston and Stewart, 1971). Although pedigree studies may produce a good deal of insight into the genetic etiology of a disease, they involve certain practical limitations—primarily, the difficulty of collecting enough data on each pedigree and the complexity of the statistical analysis (e.g., see El-ston and Rao, 1978; Elston and Stewart, 1971; Elston and Sobel, 1979).

**5.4
COMPARING
OBSERVA-
TIONAL
DESIGNS**

In this chapter, we have described 15 types of designs used for investigat-ing the etiology of a disease. To develop the methodological topics in the remainder of this book, we will focus on only 4 of these designs: cohort, cross-sectional, case-control, and ambidirectional studies. Nevertheless, the researcher should recognize the full range of design alternatives and should appreciate the importance of study design as the link between observations and ideas. Indeed, the future of epidemiology depends, to some extent, on the development of new design approaches (Greenhouse, 1980), ranging from innovative data collection and record linkage systems to specific adaptations of our current methods for studying previously unexplored health problems.

In Sections 5.1, 5.2, and 5.3, numerous references were made to the relative advantages and limitations of each type of study. We will review, briefly, in this section the general criteria for comparing observational designs. These criteria are grouped under three headings: (1) the *type* of information sought by the investigator, (2) the *quality* of the information expected in the data, and (3) the *cost* of acquiring this information. Many of the issues in the following subsections will be elaborated and expanded in subsequent chapters.

**5.4.1
Type of
Information**

In recent years, epidemiologic methods have been applied to a large array of substantive research areas, including occupational and environmental health (Hernberg, 1974; Saracci, 1978; Kilian and Barna-Lloyd, 1979), genetics (Murphy, 1978; Omenn, 1979), medical and health services (Henderson, 1976); Hulka, 1978; World Health Organization, 1980), and public health policy (Griffith, 1979; Holland and Wainwright, 1979; Ter-ris, 1980). Despite indications to the contrary, no one study design is uni-formly superior to all others in every situation. The preferred design should meet specific objectives and constraints, which vary considerably among studies. Table 5.1 lists the designs described in the previous sections of this chapter, according to selected study objectives. In many situations, the preferred design also depends on the particular nature of the disease— namely, the relative frequency of the disease in the target population, the length of the latent period between first exposure and clinical onset, and the duration of the disease between clinical onset and termination. In many empirical investigations, the design of choice also depends on certain constraints, such as the limited availability of data, limited knowledge of the disease etiology, and the inability to observe the candidate population.

Table 5.1   Commonly Used Designs for Selected Study Objectives

Objective of Study and Nature of Disease	Commonly Used Study Designs
Generate new etiologic hypotheses regarding environmental determinants of a specific disease	Case-control, ambidirectional, ecologic, proportional, space/ time cluster
Generate new etiologic hypotheses regarding the health effects of a specific study factor	Retrospective cohort, ecologic, proportional
Test or generate etiologic hypotheses by merging two or more large data sets to obtain information on both the study factor and the disease	Ecologic
Identify determinants of a disease for which we cannot observe the population at risk	Selective prevalence, proportional
Study the genetic etiology of a disease	Family cluster
Determine whether a disease is likely to have an infectious etiology	Space/time cluster
Identify environmental determinants of a remittent disease or study the relationship between two diseases	Repeated follow-up
Identify environmental determinants of a specific rare disease with a long latent period	Retrospective cohort, case-control, ambidirectional
Study the relationship between a chronic health effect and acute responses to a specific factor	Intervention follow-up
Identify the determinants of a relatively frequent disease with a long duration, which often goes undiagnosed or unreported	Cross-sectional, prospective cohort
Study the health effect of a specific study factor, which is likely to be influenced by the occurrence of the disease, or study the effect of a specific study factor on a disease, whose detection is likely to be influenced by the study factor	Prospective cohort, repeated follow-up
Assess the impact of a planned intervention on the health status of a target population	Repeated survey, ecologic
Assess the need for health services and facilities in a target population	Cross-sectional, survey follow-up, repeated survey, ecologic

As we will show in Chapters 6 and 7, the various study designs permit the estimation of different parameters. For example, one cannot directly estimate any measure of disease frequency in a case-control or a proportional study; the other designs allow one to estimate either prevalence, incidence, mortality, or some combination of these measures. Furthermore, one can only directly estimate an individual's risk of developing the disease, conditional on study factor level, in a cohort, ambidirectional, repeated follow-up, or intervention follow-up study.

5.4.2 Quality of Information

Quality of information refers to the relevance and accuracy of the data for making specific inferences about the target population. When making causal inferences, the investigator must attempt to demonstrate that (1) there is a statistical association between the study factor and the disease, (2) the presence of the study factor (or its deleterious level) preceded the occurrence of the disease, and (3) the observed association is not entirely due to any sources of error (see Section 2.2.1). All the designs described in Sections 5.1–5.3 allow the investigator to estimate the magnitude of the observed association by making a comparison, either between groups (e.g., exposed versus unexposed, or cases versus noncases), between geographic areas, or between time periods for the same population. The ability of the investigator to distinguish antecedent from consequent depends primarily on the directionality of the design. Forward designs are best, because the study factor level is measured before the disease occurs and because the designs involve incident cases; nondirectional designs are least desirable, because there is no way to ascertain from the data which came first, the hypothesized cause or the disease.

To make a causal inference, the investigator must also seek to eliminate possible sources of error as alternative explanations for his or her findings. Thus, causal inference in epidemiologic research depends on an understanding of what can go wrong with the study; consequently, the investigator must plan each empirical study according to these considerations (Cochran, 1965; McKinlay, 1975). The relative lack of error in estimating a population parameter is called *accuracy* or informativeness (Miettinen, 1975). In all phases of empirical research, it is convenient to divide estimation error into two types: random (or sampling) errors and nonrandom (or systematic) errors. *Precision* refers to the relative lack of random error, and *internal validity* refers to the lack of nonrandom error (or bias). These concepts and their application to causal inference will be elaborated in Chapters 10–14. *For now, it is important to recognize that internal validity is the sine qua non of etiologic research; thus, it is more important that an estimate be valid than that it be precise.* Moreover, establishing the validity of an observed association is based on nonstatistical as well as statistical considerations, relying on our a priori knowledge of the disease and on a careful consideration of our methods for selecting and observing subjects.

In general, incidence data are preferred for testing etiologic hypotheses, because prevalence and mortality depend on both the duration of the disease and incidence. Prospective data are usually preferable to retrospective data, since the latter are more subject to errors of measurement (or misclassification), which can lead to invalid results (see Chapter 12). As we mentioned above, a forward design is preferable to a backward, nondirectional, or ambidirectional design for distinguishing the antecedent from the consequent. Coupling these desired features with the objective of reducing attrition, we may conclude that, in general, a prospective cohort study involving incident cases and a short follow-up period is the most informative observational design for testing an etiologic hypothesis. Conversely, incomplete designs involving secondary data sources are the least informative. Since the most informative design is not often the most feasible, the investigator normally must make certain trade-offs. The net result of these trade-offs is an increase in the number of assumptions required to support a causal interpretation. It is, therefore, the responsibility of the investigator to make these key assumptions explicit so that the reader can judge how critical they are for reaching the stated conclusions (Bross, 1976).

5.4.3 Cost of Information

In practice, cost criteria should not be separated from the criteria listed above, because the ultimate worth of a study is its *cost effectiveness*—i.e., the total value of the derived information (now and in the future) relative to the amount of the actual expenditure in time, money, and other resources (Miettinen, 1975). Of course, the optimal solution for a given study—i.e., the design with the maximum cost effectiveness—is never obtainable. In planning a study, we can only hope to obtain the most accurate information for a given expected cost or, conversely, to spend the least time and money for a desired amount and quality of information. Naturally, attempting to meet either one of these goals is never a simple or unambiguous task, because it depends on several unknown parameters, such as the amount of expected bias, and because it depends on certain external constraints, such as the political climate and available funding.

In general, a study is more expensive if it includes a follow-up period, the use of primary data, or probability-sampling procedures. The least expensive studies are typically the incomplete designs, especially those done with secondary data. The total cost of conducting a study that does not use secondary data entirely is usually directly proportional to the total sample size. Yet increasing the sample size usually increases the accuracy of our estimation by enhancing precision. Thus, the critical issue in the design phase of an investigation is how to make an appropriate trade-off between expected accuracy and direct study costs. Probably, the greatest trade-offs are required when the expected effect of the study factor is weak, when the disease is very rare or has a long latent period, and when cases of the disease do not get routinely diagnosed or reported. For a given sample size, we can often enhance precision by fixing the ratio of subjects in the compared groups—i.e., by making the sizes of groups approximately equal (or more equal than they are in the target population). We achieve this result in case-control, ambidirectional, and proportional studies by stratifying on disease status before subject selection; thus, these designs are well suited for studying rare diseases (i.e., diseases with low prevalence, incidence, or mortality). We can achieve precision enhancement also in cohort and cross-sectional studies (or their hybrid derivatives) by stratifying on study factor level before selection; thus, these latter designs are well suited for studying rare exposures (i.e., study factor levels with a low prevalence in the target population). In all these designs, precision of estimation, for a given sample size, also may be enhanced if complete restriction or matching is used in the selection of subjects. However, these options often impose added costs, or they may seriously limit the number of potential subjects in one group. The investigator, therefore, must justify such methods in terms of the expected cost effectiveness of conducting a study.

5.5 CON-CLUDING REMARKS

To facilitate the presentation of epidemiologic principles and to enhance the communication of results from specific studies, we have created a typology of 15 observational designs that are grouped into three broad categories: basic designs, hybrid designs, and incomplete designs. The three basic designs are cohort, cross-sectional, and case-control studies, which may be modified and combined in various ways to define 8 (or more) hybrid designs. The most important hybrid design in etiologic research is the ambidirectional study, which combines some of the positive features of both cohort and case-control studies. The incomplete designs include ecologic, proportional, space/time cluster, and family cluster studies; these are characterized by missing information on either the study factor, the disease, or their joint distribution in the study population.

The prospective cohort study or one of its hybrid derivatives (i.e., repeated or intervention follow-up studies) is preferred, in theory, for testing an etiologic hypothesis regarding a nongenetic study factor, because this type of observational study most closely resembles an experiment. Nevertheless, other design types may offer certain practical advantages that make them especially attractive under special conditions. Moreover, a few designs are useful for other purposes, such as generating new hypotheses, describing the frequency of disease in a population, understanding the genetic component of disease etiology, evaluating the impact of an intervention, and assessing the need for health services.

We conclude that the study design must be carefully tailored to the objectives of the investigation, to the nature of the disease being studied, to the availability of time, money, and human resources, and to certain sociopolitical constraints. Failure to consider the implications of design decisions in the early stages of a study may result in problems that cannot be corrected in subsequent stages. We will discuss many of these problems in more detail in Part II.

REFERENCES

British Medical Journal. 1979. The case-control study (editorial). 2: 884–886.

Bross, I. D. J. 1976. Right answers from wrong assumptions (editorial). *Prev. Med.* 5: 203–206.

Cochran, W. G. 1965. The planning of observational studies of human populations. *J.R. Stat. Soc. A* 138: 234–265.

Cole, P. 1979. The evolving case-control study. *J. Chronic Dis.* 32: 15–27.

Cornfield, J., and Haenszel, W. 1960. Some aspects of retrospective studies. *J. Chronic Dis.* 11: 523–534.

Decouflé, P.; Thomas, T. L.; and Pickle, L. W. 1980. Comparison of the proportionate mortality ratio and standardized mortality ratio risk measures. *Am. J. Epidemiol.* 111: 263–269.

Durkheim, E. 1951. *Suicide.* New York: Free Press.

Elston, R. C., and Rao, D. C. 1978. Statistical modeling and analysis in human genetics. *Annu. Rev. Bioeng.* 7: 253–286.

Elston, R. C., and Sobel, E. 1979. Sampling considerations in the gathering and analysis of pedigree data. *Am. J. Hum. Genet.* 31: 62–69.

Elston, R. C., and Stewart, J. 1971. A general model for the genetic analysis of pedigree data. *Hum. Hered.* 21: 523–542.

Feinstein, A. R. 1978. XLIII. The architecture of cross-sectional research (conclusion). *Clin. Pharm. & Therapeut.* 23: 481–493.

Firebaugh, G. 1978. A rule for inferring individual-level relationships from aggregate data. *Am. Sociol. Rev.* 43: 557–572.

Freedman, L. S. 1979. The use of a Kolmogorov-Smirnov type statistic in testing hypotheses about seasonal variation. *J. Epidemiol. Community Health* 33: 223–228.

Friedman, G. D. 1980. *Primer of epidemiology.* 2nd ed. New York: McGraw-Hill; Chaps. 5–8.

Friedman, M., and Rosenman, R. H. 1971. Type A behavior pattern: Its association with coronary heart disease. *Ann. Clin. Res.* 3: 300–312.

Goodman, L. A. 1953. Ecological regressions and behavior of individuals. *Am. Sociol. Rev.* 18: 663–664.

——————. 1959. Some alternatives to ecological correlations. *Am. J. Sociol.* 64: 610–625.

Greenhouse, S. W. 1980. Some epidemiologic issues for the 1980s. *Am. J. Epidemiol.* 112: 269–273.

Griffith, J. 1979. Significance of epidemiology as viewed by a government scientist. *Fed. Proc.* 38: 1888–1890.

Harlap, S. 1974. A time-series analysis of the incidence of Down's syndrome in West Jerusalem. *Am. J. Epidemiol.* 99: 210–217.

HENDERSON, M. 1976. The engagement of epidemiologists in health services research. *Am. J. Epidemiol.* 103: 127–137.

HERNBERG, S. 1974. Epidemiologic methods in occupational health research. *Work-Environ.-Health* 11: 59–68.

HILL, A. B. 1971. *Principles of medical statistics.* 9th ed. New York: Oxford University Press; Chap. 22.

HOLLAND, W. W., and WAINWRIGHT, A. H. 1979. Epidemiology and health policy. *Epidemiol. Rev.* 1: 211–232.

HULKA, B. S. 1978. Epidemiological applications to health services research. *J. Community Health* 4: 140–149.

IBRAHIM, M. A., ed. 1979. The case-control study: Consensus and controversy. *J. Chronic Dis.* 32: 1–190.

KALIMO, E., and BICE, T. W. 1973. Causal analysis and ecological fallacy in cross-national epidemiological research. *Scand. J. Social Med.* 1: 17–24.

KEYS, A. 1970. Coronary heart disease in seven countries: Summary. *Circulation* (Suppl. 1) 41: 186–198.

KILIAN, D. J., and BARNA-LLOYD, G. 1979. Industrial epidemiology. *Fed. Proc.* 38: 1883–1887.

KUPPER, L. L.; MCMICHAEL, A. J.; and SPIRTAS, R. 1975. A hybrid epidemiologic study design useful in estimating relative risk. *J. Am. Stat. Assoc.* 70: 524–528.

KUPPER, L. L.; MCMICHAEL, A. J.; SYMONS, M. J.; and MOST, B. M. 1978. On the utility of proportional mortality analysis. *J. Chronic Dis.* 31: 15–22.

LANGBEIN, L. I., and LICHTMAN, A. J. 1978. *Ecological inference.* Beverly Hills, Calif.: Sage.

LILIENFELD, A. M., and LILIENFELD, D. E. 1979. A century of case-control studies: Progress? *J. Chronic Dis.* 32: 5–13.

MCKINLAY, S. M. 1975. The design and analysis of the observational study—A review. *J. Am. Stat. Assoc.* 70: 503–523.

MACMAHON, B., and PUGH, T. F. 1970. *Epidemiology: Principles and methods.* Boston: Little, Brown.

MANCUSO, T. F.; STEWART, A.; and KNEALE, G. 1977. Radiation exposures of Hanford workers dying from cancer and other causes. *Health Phys.* 33: 369–385.

MANN, J. I., and VESSEY, M. P., JONES, R., YOUNG, D. 1979. The case-control study and retrospective controls (three letters to the editor). *Br. Med. J.* 2: 1507–1508.

MARMOT, M. G.; SYME, S. L.; KAGAN, A.; KATO, H.; COHEN, J. B.; and BELSKY, J. 1975. Epidemiological studies of coronary heart disease and stroke in Japanese men living in Japan, Hawaii and California: Prevalence of coronary and hypertensive heart disease and associated risk factors. *Am. J. Epidemiol.* 102: 514–525.

MIETTINEN, O. S. 1975. Principles of epidemiologic research. Unpublished manuscript. Cambridge, Mass.: Harvard University.

——— . 1976. Estimability and estimation in case-referent studies. *Am. J. Epidemiol.* 103(2): 226–236.

MIETTINEN, O. S., and WANG, J. D. 1981. An alternative to the proportionate mortality ratio. *Am. J. Epidemiol.* 114: 144–148.

MURPHY, E. A. 1978. Epidemiological strategies and genetic factors. *Int. J. Epidemiol.* 7: 7–14.

OMENN, G. S. 1979. Genetics and epidemiology: Medical interventions and public policy. *Social Biol.* 26: 117–125.

OREGLIA, A., and DUNCAN, R. P. 1977. Health planning and the problem of the ecological fallacy. *Am. J. Health Planning* 2(2): 1–6.

PEARSON, R. J. C. 1979. Significance of retrospective studies. *Fed. Proc.* 38: 1880–1882.

PERCY, C.; STANEK, E.; and GLOECKLER, L. 1981. Accuracy of cancer death certificates and its effect on cancer mortality statistics. *Am. J. Public Health* 71: 242–250.

PIKE, M. C., and SMITH, P. G. 1968. Disease clustering: A generalization of Knox's approach to the detection of space-time interactions. *Biometrics* 24: 541–556.

ROBINSON, W. S. 1950. Ecological correlations and the behavior of individuals. *Am. Sociol. Rev.* 15: 351–357.

SARACCI, R. 1978. Epidemiological strategies and environmental factors. *Int. J. Epidemiol.* 7: 101–111.

SARTWELL, P. E. 1974. Retrospective studies: A review for the clinician. *Ann. Intern. Med.* 81: 381–386.

SCHNEIDERMAN, M. A., and LEVIN, D. L. 1973. Parallels, convergences, and departures in case-control studies and clinical trials. *Cancer Res.* 33: 1498–1503.

SELVIN, H. C. 1958. Durkheim's suicide and problems of empirical research. *Am. J. Sociol.* 63: 607–619.

SNEDECOR, G. W., and COCHRAN, W. F. 1967. *Statistical methods.* 6th ed. Ames: Iowa State University Press; pp. 294–296.

STAVRAKY, K. M. 1976. The role of ecologic analysis in studies of the etiology of disease: A discussion with reference to large bowel cancer. *J. Chronic Dis.* 29: 435–444.

SUSSER, M. 1973. *Causal thinking in the health sciences.* New York: Oxford University Press; Chap. 9.

TERRIS, M. 1980. Epidemiology as a guide to health policy. *Am. Rev. Public Health* 1: 323–344.

VALKONEN, T. 1969. Individual and structural effects in ecological research. In *Social ecology,* edited by M. Dogan and S. Rokkan, Chap. 3, pp. 53–68. Cambridge, Mass.: MIT Press.

WORLD HEALTH ORGANIZATION. 1980. Use of epidemiology in primary health care. *WHO Chronicle* 34: 16–19.

6

Measures of Disease Frequency: Incidence

CHAPTER OUTLINE

The purpose of the next four chapters is to describe the basic measures used in epidemiologic research. This chapter and the next focus on a class of measures used to quantify the relative frequency of disease occurrence in a population—i.e., *measures of disease frequency*. The proper choice and the estimation of such measures are fundamental requirements for drawing meaningful causal inferences from our observations and must be considered at both the design and analysis stages of a study. For each measure considered, we will provide conceptual and intuitive descriptions, computational techniques for estimation, a discussion of relationships with certain other measures, and applications to specific study designs described in Chapters 4 and 5. Our emphasis in this chapter and those that follow is the treatment of categorical variables, particularly study factors and disease indicators that are dichotomous.

6.0 PREVIEW

As a background to our discussion of specific epidemiologic measures, we will first review three general classes of mathematical quantities that can be employed to describe empirical results involving discrete events (Elandt-Johnson, 1975; Morgenstern et al., 1980). Each frequency measure discussed in this chapter and the next falls into one of these three classes.

6.1 MEASURES IN GENERAL

The simplest of these quantities is a *proportion,* which is a fraction in which the numerator is included within the denominator. A proportion is often expressed as a percentage—i.e., the decimal representation of the proportion multiplied by 100. For example, we might describe the overall amount of smoking in a population as the proportion of people in the population who smoke at least one pack per month. Proportions are dimensionless quantities (i.e., they have no units of measurement), and their values must range between zero and one.

The second type of mathematical quantity is a *rate,* which is a more complex concept than a proportion and is often confused with the latter (sometimes to conform with common usage). A true rate is an instantaneous change (actually a potential for change) in one quantity per unit change in another quantity, where the latter quantity is usually time. For example, the velocity of an automobile at a given instant is a rate expressed as distance per unit of time (e.g., miles per hour). Thus, a rate is not dimensionless and has no finite upper bound—i.e., theoretically, a rate can approach infinity. Since some knowledge of calculus is necessary for a detailed understanding of an instantaneous rate, we will restrict our focus to *average rates,* which are more easily operationalized in epidemiology. For instance, an average velocity for a given period of travel is called speed and is calculated by dividing the total distance traveled by the total travel time.

Lastly, a *ratio* is a fraction in which the numerator is not included in the denominator, thereby distinguishing it from a proportion. In practice, there are two kinds of ratios: one that has dimensions and one that is

6.1.1 Proportions, Rates, and Ratios

dimensionless. Examples of the former are the number of hospital beds per 100,000 persons in the population and the number of infant deaths in a population during one year per 1,000 live births during that same year. We will see in Section 7.2 that the second example of a ratio is also an *estimate* of an average rate—i.e., the infant mortality rate in the population. Dimensionless ratios are formed by dividing one proportion or rate by another proportion or rate. This type of ratio refers either to one population—e.g., the proportion of smokers divided by the proportion of nonsmokers (called odds)—or to the comparison of two populations—e.g., the proportion of smokers in one group divided by the proportion of smokers in another group.

**6.1.2
Types of
Epidemiologic
Measures**

The principal measures used in epidemiologic research can be grouped into three categories: measures of disease frequency, measures of association, and measures of potential impact. *Frequency measures* characterize the occurrence of disease, disability, or death in human populations and therefore are fundamental to descriptive and etiologic investigations. They enable us to describe how common an illness or health event is in reference to the size of a particular candidate population (i.e., population at risk). For example, we might wish to know the average incidence rate of coronary heart disease (CHD) for 60-year-old white females with hypertension.

Measures of association assess the strength of the statistical relationship between a given study factor and a disease. Either implicitly or explicitly, a measure of association reflects a comparison of frequency measures for two or more categories (or values) of the study factor. For example, we might compare the average incidence rate of CHD for 60-year-old white females with hypertension to the corresponding rate for 60-year-old white females without hypertension. In this way, we can make an inference about the possible causal association between high blood pressure and CHD among white women.

Measures of potential impact reflect the expected contribution of a study factor to the frequency of a disease in a particular population. These measures are especially useful in public health practice for predicting the efficacy or effectiveness of therapeutic maneuvers and intervention strategies within specific populations. For example, we might wish to know the proportion or number of all new CHD cases among white women in a given year that are attributable or due to high blood pressure. Then we could project the potential impact of a hypertension control program on the frequency of disease in the population. Essentially, potential impact measures are a combination of frequency and association measures.

The remainder of this chapter and all of Chapter 7 will be devoted to frequency measures; measures of association and of potential impact will be discussed in Chapters 8 and 9. Measures of disease frequency may express the degree of (relative) *morbidity* or *mortality* in a population. Furthermore, in epidemiologic research, it is most important to distinguish between two types of morbidity measures: *incidence,* which reflects the number of new cases within a given period, and *prevalence,* which reflects the number of existing cases at a point in time. These three types of frequency measures—incidence, prevalence, and mortality—will be elaborated in this chapter and the next. We focus on incidence in the following sections.

Frequency measures based on new or incident cases reflect a *change* in disease status—i.e., becoming a case—and, therefore, such measures are particularly suited to identifying risk factors. Typically, incidence measures are estimated from cohort or ambidirectional studies, which involve the follow-up of either fixed or dynamic populations (Chapter 5). Many cluster studies also involve incidence data, although information about the corresponding candidate populations is not available. For most chronic diseases, especially incurable conditions, we are concerned with the first occurrence of the disease for each subject at risk. When studying acute diseases, however, especially in the absence of acquired immunity, we might be interested in multiple occurrences of disease within individuals (i.e., total incidence).

**6.2
BASIC
INCIDENCE
MEASURES:
RISK AND
RATE**

As we discussed in Chapter 2, we generally cannot specify precisely the time at which a noninfectious disease becomes irreversible. Consequently, our observation of disease incidence depends entirely on existing practices of medical diagnosis and community surveillance. In subsequent chapters, we will see how these procedures can affect the accuracy of our estimates.

As we suggested in Chapter 1, there are two distinct measures of disease incidence, risk and rate. Each can be estimated in different ways, and the method of estimation depends on certain features of the study design (Morgenstern et al., 1980; Miettinen, 1976). *Risk* is defined as the probability of a disease-free individual's developing a given disease over a specified period, conditional on that individual's not dying from any other disease during the period. As a *conditional probability,* risk can vary between zero and one and is dimensionless. Moreover, it usually refers to the first occurrence of the disease for each disease-free person, although it is possible to consider the risk of developing the disease twice (or more) within a given period.

The concept of risk, as defined above, requires a period referent that describes the time (or age) span over which new cases are detected. This period may be arbitrarily fixed, such as the five-year risk of developing CHD, or it may vary among individuals, such as the lifetime risk of developing CHD. Frequently, a fixed time referent is implicitly determined by the nature of the disease being studied. In the investigation of a local outbreak of a communicable disease, for example, the period may be conveniently defined as the duration of the epidemic or the time during which primary cases occur. In this situation, the risk is often called an "attack rate" (MacMahon and Pugh, 1970, Chap. 5) (though it is not actually a true rate).

A related frequency measure is the *risk odds,* which is the conditional probability of developing the disease divided by the conditional probability of not developing it. In other words, the risk odds is the ratio of the risk for an individual to one minus the risk. We will see the utility of odds measures in Chapter 8.

The incidence *rate* of disease occurrence is the instantaneous potential for change in disease status (i.e., the occurrence of new cases) per unit of time at time t, relative to the size of the candidate (i.e., disease-free) population at time t (Morgenstern et al., 1980).* Others have referred to this concept as an "instantaneous risk" (or probability) (Haberman, 1978), a "hazard" (especially when death is the event of interest) (Gehan, 1969), a "person-time incidence rate" (Schlesselman, 1982), and a "force of morbidity" (Miettinen, 1976). The last term suggests that an incidence rate refers strictly to a population and therefore has no direct interpretation on the individual level, as does risk. Also, in contrast to the concept of risk, the incidence rate, as an instantaneous measure, refers to a "point in time" and has no period referent. While risk is dimensionless and has an upper limit of one, the incidence rate is expressed in units of 1/time (e.g., years^{-1}) and can exceed one simply by changing the units (e.g., to days^{-1}).

6.3 ESTIMATION OF AVERAGE RATES

Because we generally cannot express the size of the candidate population as a mathematical function of time, we seldom obtain instantaneous incidence rates (see the first footnote below). Instead, we estimate an *average rate* for a given period, analogous to the use of speed as an estimate of average velocity. We will refer to this average rate[†] for a given follow-up period (t_0, t), of duration Δt, as the *incidence density* (ID) (Miettinen, 1976), which is estimated as follows:

$$\hat{\mathrm{ID}}_{(t_0, t)} = I/\mathrm{PT} \tag{6.1}$$

where I is the number of new cases that occur during the calendar period (t_0, t), PT is the amount of population-time accrued by the observed candidate population during that period (expressed in person-years, per-

---

*In mathematical terms, where the size of the fixed candidate population (N_t') is regarded as a function of time, the instantaneous incidence rate is equal to (-1) times the first derivative of N_t' at time t, divided by N_t' at time t—i.e., $[-d(N_t')/dt]/N_t'$ (Elandt-Johnson, 1975).

†In mathematical terms, the average rate (ID) for the period (t_0, t) is equal to the number of new cases (I) occurring in a candidate population (of size N_t') during the period, divided by the integral of $N_t'(dt)$ from t_0 to t—i.e., $\mathrm{ID}_{(t_0, t)} = I/\int_{t_0}^{t} N_t'(dt)$. Expression 6.1 represents an approximation of this quantity. The term "incidence density" reflects an intuitive interpretation of an average incidence rate—i.e., the concentration or density of new case occurrences in an accumulation (or sea) of population-time (see Morgenstern et al., 1980).

son-days, etc.), and $\hat{\text{ID}}$ is expressed in units of time^{-1}. For example, a fixed cohort of 101 disease-free people followed for two years (Δt) will contribute 202 person-years of experience if none of them develop the disease or are withdrawn from observation. If, on the other hand, two new cases occur exactly at the midpoint of the observation period, there will be $99(2) + 2(1) = 200$ person-years, and the estimated incidence density will be $2/200 = .01/\text{year} = 10 \times 10^{-3}/\text{year}$.

The amount of population-time (PT) in the denominator of expression 6.1 can be calculated in either of two ways; the method of calculation depends on certain features of the study design. If the durations of the individual follow-up periods for all N' disease-free subjects are known (or assumed by the investigator), PT may be computed by summing over subjects, as follows:

$$\text{PT} = \sum_{i=1}^{N'} \Delta t_i \qquad (6.2)$$

where Δt_i is the duration of the observed follow-up period for the ith individual from entry into the study until either disease detection or withdrawal. *Withdrawals* can occur for any of four reasons: (1) follow-up loss due to migration, lack of cooperation, etc.; (2) death from another cause (not the disease of interest); (3) termination of the study, thereby cutting short the follow-up period for individuals who entered after the start of the study; and (4) use of certain medical procedures that remove the person from the candidate population (e.g., hysterectomy and uterine cancer).

EXAMPLE 6.1

As an illustration of the method for estimating the ID, consider a hypothetical dynamic cohort of 12 subjects followed for a total duration (Δt) of 5.5 years, diagramed in Figure 6.1. Notice that 3 subjects enter the study at the beginning of each of the first 4 years (say, after being exposed for the first time) and that all subsequent events of interest occur at interval midpoints. There are 7 withdrawals among the noncases, including 3 who are lost to follow-up (persons 7, 8, and 12), 2 who die (persons 3 and 4), and 2 who are terminated by the end of the study (persons 5 and 10). The individual follow-up periods (Δt_i), until either disease occurrence or withdrawal, are given on the right side of Figure 6.1. Using Equations 6.1 and 6.2, we find the average incidence rate for the cohort during the entire study period to be $5/(2.5 + 3.5 + \cdots + 1.5) = .192/\text{year}$.

For health events that may occur more than once within an individual (e.g., myocardial infarctions), the investigator may wish to estimate the *total incidence* for a population. In this situation, Δt_i would include the

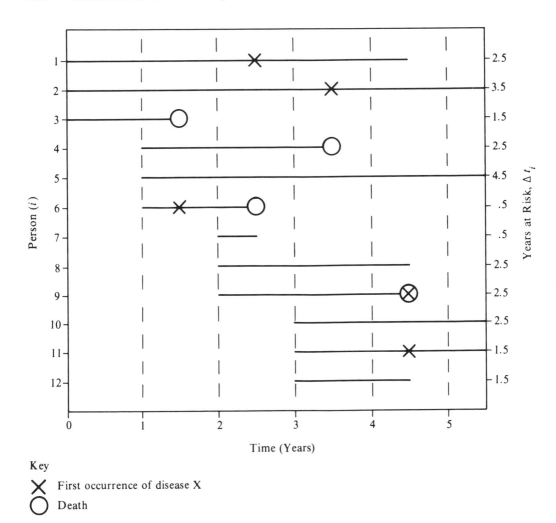

Figure 6.1 Diagrammatic Representation of the 5.5-Year Follow-up of a Hypothetical Cohort of 12 Subjects Initially Free of Disease X

follow-up experience of cases who remained in the study long enough to reenter the candidate population. For example, if the disease portrayed in Figure 6.1 has a very short duration and does not confer subsequent immunity, person 1 would contribute 4.5 years (instead of 2.5 years) to the denominator of the total ID estimate.

A practical limitation to the estimation of IDs using Equations 6.1 and 6.2 is that we must know the exact time of disease onset and/or withdrawal for every subject in order to ascertain Δt_i. Thus, we generally assume that disease onset occurs either on the day of reported diagnosis or at the midpoint of an interval between exams, involving a change in disease status.

The second method for calculating the amount of population-time does not require knowledge of the individual follow-up periods (Δt_i). In an ambidirectional study, for example, estimation of the average rate is still possible if we assume that the dynamic population is stable over time— i.e., that the size and age distribution remain constant. PT is then computed by multiplying the size (N') of the stable, disease-free population by the actual duration (Δt) of follow-up (Morgenstern et al., 1980):

$$PT = N' (\Delta t) \qquad (6.3)$$

With rare diseases, N' is approximately equal to the size (N) of the total population, including prevalent cases, as enumerated in a census. For instance, suppose we follow a stable population of 100,000 men for a period of 5 years (Δt), during which time we detect 500 new cases of bladder cancer. The average incidence rate for the study period is then approximately $500/100,000(5) = .001/\text{year}$.

Since Expression 6.1 is an estimate of an *average* rate, any fluctuations in the (instantaneous) rate over the follow-up period are obscured, with possible misleading consequences. For example, 1,000 people followed for 1 year after first exposure produce the same number of person-years as 100 persons followed for 10 years. If the average duration between first exposure and disease onset is 5 years, we would expect the estimated ID to be lower in the larger cohort, because it is not followed long enough to result in as many exposure-related cases.

Three methods of risk estimation will be described in the following subsections: the simple cumulative method, the actuarial method, and the density method. Multiple approaches are needed to handle a variety of design situations. Although the simple cumulative method is a special case of the actuarial method, the former is presented first because it is the easiest and most widely used approach for estimating risk.

6.4 ESTIMATION OF RISK

For a cohort of subjects followed for Δt years, we may often estimate the risk by calculating the proportion of candidate subjects who develop the disease during the observation period (t_0, t). We will refer to this proportion as the *cumulative incidence* (CI) (Morgenstern et al., 1980; Miettinen, 1976). Generally, the CI is estimated only for first occurrence of the disease; thus, the candidate population consists of disease-free subjects at the beginning of the follow-up period or upon inclusion in the study. If the durations (Δt_i) of the individual follow-up periods for all noncases are equal, the CI is equivalent to the average risk for members of the cohort. In practice, however, this special condition seldom occurs because of withdrawals from the study population (see Section 6.3). However, if the cohort is fixed and there is little attrition during the follow-up period (so that $\Delta t_i \approx \Delta t$ for

6.4.1 Simple Cumulative Method

all noncases), the Δt-year CI—and, therefore, the Δt-year risk (R)—can be estimated as follows:

$$\hat{R}_{(t_0,t)} = \hat{CI}_{(t_0,t)} = I/N_0' \tag{6.4}$$

where I is the number of new cases diagnosed during the period (t_0, t) and N_0' is the number of disease-free subjects at t_0.

Because risk is, by definition, a *conditional* probability, the $\hat{CI}$ is not an accurate estimate of risk unless all subjects in the observed candidate population are followed for the entire follow-up period or are known to develop the disease during the interval. Unfortunately, even with perfect follow-up information of a fixed cohort, we are not able to avoid deaths from other (competing) causes—i.e., from diseases other than the one of interest. For example, according to Equation 6.4, the 5-year* $\hat{CI}$ for subjects 1–3 in Figure 6.1 is $2/3 = .67$. But since subject 3, the one noncase, died after 1.5 years, we cannot know whether this person would have developed the disease in the remaining 3.5 years. We conclude, therefore, that Expression 6.4 is suitable for estimating risk only under very restricted conditions that frequently do not exist, particularly with long follow-up periods.

**6.4.2
Actuarial
Method**

When the durations (Δt_i) of the individual follow-up periods for noncases vary substantially in either fixed or dynamic populations,[†] we often use an *actuarial* (or life table) *method* to calculate the cumulative incidence. While this method is typically used to estimate the probability of death from any disease (Cutler and Ederer, 1958; Elveback, 1958; Fleiss et al., 1976), it is easily adapted to incidence estimation. In this regard, it is most applicable when the beginning of an individual's follow-up period is characterized by a discrete event, such as first diagnosis of a disease, the start of treatment, surgery, first use of a preventive measure, or first exposure to a suspected risk factor.

In the actuarial method, the CI for a given period (t_0, t)—and, therefore, the risk (R)—is estimated as follows:

$$\hat{R}_{(t_0,t)} = \hat{CI}_{(t_0,t)} = \frac{I}{N_0' - (W/2)} \tag{6.5}$$

where W is the number of withdrawals from the study population during the period (t_0, t) of duration Δt. The denominator of Expression 6.5, $[N_0' - (W/2)]$, may be regarded as the "effective number" of persons at

---

*For all risk estimates that involve the hypothetical cohort in Figure 6.1, we will consider no more than 5 years (not 5.5 years) of individual follow-up experience, because no subject was observed to be at risk of developing the disease for more than 5 years; i.e., $\Delta t_i < 5$ for every subject.

[†]In a dynamic population, Δt_i nearly always varies among noncases.

risk of developing the disease, assuming the mean withdrawal time occurs at the midpoint of the follow-up period (Littell, 1952; Elandt-Johnson, 1977). That is, it represents the number of disease-free persons that would be expected to produce I new cases if all persons could be followed for the entire period. In this sense, Expression 6.5 is a refinement of Expression 6.4—or, equivalently, the simple cumulative method is a special case of the actuarial method.

If the study population is dynamic, the actuarial method works by artificially converting the design to a fixed cohort for which the common starting time for each subject corresponds to entry into the study.

EXAMPLE 6.2

Consider the hypothetical dynamic cohort of 12 subjects, diagramed in Figure 6.1. To calculate the ĈI for any given period of 5.5 years or less, we can imagine that each subject "line" is shifted to the left margin (time $= t_0$) and that the total observation period is divided into 5 consecutive 1-year intervals (t_{j-1}, t_j), where $j = 1, \ldots, 5$. Thus, for example, subject 6 develops the disease in the first year ($j = 1$), and subject 12 is lost to follow-up in the second year ($j = 2$). As a result of disease occurrence and withdrawals, the size (N'_{0j}) of the disease-free cohort at the beginning of the jth interval decreases from 12 ($j = 1$) to 10 ($j = 2$), to 7 ($j = 3$), to 2 ($j = 4$), to 1 ($j = 5$). Using Expression 6.5, we may compute the 1-year cumulative incidence $(\hat{\text{CI}}_j)$ for the jth interval. For example, we would estimate the risk ($R_1 = \text{CI}_1$) of developing the disease for the first year after exposure to be $1/(12 - 1/2) = .087$. Computed results for all 5 intervals are presented in Table 6.1.

To estimate the risk for an accumulated period (t_0, t_j) of Δ years $(\Delta \leq \Delta t)$, we combine 1-year estimates of risk $(R_j = \text{CI}_j)$ by using the following formula (Elveback, 1958):

$$\hat{R}_{(t_0, t_j)} = \hat{\text{CI}}_{(t_0, t_j)} = 1 - \prod_{j'=1}^{j} (1 - \hat{\text{CI}}_{j'}) \qquad (6.6)$$

where $\hat{\text{CI}}_j$ is the Δ_j-year cumulative incidence for the jth age (time) interval (t_{j-1}, t_j), according to Expression 6.5, $\Delta = \Sigma_{j'=1}^{j} \Delta_{j'} = t_j - t_0$, $\Delta_j = t_j - t_{j-1}$ (equal to 1 year for each interval in the example), and j' is a dummy subscript for the jth stratum (so that we may accumulate time from the beginning of the first age interval to the end of the jth age interval). Notice the distinction between Δt and Δ: the former refers to *calendar time*—i.e., the number of years that a population is actually followed (e.g., 1970 to 1979)—and the latter refers to *age time*—i.e., a designated number of years in the life of an individual (e.g., age 50 to age 59). In following a

Table 6.1   Estimation of the Risk (R) of Developing Disease X for the Hypothetical Cohort of 12 Subjects (Figure 6.1), by 1-Year Interval (t_{j-1}, t_j), Using the Actuarial Method (Equations 6.5 and 6.6)

j	(t_{j-1}, t_j)	N'_{0j}	I_j	W_j	$\hat{R}_j$	$\hat{R}_{(t_0, t_j)}$
1	(0, 1)	12	1	1	.087	.087
2	(1, 2)	10	1	2	.111	.188
3	(2, 3)	7	2	3	.364	.484
4	(3, 4)	2	1	0	.500	.742
5	(4, 5)	1	0	1	.000	.742
Total	(0, 5)	—	5	7	—	—

Note: $\hat{R}_j$ is the 1-year risk estimate for the jth interval (t_{j-1}, t_j). $\hat{R}_{(t_0, t_j)}$ is the Δ-year risk estimate for the accumulated period (t_0, t_j), where $\Delta = t_j - t_0$.

narrow age-specific cohort (e.g., all 50-year-olds between 1970 and 1979), the two time dimensions are identical for subjects not withdrawn from observation.

Applying Expression 6.6 to the data in Table 6.1, we estimate the 2-year risk of developing the disease after first exposure to be

$$1 - (1 - .087)(1 - .111) = .188$$

Similarly, the estimated 5-year-risk of developing the disease is .742 (see Table 6.1).

Implicit in the application of Expression 6.6 for risk estimation is the assumption that all withdrawals occur, on the average, at the midpoints of the intervals. If the intervals are short enough (say $\Delta_j \leq 1$ year) or if there are relatively few withdrawals, violation of this assumption will not seriously affect the risk estimates. Nevertheless, even if all withdrawals were to occur at the interval midpoints, the actuarial method described above results in biased estimates of risk (Cutler and Ederer, 1958; Fleiss et al., 1976). Because of this problem, several alternative approaches have been proposed; all produce approximately the same results for large study populations (Elandt-Johnson, 1977).

**6.4.3
Density
Method**

The last method for estimating risk is based on the estimation of average rates (i.e., IDs) and thus depends on the functional relationship between a risk and a rate. To appreciate this relationship, consider a fixed cohort of N'_0 disease-free subjects (at time t_0) that is followed for Δt years for subsequent detection of a disease (first incidence). Let N'_t be the number of healthy subjects remaining at time t during the follow-up period. Figure 6.2 represents how N_t' changes over time, assuming that the (instantaneous) incidence rate remains constant (equal to ID) during the entire period (t_0, t_2).* Mathematically, then, given a constant rate (ID), the number of healthy subjects (N_t') at time t is an exponential function with a negative slope (Elandt-Johnson, 1975; Morgenstern et al., 1980). That is,

$$N_t' = N_0' \exp[-\text{ID}(\Delta)]$$

where $\Delta = t - t_0$ is the elapsed time (or age) between the start of follow-up and time t, and $\Delta \leq \Delta t$ is the duration of the observed follow-up period. Thus, we can estimate the Δ-year risk, $R_{(t_0, t)}$, as a function of the estimated average rate $(\hat{\text{ID}})$ by using the following expression:

$$\hat{R}_{(t_0, t)} = 1 - (N_t'/N_0') = 1 - \exp[-\hat{\text{ID}}(\Delta)] \qquad (6.7)$$

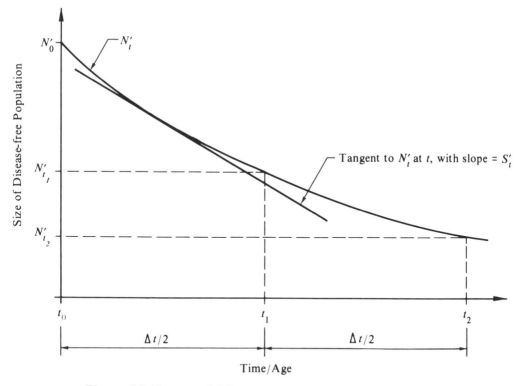

Figure 6.2 Exponential Reduction in the Size (N_t') of a Fixed, Disease-free Population During a Period (t_0, t_2), with a Constant Rate of Disease Incidence (ID)

---

*In mathematical terms, $-\text{ID} = S_t'/N_t'$, where $S_t' = $ slope of N_t' curve at time $t = d(N_t')/dt$. Refer to the first footnote on page 100.

When the quantity $\hat{ID}(\Delta)$ is small (say less than .10), Expression 6.7 is approximately equal to $\hat{ID}(\Delta)$. Under these conditions, the annual risk (i.e., $\Delta = 1$ year) is approximately equal to the average rate ($\hat{ID}$) times 1 year.

EXAMPLE 6.3

As an illustration of the density method for estimating risk, consider the hypothetical cohort of 12 subjects diagramed in Figure 6.1. In Example 6.1, we found that the $\hat{ID}$ for the cohort during the entire study period was .192/year. Using Expression 6.7, we estimate the 5-year risk to be $1 - \exp[-.192(5)] = .618$. However, as shown in Table 6.2, the incidence rate does not remain constant during the follow-up period. Shifting every subject line in Figure 6.1 to the left margin (t_0) (as we did in the actuarial method) and computing the amount of population-time (PT_j) for each 1-year interval, we find that the estimated average rate ($\hat{ID}_j$) for the jth interval varies considerably, increasing from .091/year in the first interval ($j = 1$) to .667/year in the fourth interval ($j = 4$) and falling to 0 in the fifth interval ($j = 5$). Consequently, we must conclude that the previous 5-year risk estimate is wrong. The correct procedure is to estimate the 1-year risks (R_j) separately for each interval, using interval-specific rate estimates ($\hat{ID}_j$) and Expression 6.7, and to combine them by using Expression 6.6. Using that procedure, we need only assume that the rate is constant within each 1-year interval.

In general, we can represent the procedure described in Example 6.3 as

$$\hat{R}_{(t_0,t_j)} = 1 - \prod_{j'=1}^{j} (1 - \hat{R}_{j'})$$

where $\hat{R}_j = 1 - \exp[-\hat{ID}_j(\Delta_j)]$, $\Delta = t_j - t_0 = \sum_{j'=1}^{j} \Delta_{j'}$ and $\Delta_j = t_j - t_{j-1}$. Or, equivalently, we can express the above risk estimate as

$$\hat{R}_{(t_0,t_j)} = 1 - \exp[-\sum_{j'=1}^{j} \hat{ID}_{j'}(\Delta_{j'})] \tag{6.8}$$

Note that Δ in Expression 6.8 can exceed Δt (the duration of observed follow-up).

Returning to Example 6.3, we find that the estimated 5-year risk of developing the disease, according to Expression 6.8, is

$$1 - \exp[-.091(1) - .118(1) - .444(1) - .667(1) - 0(1)] = .733$$

(see Table 6.2). Notice that this estimate is substantially different from the previous estimate (.618), for which the rate was assumed constant through-

**Table 6.2   Estimation of the Risk (R) of Developing Disease
X for the Hypothetical Cohort of 12 Subjects (Figure 6.1),
by 1-Year Interval, Using the Density Method
(Expressions 6.7 and 6.8)**

j	(t_{j-1}, t_j)	PT_j	I_j	$\hat{ID}_j$	$\hat{R}_j$	$\hat{R}_{(t0, tj)}$
1	(0, 1)	11.0	1	.091	.087	.087
2	(1, 2)	8.5	1	.118	.111	.188
3	(2, 3)	4.5	2	.444	.359	.480
4	(3, 4)	1.5	1	.667	.487	.733
5	(4, 5)	.5	0	.000	.000	.733
Total	(0, 5)	26.0	5	.192	—	—

Note: See the note in Table 6.1.

out the 5-year period. Using Expression 6.8, we must assume that the rate is constant within each interval (t_{j-1}, t_j) of duration Δ_j. By dividing Δ into enough intervals (so that the Δ_j are "small"), we can be reasonably sure that this assumption is not violated enough to affect the risk estimate substantially.

EXAMPLE 6.4

Since age is a risk factor for most diseases, average rates should be estimated for age categories that are as narrow as possible for the available data. Consider another hypothetical study in which a stable population of 1,000,000 people, divided into exposed and unexposed groups, is followed for 2 years (Δt) for detection of a disease. As summarized in Table 6.3, the total population for each exposure group is distributed into four age decades ($j = 1, \ldots, 4$), and about 18,000 new cases are observed during the 2-year period. Also given in Table 6.3 are the numbers of prevalent cases (C) within each age-exposure category, enabling us to estimate the number ($N' = N - C$) of disease-free persons in each category. Computational results are presented in Table 6.4 by age and exposure categories. For example, the estimated 10-year risk for an unexposed 40-year-old person in the population is

$$1 - \exp[-.0005(10)] \cong .005$$

where

EXAMPLE 6.4 (*continued*)

$$\hat{ID}_1 = \frac{240}{(240,000 - 600)(2)} \approx .0005/year$$

(which is assumed fixed for the entire age decade 40–49). Using Expression 6.8, we find the estimated 40-year (Δ) risk for an unexposed 40-year-old person to be

$$1 - \exp[-.0005(10) - .0025(10) - .0100(10) - .0250(10)] \approx .3162$$

where Δ_j is 10 years for each interval.

This method of risk estimation is closely related to the calculation of life expectancy in demographic life table analysis, where the outcome event of interest is usually death from any cause (Mausner and Bahn, 1974). The objective of the latter approach is to estimate the expected number of years remaining in the life of a person at age x (i.e., $\mathring{e}_x$), rather than to estimate the conditional probability of dying within Δ years at age x.

By combining information from consecutive age intervals, as we did in Example 6.4, we can estimate risk for a much longer duration (Δ) than the actual follow-up period (Δt). To combine risk estimates in this way, however, we must assume that there is no "secular trend" in the disease rate. Specifically, this assumption requires that each age-specific rate (ID_j) not change for a period of ($\Delta + \Delta t$) years. For example, if the 2-year (Δt) study resulting in the data of Table 6.3 began in 1950, we assume no change in ID for the youngest age decade (40–49) between 1950 and 1992.

Table 6.3   Number of Prevalent Cases (*C*) and Incident Cases (*I*) During a 2-Year Follow-up of a Hypothetical Stable Population (Size *N*), by Exposure Status and Age ($j = 1, \ldots, 4$)

	EXPOSED			UNEXPOSED		
Age	N_j	C_j	I_j	N_j	C_j	I_j
40–49	35,000	175	70	240,000	600	240
50–59	50,000	1,220	488	230,000	2,840	1,136
60–69	60,000	5,455	2,182	200,000	9,525	3,810
70–79	55,000	11,000	4,400	130,000	14,445	5,778
Total	200,000	17,850	7,140	800,000	27,410	10,964

Table 6.4   Estimation of Average Incidence Rates (ID) and Risks (R), Using the Density Method (Expressions 6.7 and 6.8), for the Data in Table 6.3, by Exposure Status and Age

Age	EXPOSED			UNEXPOSED		
	$\hat{ID}_j$	$\hat{R}_j$	$\hat{R}_{(t_0,t_j)}$	$\hat{ID}_j$	$\hat{R}_j$	$\hat{R}_{(t_0,t_j)}$
40–49	.0010	.0100	.0100	.0005	.0050	.0050
50–59	.0050	.0488	.0583	.0025	.0247	.0296
60–69	.0200	.1813	.2290	.0100	.0952	.1219
70–79	.0500	.3935	.5324	.0250	.2212	.3162
Total	.0179	—	—	.0069	—	—

Note: $\hat{ID}_j$ is the estimated rate for the jth 10-year interval ($j = 1, \ldots , 4$), using Expressions 6.1 and 6.3. $\hat{R}_j$ is the 10-year risk estimate for the jth interval (t_{j-1}, t_j). $\hat{R}_{(t_0,t_j)}$ is the Δ-year risk estimate for the accumulated period (t_0, t_j), where $\Delta = t_j - t_0$.

Analogously, we assume no change in ID for the oldest age decade (70–79) between 1910 and 1952. In summary, the use of Expression 6.8 to estimate risk requires two time-related assumptions: (1) the rate is constant within each age interval ($j = 1, \ldots$) and (2) each age-specific rate (ID_j) remains constant over (calendar) time.

6.5 CHOOSING AN INCIDENCE MEASURE

As we demonstrated in the two previous sections, we can quantify disease incidence in different ways; the method used depends on particular features of the study design. The basic procedures and the central issues discussed in those sections are summarized in Figure 6.3 and in the accompanying notes. Essentially, there are two related decisions required for estimating incidence measures in a follow-up study: (1) choosing the proper empirical measure—i.e., CI versus ID—and (2) choosing the desired theoretical measure—i.e., risk versus rate. The former decision has been discussed throughout this chapter (see Figure 6.3), but the latter decision needs further clarification. As suggested in Figure 6.3, theoretically, $\hat{ID}$s can be used to estimate either rates or risks; CIs usually are limited to estimating risks. Which theoretical measure should be estimated in practice? The principal criterion for selecting an appropriate incidence measure is the objective of the study—i.e., whether the purpose of the investigation is to predict individual disease occurrence or to test an etiologic hypothesis.

To predict an individual's change in health status on the basis of certain known characteristics (e.g., exposures or behaviors), we must know the risk (i.e., conditional probability) of developing the outcome event. Recall that an incidence rate has no useful interpretation at the

Figure 6.3 A Decision Flow Chart for Choice and Estimation of Incidence Measures in Epidemiologic Research

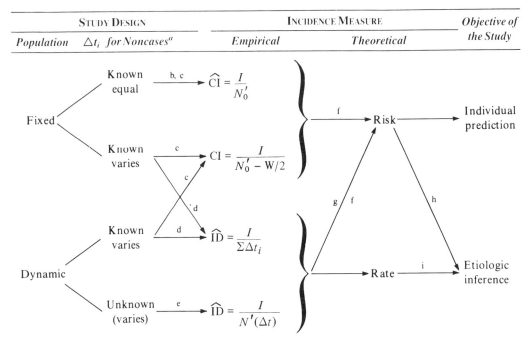

[a] Δt_i is the duration of the observed follow-up period for the i th individual from entry into the study until either disease detection or withdrawal.

[b] In the *simple cumulative method*, we assume that there are no withdrawals (W) from observation. That is, the simple cumulative method (upper expression for $\widehat{CI}$) is a special case of the actuarial method (lower expression for $\widehat{CI}$).

[c] In the *actuarial method*, CI usually is estimated for first occurrence of disease. Typically, this method is used only if the start of the follow-up period for each subject is marked by a discrete event (e.g., diagnosis of a disease or first exposure to a potential risk factor).

[d] The durations (Δt_i) of the individual follow-up periods are known (or assumed) for all cases and noncases—i.e., we must know (or assume) the time of disease onset and withdrawal from observation.

[e] We assume that the (dynamic) disease-free population is stable—i.e., the size (N') and age distributions remain constant over time.

[f] If we combine risk estimates from consecutive age intervals, using Expressions 6.6 or 6.8, we assume no secular trends in the age-specific rates (ID_j).

[g] In the *density method* of estimating risk, we assume that the average incidence rate (ID) is constant over the age/time duration (Δ) of the observed follow-up period.

[h] The disease has a *restricted risk period* relative to the observation period (true for most acute diseases).

[i] The disease has an *extended risk period* relative to the observation period (true for most chronic diseases).

individual level. Risk estimation is most relevant for assessing the prognosis of a patient, for selecting an appropriate treatment strategy, and for making personal decisions about health-related behaviors.

On the other hand, if we wish to test specific etiologic hypotheses regarding the possible effects of one or more factors, the choice of an incidence measure depends on the nature of the disease and the way in which we observe new case occurrences (Morgenstern et al., 1980; Miettinen, 1976). In theory, hypothesis testing requires estimation of rates for most chronic diseases with long latent periods. In this situation, the actual follow-up period for each subject represents only a part of the total time that the person is at risk of developing the disease. We will refer to such diseases as having *extended risk periods,* since the actual period of disease susceptibility extends beyond (i.e., before and after) the observed follow-up period. However, if the disease has a short latent period and the study factor represents an event, an exposure of short duration, or a fixed attribute (e.g., race), the entire risk period for each subject typically is included within the actual follow-up period. For example, in the investigation of a local "point source" epidemic of an acute disease, the investigator may identify all cases that were attributable to the source of the outbreak. In this situation, the disease has a *restricted risk period* and calls for the estimation of risks to make causal inferences. Notice that the (instantaneous) rate in such an investigation will change extensively during the course of the epidemic.

We have presented two distinct measures to quantify the occurrence of incident events: risk (which is a dimensionless quantity) and rate (which is expressed in units of 1/time). Risk is the conditional probability of developing a disease during a given period and is used both to predict individual changes in disease status and to test etiologic hypotheses for diseases with restricted risk periods (typically, acute conditions). Rate, on the other hand, is the instantaneous potential for disease occurrence per unit of time, relative to the size of the candidate population, and is used to test etiologic hypotheses for diseases with extended risk periods (typically, chronic conditions).

6.6 CONCLUDING REMARKS

An average incidence rate for a given period is estimated in follow-up studies by calculating the incidence density—i.e., the number of new cases divided by the amount of population-time of follow-up experience. The amount of population-time can be estimated either directly by summing individual contributions for members of the candidate population over the entire follow-up period or indirectly for a stable candidate population by multiplying the size of the population by the duration of follow-up.

Risks are estimated in one of three ways: (1) by calculating the proportion (i.e., cumulative incidence) of candidate persons who develop the disease during a given period, if there are few withdrawals during the period; (2) by extending the first approach to handle withdrawals from follow-up—i.e., the actuarial method; and (3) by using estimated age-specific incidence densities to estimate risk for a specified age (time) interval—i.e., the density method. To combine risk estimates from consecutive age intervals when using the density method, we must assume that the incidence rate is constant within each age interval and that each age-specific rate remains constant over (calendar) time. If the times of disease detection and withdrawal are known, the actuarial and density methods produce approximately the same results. Moreover, if the incidence rate (ID) is small and/or if the duration (Δ) is short [so that ID(Δ) is less than .10], the estimated Δ-year risk is approximately equal to ID(Δ).

NOTATION   The following list summarizes the key notation introduced in this chapter.

N_t	Size of total population at time t.
N_t'	Size of candidate population at time t—i.e., size of disease-free population if concerned with first occurrence of disease.
N_0'	Size of candidate population at start of follow-up (time t_0).
I	Number of new incident cases occurring or detected during period (t_0, t).
I_j	Number of incident cases occurring in jth age (time) interval (t_{j-1}, t_j).
PT	Amount of population-time (e.g., person-years) accrued by candidate population during period (t_0, t).
W	Number of withdrawals from candidate population during period (t_0, t).
$\Delta t = t - t_0$	Duration of observed follow-up period (t_0, t) for a population (in calendar time).
Δt_i	Duration of observed follow-up period for ith individual from entry into study until either disease detection or withdrawal.
$\Delta = t_j - t_0$	Width of accumulated age (time) interval (t_0, t_j) for individuals in an age-specific cohort—i.e., duration of a hypothetical follow-up period $(t_0, t_j) = \sum_{j'=1}^{j} \Delta_{j'}$.
$\Delta_j = t_j - t_{j-1}$	Width of jth age (time) interval (t_{j-1}, t_j).
$\hat{\text{ID}} = I/\text{PT}$	Incidence density (or average incidence rate) for calendar period (t_0, t) of duration Δt.
ID_j	Incidence density for jth age interval (t_{j-1}, t_j) of duration Δ_j.
$R_{(t_0, t)}$	Δt-year risk of developing disease during observed follow-up period (t_0, t).
$R_{(t_0, t_j)}$	Δ-year risk of developing disease during age (time) interval (t_0, t_j).
R_j	Δ_j-year risk of developing disease during age (time) interval (t_{j-1}, t_j).
CI	Cumulative incidence of disease for a given period (corresponding to the above risk measures).

PRACTICE EXERCISES   **6.1** The accompanying hypothetical data (Exercise Table 6.1) represent the 5-year follow-up experience of 1,000 newly diagnosed cases of ovarian cancer. As-

Exercise Table 6.1

Year After Diagnosis, j	No. of Cases at Start of Period, N_{0j}	No. of Deaths During Period, D_j	No. of Withdrawals During Period, W_j
1	1000	214	55
2	731	117	63
3	551	57	47
4	447	30	45
5	372	16	38

sume that all deaths and withdrawals occur uniformly throughout the 1-year intervals.

a. Using the actuarial method, estimate the 5-year risk that a new case will die with ovarian cancer.

b. Using the density method, estimate the 5-year risk that a new case will die with ovarian cancer.

6.2 Using the data in Table 6.3, estimate the following parameters for the exposed group:

a. the 2-year risk for a 55-year-old person

b. the 10-year risk for a 55-year-old person

c. the 20-year risk for a 55-year-old person

REFERENCES

CUTLER, S. J., and EDERER, F. 1958. Maximum utilization of the life table method in analyzing survival. *J. Chronic Dis.* 8: 699–712.

ELANDT-JOHNSON, R. C. 1975. Definition of rates: Some remarks on their use and misuse. *Am. J. Epidemiol.* 102: 267–271.

———. 1977. Various estimators of conditional probabilities of death in follow-up studies: Summary of results. *J. Chronic Dis.* 30: 247–256.

ELVEBACK, L. 1958. Estimation of survivorship in chronic disease: The "actuarial" method. *J. Am. Stat. Assoc.* 53: 420–440.

FLEISS, J. L.; DUNNER, D. L.; STALLONE, F.; and FIEVE, R. R. 1976. The life table: A method for analyzing longitudinal studies. *Arch. Gen. Psychiat.* 33: 107–112.

GEHAN, E. A. 1969. Estimating survival functions from the life table. *J. Chronic Dis.* 21: 629–644.

HABERMAN, S. 1978. Mathematical treatment of the incidence and prevalence of disease. *Social Sci. & Med.* 12: 147–152.

LITTELL, A. S. 1952. Estimation of the t-year survival rate from follow-up studies over a limited period of time. *Hum. Biol.* 24: 87–116.

MACMAHON, B., and PUGH, T. F. 1970. *Epidemiology: Principles and methods.* Boston: Little, Brown.

MAUSNER, J. S., and BAHN, A. K. 1974. *Epidemiology: An introductory text.* Philadelphia: Saunders; App. 9.1, pp. 206–212.

MIETTINEN, O. S. 1976. Estimability and estimation in case-referent studies. *Am. J. Epidemiol.* 103(2): 226–235.

MORGENSTERN, H.; KLEINBAUM, D. G.; and KUPPER, L. L. 1980. Measures of disease incidence used in epidemiologic research. *Int. J. Epidemiol.* 9:97–104.

SCHLESSELMAN, J. J. 1982. *Case-control studies: Design, conduct, analysis.* New York: Oxford University Press.

7

Other Measures of Disease Frequency

CHAPTER OUTLINE

**7.0
PREVIEW**

In this chapter, we present the two other major types of frequency measures, *prevalence* and *mortality,* both of which depend on disease incidence, which was described in Chapter 6. In addition, we will discuss the general approach for analyzing changes in disease frequency over long periods, a methodology called *cohort analysis.*

**7.1
PREVA-
LENCE
MEASURES**

Observation of existing (i.e., prevalent) cases of disease in a population is the primary design feature of cross-sectional studies. Because prevalent cases represent survivors of a disease, they are not as well suited to identifying risk factors as are incident cases identified from a well-defined candidate population. Yet it is sometimes more feasible and/or less costly to use a set of prevalent cases rather than a set of incident cases to test an etiologic hypothesis. Of course, causal inference is not the only goal of epidemiologic research. Knowledge of disease prevalence is most important in planning health services and administering medical care facilities, since the number of prevalent cases at any time is one determinant of the demand for health care. In addition, we will see that prevalence measures are useful for describing the frequency of remittent diseases—i.e., conditions that recur within individuals and that are characterized by alternating periods of clinical symptoms and remission.

**7.1.1
Point and
Period
Prevalence**

We use two basic types of measures to quantify disease prevalence in a population: point prevalence and period prevalence (MacMahon and Pugh, 1970; Mausner and Bahn, 1974; Zeighami et al., 1979). The most common of these measures is the simple *point prevalence* (usually called prevalence), which is the probability that an individual in a population will be a case at time t. A function of point prevalence is the *prevalence odds,* which is the probability of being a case divided by the probability of not being a case at time t. Another variation of point prevalence is *lifetime prevalence,* which is the probability that an individual at time t has ever been a case. The latter measure might be employed to describe the overall occurrence of a remittent disease (e.g., arthritis) in a population.

Perhaps a more useful measure for studying remittent diseases is *episodic prevalence,* another variation of point prevalence, which has also been called "protep" (i.e., *pro*portion of *t*ime in *ep*isode) (Cobb, 1962) and "sick-day proportion" (Von Korff and Parker, 1980). Episodic prevalence treats an individual's disease status as a source of variation; it may be defined as the probability that a particular individual is clinically ill at time t. Very often, this measure is restricted to persons who are known to have suffered from the disease.

A second and less frequently used prevalence measure is *period prevalence,* which is the probability that an individual in a population will be a case anytime during a given period (t_0, t) of duration Δt. Period prevalence is most often used as a substitute for risk when the exact time of onset for individual cases is not known, a situation that is likely to occur in certain psychiatric illnesses. In this situation, the investigator normally would not be able to distinguish an incident case from a prevalent case.

Simple point prevalence (P_t) at time t is estimated as the proportion of persons in the study population of size N at time t that have the disease:

$$\hat{P}_t = C_t/N_t \qquad (7.1)$$

where $C_t = N_t - N_t'$ is the number of prevalent cases at time t. For example, estimates of the age-exposure-specific prevalences for the data in Table 6.3 are given in Table 7.1. The crude prevalence for unexposed subjects (ignoring age) is $27,410/800,000 = .0343$. This deceptively simple procedure for estimating prevalence belies the true complexity of the measure, a fact that should be considered when interpreting such results. These issues will be discussed further in the next section and in subsequent chapters.

Lifetime prevalence at time t is estimated from Expression 7.1, where C_t includes persons who have the disease at time t, persons who were previously cured of the disease, and persons who are in remission at time t. Since lifetime prevalence is a retrospective measure, it must be estimated by using subject recall and/or medical records.

Episodic prevalence for an individual is estimated as the proportion of time that the person is clinically ill (i.e., in episode). For remittent diseases, a full description of disease prevalence in the population at time t is provided by a frequency distribution of all persons, according to this measure (Cobb, 1962). Unfortunately, the information required to specify

**Table 7.1   Estimation of Average Incidence Rates (ID), Using
the Density Method (Expressions 6.7 and 6.8), and Prevalences (P)
for the Data in Table 6.3, by Exposure Status and Age**

	EXPOSED		UNEXPOSED	
Age	$\hat{ID}_j$	$\hat{P}_j$	$\hat{ID}_j$	$\hat{P}_j$
40–49	.0010	.0050	.0005	.0025
50–59	.0050	.0244	.0025	.0123
60–69	.0200	.0909	.0100	.0476
70–79	.0500	.2000	.0250	.1111
Total	.0179	.0893	.0069	.0343

Note: $\hat{ID}_j$ is the estimated rate for the jth 10-year interval ($j = 1, \ldots, 4$), using Expressions 6.1 and 6.3. $\hat{P}_j$ is the estimated average prevalence for the jth 10-year interval, using Expression 7.1.

this distribution from a single survey or examination may not be too reliable. But two successive examinations of the same population are adequate to determine the frequency distribution, if we assume a general mathematical model (Beall and Cobb, 1961); with additional examinations, the model may be derived from the data.

Period prevalence (PP) for a stable (dynamic) population is estimated as the ratio* of the number $(C_{(t_0,t)})$ of persons who were observed to have the disease anytime during the follow-up period (t_0, t) to the size $(N)^{\dagger}$ of the population:

$$\hat{\mathrm{PP}}_{(t_0,t)} = C_{(t_0,t)}/N = (C_0 + I)/N \tag{7.2}$$

where $C_{(t_0,t)}$ includes both prevalent cases (C_0) at t_0 and incident cases (I) detected during the period. If the study population is a fixed cohort, the denominator of Expression 7.2 should be replaced by the size (N_0) of the cohort at t_0. However, if the (dynamic) study population is unstable, any choice of a denominator will probably lead to an estimate of PP that has little practical value. For example, if we use the total number of subjects observed during the period as the denominator, the 5.5-year PP for the 12 subjects in Figure 6.1 is $5/12 = .417$. (Note that the numerator includes only incident cases.) In this example, it is doubtful whether such an estimate has any meaningful interpretation, since P_t changes considerably over the follow-up period and Δt_i varies among subjects. It is preferable, in such situations, to estimate (cumulative) incidence and prevalence separately, if the two can be distinguished.

**7.1.3
Prevalence and
Incidence**

While it is evident that the (point) prevalence of a disease in a dynamic population depends, in part, on the incidence rate of the disease, the functional relationship is rather complex. However, a simple mathematical relationship can be derived if we assume that the population is in a state of equilibrium—i.e., that the population is stable and that both the prevalence and incidence rates remain constant (Miettinen, 1976; Morrison, 1979). Under these *steady-state conditions,* the number of new case occurrences (I) within a period (t_0, t) of duration Δt is equal to the number of *terminated cases* (TC) during the same period. The latter quantity includes cases who die of the disease, cases who die of other causes, and cases who recover.[‡] From Equations 6.1 and 6.3, we can express I as $\mathrm{ID}(N')(\Delta t)$.

---

*The estimated PP is a ratio, not a proportion, because some cases counted in the numerator may not have been in the population for the entire observation period (t_0, t).

[†]Use of the symbols C and N without subscripts indicates values for these quantities that we assume are stable over time.

[‡]TC could also include those prevalent cases who migrate from the population. However, to avoid the complexities of selective case migration, we will assume that the numbers of diseased immigrants and emigrants are equal and, thus, cancel each other out.

Similarly, TC is equal to TD(C)(Δt), where TD is the *termination rate* (or density) and $C = N' - N = P(N)$ is the number of prevalent cases (i.e., the population at risk of terminating). Thus, we can express the steady-state relationship as ID(N')(Δt) = TD(C)(Δt). Dividing both sides of this equation by $N'(\Delta t)$ and solving for P (which is equal to C/N), we get

$$P = \frac{ID}{ID + TD} = \frac{1}{(TD/ID) + 1} \qquad (7.3)$$

Since terminations of the disease can be represented as a Poisson process, as is implied by Equation 6.7, the termination rate is equal to the reciprocal of the *mean duration* of the disease ($\overline{T}$) from first occurrence to termination, under steady-state conditions—i.e., TD = $1/\overline{T}$ (Lindgren, 1976). Substituting this expression for TD in Expression 7.3 results in the following relationship:

$$P = ID(\overline{T})/[ID(\overline{T}) + 1] \qquad (7.4)$$

Thus, P is directly proportional to both ID and $\overline{T}$ under steady-state conditions. If the disease is rare—and, especially, if it is highly fatal*—ID will be much smaller than TD (i.e., ID $\ll$ TD); therefore, P will be approximately equal to ID($\overline{T}$).

Equation 7.4 enables us to estimate the prevalence (or incidence) of a disease in a population, assuming equilibrium conditions, from estimates of both the incidence rate (or prevalence) and the mean duration of the disease. Unfortunately, a complete and lifelong follow-up of many incident cases is a very impractical method for estimating $\overline{T}$ for chronic diseases with long durations. Recently, however, a group of researchers (Visscher et al., 1980) found that $\overline{T}$ can be estimated quite accurately by following a group of prevalent cases for a short period (e.g., one or two years). From information about the date of first onset, recalled by relatives or abstracted from records, $\overline{T}$ is estimated by averaging the individual durations for all case deaths during the observation period.

Another method for estimating $\overline{T}$ is based on the steady-state relationship between the mean durations of an incidence and a prevalence series. In general, a prevalence series includes a larger proportion of chronic cases than does an incidence series. Freeman and Hutchison (1980) have shown that $\overline{T}$ (for incident cases), as well as the distribution of durations, can be estimated from the reported durations-to-date in a representative series of prevalent cases.

Alternatively, if estimates of P and ID are available, we can estimate $\overline{T}$ as a function of these values by rearranging Equation 7.4:

$$\overline{T} = P/[ID(1 - P)] \qquad (7.5)$$

---

*In fact, for the approximation to hold, it is not necessary that the disease be highly fatal, because every case eventually dies with the disease or recovers.

Consider, for example, the frequency estimates for the stable population given in Table 7.1. The estimated mean duration $(\overline{T}_1)$ of all exposed cases, ignoring age, is $.0893/.0179(1 - .0893) = 5.5$ years; similarly, the mean duration $(\overline{T}_0)$ of all unexposed cases is 5.2 years. A puzzling result emerges, however, if one estimates $\overline{T}$ in this manner within each age-exposure category: $\overline{T}$ is found to be 5.0 years in every category. The discrepancy occurs because Equations 7.4 and 7.5 are not applicable within narrow age categories, even under equilibrium conditions. However, if the disease is irreversible and if it does not affect the probability of dying (e.g., glaucoma), we can estimate the Δ_j-year risk (R_j) from age-specific prevalence estimates (Leske et al., 1981) as follows:

$$\hat{R}_j = (\hat{P}_{j+1} - \hat{P}_j)/(1 - \hat{P}_j) \tag{7.6}$$

where $\hat{P}_j$ is the estimated prevalence at the start of the jth interval, $\hat{P}_{j+1}$ is the estimated prevalence at the start of the $(j + 1)$th interval, and $\Delta_j = t_{j+1} - t_j$. We may then combine these risk estimates by using Expression 6.6. In addition, we may estimate average rates (ID_j) from the age-specific risks if we know the probability of dying within each age interval (Leske et al., 1981).

The steady-state relationship between incidence and prevalence also applies to remittent diseases. Von Korff and Parker (1980) have shown that point prevalence is equal to *lifetime episodic prevalence,* defined as the average number of years lived with the disease for the entire population divided by the life expectancy. The average number of years with the disease depends on the average number of episodes in a lifetime and the average episode duration, neither of which is generally estimable directly from available data. However, methods for approximating both parameters, using mathematical-modeling techniques, have been suggested by Von Korff and Parker.

The relationship between period prevalence (PP) and incidence in stable populations is even more complex than those steady-state functions presented above, because prevalent and incident cases are combined. However, reference to Expression 7.4 leads to a straightforward approximation of PP if the point prevalence (P) is small and constant over the follow-up period (t_0, t):

$$PP = (C_0 + I)/N \approx P + ID(\Delta t) \tag{7.7}$$

where $ID \approx N(\Delta t)$ if P is small. Thus, in general, period prevalence depends on both point prevalence and the (average) incidence rate of the disease.

**7.2
MORTALITY
MEASURES**

Frequency measures based on mortality are obtained primarily from the same types of designs that generate incidence data—i.e., cohort and ambidirectional studies. In addition, ecologic and proportional studies typically incorporate mortality data, although the latter do not include appropriate information about the candidate population (see Chapters 4 and 5).

Because mortality data are often much easier to collect and are generally more reliable than incidence data, the former are sometimes used in place of the latter to generate and test etiologic hypotheses, especially with highly fatal rare diseases. Another use of mortality data is as "hard" outcome information—the ultimate endpoint—for evaluating therapeutic and preventive interventions. We will see in Chapter 8, however, that such approaches may not be very sensitive for comparing group experiences (e.g., exposed and unexposed), since the observed exposure effect on death can easily become diluted, thereby resulting in misleading conclusions.

Mortality measures are analogous to incidence measures where the outcome event of interest is death instead of the occurrence of a new case. To develop the basic principles of these frequency measures, we will consider three mutually exclusive classes of mortality events: (1) death due to disease X (the disease of interest)—i.e., X is the immediate cause of death; (2) death due to other causes (Y) among cases of disease X—i.e., X is the underlying or contributing cause of death; and (3) death due to other causes (Y) among persons who do not have disease X. The numbers of these events occurring in a stable population for a period (t_0, t) will be represented by the symbols D_x, D_{xy}, and D_y, respectively. The total number of deaths in the period is therefore $D_x + D_{xy} + D_y = D$.

7.2.1 Mortality, Fatality, and Death

There are two fundamental concepts for expressing the frequency of death in a population: the rate or "force of mortality" (Miettinen, 1976) and the risk of dying or probability (see Section 6.2). Beginning with the former, we can further designate three types of frequency measures; these categories depend on how we define the event of interest and how we define the candidate population. First, the *mortality rate* refers to the force of mortality of a particular disease X in the total population. This measure can refer either to deaths *due to* X (i.e., D_x) or to deaths *with* X (i.e., $D_x + D_{xy}$). With most chronic diseases, we may not wish (or be able) to distinguish between D_x and D_{xy}, so the mortality rate with disease X becomes the more relevant measure. Second, the *fatality rate* refers to the force of mortality among cases of disease X. This measure can also refer to either deaths due to X or deaths with X, where the latter is more relevant to the study of chronic diseases. Third, the total *death rate* refers to the total force of mortality for all diseases among the total population.

All the above measures have corresponding risk measures, as described for incidence in Section 6.2. Mortality and fatality risks due to disease X and mortality risks with disease X are conditional probabilities; the other risks are unconditional probabilities (i.e., they are not conditional on surviving). *Survival,* which is the probability of not dying with disease X, is equivalent to one minus the risk of a case dying with disease X during a given period.

7.2.2
Estimation of
Mortality

We may estimate the various rates described in the previous section by calculating average rates or densities, in a manner similar to the way we estimated incidence rates. The estimated *mortality density* (MD$_x$) *due to disease* X for a given follow-up period (t_0, t) is

$$\hat{MD}_{x(t_0,t)} = D_x/PT \tag{7.8}$$

where PT is the amount of population time experienced by the candidate population during the period (t_0, t). Since a person is at risk of dying after disease onset, PT in Expression 7.8 is calculated differently for mortality than it is for incidence (see Equations 6.2 and 6.3). If the durations of individual follow-up periods (Δt_i) for all subjects are known, PT may be computed by summing over all persons as follows:

$$PT = \sum_{i=1}^{N} \Delta t_i \tag{7.9}$$

where N is the size of the total observed candidate population (including prevalent cases) and Δt_i is the duration from start of follow-up to withdrawal (i.e., death, loss to follow-up, or termination of the study). If the individual follow-up periods are not known, PT for a stable (dynamic) population of size N is

$$PT = N(\Delta t) \tag{7.10}$$

The *mortality density* (MD) *with disease* X for a given period (t_0, t) is estimated in a similar manner:

$$\hat{MD}_{(t_0,t)} = (D_x + D_{xy})/PT = \hat{MD}_{x(t_0,t)} + \hat{MD}_{xy(t_0,t)} \tag{7.11}$$

where PT is computed from Expression 7.9 or 7.10.

EXAMPLE 7.1

Consider the cohort of 12 subjects in Figure 6.1. The average mortality rates ($\hat{MD}_j$) for the five 1-year intervals are presented in Table 7.2. Also given in this table are the corresponding risk (R) estimates for each interval (t_{j-1}, t_j) and for an accumulated period (t_0, t_j), using both the actuarial and density methods. The only difference between estimating the risk of dying and estimating the risk of developing the disease (aside from the outcome event) is that the size of the candidate population for the former is the total population (N), while, for the latter, it is the number of disease-free subjects (N'). To see this difference, compare the number of person-years (PT$_j$) observed for each 1-year interval for the incidence data (Table 6.2) with the corresponding values for the mortality data (Table 7.2).

**Table 7.2   Estimation of the Risk (R) of Dying with Disease X
for the Hypothetical Cohort of 12 Subjects (Figure 6.1), by 1-Year Interval
(t_{j-1}, t_j), Using the Actuarial Method (Expressions 6.5 and 6.6)
and the Density Method (Expressions 6.7 and 6.8)**

j	N_{0j}	PT_j	No. of Deaths, $(D_x + D_{xy})_j$	W_j	$\hat{MD}_j$	ACTUARIAL $\hat{R}_j$	$\hat{R}_{(t_0,t_j)}$	DENSITY $\hat{R}_j$	$\hat{R}_{(t_0,t_j)}$
1	12	11.5	0	1	.000	.000	.000	.000	.000
2	11	9.5	1	2	.105	.100	.100	.100	.100
3	8	5.5	1	4	.182	.167	.250	.166	.250
4	3	3.0	0	0	.000	.000	.250	.000	.250
5	3	2.0	0	2	.000	.000	.250	.000	.250
Total	—	31.5	2	9	.063	—	—	—	—

Note: $\hat{R}_j$ is the 1-year risk estimate for the jth interval (t_{j-1}, t_j). $\hat{R}_{(t_0,t_j)}$ is the Δ-year risk estimate for the accumulated period (t_0, t_j), where $\Delta = t_j - t_0$.

The *fatality density* (FD$_x$) *due to disease* X is estimated from Equation 7.8, where PT refers strictly to the follow-up experience of new cases.* Similarly, the *fatality density* (FD) *with disease* X is estimated from Expression 7.11. Returning to the hypothetical cohort in Figure 6.1, there are two case fatalities (subjects 6 and 9) observed for 6 person-years of follow-up; thus, $\hat{FD}$ is 2/6 = .33/year.

The *average death rate* or density (DD) due to all diseases for the period (t_0, t) is estimated in a manner similar to that for the disease-specific mortality rates. Thus, we have

$$\hat{DD}_{(t_0,t)} = (D_x + D_{xy} + D_y)/PT = D/PT \qquad (7.12)$$

where PT is computed from Equation 7.9 or 7.10.

EXAMPLE 7.2

The average 1-year death rates ($\hat{DD}_j$) for the hypothetical cohort of Figure 6.1 are given in Table 7.3; the table also gives their corresponding risk estimates, calculated from both the actuarial and the density method. Also provided in Table 7.3 are the Δ-year risk estimates, $\hat{R}_{(t_0,t_j)}$, for accumulated

---

*In practice, PT may be calculated for a combination of incident and prevalent cases.

EXAMPLE 7.2 (*continued*)

periods (t_0, t_j) of 1 to 5 years. As was true for incidence estimation, combining consecutive interval-specific risk estimates by using Expression 6.6 assumes there are no secular trends in the postexposure rates. (Note that the 12 subjects enter the study over a span of 3 years.)

Table 7.3 Estimation of the Risk (R) of Dying from Any Cause for the Hypothetical Cohort of 12 Subjects (Figure 6.1), by 1-Year Interval (t_{j-1}, t_j), Using the Actuarial Method (Expressions 6.5 and 6.6) and the Density Method (Expressions 6.7 and 6.8)

						ACTUARIAL		DENSITY	
j	N_{0j}	PT_j	*No. of Deaths, D_j*	W_j	$\hat{DD}_j$	$\hat{R}_j$	$\hat{R}_{(t0,tj)}$	$\hat{R}_j$	$\hat{R}_{(t0,tj)}$
1	12	11.5	0	1	.000	.000	.000	.000	.000
2	11	9.5	2	1	.211	.190	.190	.190	.190
3	8	5.5	2	3	.364	.308	.440	.305	.437
4	3	3.0	0	0	.000	.000	.440	.000	.437
5	3	2.0	0	2	.000	.000	.440	.000	.437
Total	—	31.5	4	7	—	—	—	—	—

Note: See the note in Table 7.2.

7.2.3 Mortality and Incidence

We begin our treatment of the steady-state relationships between mortality and incidence by considering death due to disease X in a stable population. Using the approach described in Section 7.1.3 for prevalence, we can show that the mortality rate (MD_x) due to disease X is

$$MD_x = \frac{ID(FD_x)}{ID + TD} = \frac{ID(FD_x)(\overline{T})}{ID(\overline{T}) + 1} = FD_x(P) \tag{7.13}$$

where $TD = FD_x + FD_{xy} + RD_x = 1/\overline{T}$, and RD_x is the *recovery rate* for cases. If the disease is rare (i.e., $ID \ll TD$), Equation 7.13 reduces to the following approximation:

$$MD_x \approx ID(FD_x)(\overline{T}) = ID(LF_x) \tag{7.14}$$

where LF_x is the *cumulative lifetime fatality* due to disease X (i.e., the proportion of new cases who eventually die of the disease) and is equal to $D_x/I = D_x/TC = FD_x/TD = FD_x(\overline{T})$. Notice that for a highly fatal rare disease (i.e., FD_x is large)—and particularly for an acute disease (where

FD_{xy} is likely to be very low)—MD_x is approximately equal to the incidence rate (ID).

Next, we will consider death with disease X, which is more common in chronic disease epidemiology. Proceeding as before, we can show that the steady-state relationship between the mortality rate (MD) with disease X and the incidence rate (ID) is

$$MD = \frac{ID(FD)}{ID + TD} = \frac{ID(FD)(\overline{T})}{ID(\overline{T}) + 1} = FD(P) \qquad (7.15)$$

Assuming the disease is irreversible (i.e., there is no recovery from the disease, so that $FD = FD_x + FD_{xy} = TD$), which is true for most chronic diseases, Expression 7.15 reduces to

$$MD = ID/[ID(\overline{T}) + 1] = P/\overline{T} \qquad (7.16)$$

Thus, we see that MD varies indirectly with $\overline{T}$. If, in addition to assuming that the disease is irreversible, we assume that the disease is rare (i.e., $ID \ll TD$), the steady-state mortality rate (MD) is approximately equal to the incidence rate (ID). Thus, for most chronic diseases, any change in the fatality rate (FD) will have little or no effect on the steady-state mortality rate. Suppose, for example, that a new miraculous treatment suddenly extends the average survival of pancreatic cancer patients from less than 1 year to 20 years. Although the average fatality rate will decrease substantially, there will be very little change in the mortality rate, when we compare steady-state conditions before and after the treatment is introduced. However, during the transition period, the mortality rate will decline temporarily as the new treatment begins to postpone death for early cases.

An implicit assumption of the steady-state relationship of Equation 7.15 is that the mortality rate for all other diseases (MD_y) remains fixed. This assumption is necessary because a change in MD_y would have a direct effect on FD_{xy}, which, in turn, would alter TD. Consequently, for a fixed value of ID, an increase in MD_y will result in a decrease in prevalence (see Expression 7.4) and an increase in the cause-specific mortality rate (see Expression 7.15) (Zeighami et al., 1979). So, for example, if the incidence rate for a disease is identical for men and women, the prevalence will be slightly greater for women, and the mortality rate will be greater for men (because MD_y is greater for men).

Although it might seem that the average all-causes death rate (DD) cannot be expressed as a function of an index disease X, there is such a relationship under steady-state conditions (Zeighami et al., 1979) if we consider an index disease that is relatively rare. First, we must introduce a new parameter, *lifetime risk* (LR), which is the probability of developing the disease in one's lifetime. Letting N_0 be the fixed number of persons born during the period (t_0, t) within a stable population of size N, we may express LR as I/N_0. Using standard demographic life table methods (e.g., see Mausner and Bahn, 1974), we can express the life expectancy at birth ($\overset{\circ}{e}$) for the cohort as PT/N_0, where PT is the total number of person-years experienced by the birth cohort and is equal to the total number of person-years experienced by the stable population during the period (t_0, t). Thus, the ratio of LR to $\overset{\circ}{e}$ is I/PT, which is approximately equal to ID for a rare disease. Since DD is equal to the reciprocal of $\overset{\circ}{e}$ (Lindgren, 1976), we may express DD with the following approximation:

$$DD \approx ID/LR \tag{7.17}$$

If the disease is irreversible (i.e., FD = TD), then the number of new cases (I) occurring during the period will equal the number of deaths $(D_x + D_{xy})$ with the disease. Therefore, the death rate (DD) can be expressed as a function of the mortality rate (MD), under steady-state conditions:

$$DD = MD/LR \tag{7.18}$$

Notice that Equation 7.18 does not assume that the disease is rare.

In this chapter, we have presented the basic theoretical measures used for quantifying disease occurrence in a population, alternative methods for estimating these parameters, and functional relationships among certain theoretical measures under steady-state conditions. We emphasize that these latter relationships, summarized in Table 7.4, assume a very special

Table 7.4 Steady-State Relationships Between Selected Frequency Measures and Incidence, by Frequency Measure and Type of Disease

Frequency Measure	General Formulation	TYPE OF DISEASE		
		Irreversible	*Rare*	*Irreversible and Rare*
Point prevalence (P)	$\dfrac{\text{ID}(\bar{T})}{\text{ID}(\bar{T}) + 1}$	$\dfrac{\text{ID}}{\text{ID} + \text{FD}}$	$\text{ID}(\bar{T})$	$\dfrac{\text{ID}}{\text{FD}} = \text{ID}(\bar{T})$
Period prevalence (PP)	$\dfrac{C_0 + I}{N}$	$\dfrac{C_0 + I}{N}$	$P + \text{ID}(\Delta t)$	$P + \text{ID}(\Delta t)$
Mortality rate due to the disease (MD_x)	$\dfrac{\text{ID}(\bar{T})(\text{FD}_x)}{\text{ID}(\bar{T}) + 1}$	$\dfrac{\text{ID}(\text{FD}_x)}{\text{ID} + \text{FD}}$	$\text{ID}(\bar{T})(\text{FD}_x)$	$\dfrac{\text{ID}(\text{FD}_x)}{\text{FD}}$
Mortality rate with the disease (MD)	$\dfrac{\text{ID}(\bar{T})(\text{FD})}{\text{ID}(\bar{T}) + 1}$	$\dfrac{\text{ID}}{\text{ID}(\bar{T}) + 1}$	$\text{ID}(\bar{T})(\text{FD})$	ID
All-causes death rate (DD)	—	$\dfrac{\text{MD}}{\text{LR}}$	$\dfrac{\text{ID}}{\text{LR}}$	$\dfrac{\text{MD}}{\text{LR}} \approx \dfrac{\text{ID}}{\text{LR}}$

Note: ID = average incidence rate; $\bar{T}$ = average duration of the disease; FD_x = average fatality rate due to the disease; FD = average fatality rate with the disease; LR = lifetime risk of developing the disease; I = number of new cases occurring during a period (t_0, t) of duration Δt; C_0 = number of prevalent cases at t_0; N = size of the stable population. A rare disease for all measures (except PP) indicates that the ID is small, so that ID $\ll$ TD (termination rate). For PP, a rare disease indicates that P is small, so that the ID is approximately equal to $I/N(\Delta t)$. If the disease is irreversible (i.e., there is no recovery), then FD = TD = $1/\bar{T}$.

set of equilibrium conditions that often do not exist for more than 5 or 10 years, and they do not apply to frequency measures within narrow age categories or to weighted averages of age-specific frequency measures (see Chapter 17). Therefore, Equations 7.4, 7.7, 7.13, 7.15, 7.17, and 7.18 are not often appropriate for *estimating* one measure of disease occurrence, given available estimates of the other parameters. They are presented here to enhance your understanding of the functional relationships among various measures of disease frequency.

Figure 7.1 conveys a more comprehensive impression of these functional relationships without quantitative specification. This diagram suggests that the values of all frequency measures derive, ultimately, from the distributions of three broad categories of health determinants: *risk factors*—i.e., attributes of the environment or individuals that affect the development of disease; *prognostic factors*—i.e., attributes of the environment or individuals that affect the outcome of disease*; and *medical care*—i.e., therapeutic or preventive maneuvers that also influence the disease process. As we suggested in Chapter 2, the *estimation* of frequency measures

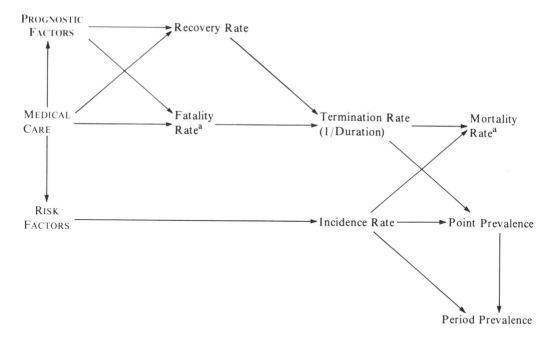

[a]Refers to death *with* disease X (i.e., due to X or other immediate causes).

Figure 7.1 Functional Relationships Among Frequency Measures

---

*It is possible, of course, for the same factor to act as both a risk factor and a prognostic factor for the same disease.

also depends on those *detection factors* (not included in Figure 7.1) that affect our observation of disease occurrence, such as incomplete case detection, changes in disease nomenclature, shifts in diagnostic custom, and
sampling errors.

**7.3
AGE,
PERIOD, AND
COHORT
EFFECTS**

Health researchers and planners frequently wish to assess the change in disease frequency over time in order to generate or test etiologic hypotheses,
to evaluate population interventions, and to predict the need for health
care. An approach for analyzing longitudinal data to achieve these objectives is called *cohort analysis*, which is a general methodological strategy
that was developed primarily by social scientists and demographers. Cohort analysis involves the (retrospective) collection of data from at least
three surveys or observation periods for a single dynamic population. The
approach may involve incidence, prevalence, or mortality data, and the
entire study period is usually spaced over a span of 20 or more years. For
example, using vital statistics and census information between 1940 and
1970, we could estimate the age-specific mortality rates for lung cancer
among male residents of New York State every 10 years—i.e., four 1-year
observation periods: 1940, 1950, 1960, and 1970. Methodologically, the
major objective of cohort analysis is the empirical separation of three time-
related effects that could provide alternative explanations for the observations; these are age, period, and (birth) cohort effects (Glenn, 1977; Blanchard, 1977). To describe and illustrate such patterns, we present data
from hypothetical cohort analyses, graphically, in Figure 7.2, displaying
the rate of disease as a function of age, by birth cohort (i.e., years of birth).

An *age effect* is present when the disease rate varies by age, regardless
of birth cohort (see Figures 7.2a, d, e). In Figure 7.2, an age effect is indicated by birth cohort (C) "curves" with either positive or negative slopes
that are independent of the period (i.e., calendar time). In fact, most diseases exhibit this characteristic, presumably because human aging reflects
a combination of biological, social, and psychological changes that influence general susceptibility to disease (Haynes and Feinleib, 1980).

A *period effect* is present when the disease rate varies by period (i.e.,
calendar time), regardless of age or birth cohort (see Figures 7.2b, d, f).
In other words, the change in disease rate uniformly affects all age groups
and birth cohorts, such that the cohort (C) "curves" in Figure 7.2 change
slope in the same period (around 1950), in the same direction, and in approximately the same amount. Note that the change in rates for birth cohorts in Figure 7.2b is temporary, returning to the same baseline level after
about five years, while the rate increases for birth cohorts in Figures 7.2d
and f do not reverse. As an illustration of a temporary period effect, consider the early part of U.S. Prohibition (1920–1933) when the average rate
of alcohol consumption decreased temporarily throughout the country. As
a result, mortality from liver cirrhosis also declined for all adult age groups

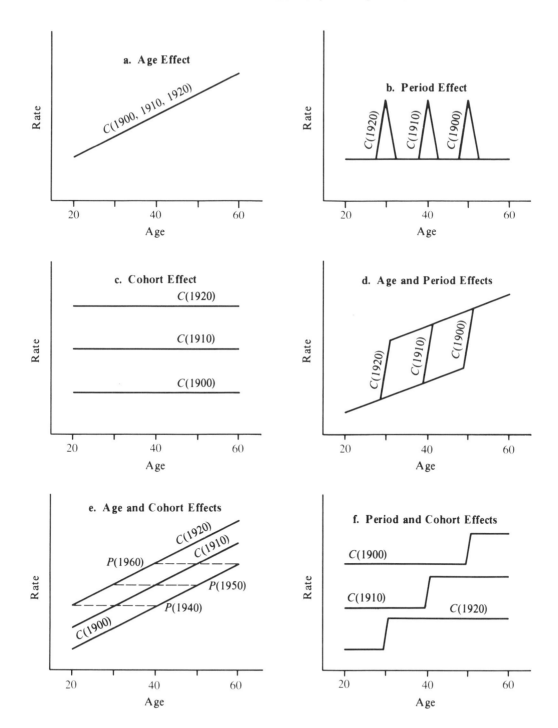

Figure 7.2 Age, Period (*P*), **and Birth Cohort** (*C*) **Effects, 1920–1980**

during the early 1920s, but it rose again during the 1930s and 1940s when alcohol consumption also increased (Terris, 1967).

A *cohort effect* is present when the disease rate varies by year of birth, regardless of age (see Figures 7.2c, e, f). That is, persons born in certain years carry with them throughout their lives a relatively higher (or lower) rate of disease, such that the cohort (C) "curves" in Figure 7.2 are separated vertically. For example, the prevalence of deafness in New South Wales, Australia, was particularly high for 10–14-year-olds in 1911, for 20–24-year-olds in 1921, and for 30–34-year-olds in 1933 (Lancaster, 1951). The most tenable explanation for these observations is the 1899 rubella epidemic in New South Wales, which resulted in congenital deafness among a large proportion of births because of maternal exposure during early pregnancy.

Another long-term pattern of disease occurrence is a *secular trend,* which is characterized by a systematic change in the age-specific rates over (calendar) time. For any single age group, a secular trend may be due to a period effect, a cohort effect, or some combination of the two (see Figures 7.2b, c, f). As we suggested above, the ability to explain age-specific changes in disease rates rests largely on the simultaneous (cohort) analysis of such trends for several age groups. We would then be able to derive the birth cohort "curves," such as those diagramed in Figure 7.2. Unfortunately, from a purely statistical perspective, there is always an inherent limitation of any cohort analysis: each set of data has at least two etiologic explanations (Glenn, 1977; Blanchard et al., 1977; Mason et al., 1973). This limitation—or "identification problem," as it is often called—is due to the linear dependency of each time-related variable on the other two. Thus, for example, if we know that a person is 70 years old in 1980, then we also know that the person was born in 1910.

The net result of the identification problem is that any attempt to separate the three effects empirically depends on a priori knowledge. As a hypothetical example, consider Figure 7.2e, which was used to illustrate the combination of age and cohort effects. An alternative explanation (in theory) is that there was a pure period effect (refer to the dotted "curves" in Figure 7.2e). That is, the variation in disease rate may have been due to a gradual increase in the prevalence of certain risk factors, affecting all age groups and birth cohorts equally. Of course, the latter explanation would not be very compelling in most epidemiologic settings, because we would have to assume no age effect. Nevertheless, the identification problem cannot be solved by statistical analysis alone. Interpretation of results depends on discovering one etiologic explanation that appears more convincing than all other conceivable explanations. This inferential ability is sometimes made possible when the duration of the suspect exposure is very *short* (e.g., the rubella epidemic in New South Wales) or when there is a gradual *reversal* in the overall exposure level (e.g., the change in alcohol consumption between 1920 and 1940 in the United States). In addition, more sophisticated statistical approaches have recently been developed for performing cohort analysis. For example, Kupper and Janis (1980) and Janis (1981) have developed a new methodology that combines descriptive and statistical modeling components for isolating adjusted age, period, and cohort effects.

In general, when observing one age group, one period, or one birth cohort, the other two effects can get mixed (i.e., confounded*) in the data. Thus, for example, the major concern in the interpretation of (age-specific) secular trends is the possible mixing of period and cohort effects, as we discussed above. Analogously, the concern with data from one period is the possible mixing of age and cohort effects.

EXAMPLE 7.3

As an illustration of the possible mixing of age and cohort effects, consider the relationship between age and lung cancer mortality among U.S. white males in the period 1949–1950 (Dorn and Cutler, 1959). As shown by the dotted curve at the top of Figure 7.3, the mortality rate appears to increase with age before 65 and to decrease after 70. This finding would seem to suggest either a reduced exposure to carcinogens late in life or enhanced resistance to the disease after age 70. However, combining data from several periods reveals a different picture. The solid curves in Figure 7.3 display the mortality rates by age for different birth cohorts, spanning the years from 1850 to 1890. We observe an increasing rate with age for every birth cohort, suggesting no decline in mortality late in life. Also, the more recent birth cohorts experience higher mortality rates at each age, an effect that possibly is related to marked increases in cigarette smoking before 1950 in the United States. Of course, this interpretation of a temporal relationship between smoking and lung cancer mortality depends on the validity of other information relating cigarette smoking to this disease.

In Section 6.4, we described two methods of risk estimation for any age span of duration Δ for data from one observation period (t_0, t) of duration Δt. Since the average disease rate (ID) generally varies with age and since we often want Δ to be greater than Δt, we must combine risk estimates from consecutive age intervals (t_{j-1}, t_j), using Expression 6.6 or 6.8. However, the validity of these risk estimates depends on the assumption of no age-specific secular trends or, equivalently, no period and/or cohort effects. That is, we must assume that the observed age effect did not get mixed with possible period or cohort effects.

---

*The general concept of confounding will be discussed in Chapter 13.

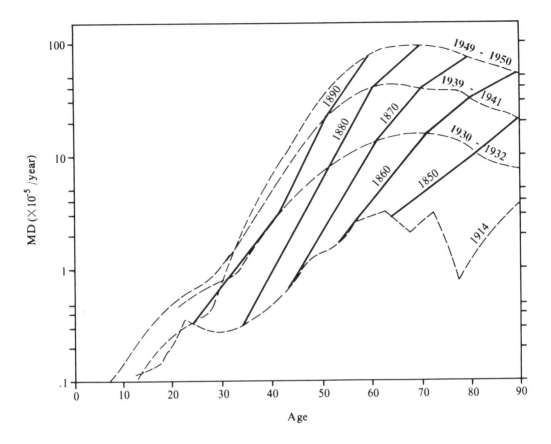

Source: Dorn and Cutler (1959).

**Figure 7.3 Lung Cancer Mortality Rates (MD) for U.S. White Males,
by Birth Cohort (Solid Lines) and Current Age (Dotted Lines),
1914–1950**

**7.4
CON-
CLUDING
REMARKS**

We have seen that there are three basic types of measures for describing the frequency of disease in a population: incidence, prevalence, and mortality. As we suggested in Chapter 6, incidence measures (dealing with new case occurrences) are preferred for making causal inferences about disease etiology.

In this chapter, we have shown how to estimate point prevalence (dealing with existing cases at a point in time), period prevalence (dealing with existing cases during a period), and three types of mortality rates or risks: disease-specific mortality, case fatality, and death from all causes. We have emphasized that prevalence and disease-specific mortality measures depend on incidence. For steady-state conditions in which the age composition of the population and all frequency measures remain constant over time, we may express, mathematically, the functional relationships between specific (crude) prevalence and mortality measures and the crude incidence rate (see Table 7.4).

For non-steady-state conditions involving observed changes in frequency measures over a long period (say 20 years or more), we have briefly described a general methodological approach (cohort analysis) for examining age, period, and birth cohort effects. Although these three effects provide alternative explanations for longitudinal data, there is a basic identification problem in making a particular inference, because of the linear dependency of each time-related variable on the other two.

The following list summarizes the key notation introduced in this chapter. **NOTATION**

N	Size of total (stable) population.
C_t	Number of persons with disease at time t—i.e., prevalent cases.
C	Number of persons with disease in a stable population—i.e., C remains constant over time.
$C_{(t_0,t)} = C_0 + I$	Number of persons observed to have had disease anytime during follow-up period (t_0, t).
C_0	Number of persons with disease at start (time t_0) of follow-up period (t_0, t).
TC	Number of terminated cases during period (t_0, t)—i.e., persons who die with disease X (disease of interest) and cases who recover.
D_x	Number of deaths due to disease X during period (t_0, t)—i.e., X is the immediate cause of death.
D_{xy}	Number of deaths due to other causes (Y) among cases of disease X during period (t_0, t) —i.e., X is the underlying or contributing cause of death (but not the immediate cause).
D_y	Number of deaths due to other causes (Y) among persons who do not have disease X during period (t_0, t).
D	Total number of deaths during period $(t_0, t) = D_x + D_{xy} + D_y$.
$\hat{P}_t = C_t/N_t$	Point prevalence of disease in population at time t.

$\hat{PP}_{(t_0,t)} = C_{(t_0,t)}/N$	Period prevalence of disease for period (t_0, t).
$\hat{P} = C/N$	Prevalence of disease, assumed constant over time—i.e., under steady-state conditions.
P_j	Prevalence of disease (at time t) for persons in jth age interval (or at start of jth age interval).
TD	Termination density (or average termination rate) among persons with disease—i.e., due to death or recovery.
$\bar{T}$	Mean duration of disease from first occurrence (or detection) to termination.
$MD_{x(t_0,t)}$	Mortality density (or average mortality rate) due to disease X during period (t_0, t).
$MD_{xy(t_0,t)}$	Mortality density due to other diseases (Y) among cases of disease X during period (t_0, t).
$MD_{y(t_0,t)}$	Mortality density due to other diseases (Y) among persons who do not have disease X.
$MD_{(t_0,t)}$	Mortality density with disease X during period (t_0, t) = $MD_{x(t_0,t)} + MD_{xy(t_0,t)}$.
MD_j	Mortality density for jth age interval.
FD_x	Case fatality density (or average fatality rate) due to disease X.
FD_{xy}	Fatality density due to other diseases (Y) among cases of disease X.
FD	Fatality density with disease X = $FD_x + FD_{xy}$.
RD_x	Recovery density (or average recovery rate) among cases of disease X.
LF_x	Cumulative lifetime case fatality due to disease X.
DD	Death density (or average death rate) due to all diseases = $MD_x + MD_{xy} + MD_y$.
LR	Lifetime risk of developing disease.

PRACTICE EXERCISES

7.1 Indicate whether each of the following computed indices is an incidence density, a cumulative incidence, a point prevalence, a period prevalence, or an odds for the disease of interest.

  a. The number of adult men in Delaware identified with psychiatric problems during 1980, divided by the total number of adult men in Delaware in 1980.

  b. The number of sudden infant deaths in Delaware in 1980, divided by the number of live births in Delaware in 1980.

c. The number of children born with congenital heart defects in Delaware in 1980, divided by the number of live births in Delaware in 1980.

d. The number of persons who resided in Delaware on January 1, 1980, and who developed colon cancer during 1980, divided by the total number of disease-free persons who were Delaware residents on January 1, 1980.

e. The number of myopic children under the age of 13 in Delaware on July 1, 1980, divided by the total number of children under the age of 13 in Delaware on July 1, 1980.

f. The number of legally deaf males in Delaware in 1980, divided by the number of males who were not legally deaf in Delaware in 1980.

g. The number of 60–64-year-old Delaware residents who had a stroke in 1980, divided by the total number of 60–64-year-old Delaware residents on July 1, 1980.

7.2 Between 1970 and 1980, the prevalence of a given exposure was substantially reduced in a particular stable population. During the same period, there was no change in the prevalence of disease X, and there was a decline in the disease-specific mortality rate (i.e., comparing the steady-state measures in 1970 and 1980). Assuming no changes in diagnostic custom and no recovery from the disease, we would most likely conclude that the exposure is which of the following?

a. a positive (i.e., causal) risk factor for the disease and a prognostic factor
b. a positive risk factor but not a prognostic factor
c. a negative (i.e., protective) risk factor and a prognostic factor
d. a negative risk factor but not a prognostic factor
e. not a risk factor but a prognostic factor

7.3 Exercise Table 7.1 lists the relative frequency of a disease by age and year in a particular population. Which one of the following measures is most likely described by the data?

Exercise Table 7.1

Age	1940	1950	1960	1970
		YEAR		
40–49	60	50	40	30
50–59	50	60	50	40
60–69	40	50	60	50
70–79	30	40	50	60

a. the incidence rate of a common viral infection
b. the prevalence of chronic ischemic heart disease
c. the prevalence of a nonfatal congenital defect

    d. the mortality rate of a highly fatal cancer

    e. the mortality rate of motor vehicle–related injuries

REFERENCES   BEALL, G., and COBB, S. 1961. The frequency distribution of episodes of rheumatoid arthritis as shown by periodic examination. *J. Chronic Dis.* 14: 291–310.

BLANCHARD, R. D.; BUNKER, J. B.; and WACHS, M. 1977. Distinguishing aging, period and cohort effects in longitudinal studies of elderly populations. *Sociol.-Econ. Planning Sci.* 11: 137–146.

COBB, S. 1962. A method for the epidemiologic study of remittent disease. *Am. J. Public Health* 52: 1119–1125.

DORN, H. F., and CUTLER, S. J. 1959. *Morbidity from cancer in the United States.* Public Health Monograph No. 56. Washington, D.C.: Government Printing Office.

FREEMAN, J., and HUTCHISON, G. B. 1980. Prevalence, incidence and duration. *Am. J. Epidemiol.* 112: 707–723.

GLENN, N. D. 1977. *Cohort analysis.* Quantitative Applications in the Social Sciences, Series No. 07-005. Beverly Hills, Calif.: Sage.

HAYNES, S. G., and FEINLEIB, M., eds. 1980. *Second conference on the epidemiology of aging.* NIH Publ. No. 80–969. Washington, D.C.: Government Printing Office.

JANIS, J. M. 1981. A descriptive and statistical age-period-cohort analysis of lung cancer mortality. Dr. P. H. dissertation, Department of Biostatistics, University of North Carolina at Chapel Hill.

KUPPER, L. L., and JANIS, J. M. 1980. The multiple classification model in age-period-cohort analysis: Theoretical considerations. University of North Carolina Institute of Statistics Mimeo Series No. 1311.

LANCASTER, H. O. 1951. Deafness as an epidemic disease in Australia. *Br. Med. J.* 2: 1429–1432.

LESKE, M. C.; EDERER, F.; PODGOR, M. 1981. Estimating incidence from age-specific prevalence in glaucoma. *Am. J. Epidemiol.* 113: 606–613.

LINDGREN, B. W. 1976. *Statistical theory.* 3rd ed. New York: Macmillan; p. 181.

MACMAHON, B., and PUGH, T. F. 1970. *Epidemiology: Principles and methods.* Boston: Little, Brown.

MASON, K. O.; WINSBOROUGH, H. H.; MASON, W. M.; and POOLE, W. K. 1973. Some methodological issues in cohort analysis of archival data. *Am. Sociol. Rev.* 38: 242–258.

MAUSNER, J. S., and BAHN, A. K. 1974. *Epidemiology: An introductory text.* Philadelphia: Saunders; App. 9.1, pp. 206–212.

MIETTINEN, O. S. 1976. Estimability and estimation in case-referent studies. *Am. J. Epidemiol.* 103(2): 226–235.

MORRISON, A. S. 1979. Sequential pathogenic components of rates. *Am. J. Epidemiol.* 109: 709–718.

TERRIS, M. 1967. Epidemiology of cirrhosis of the liver: National mortality data. *Am. J. Public Health* 57: 2076–2088.

VISSCHER, B.; MALMGREN, R.; DUDLEY, J.; VALDIVIEZO, N.; CLARK, V.; and DETELS, R. 1980. Completed course of disease: A possible substitute for long term follow-up. Paper presented at the Thirteenth Annual Meeting of the Society of Epidemiologic Research, June 18–20, in Minneapolis, Minnesota.

VON KOTFF, M. V., and PARKER, R. D. 1980. The dynamics of the prevalence of chronic episodic disease. *J. Chronic Dis.* 33: 79–85.

ZEIGHAMI, E.; SOHLER, K. B.; and DEAL, R. B. 1979. Estimators of relative disease risk—A life table simulation. *J. Chronic Dis.* 32: 589–598.

8

Measures of Association

In this chapter, we focus on another class of quantitative measures that are used to investigate the etiology, treatment, and prevention of disease. Measures of association reflect the strength of the statistical relationship between a study factor and a disease; thus, they are most instrumental for making causal inferences.

In principle, *measures of association* involve a direct comparison of frequency measures for different values or categories of the study factor. As we did in previous chapters, we will concentrate on study factors that are analyzed as categorical variables. This categorization divides the study population into two or more groups, each of which can be compared to a single category designated as the *reference group*. Although selection of a reference category is somewhat arbitrary, its choice is quite important for interpreting results. Preferably, the reference group should be large enough to provide precise frequency estimates (i.e., not too much random error), and it should be relatively homogeneous so that comparisons are meaningful. If possible, the referent should also correspond to the "natural" category or value of comparison, which typically would be the lowest risk group. For example, we might choose nonsmokers, nulliparous women, and nonusers of a health care facility as reference groups for studies involving smoking, parity, and utilization. For continuous variables, we might assign, arbitrarily, a range of values as the referent, such as all subjects who consume less than one alcoholic drink per week. Similarly, for nominal variables with many values, we may find it useful to combine categories. But we should avoid comparing each group to the total population, unless there are so many groups that each is only a very small fraction of the total.

The general data layouts or tabular notations for studies involving population-time (PT) of follow-up experience are given in Table 8.1. Table 8.1a refers to the general case of $(k + 1)$ exposure categories, and Table 8.1b refers to the special case of a dichotomous study factor. The data layouts for other types of study designs are shown in Table 8.2. While

Table 8.1   Data Layouts for Studies Involving Population-Time

a. $k + 1$ Exposure Categories

	EXPOSURE CATEGORY ($i = 0, \ldots, k$)				
	E_k	$\cdots$	E_1	E_0	Total
No. of New Cases	a_k	$\cdots$	a_1	a_0	m_1
Population-Time	L_k	$\cdots$	L_1	L_0	L

Table 8.1 (*continued*)

b. Two Exposure Categories

	No. of Exposed	No. of Unexposed	Total
No. of New Cases	*a*	*b*	m_1
Population-Time	L_1	L_0	L

Note: The reference group consists of all unexposed subjects—i.e., $i = 0$.

many statistical measures of association are available for analyzing simple contingency tables (e.g., see Hamilton, 1979), most of them can be divided into two types, ratio and difference measures; each will be discussed in the following sections.

Table 8.2   Data Layouts for Studies Involving Case-Noncase Status

a. $k + 1$ Exposure Categories

Disease Status	EXPOSURE CATEGORY ($i = 0, \ldots, k$)				
	E_k	$\cdots$	E_1	E_0	Total
No. of cases	a_k	$\cdots$	a_1	a_0	m_1
No. of noncases	c_k	$\cdots$	c_1	c_0	m_0
Total	n_k	$\cdots$	n_1	n_0	n

b.   Two Exposure Categories

Disease Status	No. of Exposed	No. of Unexposed	Total
No. of cases	*a*	*b*	m_1
No. of noncases	*c*	*d*	m_0
Total	n_1	n_0	n

Note: The reference group consists of all unexposed subjects—i.e., $i = 0$.

A *ratio measure of association* (or effect) is a frequency measure for one (the ith) exposed group (E_i) divided by a comparable frequency measure for an unexposed or reference group ($i = 0$). We will consider various classes of ratio measures, the category depending on the type of frequency measure being studied.

A ratio comparison of two average rates is called an *incidence density ratio* (IDR) or rate ratio (Miettinen, 1975, 1976) and is estimated as follows:

$$\hat{IDR}_i = \frac{\hat{ID}_i}{\hat{ID}_0} = \frac{a_i/L_i}{a_0/L_0} \tag{8.1}$$

where $\hat{ID}_i$ is the estimated rate for the ith exposure group (see Table 8.1a) and $\hat{IDR}_i$ is the estimated incidence density ratio comparing the ith exposure category with the reference group ($i = 0$). Theoretically, the IDR can range from zero, indicating a strong negative association, to infinity, indicating a strong positive association. Under the null hypothesis of no association between the exposure and the disease (i.e., no effect), the value of IDR is one,* which we call the *null value*.

EXAMPLE 8.1

Consider the data in Table 8.3 (described in Chapter 6; see Table 6.3, p. 100). The estimated crude IDR, ignoring age, for all subjects is .0179/ .0069 = 2.60, a result suggesting a positive effect. That is, the rate for exposed subjects is 2.6 times the rate for unexposed subjects. Applying the same technique to each age category, we find the estimated IDR_i to be 2.00 in every stratum. This discrepancy occurs because the mean age of exposed subjects is greater than the mean age of unexposed subjects; since age is a (positive) risk factor for the disease (see Table 8.3), the crude exposure effect is distorted or confounded by age. Thus, the age-specific estimates of effect should be used to make a causal inference about the possible relationship between the exposure and the disease. More will be said about the issue of confounding in Chapters 13 and 14.

A ratio comparison of two risk estimates is called a *risk ratio* (RR) (Miettinen, 1975, 1976) or relative risk, which may be computed directly from the ratio of two cumulative incidence measures as follows:

$$\hat{RR}_i = \frac{\hat{R}_i}{\hat{R}_0} = \hat{CIR}_i = \frac{\hat{CI}_i}{\hat{CI}_0} = \frac{a_i/n_i}{a_0/n_0} \tag{8.2}$$

---

*The *estimated value* of the IDR may differ from one under the null hypothesis because of random and nonrandom estimation errors (see Chapter 10).

**Table 8.3   Estimation of Average Incidence Rates (ID) and Risks (R),
Using the Density Method (Equations 6.7 and 6.8), and Prevalences (P)
for the Data in Table 6.3, by Exposure Status and Age**

	EXPOSED				UNEXPOSED			
Age	$\hat{ID}_j$	$\hat{R}_j$	$\hat{R}_{(t_0,t_j)}$	$\hat{P}_j$	$\hat{ID}_j$	$\hat{R}_j$	$\hat{R}_{(t_0,t_j)}$	$\hat{P}_j$
40–49	.0010	.0100	.0100	.0050	.0005	.0050	.0050	.0025
50–59	.0050	.0488	.0583	.0244	.0025	.0247	.0296	.0123
60–69	.0200	.1813	.2290	.0909	.0100	.0952	.1219	.0476
70–79	.0500	.3935	.5324	.2000	.0250	.2212	.3162	.1111
Total	.0179	—	—	.0893	.0069	—	—	.0343

Note: $\hat{ID}_j$ is the estimated rate for the jth 10-year interval ($j = 1, \ldots, 4$), using Expressions 6.1 and 6.3. $\hat{R}_j$ is the 10-year risk estimate for the jth interval (t_{j-1}, t_j). $\hat{R}_{(t_0,t_j)}$ is the Δ-year risk estimate for the accumulated period (t_0, t_j), where $\Delta = t_j - t_0$.

where $\hat{R}_i$ is the risk estimate for the ith exposure category (see Table 8.2a) and $\hat{CIR}_i$ is the estimated *cumulative incidence ratio*, comparing the ith exposure category with the reference group ($i = 0$).

EXAMPLE 8.2

As a simple example involving a dichotomous study factor, consider the hypothetical data in Table 8.4. If we assume we have a fixed cohort design with little attrition over the follow-up period, $\hat{RR}$ is $(40/120)/(60/380) = 2.11$. Thus, we would infer that exposed subjects were more than twice as likely to develop the disease during the follow-up period as were unexposed subjects.

We can also estimate the Δ-year RR from average rates, using the actuarial or density method of risk estimation for each exposure category (see Chapter 6). For example, if we assume the hypothetical data in Table 8.3 were taken from a stable population, the 40-year $\hat{RR}$, comparing a 40-year-old exposed person with a 40-year-old unexposed person, is $.5324/.3162 = 1.68$, which is less than both the crude estimate of the IDR (2.60) and the age-specific estimates of the IDR (2.00). This time, however, the difference is not due to the confounding effect of age but to the inherent difference between the incidence rate and risk.

**Table 8.4   Number of Subjects, by Exposure Category
and Disease Status (Hypothetical Data)**

Disease Status	EXPOSURE CATEGORY		
	Exposed	Unexposed	Total
Cases	40	60	100
Noncases	80	320	400
Total	120	380	500

Given a fixed rate ratio over time, we can show that the theoretical limit of the RR, as Δ approaches zero, is the IDR (Miettinen, 1975; Morgenstern et al., 1980). That is,

$$\lim_{\Delta \to 0} RR_{(t_0, t)} = IDR \qquad (8.3)$$

where Δ is the age/time span of follow-up and is equal to $t - t_0$. Conversely, the limit of RR, as Δ becomes infinitely large, is one:

$$\lim_{\Delta \to \infty} RR_{(t_0, t)} = 1 \qquad (8.4)$$

In other words, if a cohort could be followed for an infinite period of time, the risk of disease would be one in all exposure groups, since no one could die of any other disease. (Recall that risk is a *conditional* probability.) Consequently, as Δ increases for any fixed ID_i, the value of the RR becomes closer to the null value (one).

In a case-control study involving incident cases, we cannot estimate exposure-specific rates or risks without additional information. However, we can estimate the *ratio* of these rates or risks from the available data (Cornfield, 1951; Miettinen, 1976). If the disease involves an extended risk period relative to the observation period (e.g., chronic diseases), the parameter of interest is the rate ratio. For a dichotomous exposure (i.e., $k = 1$), if we assume that the candidate population is stable, the exposed incidence rate is $I_1/[N_1'(\Delta t)]$, and the unexposed rate is $I_0/[N_0'(\Delta t)]$, where I_i is the number of new cases detected in the ith exposure category during the follow-up period of duration Δt, and N_i' is the size of the disease-free population for the ith exposure category. Thus, the IDR is $\hat{ID}_1/\hat{ID}_0$, which is equal to $(I_1/I_0)/(N_1'/N_0')$. The numerator of this expression gives the odds of being exposed among new cases and can be estimated from case-control data as a/b (see Table 8.2b). Similarly, the odds of being exposed among noncases (N_1'/N_0') can be estimated as c/d. Dividing the former by the latter, we get the quantity ad/bc, which is an estimate of the *exposure odds* *ratio* (EOR). Thus, if the noncases in a case-control study are representative of the stable candidate population from which the observed cases developed, the EÔR is equal to the IDR (Miettinen, 1976).*

EXAMPLE 8.3

Suppose that the data in Table 8.4 were taken from a case-control study. The estimated EOR is then $40(320)/[80(60)] = 2.67$. Thus, we would infer that the average incidence rate of the disease is 2.67 times as great in the exposed group as in the unexposed group.

If the disease in a case-control study involves a restricted risk period relative to the observation period (e.g., acute diseases), the risk ratio is usually the parameter of interest. In terms of conditional probabilities (pr), we may express RR as $pr(D|E)/pr(D|\overline{E})$, where $pr(D|E)$ is the probability of developing the disease conditional on being exposed and $pr(D|\overline{E})$ is the probability of developing the disease conditional on not being exposed. Using Bayes' theorem (Neutra and Drolette, 1978), we can express these two risks as follows:

$$pr(D|E) = \frac{pr(D)\,pr(E|D)}{pr(D)\,pr(E|D) + pr(\overline{D})\,pr(E|\overline{D})}$$

$$pr(D|\overline{E}) = \frac{pr(D)\,pr(\overline{E}|D)}{pr(D)\,pr(\overline{E}|D) + pr(\overline{D})\,pr(\overline{E}|\overline{D})}$$

where $pr(E|D)$ is the probability of a new case being exposed, etc. Thus,

$$RR = \frac{pr(E|D)}{pr(\overline{E}|D)}\left[\frac{pr(D)\,pr(\overline{E}|D) + pr(\overline{D})\,pr(\overline{E}|\overline{D})}{pr(D)\,pr(E|D) + pr(\overline{D})\,pr(E|\overline{D})}\right]$$

If the overall risk of the disease is low, so that $pr(D) \approx 0$, the above expression simplifies to

$$RR \approx \frac{pr(E|D)/pr(\overline{E}|D)}{pr(E|\overline{D})/pr(\overline{E}|\overline{D})}$$

Notice that the numerator of the simplified expression represents the odds of being exposed among new cases and the denominator represents the odds of being exposed among noncases. If we assume the noncases are representative of the candidate population from which the observed cases developed, the RR is approximately equal to the EOR. Thus, in a case-control study of a rare disease,[†] the RR is estimated by the quantity ad/bc.

---

*Note that it is not necessary to assume that the disease is rare.

[†]The approximation holds fairly well if $pr(D) < .10$.

We may conclude that, in any type of case-control study involving incident cases, the EOR (or simply the OR) is used to quantify the magnitude of the association between the exposure and the disease. However, the interpretation of the EOR depends on whether the disease has an extended or a restricted risk period. For chronic diseases (usually involving extended risk periods), the parameter of interest is the IDR. For acute diseases (usually involving restricted risk periods), the parameter of interest is the RR.

In a fixed cohort study, the EOR is equal (under Bayes' theorem) to the *risk odds ratio* (ROR). That is,

$$ \text{ROR} = \frac{R_1/(1 - R_1)}{R_0/(1 - R_0)} = \text{RR} \left(\frac{1 - R_0}{1 - R_1} \right) = \text{EOR} $$

where ROR (equal to EOR) is also estimated by the quantity ad/bc. Whenever the RR is not equal to one (the null value), the ROR is further from the null value than is the RR. For example, the estimated RR for the data in Table 8.4 is 2.11, and the estimated ROR is 2.67. Nevertheless, even with a chronic disease, the ROR obtained from a cumulative incidence study is not a valid estimate of the IDR. In fact, the ROR and the IDR are approximately equal only if the disease is rare enough so that the RR is approximately equal to the ROR.

8.1.2 Prevalence Comparisons

In cross-sectional studies, the *prevalence ratio* ($PR_i = P_i/P_0$) is estimated in a manner similar to the estimation of the CIR in cohort studies (see Expression 8.2), where $\hat{P}_i = a_i/n_i$ is the estimated prevalence for the ith exposure category (see Table 8.2) and n_i refers to the size of the total population in the ith group. So, for example, if the data in Table 8.4 were taken from a cross-sectional study, the PR would be estimated as 2.11. That is, exposed subjects are more than twice as likely to have the disease as are unexposed subjects.

In a cross-sectional study with an extended risk period or in a case-control study with prevalent cases and an extended risk period (e.g., most chronic diseases), the parameter of primary interest for making causal inferences is the IDR. Under steady-state conditions, we can express the average rate (ID_i) in the ith exposure category as $P_i/[\bar{T}_i(1 - P_i)]$, where $\bar{T}_i$ is the mean duration of the disease among cases in the ith group (see Equation 7.5). Substituting this expression for each exposure-specific rate, we get the following expression for the IDR, comparing two groups (i.e., $k = 1$):

$$ \text{IDR} = \frac{ID_1}{ID_0} = \frac{\bar{T}_0}{\bar{T}_1} \left[\frac{P_1/(1 - P_1)}{P_0/(1 - P_0)} \right] $$

or, equivalently,

$$ \text{POR} = \text{IDR} \left(\frac{\bar{T}_1}{\bar{T}_0} \right) \tag{8.5} $$

where POR is the *prevalence odds ratio* and is equal to the EOR, and the estimated POR is ad/bc (see Table 8.2b). If the mean duration of the disease is identical for exposed and unexposed cases (i.e., the exposure is not a prognostic factor) and if the disease does not affect exposure status, the POR estimated from either a cross-sectional or a case-control study is equal to the IDR (Miettinen, 1976; Morrison, 1979). As we pointed out in Chapter 7, however, the steady-state relationship between prevalence and incidence—and thus Expression 8.5—does not apply exactly within narrow age categories.

Using the same approach that we used above, we find that the PR is

$$PR = \frac{P_1}{P_0} = IDR\left(\frac{\overline{T}_1}{\overline{T}_0}\right)\left[\frac{ID_0(\overline{T}_0) + 1}{ID_1(\overline{T}_1) + 1}\right] \tag{8.6}$$

Thus, even if $\overline{T}_1 = \overline{T}_0 = \overline{T}$,

$$PR = IDR\left[\frac{ID_0(\overline{T}) + 1}{ID_1(\overline{T}) + 1}\right] < IDR \tag{8.7}$$

if IDR > 1. That is, if the exposure is not a prognostic factor and if the disease does not affect exposure status, the PR in a cross-sectional study will be closer to the null value (one) than will the IDR. Only if the incidence rate is much less than the termination rate (equal to $1/\overline{T}$) will the PR be approximately equal to the IDR. For example, the crude $\hat{PR}$ for the hypothetical data in Table 8.3 is $.0893/.0343 = 2.60$, which is equal to the crude $\hat{IDR}$. In practice, however, this approximation does not often hold, because rare diseases, especially highly fatal rare diseases, are not usually investigated with cross-sectional studies.

In a cross-sectional study involving a restricted risk period and in a case-control study involving prevalent cases and a restricted risk period (or in any of their corresponding hybrid derivatives), the parameter of etiologic interest is the RR.* For example, we might compare the prevalence of a certain (birth) defect for newborns who were exposed in utero with the corresponding prevalence for newborns who were not exposed. As suggested in Chapter 4, we cannot observe the total candidate population for either exposure group, since many pregnancies do not terminate in live births and therefore go unrecognized. However, if the outcome event is unrelated to the probability of a fetus's surviving, conditional on exposure status, and if the outcome event does not affect exposure status, then the PR among live births is equal to the RR among all pregnancies.[†] In the more probable situation where "defective" fetuses are less likely to survive

---

*Of course, in both types of prevalence studies, subjects are not observed for their (restricted) risk periods. Rather, survivors are observed at the end of their risk periods (e.g., the investigation of birth outcome following intrauterine exposure).

[†]Although this condition is sufficient for having the PR equal the RR, it is not a necessary condition. Refer to Chapter 11 for a more thorough discussion of this topic.

than "nondefective" fetuses, the PR may be greater or less than the RR, depending on how exposure status affects survival (see Chapter 11). If, on the other hand, we select a case-control design to study the etiology of birth defects, the POR will be further from the null value than will the PR, and, thus, the estimated POR may also differ from the desired RR. However, when the overall prevalence is very small (so that POR $\approx$ PR), when the outcome event is conditionally unrelated to survival, and when the outcome event does not affect exposure status, then the estimated POR in a case-control study serves as an approximation to the RR.

Ratio measures of association involving mortality data are estimated in a manner similar to that for incidence comparisons, both for rates (Equation 8.1) and for risks (Equation 8.2). The only such measure that we will deal with in this section is the *mortality density ratio* (MDR), referring to death *with* the disease in the total population. Using the notation of Table 8.1a, we have

8.1.3 Mortality Comparisons

$$\hat{\text{MDR}}_i = \frac{\hat{\text{MD}}_i}{\hat{\text{MD}}_0} = \frac{a_i/L_i}{a_0/L_0} \tag{8.8}$$

where $\hat{\text{MD}}_i$ is the estimated mortality rate for the ith exposure category. As we noted in Chapter 7, the computation of L_i differs for mortality and incidence.

To derive the steady-state relationship between the MDR and the IDR, we will use the same procedure that we used in the previous section for the PR. Taking the ratio of two steady-state expressions for the exposure-specific MDs (see Expression 7.15) and simplifying, we get the following general expression for the MDR, comparing exposed with unexposed subjects:

$$\text{MDR} = \text{IDR(FDR)}\left(\frac{\overline{T}_1}{\overline{T}_0}\right)\left[\frac{\text{ID}_0(\overline{T}_0) + 1}{\text{ID}_1(\overline{T}_1) + 1}\right] \tag{8.9}$$

where FDR $= \text{FD}_1/\text{FD}_0$ is the *fatality density ratio* among cases. If the disease is irreversible (i.e., $\text{FD}_i = \text{TD}_i$), and if the exposure is not a prognostic factor (i.e., $\overline{T}_1 = \overline{T}_0 = \overline{T}$), Expression 8.9 simplifies to

$$\text{MDR} = \text{IDR}\left[\frac{\text{ID}_0(\overline{T}) + 1}{\text{ID}_1(\overline{T}) + 1}\right] < \text{IDR} \tag{8.10}$$

if IDR > 1. Thus, for most chronic disease risk factors that are not prognostic factors, the MDR will be closer to the null value than will the IDR (Morrison, 1979). It also follows from Equations 8.9 and 8.10 that the MDR is approximately equal to the IDR (the parameter of etiologic interest) under steady-state conditions if the exposure is not a prognostic factor, if the disease is irreversible and does not affect exposure status (before selection), and if the disease is rare and/or highly fatal (so that ID $\ll$ TD).

**8.2
DIFFERENCE
MEASURES**

A *difference measure of association* (or effect) is calculated by subtracting the frequency estimate for the reference group from the comparable estimate for the *i*th exposure group. We will briefly consider three classes of difference measures, the classification depending on the type of frequency measure being studied. Unlike ratio measures of association, difference measures cannot be estimated from case-control data without additional information.

**8.2.1
Incidence
Comparisons**

The *incidence density difference* (IDD) or average rate difference for the *i*th exposure category is estimated as follows:

$$\hat{\text{IDD}}_i = \hat{\text{ID}}_i - \hat{\text{ID}}_0 = (a_i/L_i) - (a_0/L_0) \qquad (8.11)$$

(see Table 8.1a). The null value of the IDD is zero, and the theoretical limits are negative infinity, indicating a strong negative association, and positive infinity, indicating a strong positive association. Thus, a value of zero for the IDD corresponds to a value of one for the IDR. Using the data in Table 8.3, we find the crude $\hat{\text{IDD}}$ to be .0179 − .0069 = .011/year. While IDR remains constant (equal to 2) over age, the age-specific $\hat{\text{IDD}}$ increases from .0005/year for the youngest group to .0250/year for the oldest group.

Since $\text{ID}_i = \text{IDR}_i(\text{ID}_0)$, we can express the average rate difference as a function of the average rate ratio:

$$\text{IDD}_i = \text{ID}_0(\text{IDR}_i - 1) \qquad (8.12)$$

For example, for the data in Table 8.3, $\hat{\text{IDD}}$ is .0069(2.60 − 1) = .011/year, as shown above.

The *risk difference* (RD)—also called the "attributable risk" or the "excess risk" (MacMahon and Pugh, 1970)—can be estimated directly from the *cumulative incidence difference* (CID):

$$\hat{\text{RD}}_i = \hat{R}_i - \hat{R}_0 = \hat{\text{CID}}_i = (a_i/n_i) - (a_0/n_0) \qquad (8.13)$$

(see Table 8.2a). For example, if we treat the hypothetical data in Table 8.4 as the results of a fixed cohort study, $\hat{\text{RD}}$ = (40/120) − (60/380) = .175, or 17.5%.

EXAMPLE 8.4

We may also estimate the Δ-year RD by applying either the actuarial or the density method described in Chapter 6 to each exposure category and computing the difference. Using the density method, for example, we find the 40-year $\hat{\text{RD}}$ for a 40-year-old person in Table 8.3 to be .5324 − .3162 = .216. Thus, a 40-year-old exposed person without the disease is 21.6%

EXAMPLE 8.4 (*continued*)

more likely to develop the disease before age 80 than is a 40-year-old unexposed person, conditional on the person's not dying from any other
cause during that period.

Since $R_i = \text{RR}_i(R_0)$, we can express the RD as a function of the RR:

$$\text{RD}_i = R_0(\text{RR}_i - 1) \tag{8.14}$$

which is analogous to the relationship between rate measures (Equation
8.12).

The *prevalence difference* (PD) for the ith exposure category is estimated
as follows:

$$\hat{\text{PD}}_i = \hat{P}_i - \hat{P}_0 = (a_i/n_i) - (a_0/n_0) \tag{8.15}$$

8.2.2
Prevalence
Comparisons

(see Table 8.2a). For the data in Table 8.3, the crude PD is .0893 −
.0343 = .055. Thus, exposed women between the ages of 40 and 79 are
5.5% more likely to have the disease at the start of follow-up than are unexposed women in the same age group.

Like risk measures, the PD can be expressed as a function of the PR:

$$\text{PD}_i = P_0(\text{PR}_i - 1) \tag{8.16}$$

Noting that the prevalence odds ratio (POR_i) is equal to $P_i(1 - P_0)/$
$[P_0(1 - P_i)]$, we can also express the PD as

$$\text{PD}_i = \frac{(P_0 - P_0^2)(\text{POR}_i - 1)}{P_0(\text{POR}_i - 1) + 1} \tag{8.17}$$

While it is possible to compute difference estimates for all the mortality frequency measures presented in Chapter 7, we will restrict our discussion in
this section to the *mortality density difference* (MDD), referring to death
with the disease in the total population. Using the notation of Table 8.1a,
we have

8.2.3
Mortality
Comparisons

$$\hat{\text{MDD}}_i = \hat{\text{MD}}_i - \hat{\text{MD}}_0 = (a_i/L_i) - (a_0/L_0) \tag{8.18}$$

where L_i is the amount of population-time experienced by all persons in the
ith exposure category.

Following the approach of previous sections, we can express the
MDD as a function of the MDR:

$$\text{MDD}_i = \text{MD}_0(\text{MDR}_i - 1) \tag{8.19}$$

**8.3
OTHER
MEASURES
OF ASSO-
CIATION**

The measures of association discussed thus far are intended specifically for use with categorical data. For the remainder of this section, we will consider association measures that can be used with continuous data (i.e., both the study factor and the disease). We will focus, however, on adapting these measures to the familiar context of a dichotomous study factor and disease.

**8.3.1
Correlation
Coefficients**

A *correlation coefficient* is a symmetrical measure of association that reflects the degree of "shared variance" between two variables—i.e., the extent to which each variable can linearly predict the other when both are measured on standard scales (Nunnally, 1978). The most widely used correlation measure with continuous variables is the *Pearson product-moment correlation coefficient* (r), which can be estimated as follows:

$$r = \frac{\hat{\text{Cov}}(X, Y)}{\sqrt{\hat{\text{Var}}(X)\,\hat{\text{Var}}(Y)}} = b_1 \sqrt{\frac{\hat{\text{Var}}(X)}{\hat{\text{Var}}(Y)}} \tag{8.20}$$

where $\hat{\text{Cov}}(X, Y)$ is the sample *covariance* between variables X and Y, $\hat{\text{Var}}(X)$ is the sample *variance* of X, $\hat{\text{Var}}(Y)$ is the sample variance of Y, and b_1 is the estimated *slope* of the fitted line, regressing Y on X. The range of r is from -1 to $+1$, and its null value is zero. As suggested by Equation 8.20, there is a relationship between r and straight-line regression: r reflects the fit of the model—i.e., the extent to which the fitted line conforms to the joint distribution of the two variables. Without changing the slope (b_1) of the fitted line, we can alter r by changing either variance, which can be done, for example, by selecting subjects in a different manner. Therefore, causal inference regarding the magnitude of the effect of X on Y should be based on the estimated slope, not on the correlation coefficient (Blalock, 1964).

The computation of r simplifies if both variables are dichotomous, as they are in Table 8.2b. Letting X refer to exposure status and Y refer to disease status, we can estimate the covariance and variances as follows:

$$\hat{\text{Cov}}(X, Y) = (ad - bc)/n^2$$
$$\hat{\text{Var}}(X) = n_1 n_0/n^2 \qquad \hat{\text{Var}}(Y) = m_1 m_0/n^2$$

Substituting these expressions in Equation 8.20, we arrive at a measure usually called the *phi (ϕ) coefficient* (Nunnally, 1978):

$$\phi = \frac{(ad - bc)}{\sqrt{m_1 m_0 n_1 n_0}} \tag{8.21}$$

Thus, the product-moment correlation coefficient applied to dichotomous variables is ϕ. Phi-square is, therefore, the proportion of the variance in each variable "explained" by the other and is equal to χ^2/n, where χ^2 is the common, uncorrected Pearson chi-square for a 2×2 table with one degree of freedom (Fleiss, 1981). Since χ^2 can be computed for a contingency table of any dimensions, this last formulation suggests a method for calculating ϕ for a multiple-category exposure. Unfortunately, with more than one degree of freedom, the upper and lower limits of ϕ tend to approach zero (the null value) (Fleiss, 1981), creating a rather undesirable property for a measure of association.

Solving Equation 8.20 for b_1, we find that the estimated slope corresponding to a given value of ϕ is equal to $\hat{\text{Cov}}(X, Y)/\hat{\text{Var}}(X) = (ad - bc)/n_1 n_0 = (a/n_1) - (c/n_0) = \hat{\text{PD}}$ or $\hat{\text{RD}}$ (the result depends on the study design). That is, b_1 is equivalent to a difference measure of association between dichotomous variables. Using the hypothetical data in Table 8.4 as an illustration of cross-sectional results, we find that $\phi = .187$, $\phi^2 = .035$, and $b_1 = \hat{\text{PD}} = .175$.

A major problem with the phi coefficient, which does not occur with the odds ratio, is that ϕ is not invariant over different types of study designs or changes in the marginal distributions (Fleiss, 1981). Suppose, for example, that we changed the ratio of exposed to unexposed subjects in Table 8.4. Assuming the two exposure-specific prevalence estimates remain the same, ϕ would differ from the value estimated above. Consequently, it is best to restrict our use of ϕ to cross-sectional studies involving simple random sampling of a single target population.

8.3.2 Statistical Model Coefficients

Over the past several years, epidemiologists have come to depend on the use of statistical models to test hypotheses and predict the occurrence of disease. As we suggested in Section 8.3.1, estimates of the model coefficients corresponding to specific predictors are, themselves, measures of association. The application of model fitting will be covered in more detail in Chapters 20–24; we will focus here on the derivation of particular categorical measures of association from selected models. To simplify the presentation, we will consider a dichotomous exposure (X) (coded as 1 = exposed, 0 = unexposed) and a study involving incident cases.

With a simple *linear model*, the fitted line may be expressed as

$$\hat{R} = b_0 + b_1 X \tag{8.22}$$

where $\hat{R}$ is the predicted value of the disease risk (or simply the probability of being a case in the study population), b_1 is the estimated *slope*, and b_0 is the *intercept*. Given this model, we can estimate the risk difference (RD) as

$$\hat{\text{RD}} = \hat{R}_1 - \hat{R}_0 = b_1 \tag{8.23}$$

where $\hat{R}_1 = b_0 + b_1$ is the estimated risk for exposed persons and $\hat{R}_0 = b_0$ is the estimated risk for unexposed persons. Thus, assuming a linear model, we may interpret the slope as an estimate of the risk difference.

Next, consider the following nonlinear model involving a natural logarithmic (ln) transformation of $\hat{R}$:

$$\ln \hat{R} = b_0 + b_1 X$$

or, equivalently,

$$\hat{R} = \exp(b_0 + b_1 X) \tag{8.24}$$

Given this *exponential model,* we can now estimate the risk ratio (RR) as

$$\hat{RR} = \hat{R}_1/\hat{R}_0 = \exp(b_1) \tag{8.25}$$

Thus, the antilogarithm of b_1 may be interpreted as the RR, comparing exposed with unexposed subjects.

Finally, a widely used method for predicting disease involves a *logit transformation* of $\hat{R}$:

$$\ln [\hat{R}/(1 - \hat{R})] = b_0 + b_1 X$$

or, equivalently,

$$\hat{R} = \frac{1}{1 + \exp[-(b_0 + b_1 X)]} \tag{8.26}$$

With this *logistic model,* we can estimate the risk odds ratio (ROR) as

$$\hat{ROR} = \frac{\hat{R}_1/(1 - \hat{R}_1)}{\hat{R}_0/(1 - \hat{R}_0)} = \exp(b_1) \tag{8.27}$$

Thus, the antilogarithm of b_1 may be interpreted as the odds ratio, which is an estimate of the incidence density ratio in a case-control study.

In subsequent chapters, we will see that the approach discussed in the preceding paragraphs can also be applied to multiple-category or continuous exposures. Furthermore, we can extend the method to models involving several exposures (X's), for which each estimated coefficient (b_i) represents an adjusted measure of association.

8.4 CONCLUDING REMARKS

Measures of association reflect the strength of the statistical relationship between a study factor and a disease; thus, they are used for making causal inferences. For categorical study factors, there are two basic types of association (or effect) measures: those based on the ratio of frequency measures for two exposure groups and those based on the difference in frequency measures between groups. Each type of comparison may involve incidence, prevalence, or mortality data; consequently, the choice, estimation, and interpretation of an effect measure depends on the study design. Although a direct comparison of disease frequencies is not possible in a case-control study (without additional information), we can estimate the appropriate ratio measure of association with the exposure odds ratio.

On the basis of the steady-state relationships among frequency measures presented in Chapter 7, we have derived steady-state relationships among various measures of association. Using these relationships, we have delineated the assumptions necessary to make an etiologic inference for different types of observational studies. In other words, we can assess under what special conditions the comparison of prevalence, mortality, and odds measures results in a valid estimate of what we would expect to obtain from a direct comparison of incidence rates or risks.

For continuous variables, the strength of an association ordinarily is expressed with a correlation coefficient or a coefficient (slope) derived from a statistical model. Nevertheless, these measures may also be applied to categorical variables. In fact, we have shown that ratio or difference measures of association may be easily derived from model coefficients, where the type of categorical measure depends on the type of statistical model. In Chapters 20 and 21, we will show the advantages of model fitting for simultaneously treating multiple factors that predict disease status. This approach enables us to analyze efficiently both categorical and continuous variables and to adjust the observed effect of each predictor for all other predictors in the model.

The following list summarizes the key notation introduced in this chapter. **NOTATION**

E_i	ith exposure category ($i = 0, 1, 2, \ldots, k$), where E_0 refers to the reference category (typically, all unexposed subjects).
a_i	Observed number of cases in ith exposure category ($i = 0, 1, 2, \ldots, k$), where $m_1 = \Sigma_{i=0}^{k} a_i$ [for a dichotomous exposure variable (i.e., $k = 1$), $a_1 = a$ and $a_0 = b$].
L_i	Observed amount of population-time in ith exposure category, where $L = \Sigma_{i=0}^{k} L_i$.
c_i	Observed number of noncases in ith exposure category, where $m_0 = \Sigma_{i=0}^{k} c_i$ [for a dichotomous exposure variable (i.e., $k = 1$), $c_1 = c$ and $c_0 = d$].
$n_i = a_i + c_i$	Total number of subjects in ith exposure category, where $n = \Sigma_{i=0}^{k} n_i$.

Ratio Measures of Association

$IDR_i = ID_i/ID_0$	Incidence density ratio (or average incidence rate ratio), comparing persons in ith exposure category with persons in reference category ($i = 0$), where ID_i is incidence density in ith exposure group.

$$RR_i = R_i/R_0$$

Risk ratio (or relative risk), comparing persons in ith exposure category with persons in reference category, where R_i is risk for persons in ith exposure category.

$$CIR_i = CI_i/CI_0$$

Cumulative incidence ratio, comparing persons in ith exposure category with persons in reference category, where CI_i is cumulative incidence in ith exposure group; $CIR_i = RR_i$.

$$EOR_i = \frac{pr(E_i|D)/pr(E_0|D)}{pr(E_i|\overline{D})/pr(E_0|\overline{D})}$$

Exposure odds ratio, comparing persons in ith exposure category with persons in reference category, where $pr(E_i|D)$ is the probability of being in the ith exposure category, given that one is a case, etc.

$$ROR_i = \frac{R_i/(1 - R_i)}{R_0/(1 - R_0)}$$

Risk odds ratio, comparing persons in ith exposure category with persons in reference category, where R_i is risk for persons in ith exposure category.

$$POR_i = \frac{P_i/(1 - P_i)}{P_0/(1 - P_0)}$$

Prevalence odds ratio, comparing persons in ith exposure category with persons in reference category, where P_i is prevalence in ith exposure category.

$$PR_i = P_i/P_0$$

Prevalence ratio, comparing persons in ith exposure category with persons in reference category, where P_i is prevalence in ith exposure category.

$$MDR_i = MD_i/MD_0$$

Mortality density ratio (or average mortality rate ratio), comparing persons in ith exposure category with persons in reference category, where MD_i is mortality density in ith exposure category.

$$FDR_i = FD_i/FD_0$$

Fatality density ratio (or average fatality rate ratio), comparing persons in ith exposure category with persons in reference category, where FD_i is fatality density in ith exposure category.

Difference Measures of Association

$$IDD_i = ID_i - ID_0$$

Incidence density difference (or average incidence rate difference), comparing persons in ith exposure category with persons in reference category.

$$RD_i = R_i - R_0$$

Risk difference (or attributable risk), comparing persons in ith exposure category with persons in reference category.

$\mathrm{CID}_i = \mathrm{CI}_i - \mathrm{CI}_0$ $\quad\quad = \mathrm{RD}_i$	Cumulative incidence difference, comparing persons in ith exposure category with persons in reference category.
$\mathrm{PD}_i = P_i - P_0$	Prevalence difference, comparing persons in ith exposure category with persons in reference category.
$\mathrm{MDD}_i = \mathrm{MD}_i - \mathrm{MD}_0$	Mortality density difference (or average mortality rate difference), comparing persons in ith exposure category with persons in reference category.
$r = \dfrac{\hat{\mathrm{Cov}}(X,\,Y)}{\sqrt{\hat{\mathrm{Var}}(X)\ \hat{\mathrm{Var}}(Y)}}$	Pearson product-moment correlation coefficient between two variables (X and Y) in study population, where $\hat{\mathrm{Cov}}(X,\,Y)$ is sample covariance between variables X and Y, $\hat{\mathrm{Var}}(X)$ is sample variance of X, and $\hat{\mathrm{Var}}(Y)$ is sample variance of Y.
ϕ	Phi coefficient, which is the correlation coefficient (r) between two dichotomous variables.
$\hat{Y} = b_0 + b_1 X$	Fitted value of Y (e.g., disease risk or prevalence) regressing Y on X (e.g., exposure level), where b_1 is estimated slope and b_0 is estimated Y-intercept.

REFERENCES

BLALOCK, H. M., JR. 1964. *Causal inferences in nonexperimental research.* New York: Norton.

CORNFIELD, J. 1951. A method of estimating comparative rates from clinical data. Applications to cancer of the lung, breast, and cervix. *J. Natl. Cancer Inst.* 11: 1269–1275.

FLEISS, J. L. 1981. *Statistical methods for rates and proportions.* 2nd ed. New York: Wiley; pp. 59–61.

HAMILTON, M. A. 1979. Choosing the parameter for a 2 × 2 table or a 2 × 2 × 2 table analysis. *Am. J. Epidemiol.* 109: 362–375.

MACMAHON, B., and PUGH, T. F. 1970. *Epidemiology: Principles and methods.* Boston: Little, Brown.

MIETTINEN, O. S. 1975. Principles of epidemiologic research. Unpublished manuscript. Cambridge, Mass.: Harvard University.

———. 1976. Estimability and estimation in case-referent studies. *Am. J. Epidemiol.* 103(2): 226–235.

MORGENSTERN, H.; KLEINBAUM, D. G.; and KUPPER, L. L. 1980. Measures of disease incidence used in epidemiologic research. *Int. J. Epidemiol.* 9: 97–104.

MORRISON, A. S. 1979. Sequential pathogenic components of rates. *Am. J. Epidemiol.* 109: 709–718.

NEUTRA, R. R., and DROLETTE, M. E. 1978. Estimating exposure-specific disease rates from case-control studies using Bayes' Theorem. *Am. J. Epidemiol.* 108: 214–222.

NUNNALLY, J. C. 1978. *Psychometric theory.* 2nd ed. New York: McGraw-Hill; pp. 121–133.

9

Measures of Potential Impact and Summary of the Measures

**9.0
PREVIEW**

In this chapter, we discuss the third class of quantitative measures, potential impact measures, which may be expressed as functions of either frequency measures or measures of association. As a summary of Part I, we also present an overview of all three types of measures used in epidemiologic research.

**9.1
MEASURES
OF
POTENTIAL
IMPACT**

Measures of potential impact reflect the expected effect of changing the distribution of one or more risk factors in a particular population. Once we have established that a factor is a determinant of the disease, we might wish to ascertain what proportion of all new cases purportedly are (or were) due to the risk factor—i.e., the proportion of cases that developed the disease as a result of the purported influence of the exposure.

In this section, we will discuss two types of potential impact measures: the etiologic fraction, which deals with positive risk factors (i.e., IDR > 1); and the prevented fraction, which deals with negative or protective risk factors (i.e., IDR < 1) (Miettinen, 1974). The calculations and interpretations of these measures differ; therefore, they will be treated separately in the next two sections. In Section 9.1.3, we will provide a generalized framework for viewing both measures and the practical value of potential impact measures in public health practice.

**9.1.1
Etiologic
Fractions**

The *etiologic fraction* (EF) for a dynamic population is the proportion of all new cases in a given period that are attributable to the risk factor of interest. Other names for this measure include "attributable risk" (Levin, 1953), "population attributable risk" (MacMahon and Pugh, 1970), "population attributable risk percent" (Cole and MacMahon, 1971), and "attributable fraction" (Ouellet et al., 1979b). For a given period (t_0, t) of duration Δt, EF may be expressed conceptually as

$$EF = I^*/I \qquad (9.1)$$

where I^* is the number of new cases occurring during the period (t_0, t) that are attributable or due to the risk factor. The EF may also be interpreted as the probability that a randomly selected case from the population developed the disease as a result of the risk factor. I^* can be quantified as the number of new cases that occurred during the period (t_0, t) minus the number of new cases that would have occurred in the candidate population of size N' in the absence of the exposure. Thus, for a stable candidate population,

$$I^* = ID(N')\,(\Delta t) - ID_0\,(N')\,(\Delta t) = N'\,(\Delta t)\,(ID - ID_0)$$

where $ID = I/[N'\,(\Delta t)]$ is the rate in the total candidate population, $ID_0 = I_0/[N'\,(\Delta t)]$ is the rate in the reference population, and I_0 is the number of unexposed cases observed during (t_0, t). Substituting the above expression for I^* in Equation 9.1 and noting that $I = ID(N')$ (Δt), we arrive at the following expression for estimating the EF:

$$\hat{EF} = (\hat{ID} - \hat{ID}_0)/\hat{ID} \qquad (9.2)$$

where $\hat{ID} > \hat{ID}_0$ and both rates are estimated by using one of the methods described in Chapter 6.

Next, let p equal the *proportion* of the candidate population that is exposed (to a dichotomous study factor). Since the population is stable, $\hat{p} = L_1/(L_1 + L_0)$ (see Table 8.1b, p. 142). Therefore,

$$\hat{ID} = \hat{p}(\hat{ID}_1) + (1 - \hat{p})\hat{ID}_0 \qquad (9.3)$$

Substituting this expression for $\hat{ID}$ in Equation 9.2 and dividing both numerator and denominator by $\hat{ID}_0$, we have a second expression for estimating the EF:

$$\hat{EF} = \frac{\hat{p}(\hat{IDR} - 1)}{\hat{p}(\hat{IDR} - 1) + 1} \qquad (9.4)$$

where $\hat{IDR} > 1$. Thus, we can estimate the EF without knowing the incidence rate in the population. For example, for the data in Tables 6.3 and 8.3 (p. 110 and p. 144), $\hat{EF}$ for persons between the ages of 40 and 49 is

$$\hat{EF} = \frac{(35/275)(2 - 1)}{(35/275)(2 - 1) + 1} = .113$$

where $\hat{IDR} = .001/.0005 = 2$ and $\hat{p} = 35,000/(35,000 + 240,000) = 35/275$. Thus, assuming the exposure is a risk factor, we estimate that 11.3% of the incident cases for this age decade were due to the factor.

Notice that the EF is a function of two types of information: (1) the magnitude of the association between the risk factor and the disease and (2) the prevalence of the study factor in the candidate population. It is chiefly the latter quantity that makes the EF specific to a particular population.

Now, let p_c equal the proportion of new cases that are exposed. Noting that $L_1 = a/\hat{ID}_1$ and $L_0 = b/\hat{ID}_0$, we can express $\hat{p}$ as

$$\hat{p} = \frac{L_1}{L_1 + L_0} = \frac{\hat{p}_c}{\hat{p}_c + (1 - \hat{p}_c)\hat{IDR}}$$

Substituting this value for $\hat{p}$ in Equation 9.4, we get a third expression for estimating the EF:

$$\hat{EF} = \hat{p}_c[(\hat{IDR} - 1)/\hat{IDR}] \qquad (9.5)$$

where $\hat{IDR} > 1$. For the data of Tables 6.3 and 8.3, $\hat{EF}$ for 40–49-year-olds, according to Expression 9.5, is $(70/310)[(2 - 1)/2] = .113$ (as before), where $\hat{p}_c = 70/(70 + 240) = 70/310$. An advantage of Expression 9.5 over Expression 9.4 for estimating the EF is that Expression 9.5 can be easily modified to adjust for the confounding effect of extraneous risk factors (Miettinen, 1974).

The above formulas for $\hat{\text{EF}}$, which have been cast in terms of incidence density measures, are appropriate for most chronic diseases (and certain endemic acute diseases) with extended risk periods, for a stable population. For acute diseases with restricted risk periods, however, $\hat{\text{EF}}$ should be based on estimates of the risk ratio. For example, if we assume the data in Table 9.1 were taken from a fixed cohort study, in which the study population is representative of the target population, p is estimated as n_1/n and p_c is estimated as a/m_1 (see Table 8.2b, p. 142). $\hat{\text{EF}}$ would then be

$$\hat{\text{EF}} = \frac{(120/500)(2.11 - 1)}{(120/500)(2.11 - 1) + 1} = .211$$

according to Expression 9.4, or $(40/100)[(2.11 - 1)/2.11] = .211$, according to Expression 9.5, where $\hat{\text{RR}} = 2.11$. If this fixed cohort study involved a chronic disease with an extended risk period, $\hat{\text{EF}}$, based on $\hat{\text{RR}}$, would be only an *approximation* of the desired potential impact measure, which should be based on $\hat{\text{IDR}}$. Even if the study population is representative of the target population *at the time of selection,* as the follow-up period progresses, new cases will become increasingly unrepresentative of (i.e., older than) the cases that are developing concurrently in the target population (Morgenstern et al., 1980).

In a case-control study involving a disease with an extended risk period and incident cases, the computed odds ratio ($\hat{\text{OR}}$) is an estimate of the IDR (see Section 8.1.1). Assuming noncases are representative of the target disease-free population, p is estimated as c/m_0. Assuming cases are representative of all new cases in the target population, p_c is estimated as a/m_1.

EXAMPLE 9.1

If we assume the data in Table 9.1 were taken from a case-control study, $\hat{\text{EF}}$ is

$$\hat{\text{EF}} = \frac{(80/400)(2.67 - 1)}{(80/400)(2.67 - 1) + 1} = .250$$

according to Expression 9.4, or $(40/100)[(2.67 - 1)/2.67] = .250$, according to Expression 9.5, where $\hat{\text{OR}} = 2.67$. Given that m_1 represents all new cases that occur in the population during (t_0, t), the estimated number $(\hat{I}*)$ of new cases attributable to the exposure during the follow-up period is $\hat{\text{EF}}(I) = .250(100) = 25$.

Table 9.1   Number of Subjects, by Exposure Category and Disease Status (Hypothetical Data)

| *Disease Status* | EXPOSURE CATEGORY | | *Total* |
	Exposed	*Unexposed*	
Cases	40	60	100
Noncases	80	320	400
Total	120	380	500

In cross-sectional studies, estimation of the EF depends on the nature of the disease under investigation. If the disease has an extended risk period (e.g., most chronic diseases), the EF should be estimated as described above for a case-control study, substituting $\hat{\text{POR}}$ for $\hat{\text{IDR}}$ in Equation 9.4 or 9.5. If, on the other hand, the disease has a restricted risk period (e.g., birth defects), the EF should be estimated as described above for a fixed cohort study, substituting $\hat{\text{PR}}$ for $\hat{\text{IDR}}$ in Equation 9.4 or 9.5.

To estimate the EF for a multiple-category exposure, we extend Equation 9.4 as follows (Walter, 1976):

$$\hat{\text{EF}} = \frac{\sum_{i=0}^{k} \hat{p}_i(\hat{\text{IDR}}_i - 1)}{\sum_{i=0}^{k} \hat{p}_i(\hat{\text{IDR}}_i - 1) + 1} = 1 - \frac{1}{\sum_{i=0}^{k} \hat{p}_i(\hat{\text{IDR}}_i)} \qquad (9.6)$$

where $\hat{p}_i$ is the estimated proportion of the candidate population in the ith exposure category $(i = 0, \ldots, k)$, $\sum \hat{p}_i = 1$, $\hat{\text{IDR}}_0 = 1$ (for the reference group), and $\hat{\text{EF}} > 0$. Note that $\hat{\text{IDR}}_i$ may be less than one for one or more exposure categories, as long as $\hat{\text{EF}}$ is greater than zero.

Expression 9.5 can also be extended to deal with multiple-category exposures (Miettinen, 1974):

$$\hat{\text{EF}} = \sum_{i=0}^{k} \hat{p}_{ci}\left(\frac{\hat{\text{IDR}}_i - 1}{\hat{\text{IDR}}_i}\right) = 1 - \sum_{i=0}^{k} \frac{\hat{p}_{ci}}{\hat{\text{IDR}}_i} \qquad (9.7)$$

where $\hat{p}_{ci}$ is the estimated proportion of the cases in the ith exposure category $(i = 0, \ldots, k)$ and $\hat{\text{EF}} > 0$. A procedure equivalent to that in Equation 9.6 or 9.7, assuming no stratification, is to combine all nonreference exposure categories into one group and to compare that combined group with the reference group, using either Expression 9.4 or 9.5.

The etiologic fraction may also be defined specifically for the exposed population as the proportion of exposed cases that are due to the risk factor. This measure, called the *etiologic fraction among the exposed* (EF$_e$) (Miettinen, 1974) or the "attributable risk percent" (Cole and MacMahon, 1971), can be expressed as

$$EF_e = I*/I_1 \tag{9.8}$$

where $I_1 = ID_1(N_1')(\Delta t)$ is the number of exposed new cases occurring during the period (t_0, t). The EF_e may also be interpreted as the probability that an exposed case developed the disease as a result of the risk factor. Using the same approach we used above, we can derive the following expression for estimating the EF_e:

$$\hat{EF}_e = (I\hat{D}R - 1)/I\hat{D}R = \hat{EF}/\hat{p}_c \tag{9.9}$$

Thus, the EF_e is a function of only one parameter, the IDR, and, therefore, is not dependent on the prevalence of the risk factor in the population. For example, assuming the data in Table 9.1 to be taken from a case-control study, $\hat{EF}_e$ is $(2.67 - 1)/2.67 = .625$. That is, we would estimate the probability that an exposed case developed the disease as a result of the risk factor to be 62.5%. Notice that a value of one for the EF_e corresponds to an infinite IDR, which would indicate that the exposure is a necessary cause of the disease. The value of the (total) EF for a necessary cause would also be one.

The etiologic fraction has received considerable attention in recent years as researchers have begun to appreciate its importance to public health practice. This interest has led to several methodological developments, including use of the EF for partitioning the total effect of two risk factors on a disease (Enterline, 1980; Walker, 1981). We might wish, for example, to estimate the proportion of lung cancer cases in the asbestos industry that are due to smoking and/or asbestos exposure. With such an approach, we can provide a basis for making decisions about personal behaviors and public health interventions. Another recent development is the extension of the EF for recurrent events, such as repetitive diseases, fertility, and medical care utilization (Park, 1981). This measure includes an extra parameter: the ratio of the average duration between two successive events for the unexposed group to the corresponding duration for the exposed group. Equation 9.4 can be modified to include this feature by replacing each $I\hat{D}R$ with the product of $I\hat{D}R$ and the above ratio.

**9.1.2
Prevented
Fractions**

When the disease rate is greatest in the reference group, the EF becomes negative and, therefore, is uninterpretable. The analogous measure in this situation, where IDR < 1, is the *prevented fraction* (PF), which is the proportion of potential new cases that would have occurred in the absence of exposure but did not occur. Stated another way, the PF is the proportion of potential cases that actually were prevented by the exposure in the population. For a given period (t_0, t) of duration Δt, PF might be expressed conceptually as

$$PF = I^{**}/(I^{**} + I) \tag{9.10}$$

where $I^{**} = N'(\Delta t)(ID_0 - ID)$ is the number of new cases purportedly prevented by the exposure, which is the number of cases that would have occurred in the absence of the exposure minus the number of cases that did occur, and $I = N'(\Delta t)(ID)$ is the number of cases that did occur. Substitution of these expressions for I^{**} and I in Equation 9.10 yields the following expression for estimating the PF:

$$\hat{PF} = (\hat{ID}_0 - \hat{ID})/\hat{ID}_0 \tag{9.11}$$

where $\hat{ID}_0 > \hat{ID}$.

Substitution of Expression 9.3 for $\hat{ID}$ in Equation 9.11, assuming a dichotomous factor, yields the following expression for estimating PF, which is independent of the incidence rate in the population:

$$\hat{PF} = \hat{p}(1 - \hat{IDR}) \tag{9.12}$$

where $\hat{p} = L_1/L$, if the population is stable, and $\hat{IDR} < 1$. We estimate p and IDR for various study designs by using the procedures described in the previous section for etiologic fractions.

Using the same approach we used before, we can derive a third expression for $\hat{PF}$ as a function of the case fraction (p_c) (Miettinen, 1974):

$$\hat{PF} = \frac{\hat{p}_c(1 - \hat{IDR})}{\hat{p}_c(1 - \hat{IDR}) + \hat{IDR}} \tag{9.13}$$

where $\hat{p}_c$ is the estimated proportion of cases that are exposed and $\hat{IDR} < 1$. For an exposure with more than two categories, $\hat{PF}$ has the following general forms (Miettinen, 1974):

$$\hat{PF} = 1 - \sum_{i=0}^{k} \hat{p}_i(\hat{IDR}_i) = 1 - \left(1 / \sum_{i=0}^{k} \frac{\hat{p}_{ci}}{\hat{IDR}_i}\right) \tag{9.14}$$

where $\hat{p}_i$ is the estimated proportion of the candidate population in the ith exposure category, $\hat{p}_{ci}$ is the estimated proportion of the cases in the ith exposure category, $\hat{IDR}_0 = 1$ (for the reference group), and $\hat{PF} > 0$.

As was true for the etiologic fraction, we might want to estimate the *prevented fraction among the exposed* (PF_e). The PF_e is the proportion of potential exposed cases that were prevented by the exposure and can be expressed conceptually as

$$PF_e = I^{**}/(I^{**} + I_1) \tag{9.15}$$

where $I_1 = N_1'(\Delta t)(ID_1)$. Making the same substitutions we made before and noting that $p = N_1'/N'$, we arrive at the following expression for estimating the PF_e:

$$\hat{PF}_e = 1 - I\hat{D}R = \hat{PF}/\hat{p} \qquad (9.16)$$

where $I\hat{D}R < 1$. Thus, the PF_e is independent of the exposure prevalence in the population, just as EF_e was a simple function of the IDR.

EXAMPLE 9.2

Suppose that the data in Table 9.1 were taken from a case-control study and that the two exposure categories were switched—i.e., 60 cases and 320 noncases are exposed, etc. The estimated odds ratio would then be $60(80)/[40(320)] = .375$, and $\hat{PF}$ would be $(320/400)(1 - .375) = .50$, according to Equation 9.12, or

$$\hat{PF} = \frac{(60/100)(1 - .375)}{(60/100)(1 - .375) + .375} = .50$$

according to Expression 9.13. Thus, 50% of all potential cases that would have occurred in the absence of the exposure were actually prevented by the factor in the population. $\hat{PF}_e$, according to Equation 9.16, is $(1 - .375) = .625$. Rearranging Equation 9.10, we can express I^{**} as $I(PF)/(1 - PF)$, where $I = m_1$, assuming a total of m_1 cases occurred in the population during the period (t_0, t). Therefore, the number of cases purportedly prevented by the exposure in this example is $100(.5)/(1 - .5) = 100$.

**9.1.3
Generalized
Impact
Fractions**

Perhaps the most important application of potential impact measures is to health planning—i.e., for predicting and evaluating the effect of intervention strategies and other changes on the health status of a target population (Walter, 1978; Ouellet et al., 1979a; Morgenstern and Bursic, in press). It follows from Section 9.1.1 that the total EF can be interpreted as the *expected* proportional reduction in disease incidence resulting from the optimal shift in the population distribution of a given risk factor. The risk reduction program is "optimal," of course, if all persons can be shifted to the lowest risk category (i.e., the reference group).

EXAMPLE 9.3

Suppose the EF corresponding to the association between cigarette smoking and lung cancer mortality were .80. As we suggested in Section 9.1.1,

EXAMPLE 9.3 (*continued*)

this result means that an estimated 80% of all lung cancer deaths are due to cigarette smoking. In addition, we would predict a maximum reduction in the lung cancer mortality rate by 80%, if smoking were totally abolished. Naturally, this inference assumes that the postintervention rate experienced by exsmokers will be equal to the preintervention rate experienced by nonsmokers. Furthermore, it assumes that our estimates of the population parameters (e.g., IDR and p) are valid, and that there are no secular trends in either the effect measure or the age-specific rates resulting from changes that are unrelated to the risk factor.

Analogously, we can interpret the total PF as the *actual* proportional reduction in disease incidence resulting from the current exposure level in the population.

EXAMPLE 9.4

Suppose the PF corresponding to the association between fluoride exposure and dental decay in children is .50. We would therefore estimate the rate of dental decay to have decreased by 50% in the last few decades as a result of new mass fluoride exposures, including water supplies and toothpastes. With available data, we could also estimate the *observed* proportional change in the rate of dental decay among children since the beginning of fluoride exposures and compare this estimate with the PF. If there were no changes in other risk factors for dental decay over the past few decades, we would expect the two estimates to be approximately equal.

The above examples suggest a common formulation for both the EF and the PF: each may be interpreted as a proportional reduction in disease incidence resulting from a particular change—either a decrease in the prevalence of a positive risk factor (EF) or an increase in the prevalence of a negative risk factor (PF). The EF refers to a potential for future benefits as a result of eliminating the current exposure; the PF refers to past benefits as a result of introducing the exposure (at the current level). From a public health perspective, we see that the full range of this general formulation has not been realized by the two measures already presented. For example, we might wish to predict the reduction in lung cancer mortality if smoking were reduced but not eliminated; or we might wish to predict the reduction in coronary heart disease (CHD) as a result of increased levels of physical activity (a negative risk factor). For this broader application, the following expression for a generalized *impact fraction* (IF) may be used (Walter,

1980; Morgenstern and Bursic, in press):

$$\hat{\text{IF}}_r = \sum_{i=0}^{k} (\hat{p}_i' - \hat{p}_i'') \, \hat{\text{IDR}}_i \Bigg/ \sum_{i=0}^{k} \hat{p}_i' \, (\hat{\text{IDR}}_i) \qquad (9.17)$$

where $\hat{\text{IF}}_r$ is the estimated impact fraction reflecting a reduction in the disease rate as a result of a change in the distribution of a risk factor in the population, $\hat{p}_i'$ is the estimated proportion of the candidate population in the ith exposure category *before* the planned intervention or change, $\hat{p}_i''$ is the estimated proportion of the candidate population in the ith exposure category *after* the change, and $\hat{\text{IF}}_r > 0$. For a dichotomous positive risk factor (i.e., $k = 1$ and $\hat{\text{IDR}} > 1$) and a postintervention state in which no one is exposed (i.e., $\hat{p}_1'' = 0$), Equation 9.17 reduces to $\hat{\text{EF}}$ (Expression 9.4). Similarly, for a dichotomous negative risk factor (i.e., $k = 1$ and $\hat{\text{IDR}} < 1$) and a preintervention state in which no one is exposed (i.e., $\hat{p}_1' = 0$), Equation 9.17 reduces to $\hat{\text{PF}}$ (Expression 9.12).

Expression 9.17 may be applied not only to a single risk factor with multiple categories ($i = 0, \ldots, k$) but also to combinations of two or more risk factors, where one joint category is selected as the reference group. For example, we might wish to predict the proportional reduction in the incidence of oral cancer resulting from certain changes in cigarette smoking and alcohol consumption. In this example, potential estimates would require the combined treatment of both factors, since their effects on the disease are not independent (Rothman, 1975).* Although estimation of the EF and PF was originally presented in the context of a single epidemiologic study, researchers and planners can derive estimates of potential impact fractions by combining results from different data sources, such as epidemiologic studies, community surveys, disease registries, and vital statistics.

We can extend the concept of a generalized fraction to deal with the actual or predicted *increase* in disease frequency. For example, we might wish to predict the proportional increase in breast cancer incidence as a result of delayed childbearing (i.e., postponement of first pregnancy to the late twenties and early thirties). Or we might wish to estimate the extent to which the recent increase in the rate of benign breast disease is due to a decrease in the use of oral contraceptives. The mathematical expression for such a measure is

$$\hat{\text{IF}}_s = \frac{\displaystyle\sum_{i=0}^{k} (\hat{p}_i'' - \hat{p}_i') \, \hat{\text{IDR}}_i}{\displaystyle\sum_{i=0}^{k} \hat{p}_i' \, (\hat{\text{IDR}}_i)} \qquad (9.18)$$

where $\hat{\text{IF}}_s$ is the estimated impact fraction reflecting an increase in the disease rate as a result of a change in the distribution of a risk factor in the

---

*The general concepts of synergism and effect modification will be discussed in Chapter 19.

population, and $\hat{IF}_s > 0$. As the complement of $\hat{IF}_r$, Expression 9.18 is used when there is an increase in the prevalence of a positive risk factor or when there is a decrease in the prevalence of a negative risk factor.

In Chapters 6–8 and in this chapter, we have presented a comprehensive overview of the fundamental measures used in epidemiologic research involving categorical variables. In this section we will compare the interpretations of selected measures and review the specific applications of certain measures to the more important study designs discussed in Chapter 5.

**9.2
SUMMARY
OF
EPIDEMIO-
LOGIC
MEASURES**

Given the wide variety of measures used to convey the results of epidemiologic analyses, the choice of a particular measure should depend on the researcher's specific objectives. As a partial review of the last few chapters, we will refine the meanings of selected measures by comparing them for two diseases in the same population.

**9.2.1
Relative
Interpretations**

EXAMPLE 9.5

The approximate number (I) of new lung cancer and CHD cases in the United States in 1976 is presented in Table 9.2 by smoking status of the candidate population (of size N'). The average incidence rates ($\hat{ID}$) for both diseases, assuming a stable population, are also given in the table. Note that the CHD rate is more than seven times as great as the lung cancer rate in the United States. For each disease, four measures are estimated and presented in Table 9.3: the incidence density ratio ($\hat{IDR}$), comparing smokers to nonsmokers; the incidence density difference ($\hat{IDD}$); the etiologic fraction ($\hat{EF}$); and the number ($\hat{I}^*$) of new cases attributable to smoking in 1976.

The results in Table 9.3 suggest an interesting contrast between the two diseases. While $\hat{IDR}$ and $\hat{EF}$ are greater for lung cancer, $\hat{IDD}$ and $\hat{I}^*$ are greater for CHD. In fact, this reversal is due to the marked difference in overall disease frequency observed in Table 9.2. The larger $\hat{IDR}$ for cancer suggests that smoking is more strongly related to lung cancer than to CHD. Thus, we would be more likely to infer that smoking is a risk factor for lung cancer than to infer that smoking is a risk factor for CHD. The larger $\hat{EF}$ for cancer simply reflects the relative magnitudes of the $\hat{IDR}$s, since we are dealing with one population. Yet, because CHD is a much more common disease, the absolute difference in rates between smokers and nonsmokers is greater for CHD than for lung cancer. As a result, more cases of CHD are attributable to smoking, despite the greater $\hat{IDR}$ for lung cancer. This result illustrates that, while the EF reflects the

EXAMPLE 9.5 (*continued*)

proportion of cases attributable to the exposure, the IDD reflects the absolute *number* of cases attributable to the exposure.

The public health implication of these results is that we could prevent more cases of CHD than lung cancer by reducing the level of cigarette smoking in the United States. Nevertheless, these same results also lend more support to a causal relationship between smoking and lung cancer than to one between smoking and CHD (refer to Section 2.2.3).

Table 9.2   Approximate Number (I) of New Cases and Incidence Rate ($\hat{ID}$) of Lung Cancer and Coronary Heart Disease (CHD) for the U.S. Population (of Size N') in 1976, by Smoking Status

		LUNG CANCER		CHD	
Status	N' ($\times 10^6$)	I ($\times 10^3$)	$\hat{ID}$ ($\times 10^{-5}/Year$)	I ($\times 10^3$)	$\hat{ID}$ ($\times 10^{-5}/Year$)
Smoker	70	60	85.7	250	371.1
Nonsmoker	150	10	6.7	250	166.7
Total	220	70	31.8	500	227.3

Note: We assume that N' is stable and represents the candidate population for both diseases.

Table 9.3   Estimated Measures of Association for Smokers Versus Nonsmokers and Potential Impact for the U.S. Population in 1976 (Table 9.2), by Disease

Measure	*Lung Cancer*	*CHD*
$\hat{IDR}$	12.86	2.14
$\hat{IDD}$ ($\times 10^{-5}/year$)	79.1	190.5
$\hat{EF}$ (%)	79.0	26.7
$\hat{I}^* = \hat{EF}(I)$	53,333	133,333

Note: We assume that smokers and nonsmokers had similar distributions on all other risk factors for both diseases (e.g., age, race, gender).

Thus far, the chapter has been organized around the various types of epidemiologic measures first presented in Chapter 6. Although it is evident that estimation procedures differ by study design, some of the differences may have been obscured in the previous sections. Many of the more important differences in estimability are presented in Table 9.4, which summarizes the types of frequency and association measures that are appropriate to each of the study designs discussed in Chapter 5. The table does not include potential impact fractions (e.g., EF or PF), which can be

9.2.2
Applicability to
Study Designs

Table 9.4   Estimable Parameters (X) in Epidemiologic Studies, by Type of Design (O=Optional, Depending on the Study Design)

| Study Design[a] | FREQUENCY MEASURES | | MEASURES OF ASSOCIATION[b,c] | |
	Prevalence	Incidence or Mortality	Ratio	Difference
Cohort		X	X	X
Cross-sectional	X		X	X
Case-control			X	
Ambidirectional		X	X	X
Follow-up prevalence	X		X	X
Selective prevalence	X		X	X
Backward prevalence	X		X	X
Repeated survey	X		X	X
Survey follow-up	X	X	X	X
Repeated follow-up	O	X	X	X
Intervention follow-up	O	X	X	X
Ecologic[d]	X or	X	X or	X
Proportional			X	
Space/time cluster[d,e]	O or	O	X or	X
Family cluster[e,f]	O or	O	(heritability indices)	

[a]Refer to Chapter 5 for a discussion of study design.

[b]Correlation coefficients may be calculated for all study designs, but they are most appropriate for prevalence studies involving simple random sampling and for ecologic comparison studies.

[c]We can estimate potential impact measures (e.g., EF or PF) from any ratio measure of association; preferably, though, we use the IDR or the RR, depending on the type of disease.

[d]In ecologic and space/time cluster studies, we can derive measures of association indirectly, using mathematical models that have been fitted to the data.

[e]In cluster studies, the estimation of frequency measures is optional and depends on whether we know the size of the candidate population. In twin and pedigree studies, such estimation is seldom possible.

[f]In family cluster studies, we estimate the proportion of the variability in disease occurrence that is due to genetic factors—i.e., heritability.

derived from estimates of the risk factor distribution in the population (i.e., p_i or p_{ci}) and any ratio measure of effect presented in this chapter. However, for reasons discussed in Section 9.1.1, the desired effect parameter for these estimations is the IDR for diseases with extended risk periods or the RR for diseases with restricted risk periods.

To conclude this chapter, we will highlight, in the following subsections, the estimation issues and procedures for the four study designs that form the basis of all subsequent chapters: cohort, cross-sectional, case-control, and ambidirectional studies.

Cohort Studies

The estimated frequency measure in cohort studies is the incidence or mortality rate or risk. As we suggested in Chapter 6 (see Figure 6.3, p. 112), cohort designs may involve a fixed cohort or a dynamic population. In both cases, we must know the durations (Δt_i) of the individual follow-up periods for all noncases, or we must assume them to be equal; otherwise, we cannot designate appropriate denominators for estimating incidence measures. If Δt_i are known (or assumed) to be equal for noncases—i.e., there are no withdrawals from a fixed cohort—we can estimate the cumulative incidence (CI) and thus the risk of disease as a simple proportion (refer to Chapter 6). In the more general situation where withdrawals do occur, we can estimate risk with the actuarial method. Alternatively, for a dynamic population, we generally estimate average rates or incidence densities (ID) if Δt_i are known for all subjects, including cases. This latter requirement indicates that we must know (or assume) the time of disease occurrence in addition to the time of withdrawal. We may then use the density method to derive risk estimates from this set of age-specific rate estimates.

The choice of risk versus rate as a desired incidence measure was discussed in Section 6.5. Perhaps the most relevant issue here for etiologic research is whether the disease has an extended or restricted risk period, relative to the actual period of observation. Most chronic diseases have extended risk periods, suggesting the use of incidence rates for making causal inferences. Thus, in this situation, we prefer the *density type of cohort study* described above, typically involving a dynamic population. On the other hand, most acute diseases have restricted risk periods, suggesting the estimation of risks. In this situation, we prefer the *cumulative type of cohort study,* involving a fixed population (or a dynamic population that is treated as fixed). Since the estimation of risks or rates often depends on practical considerations, it is important to recognize that the estimated rate ratio (I$\hat{D}$R) will be approximately equal to the estimated risk ratio (R$\hat{R}$) whenever the disease is rare and/or the duration (Δ) of the follow-up period is short—i.e., when I$\hat{D}(\Delta) < .10$. For example, the average 10-year R$\hat{R}$ for the youngest age group in Table 8.3 is $.0100/.005 = 2.00$, which is nearly the same as I$\hat{D}$R.

In a cohort design involving mortality with the disease as the outcome event, the mortality density ratio (MD̂R) is an appropriate estimate of the IDR under certain conditions. Specifically, the MDR is approximately equal to the IDR under steady-state conditions if the exposure is unrelated to the mean duration of the disease, if the disease is rare and/or highly fatal, if there is no recovery from the disease, and if the disease does not affect exposure status (before selection).

Cross-sectional Studies

Although there is no actual follow-up period in a cross-sectional study, we can regard the disease as having either an extended or a restricted risk period. The former type refers to a density type of study in which noncases are still at risk of developing the disease after the study (e.g., most chronic diseases and certain acute diseases); therefore, the primary effect parameter of etiologic interest is the IDR. The latter type refers to a cumulative type of study in which surviving cases are observed at the end of their risk periods (e.g., birth defects following intrauterine exposure); therefore, the desired effect parameter is the RR.

In a density type of cross-sectional study, the prevalence odds ratio (POR) is equal to the IDR under steady-state conditions if the exposure is unrelated to the mean duration of the disease (i.e., the exposure is not a prognostic factor) and if the disease does not affect exposure status. However, this equality does not hold within narrow age categories for which the POR is only an approximation for the IDR. In a cumulative type of cross-sectional study, on the other hand, the prevalence ratio (PR) is equal to the RR if the outcome event is unrelated to the probability of surviving (before selection), conditional on exposure status, and if the disease does not affect exposure status. Of course, if the prevalence of the disease is low, the PR and the POR will be approximately equal.

Case-Control Studies

We discussed four types of case-control studies in Section 8.1: (1) an extended risk period with incident cases; (2) an extended risk period with prevalent cases; (3) a restricted risk period with incident cases; and (4) a restricted risk period with prevalent cases. In all types, the computed measure is the exposure odds ratio (EÔR)—i.e., the odds of being exposed among cases (a/b) divided by the odds of being exposed among noncases (c/d). As is true in cohort and cross-sectional designs, the primary effect parameter of etiologic interest is the IDR for an extended risk period (i.e., density-type study) and the RR for a restricted risk period (i.e., cumulative-type study). In the first type, given no other sources of error, the EOR is equal to the IDR if the population is stable. In the second type, the EOR is equal to the POR, which is equal to the IDR only if the population is stable, if the exposure is unrelated to the mean duration of the disease, and if the disease does not affect exposure status. In the third type, the EOR is equal to the risk odds ratio (ROR), which is approximately equal to the

RR if the disease is rare. In the fourth type, the EOR is equal to the POR, which is approximately equal to the RR if the prevalence is very small, if the outcome event is unrelated to survival (before selection), conditional on exposure, and if the disease does not affect exposure status.

As we pointed out in Table 9.4, case-control studies do not allow estimation of disease rates, risks, or prevalences within exposure categories. However, such estimations are possible if we have an a priori estimate of the total frequency measure in the target population from which the cases developed. Suppose we wish to estimate the incidence rates (ID_i) for all exposure groups in a density type of case-control study. Using Equation 9.3, we can show that the average rate (ID_0) in the reference group may be estimated as

$$\hat{ID}_0 = \frac{\hat{ID}}{\hat{p}(\hat{IDR} - 1) + 1} = \left(\frac{a_0/m_1}{c_0/m_0}\right)\hat{ID} \qquad (9.19)$$

where $\hat{ID}$ is the a priori estimate of the total rate, $\hat{p} = 1 - c_0/m_0$ is the proportion of noncases that are exposed (see Table 8.1a or 8.2a) ($\hat{p} = c/m_0$ for a dichotomous exposure), and the $\hat{IDR}$ refers to the comparison of all exposed groups with the referent, which is estimated by $\hat{EOR} = (\Sigma_{i=1}^{k} a_i)(c_0)/[(\Sigma_{i=1}^{k} c_i)(a_0)]$ ($\hat{EOR} = ad/bc$ for a dichotomous exposure). Similarly, the estimated rate ($\hat{ID}_i$) for the ith exposure group is

$$\hat{ID}_i = \hat{ID}_0(\hat{IDR}_i) = \left(\frac{a_i/m_1}{c_i/m_0}\right)\hat{ID} \qquad (9.20)$$

An equivalent procedure for rate estimation has been offered by Miettinen (1976), who replaces Equation 9.19 with

$$\hat{ID}_0 = \hat{ID}(1 - \hat{EF}) \qquad (9.21)$$

where $\hat{EF}$ is the total etiologic fraction, from Expression 9.6 or 9.7, and $\hat{IDR} > 1$. For protective risk factors, the following expression is used in place of Equation 9.21:

$$\hat{ID}_0 = \hat{ID}/(1 - \hat{PF}) \qquad (9.22)$$

where $\hat{PF}$ is the total prevented fraction, from Expression 9.14, and $\hat{IDR} < 1$.

EXAMPLE 9.6

Suppose the data in Table 9.1 were taken from a density type of case-control study. Assuming an a priori estimate for ID of .01/year, $\hat{ID}_0 =$

EXAMPLE 9.6 (*continued*)

$.01(1 - .25) = .0075$/year, from Equation 9.21; and $\hat{ID}_1 = .0075 (2.67) = .02$/year, from Expression 9.20, where $\hat{IDR} = \hat{EOR} = (40)(320)/(60)(80) = 2.67$.

If we wish to determine exposure-specific risks or prevalences in a cumulative type of case-control study, the above methods are not appropriate unless the disease is rare. One alternative approach is based on Bayes' theorem and, therefore, does not depend on the infrequency of disease (Neutra and Drolette, 1978). Given an a priori estimate of the total risk ($\hat{R}$) (or prevalence), the estimated risk ($\hat{R}_i$) for the ith exposure category is

$$\hat{R}_i = \frac{1}{1 + \left(\dfrac{c_i m_1}{a_i m_0}\right) \left(\dfrac{1 - \hat{R}}{\hat{R}}\right)} \qquad (9.23)$$

where $i = 0, 1, \ldots, k$ (see Table 8.2a). Treating the data in Table 9.1 as though they were taken from a cumulative type of case-control study and assuming an a priori Δ-year risk of .05, we find that $\hat{R}_1 = .095$ and $\hat{R}_0 = .038$. Thus, $\hat{RR}$ is $.095/.038 = 2.51$, which is less than $\hat{ROR}$ (which is 2.67).

Ambidirectional Studies

An ambidirectional study is essentially a case-control study in which noncases have been selected in such a way as to make them representative of the same candidate population from which the observed (incident) cases actually developed. Consequently, there are two types of ambidirectional studies: a density type and a cumulative type.

In the density type of ambidirectional study, the study population is usually dynamic, and the durations (Δt_i) of individual follow-up periods are not known by the investigator. With a stable population, however, the EOR is equal to the IDR. Moreover, the exposure-specific rates can be estimated from Expression 9.20, and the overall rate (ID) can be estimated directly from the data (see Equations 6.1 and 6.3).

In a cumulative type of ambidirectional study, the study population is usually fixed, and the durations (Δt_i) of the individual follow-up periods are generally known or assumed by the investigator. Exposure-specific risks may be estimated from Equation 9.23, and the total risk can be estimated directly from the data, using either the actuarial or the density method (see Chapter 6). Measures of association (e.g., $\hat{RR}$ or $\hat{RD}$) may then be computed from the exposure-specific risk estimates.

9.3 CONCLUDING REMARKS

In Chapters 6 through 9, we have presented several variations of three broad types of quantitative measures used in epidemiologic research. Frequency measures reflect the occurrence of the disease in a group. They are used primarily to describe the health status of populations and to construct the two other types of measures. Measures of association (or effect) express the strength of a statistical relationship between a study factor and a disease. They are used, therefore, to make causal inferences. Measures of potential impact, derived from either frequency or effect measures, reflect the expected contribution of the study factor to the frequency of a disease in a particular population. They are used to estimate the proportion of cases attributable to a given factor and thus to predict the impact of medical and public health interventions on the health status of populations. For each basic measure described, we have provided a definition, methods of estimation, and its application to specific study designs. Taken together, these measures serve as the basic tools for developing the principles and methods of epidemiologic research discussed throughout the remainder of this book.

NOTATION

The following list summarizes the key notation introduced in this chapter.

I^*	Number of new cases occurring during period (t_0, t) that are attributable or due to exposure under study (i.e., a positive risk factor).
$\mathrm{EF} = I^*/I$	Etiologic fraction in the population (or population attributable risk percent, etc.), where I is the number of new cases that occur during period (t_0, t); thus, EF is the proportion of new cases due to the exposure.
p	Proportion of the candidate population that is exposed (to a dichotomous study factor).
p_c	Proportion of new cases that are exposed (to a dichotomous study factor).
p_i	Proportion of candidate population in ith exposure category ($i = 0, 1, 2, \ldots, k$).
p_{ci}	Proportion of new cases in the ith exposure category.
$\mathrm{EF}_e = I^*/I_1$	Etiologic fraction in exposed population (or attributable risk percent), where I_1 is the number of exposed new cases that occur during the period (t_0, t); thus, EF_e is the proportion of exposed cases due to the exposure.
I^{**}	Number of new cases purportedly prevented by (negative) risk factor under study during period (t_0, t).

$\mathrm{PF} = I^{**}/(I^{**} + I)$ Prevented fraction in population, where I is the number of new cases that occur during period (t_0, t); thus, PF is the proportion of all potential cases that are actually prevented by the exposure.

$\mathrm{PF}_e = I^{**}/(I^{**} + I_1)$ Prevented fraction in exposed population, where I_1 is the number of exposed new cases that occur during period (t_0, t); thus, PF_e is proportion of potential exposed cases that are prevented by the exposure.

p_i' Proportion of candidate population in ith exposure category *before* a given intervention or change (involving the distribution of the exposure in the population).

p_i'' Proportion of candidate population in ith exposure category *after* a given intervention or change (involving the distribution of the exposure in the population).

IF_r Generalized impact fraction, reflecting a *reduction* in the disease rate as a result of a change in the distribution of the exposure in the population—resulting either from a decrease in the prevalence of a positive risk factor or from an increase in the prevalence of a negative risk factor (note that the EF and the PF are special cases of the IF_r).

IF_s Generalized impact fraction, reflecting an *increase* in the disease rate as a result of a change in the distribution of the exposure in the population—resulting either from an increase in the prevalence of a positive risk factor or from a decrease in the prevalence of a negative risk factor.

PRACTICE EXERCISES

9.1 In 1960, an investigator drew a 1% (simple) random sample of all adults in a community of 105,000 persons. An initial examination revealed 50 existing cases of a chronic disease for which there is no recovery. Forty percent of the noncases had a particular exposure, which remains unchanged over time. Within the next five years, 55 new cases of the disease occurred in the study population; 40 of these cases were exposed. Assume steady-state conditions and that the exposure is not a prognostic factor for the disease.

     a. Estimate the prevalence of the disease in the adult population in 1960 and the total number of adult cases in the community at that time.

     b. Estimate the five-year risk ratio and risk difference for exposed versus unexposed persons.

    c. Estimate the proportion of all new cases that are due to the exposure in the total adult population.

    d. Estimate the probability that a new exposed case developed the disease as a result of the exposure.

    e. Estimate the mean duration of the disease—i.e., the average time between diagnosis and death.

9.2 The first 100 premature births (i.e., birth weight less than 2500 g) in a large hospital in 1980 were compared with 300 normal births from the same hospital during the same period. It is known that 7% of all births in the population served by the hospital are premature. Exercise Table 9.1 presents the frequency distribution of subjects by prematurity status and the level of alcohol consumption of the mother during the first trimester (M/H = moderate/heavy alcohol consumption; L/O = light/occasional consumption).

    a. Estimate the two prevalence odds ratios, comparing infants of mothers who consumed alcohol during the first trimester with infants of non-drinking mothers.

    b. Estimate the three prevalences of low birth weight, by mother's alcohol consumption.

    c. Estimate the proportion of low–birth weight infants that is due to mother's consumption of alcohol during the first trimester.

    d. Estimate the probability that a low–birth weight infant, whose mother was a moderate/heavy drinker during pregnancy, weighed less than 2500 g at birth because of its mother's drinking habit.

9.3 A group of adult patients with advanced periodontitis (a common periodontal disease leading to teeth loss) from a large general dental clinic was compared with a group of adult patients with normal periodontal tissue. Thirteen percent of the cases and 22% of the noncases reported they had been routine users of dental floss for at least five years. (Denture users were questioned about the five years before denture use.)

    a. Estimate the average incidence rate ratio of advanced periodontitis, comparing dental floss users to nonusers.

    b. Given that the average incidence rate among nonusers is .02/year, estimate the incidence rate difference.

    c. Suppose that, because of other factors related to flossing, cases who do not floss live 10% longer (on the average) than cases who do floss. Assuming

Exercise Table 9.1

Status	ALCOHOL CONSUMPTION			Total
	M/H	*L/O*	*None*	
Premature	10	54	36	100
Normal	20	150	130	300
Total	30	204	166	400

steady-state conditions, estimate the incidence rate ratio, correcting for this difference in case survival.

d. Using the corrected estimate in part c, estimate the proportion of potential cases of advanced periodontitis that have been prevented by flossing in this population.

9.4 A stable population of 100,000 men, age 50–79, was followed from 1974 to 1976 (24 months) for detection of bladder cancer. During that period, 182 new cases were identified and compared with a random sample of 200 noncases from the same population. Exercise Table 9.2 presents the number of new cases and noncases by age decade and smoking (S) status (smoker versus nonsmoker).

a. Estimate the average incidence rate of bladder cancer for each age category (ignoring smoking status).

b. Estimate the average incidence rate ratio for each age category, comparing smokers with nonsmokers.

c. Estimate the etiologic fraction for each age category.

d. Estimate the average incidence rate for each smoking-age category.

e. Estimate the 30-year risk difference for a 50-year-old male.

9.5 State the general assumptions required for each of the following approximations (in addition to issues involving measurement and the distribution of extraneous risk factors):

a. Using the cumulative incidence ratio (CIR) as an estimate of the risk ratio (RR) in a fixed cohort study.

b. Using the CIR as an estimate of the incidence density ratio (IDR) in a fixed cohort study.

c. Using the prevalence odds ratio (POR) as an estimate of the IDR in a cross-sectional study.

d. Using the prevalence ratio (PR) as an estimate of the IDR in a cross-sectional study.

e. Using the exposure odds ratio (EOR) as an estimate of the IDR in an ambidirectional study.

f. Using the EOR as an estimate of the RR in a case-control study involving incident cases.

Exercise Table 9.2

Age	Population Size ($\times 10^3$)	NEW CASES			NONCASES		
		S	$\bar{S}$	Total	S	$\bar{S}$	Total
50–59	45	24	12	36	38	52	90
60–69	32	27	27	54	19	45	64
70–79	23	30	62	92	9	37	46
Total	100	81	101	182	66	134	200

g. Using the EOR as an estimate of the RR in a case-control study involving prevalent cases.

h. Using the EOR as an estimate of the POR in a case-control study involving prevalent cases.

i. Using the mortality density ratio (MDR) as an estimate of the IDR in a cohort study involving a dynamic population.

REFERENCES   COLE, P., and MACMAHON, B. 1971. Attributable risk percent in case-control studies. *Br. J. Soc. Prev. Med.* 25:242–244.

ENTERLINE, P. E. 1980. Attributability in the face of uncertainty. *Chest* 78 (Suppl.): 377–379.

LEVIN, M. L. 1953. The occurrence of lung cancer in man. *Acta Unio Int. Contra Cancrum* 9: 531–541.

MACMAHON, B., and PUGH, T. F. 1970. *Epidemiology: Principles and methods.* Boston: Little, Brown.

MIETTINEN, O. S. 1974. Proportion of disease caused or prevented by a given exposure trait or intervention. *Am. J. Epidemiol.* 99: 325–332.

MORGENSTERN, H., and BURSIC, E. S. In press. A method for using epidemiologic data to estimate the potential impact of an intervention on the health status of a target population. *J. Community Health.*

MORGENSTERN, H.; KLEINBAUM, D. G.; and KUPPER, L. L. 1980. Measures of disease incidence used in epidemiologic research. *Int. J. Epidemiol.* 9:97–104.

NEUTRA, R. R., and DROLETTE, M. E. 1978. Estimating exposure-specific disease rates from case-control studies using Bayes' Theorem. *Am. J. Epidemiol.* 108: 214–222.

OUELLET, R. P.; APOSTOLIDES, A. Y.; ENTWISLE, G.; and HEBEL, J. R. 1979a. Estimated community impact of hypertension control in a high risk population. *Am. J. Epidemiol.* 109: 531–538.

OUELLET, B. L.; ROMEDER, J. M.; and LANCE, J. M. 1979b. Premature mortality attributable to smoking and hazardous drinking in Canada. *Am. J. Epidemiol.* 109: 451–463.

PARK, C. B. 1981. Attributable risk for recurrent events: An extension of Levin's measure. *Am. J. Epidemiol.* 113: 491–493.

ROTHMAN, K. J. 1975. Alcohol. In *Persons at high risk of cancer: An approach to cancer etiology and control,* edited by J. F. Fraumeni, Jr., Chap. 9, pp. 139–150. New York: Academic Press.

WALKER, A. M. 1981. Proportion of disease attributable to the combined effect of two factors. *Int. J. Epidemiol.* 10: 81–85.

WALTER, S. D. 1976. The estimation and interpretation of attributable risk in health research. *Biometrics* 32: 829–849.

———. 1978. Calculation of "attributable risks" from epidemiological data. *Int. J. Epidemiol.* 7: 175–182.

———. 1980. Prevention for multifactorial diseases. *Am. J. Epidemiol.* 112: 409–416.

PART II

Validity of Epidemiologic Research

10

Validity: General Considerations

CHAPTER OUTLINE

**10.0
PREVIEW**

In any etiologic study, whether observational or experimental, the investigator must be concerned with avoiding spurious conclusions that are attributable to questionable methodology in study design and/or analysis. Considerations of study validity have, in fact, led to recent controversies in the epidemiologic literature, notably, the reserpine–breast cancer debate (e.g., Boston Collaborative Drug Report, 1974) and the more current estrogen–endometrial cancer controversy (e.g., Horwitz and Feinstein, 1978; Hutchinson and Rothman, 1978; and Hulka et al., 1978).

This is the first of five consecutive chapters devoted to the *conceptual characteristics* of validity as they relate to epidemiologic research. Here, we provide an overview of basic concepts, including a quantitative framework for assessing validity, which combines both epidemiologic and statistical considerations (Kleinbaum et al., 1981). In the next four chapters, we will describe in detail three important classes of validity issues, namely, selection bias, information bias, and confounding.

We will restrict our focus on validity to the consequences of questionable methodology on the estimation of an *effect measure* (e.g., risk ratio). We will not, therefore, directly consider validity in the estimation of a measure of disease frequency (see Criqui, 1979) or in the measurement of exposure and disease variables being studied, except with regard to how misrepresentation of these quantities can influence an effect estimate. When misrepresentation of effect can be identified, it will be called *bias*, which we will define later in quantitative terms. When there is no misrepresentation, we will say that our estimate of effect is "valid" or, equivalently, that there is "no bias."

Our discussion is embedded in an investigation of an etiologic hypothesis about the association of a dichotomous study factor $(E, \bar{E})$ with a dichotomous disease condition $(D, \bar{D})$. Thus, in essence, we will be considering characteristics of the standard fourfold table. The measure of effect we will consider is a ratio measure of association; the particular form of the measure will depend on the type of study design chosen (e.g., a risk, prevalence, or exposure odds ratio). We will not directly consider study designs that involve population-time experience (i.e., density types of studies, described in Chapter 5); however, the principles of validity described here carry over to such studies (e.g., when the odds ratio is used to estimate the incidence density ratio). Issues of statistical significance will also not be addressed here; in fact, they are inappropriate for the evaluation of validity in the effect estimator. (We will discuss this point later in this chapter and when we address the topic of confounding in Chapter 13.)

We wish to emphasize the distinction between validity in the estimation of effect and the more narrowly defined concept of measurement validity. The latter term refers to one source of misrepresentation in estimation of effect, namely, whether or not one or more of the variables being studied is properly measured. For example, in a study of the effect of personality type on the subsequent development of heart disease, the investigator should obtain proper (valid) measurement of personality type in order to arrive at an accurate estimate of effect. Nevertheless, in addition to measurement error, there are other sources of bias that may contribute to misrepresentation of an effect measure, and our focus here is on describing and quantifying the characteristics of each of these sources of invalidity. Our emphasis, moreover, is on identifying, in quantitative terms, the conditions under which no misrepresentation in effect will occur, determining the direction and magnitude of any distortion, and describing procedures for adjusting an estimate to remove distortion.

The most notable early conceptual work on validity was that of Berkson (1946), who demonstrated that case-control studies carried out exclusively in hospital settings are subject to potential selection bias attributable to the manner in which risks of hospitalization can combine in patients who have more than one condition. This phenomenon, which has continued to cause concern about the appropriateness of the case-control method (see Ibrahim, 1979), has been commonly referred to as Berkson's fallacy or Berkson's bias. As we will illustrate in Chapter 11, the principles of selection bias demonstrated by Berkson are generally applicable to other sources of bias in case-control studies, such as the choice of comparison groups and the death of potential subjects prior to selection, and are generalizable to follow-up and cross-sectional studies as well. Greenland (1977), for instance, has demonstrated how a loss to follow-up and/or nonresponse can lead to selection bias in follow-up studies. In a broader context, Miettinen (1976) has discussed alternative statistical definitions of validity and has offered a classification scheme upon which the quantitative approach to be described below is based. Feinstein (1977), Criqui (1979), and Sackett (1979) have each offered schemes for the classification of bias. Additional references that address particular sources of bias will be provided in subsequent chapters on specific validity issues.

10.1 BRIEF LITERATURE REVIEW

Before focusing in detail on the underlying (quantitative) features of validity, we must broadly distinguish between the terms "validity" and "precision," especially since different approaches to the assessment of each are advocated. In general, these terms are concerned with two different sources of inaccuracy that can occur when estimating an effect: systematic error (a validity problem) and random error (a precision problem). These two types of error are contrasted in Figure 10.1.

10.2 VALIDITY AND PRECISION

As illustrated in the figure, *random error* shows up as a difference between the estimate (say $\hat{\theta}$) computed from the study data and the parameter actually being estimated (say θ°). Random error is essentially attributable to sampling variation, the extent of which may depend on aspects of the study design (e.g., sample size considerations) and statistical characteristics of the estimator (e.g., its variance).

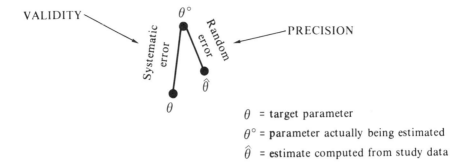

θ = target parameter

$\theta°$ = parameter actually being estimated

$\hat{\theta}$ = estimate computed from study data

Figure 10.1 Random Error Versus Systematic Error

Systematic error, on the other hand, occurs when there is a difference between what the estimator is actually estimating ($\theta°$) and the true effect measure of interest (θ). Systematic error is attributable to methodological aspects of the study design or analysis other than sampling variation, particularly the selection of subjects, the quality of information obtained, and variables of importance other than the disease (D) and study factor (E).

Figure 10.1 suggests an analogy with target shooting: validity is concerned with whether or not one is aiming at the correct bulls-eye; precision is concerned with individual variation from shot to shot, given the actual bulls-eye being considered.

Although the focus of this chapter is on validity, consideration of precision in the effect estimator is also important, particularly when we are trying to account for extraneous variables in describing the exposure-disease relationship. As we will discuss further in later chapters, we may lose precision by the indiscriminate control of variables that do not need to be considered for validity reasons. Conversely, we may gain precision by omitting such variables from control. Thus, there is often a trade-off to be considered between the potential loss of validity when controlling for too few variables and the potential loss of precision when controlling for too many variables. In practice, the recommended approach is to address problems of validity *before* trying to improve precision. In other words, we believe that validity should not be sacrificed for the sake of precision.

Problems of precision, which reflect sampling variability, generally concern statistical inferences (i.e., tests of hypotheses and interval estimation procedures) about the parameters of the population *actually* sampled. Statistical inference concepts, however, do not relate to validity issues (Miettinen, 1974; Dales and Ury, 1979).

Another distinction we need to make pertains to the terms "external validity" and "internal validity." These terms depend on the population to which inferences are made. Figure 10.2 identifies a hierarchy of (four) populations about which conclusions may be drawn regarding an etiologic

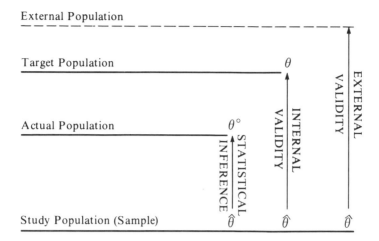

Figure 10.2 Hierarchy of Populations

hypothesis. The *study population* (previously defined in Chapter 2) is the collection of individuals from which the study data have been obtained. In ordinary statistical jargon, the study population would be called the *sample* if it were a smaller collection selected from some larger group; of course, it could also be considered a population itself in the sense that all its members, taken collectively, comprise an identifiable group. The *actual population* is defined to be the (larger) collection of individuals that the study population represents; i.e., it is an expansion of the study population to include all individuals who would meet the eligibility requirements of the study. The *target population* (see Chapter 2) is the collection of individuals of restricted interest from which one has sampled (though not necessarily in a representative manner) and about which one wishes to make statistical inferences with respect to the study objective. Due to methodological features of the study design, the study population may not be representative of the target population (i.e., there may be systematic error). The *external population* is the collection of individuals to which the study has not been restricted but to which one still wishes to generalize the study findings.

With regard to the populations defined above, the term *internal validity* concerns the validity of inferences about the target population, using information from the study population. The word "internal" thus relates to inferences that do not proceed beyond the (target) population of restricted interest. The term *external validity,* on the other hand, concerns inferences to an external population beyond the study's restricted interest. Such inferences require generalizations based on judgmental aspects, such as other findings and their connection with the study's findings, theoretical knowledge of the disease process and related factors, and biological considerations.

EXAMPLE 10.1

Consider a study carried out in North Carolina for the assessment of the relationship between personality type and pancreatic cancer. Internal validity issues would concern whether or not conclusions about the population of interest in North Carolina are spurious because of methodological flaws in the study design. External validity issues, on the other hand, would concern whether or not the study findings could be generalized to populations outside North Carolina (e.g., to the United States as a whole), to other time periods, or even in terms of a theoretical formulation of disease etiology (e.g., concluding that personality type is a cause of pancreatic cancer).

Our subsequent discussions of validity will consider only the internal type. Concerns about external validity do not lend themselves to quantification and, therefore, will not be addressed here.

10.3 DEFINITION OF INTERNAL VALIDITY

Let θ denote the (true) measure of effect in the population of interest, which we have called the target population. Let $\hat{\theta}$ denote the estimator of θ based on a subgroup (e.g., sample) from the target population; we have called this subgroup the study population. In other words, the statistical properties of $\hat{\theta}$ depend on the study population. Let $\theta°$ denote the parameter that $\hat{\theta}$ estimates in the larger population that the study population actually represents; this population has been called the actual population. Then, $\hat{\theta}$ is a *valid estimator* of θ if and only if $\theta° = \theta$. The relative *bias* in θ is defined as

$$\text{BIAS}(\hat{\theta}, \theta) = (\theta° - \theta)/\theta \tag{10.1}$$

Although other functions of $\theta°$ and θ could be used in place of Expression 10.1, we find this definition particularly useful for quantifying conditions for the existence of specific sources of bias for ratio types of estimators of effect and for indicating the direction of such bias. Expression 10.1 quantifies any distortion in effect relative to the size of the target parameter and indicates that a nonzero bias will result if the population parameter $\theta°$ actually being estimated is not equal to θ. As Miettinen (1976) has pointed out, this definition implicitly identifies a valid $\hat{\theta}$ as being a statistically *consistent* estimator; i.e., $\hat{\theta}$ must converge to θ in probability as the study size is (hypothetically) expanded, without modifying the study design itself. A definition of validity based on statistical consistency reflects only methodological aspects of study design; this type of definition is preferable to a definition based on statistical expected value theory, where statistical bias may be present solely because of mathematical properties of the estimator. For example, the sample risk ratio is *not* an un-biased estimator (in terms of its expected value) of the population risk ratio, even in the absence of any methodological flaws. Furthermore, the use of an expected value definition would necessarily imply consideration of infinite repetitions of the *same-sized study* rather than of *study size expansion*.

10.4 DIRECTION OF BIAS

In most epidemiologic studies, it may be difficult to obtain sufficient information to quantify precisely the extent (i.e., size) of the bias. However, it may be possible to determine the *direction* of the bias. "Direction" here refers to whether the effect actually being estimated ($\theta°$) either exceeds or lies below the true effect (θ), regardless of the actual size of the bias.

As we will see in the next two chapters, if certain general (mathematical) conditions hold, the bias will necessarily be in a known direction. Such conditions must be verifiable in a given study in order for the investigator to justify a conclusion regarding the direction of the bias. In any case, knowledge of the direction of the bias may be of practical importance to an investigator—e.g., when it can be shown that a very strong data-based association is not artificially high due to potential biases of concern, or when a very weak association in the data is actually weaker than it appears because of bias.

The direction of the bias may be alternatively classified as (1) positive or negative or as (2) toward the null, away from the null, or switchover. From the definition of bias given in Equation 10.1, it follows from simple algebra that the bias will be *positive* when $\theta°$ exceeds θ; when $\theta°$ is less than θ, the bias will be *negative*. Use of the terms "positive" and "negative" to characterize the direction of bias, although appropriate in the context of this chapter, has the drawback of being dependent on the specific mathematical form of our definition. A more commonly used terminology distinguishes between biases that are toward the null and away from the null. The direction of the bias is defined to be *toward the null* if $\theta°$ is closer than θ to the null value of the effect measure (e.g., closer to one if a ratio measure like the odds ratio or the risk ratio is under consideration), provided that θ and $\theta°$ are both either larger or smaller than the null value. If the bias is toward the null, then the observed effect appears (in the data) to be weaker than it really is (in the target population). The direction of the bias is *away from the null* if $\theta°$ is farther than θ from the null value of the effect measure, again provided that θ and $\theta°$ are both on the same side of the null value. Thus, if the bias is away from the null, then the observed effect appears (in the data) to be stronger than it really is (in the target population).

If $OR° = 2$ and $OR = .5$, then we cannot argue that the bias is either toward or away from the null, since the values are on either side of one. We refer to this kind of bias as a *switchover bias*. For such a bias, the exposure may appear (in the data) to be deleterious in its effect when it is truly protective, or it may appear to be protective when it is truly deleterious. Note that, by definition, a bias toward or away from the null precludes the possibility of switchover bias. Thus, for example, if we obtain an estimated odds ratio of $\hat{OR} = 1.3$, and we further determine that the bias is away from the null, then OR can be no smaller than one. Moreover, the appearance of no association in the data implies no true association (in the target population) if the bias is determined to be away from the null.

EXAMPLE 10.2

If the effect measure is the odds ratio ($\theta = OR$), and if $OR° = 8$ but $OR = 2$, then the bias would be away from the null, and it would be positive, from Equation 10.1. Thus, the effect estimate would suggest a very strong association when, in fact, the true association is only of moderate size. However, if $OR° = .50$ and $OR = .95$, the bias would also be away from the null, but it would be negative from Equation 10.1.

As another example, if $OR° = 1.3$ and $OR = 5$, then the bias would be toward the null and negative in terms of Equation 10.1. In this situation, the true effect is quite strong, even though the data would suggest essentially no association. However, if $OR° = .90$ and $OR = .35$, then the bias would also be toward the null but positive on the basis of Equation 10.1.

Before concluding this section, we point out that knowledge of the direction of the bias can have different implications, depending on the point of view of the investigator. For instance, a scientist wishing to demonstrate empirically the detrimental effect of a suspected risk factor (i.e., exposure variable) would hope to find a strong (and statistically significant) estimated association with a potential bias that can only be toward the null. On the other hand, a different scientist, charged with critiquing a study such as the one above for the purpose of setting public policy, might be more concerned about bias away from the null. In this situation, the reviewer might be worried about causing the public undue alarm over a potential health hazard if the conclusion of the study was based on inconclusive or misleading evidence.

10.5 CLASSIFICATION OF BIAS

As we previously mentioned, sources of bias resulting from methodological features of study design and analysis can be classified in a variety of ways. Of these, we have found Miettinen's (1976) terminology, which delineates selection, information, and confounding biases, to be the most conceptually appealing.

Selection bias refers to a distortion in the estimate of effect resulting from the manner in which subjects are *selected* for the study population.

Among the many sources of selection bias are flaws in the study design, most notably concerning the choice of groups to be compared (in all types of studies) and the choice of the sampling frame (particularly in case-control and cross-sectional studies); loss to follow-up or nonresponse during data collection (in follow-up studies); and selective survival (in case-control and cross-sectional studies). Also, selection bias can result in case-control studies when the procedure used to identify disease status (i.e., diagnostic surveillance) varies with exposure status. This bias is one form of what Feinstein (1977) has called "detection bias." It has also been referred to as "unmasking bias" by Sackett (1979), and it has been considered by researchers involved in the controversy about the relationship between endometrial cancer and estrogen use (Horwitz and Feinstein, 1978; Hulka et al., 1978).

Information bias refers to a distortion in the estimate of effect due to measurement error or misclassification of subjects on one or more variables. Major sources of information bias include invalid measurement, incorrect diagnostic criteria, and omissions, imprecisions, or other inadequacies in previously recorded data. Also, information bias from misclassification may result for follow-up studies when there is unequal diagnostic surveillance among exposure groups. (As we previously mentioned, however, for case-control studies, selective surveillance can lead to selection bias rather than information bias.)

Confounding is a bias that results when the study factor effect is mixed, in the data, with the effects of extraneous variables. This bias can result from causal relationships relating the study factor and the other (so-called *confounding*) variables to each other and to the disease in the population of interest, from aspects of the selection process (e.g., choice of comparison groups or self-selection patterns), or from measurement or misclassification error. Confounding may be eliminated because of selection features—e.g., when the set of values of a potential confounder is restricted to a narrow range, say by considering only persons of the same age. An important distinction between confounding bias and the other types of bias is that confounding is generally correctable at the analysis stage, whereas selection and information biases are usually difficult, if not impossible, to correct at that stage.

Specific characteristics of each of the three types of bias will be described in detail in the following four chapters, beginning with selection bias.

In this chapter, we have provided general definitions for the terms "validity" and relative "bias." We have distinguished between validity and precision, and between external and internal validity. We have also introduced terminology for describing the possible directions in bias. Finally, we have broadly classified various sources of bias; these sources will be discussed in more detail in subsequent chapters.

10.6 CONCLUDING REMARKS

NOTATION   The following list summarizes the key notation introduced in this chapter.

θ True measure of effect in the target population.

$\hat{\theta}$ Estimator of θ, whose statistical properties depend on the study and actual populations.

$\theta°$ Parameter that $\hat{\theta}$ actually estimates (in a statistical consistency sense)—i.e., $\theta°$ is a parameter in the actual population (which the study population actually represents).

PRACTICE EXERCISES   Determine if the following statements are true or false. Assume throughout that θ is a ratio type of effect measure.

10.1   There is a (nonzero) bias in the estimation of the odds ratio (OR) if the sample estimate $(\hat{OR})$ does not equal the odds ratio $(OR°)$ in the actual population being sampled.

10.2   Systematic error occurs when there is a (nonzero) difference between the true effect measure of interest (θ) and the quantity actually being estimated $(\theta°)$.

10.3   Validity is primarily concerned with random error that results from estimating an effect measure of interest, using a random sample of observations.

10.4   Internal validity concerns inferences that extend beyond the (target) population of restricted interest.

10.5   If $\hat{OR}$ = 3.5 and it is determined that there is a bias away from the null, then the (target) population association of interest, as measured by OR, is greater than 3.5.

10.6   If $\hat{OR}$ = 1.05 and it is determined that any possible bias must be toward the null, then there is essentially no association in the target population (as measured by OR).

10.7   If $\hat{OR}$ = 1.05 and it is determined that any possible bias must be negative, as defined by Equation 10.1, then there is essentially no association in the target population (as measured by OR).

10.8   If θ = 4.5 and $\theta°$ = 1.3, then the bias is toward the null and, in terms of Equation 10.1, is also negative.

10.9   If θ = .35 and $\theta°$ = .95, then the bias is toward the null and, in terms of Equation 10.1, is also positive.

10.10   If θ = 1 and $\theta°$ = 3.5, then the bias is away from the null.

10.11   If θ = 1 and $\theta°$ = .80, then the bias is away from the null.

10.12   If θ = 2.5 and $\theta°$ = .6, then the bias is toward the null and, in terms of Equation 10.1, is also negative.

10.13   Confounding is usually more difficult to correct than is selection bias.

10.14   "Detection" bias, as described by Horwitz and Feinstein (1978), is an example of information bias.

10.15 Selection bias results when the study factor effect of interest is mixed with the effects of extraneous variables.

BERKSON, J. 1946. Limitations of the application of fourfold table analysis to hospital data. *Biomet. Bull.* 2:47–53.

Boston Collaborative Drug Surveillance Program's Report on Reserpine and Breast Cancer. 1974. *Lancet* 2:669–671.

CRIQUI, M. H. 1979. Response bias and risk ratios in epidemiologic studies. *Am. J. Epidemiol.* 109:394–399.

DALES, L. G., and URY, H. K. 1979. An improper use of statistical significance testing in studying covariables. *Int. J. Epidemiol.* 7:373–375.

FEINSTEIN, A. R. 1977. *Clinical biostatistics.* St. Louis: Mosby.

GREENLAND, S. 1977. Response and follow-up bias in cohort studies. *Am. J. Epidemiol.* 106:184–187.

HORWITZ, R. I., and FEINSTEIN, A. R. 1978. Alternate analytic methods for case-control studies of estrogens and endometrial cancer. *N. Engl. J. Med.* 299:1089–1094.

HULKA, B. S.; HOGUE, C. J. R.; and GREENBERG, B. G. 1978. Methodologic issues in epidemiologic studies of endometrial cancer and exogenous estrogen. *Am. J. Epidemiol.* 107:267–276.

HUTCHINSON, G. B., and ROTHMAN, K. J. 1978. Correcting a bias. *N. Engl. J. Med.* 299:1129–1130.

IBRAHIM, M. A., ed. 1979. The case control study: Consensus and controversy. *J. Chronic Dis.* 32:1–144.

KLEINBAUM, D. G.; MORGENSTERN, H.; and KUPPER, L. L. 1981. Selection bias in epidemiologic studies. *Am. J. Epidemiol.* 113:452–463.

MIETTINEN, O. S. 1974. Confounding and effect modification. *Am. J. Epidemiol.* 100:350–353.

———. 1976. Principles of epidemiologic research. Unpublished manuscript. Cambridge, Mass.: Harvard University.

SACKETT, D. L. 1979. Bias in analytic research. *J. Chronic Dis.* 32:51–63.

11

Selection Bias

CHAPTER OUTLINE

As we described in the previous chapter, selection bias is a distortion in the estimate of effect resulting from the manner in which subjects are selected for the study population (i.e., sample). In this chapter, our focus is on specifying quantitative conditions under which selection bias is likely to occur and from which the magnitude and direction of the bias can be determined. We will also discuss and illustrate how these conditions differ by type of study design.

11.0 PREVIEW

The discussion in this chapter closely parallels that of a recent paper by Kleinbaum and colleagues (1981). In addition to previously mentioned papers by Berkson (1946) and Greenland (1977), other contributions to quantitative aspects of selection bias have been made by Roberts and colleagues (1978) and Boyd (1979). The latter two papers deal with Berkson's bias, which we will describe later in this chapter.

The influence of selection factors can be characterized conceptually by comparison of the fourfold table describing the population actually sampled (in this case, the actual population) with the corresponding fourfold table describing the larger target population of interest. This comparison is illustrated in Figure 11.1.

11.1 GENERAL FORMULATION

As the left side of this figure indicates, each of the four cell frequencies for the actual population (denoted by $\mathcal{A}°$, $\mathcal{B}°$, $\mathcal{C}°$, and $\mathcal{D}°$) represents a *subset* of the corresponding frequency for the target population. The relationship between the two tables is described through the quantities α, β, γ, and δ, which are defined as ratios of corresponding cell frequencies, as shown in the table at the right. In essence, the parameters α, β, γ, and δ represent probabilities (or relative frequencies) that a person from a given cell in the target population will be a member of the actual population from which the sample (i.e., study population) is chosen. Hence, these parameters will be referred to as the *population selection probabilities*.

When quantifying the bias in estimation of effect for this situation, we will avoid consideration of specific study designs by letting OR denote any kind of odds ratio (e.g., the risk odds ratio ROR from a follow-up study or the exposure odds ratio EOR from a case-control study) and by letting RP denote any effect measure based on a ratio of two proportions (e.g., the cumulative incidence ratio CIR or the prevalence ratio PR). From Figure 11.1, then, we can write OR = $\mathcal{A}\mathcal{D}/\mathcal{B}\mathcal{C}$ and RP = $\mathcal{A}(\mathcal{B} + \mathcal{D})/\mathcal{B}(\mathcal{A} + \mathcal{C})$, with analogous expressions involving $\mathcal{A}°$, $\mathcal{B}°$, $\mathcal{C}°$, and $\mathcal{D}°$ for OR° and RP°. Substituting these expressions for their corresponding parameters in the formula for bias given by Equation 10.1, we obtain the following results:

$$\text{BIAS}(\hat{\text{OR}}, \text{OR}) = \frac{\text{OR}° - \text{OR}}{\text{OR}} = \left(\frac{\alpha\delta}{\beta\gamma} - 1\right)$$

$$= \left(\frac{r_D - r_{\bar{D}}}{r_{\bar{D}}}\right) = \left(\frac{r_E - r_{\bar{E}}}{r_{\bar{E}}}\right) \tag{11.1}$$

and

$$\text{BIAS}(\hat{\text{RP}}, \text{RP}) = \frac{\text{RP}° - \text{RP}}{\text{RP}} = \left[\frac{\alpha(\mathscr{A} + \mathscr{C})(\beta\mathscr{B} + \delta\mathscr{D})}{\beta(\mathscr{B} + \mathscr{D})(\alpha\mathscr{A} + \gamma\mathscr{C})} - 1\right]$$

$$= \left[\frac{r_E(\mathscr{A} + \mathscr{C})(\mathscr{B}r_{\bar{E}} + \mathscr{D})}{r_{\bar{E}}(\mathscr{B} + \mathscr{D})(\mathscr{A}r_E + \mathscr{C})} - 1\right] \quad (11.2)$$

where

$$r_D = \alpha/\beta = \text{the selection odds for the diseased}$$
$$r_{\bar{D}} = \gamma/\delta = \text{the selection odds for the nondiseased}$$
$$r_E = \alpha/\gamma = \text{the selection odds for the exposed}$$
$$r_{\bar{E}} = \beta/\delta = \text{the selection odds for the nonexposed}$$
$$\alpha\delta/\beta\gamma = \text{the selection odds ratio}$$

Expressions 11.1 and 11.2 provide the quantification necessary for the assessment of selection bias in different types of studies. Using these expressions, we can state conditions for the absence of bias and for the direction of the bias, and we can describe procedures for correcting selection bias. Note that by describing the bias in terms of selection odds r_D and $r_{\bar{D}}$, or r_E and $r_{\bar{E}}$, we allow for the assessment of selection bias without having to identify all four individual selection probabilities. This capability is valuable in practice, since it may be easier to estimate the *relative* sizes of selection probabilities than to determine their absolute values.

Expressions 11.1 and 11.2 in tandem with Figure 11.1 also indicate that an understanding of selection bias requires consideration of how each

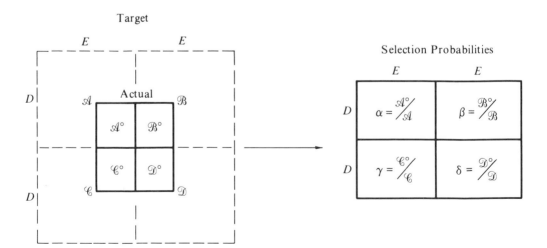

Figure 11.1 Fourfold Tables Relating E with D in Target and Actual Populations

of the cells *within* each fourfold table is altered when going from the target to the actual population. Thus, it is possible that no selection bias will result even if there are differences in all the corresponding cell frequencies (e.g., $\mathscr{A}° \neq \mathscr{A}, \mathscr{B}° \neq \mathscr{B}$, etc.). On the other hand, selection bias can result even if the corresponding distributions of *marginal frequencies* in each table are the same, i.e., $(\mathscr{A}° + \mathscr{B}°)/(\mathscr{A} + \mathscr{B}) = (\mathscr{C}° + \mathscr{D}°)/(\mathscr{C} + \mathscr{D})$ and/or $(\mathscr{A}° + \mathscr{C}°)/(\mathscr{A} + \mathscr{C}) = (\mathscr{B}° + \mathscr{D}°)/(\mathscr{B} + \mathscr{D})$.

From Equation 11.1, it follows that

$$
\text{BIAS}(\hat{\text{OR}}, \text{OR}) \gtreqless 0 \quad \text{if and only if} \quad \begin{cases} \alpha\delta/\beta\gamma \gtreqless 1 \\ \text{or} \quad r_D \gtreqless r_{\bar{D}} \\ \text{or} \quad r_E \gtreqless r_{\bar{E}} \end{cases}
$$

(11.3)

**11.2
DIRECTION
OF
SELECTION
BIAS**

Thus, the existence of selection bias in estimating OR depends on whether or not the cross product $\alpha\delta/\beta\gamma$ is different from one or, equivalently, on whether the selection odds for the diseased (or exposed) is different from the selection odds for the nondiseased (or nonexposed). In particular, the target population odds ratio will be overestimated (i.e., the bias will be positive) if, e.g., exposed cases (DE) and unexposed noncases $(\overline{D}\,\overline{E})$ are collectively overrepresented in comparison to exposed noncases $(\overline{D}E)$ and unexposed cases $(D\overline{E})$, again considered together (i.e., $\alpha\delta > \beta\gamma$). On the other hand, the target population odds ratio will be underestimated (i.e., the bias will be negative) if, among diseased subjects, the exposed and unexposed are equally likely to be selected (i.e., $r_D = 1$), whereas, among nondiseased subjects, the exposed are more likely to be selected than are the unexposed (i.e., $r_{\bar{D}} > 1$). Alternatively, there will be no bias in the odds ratio if the selection odds for exposed persons (r_E) is the same as the selection odds for unexposed persons $(r_{\bar{E}})$, even if diseased persons are overrepresented in comparison to nondiseased persons within exposure groups or overall.

Unfortunately, a statement as concise as Equation 11.3 cannot be made about selection bias in estimating RP. Moreover, despite the rare-disease assumption, there is potential danger in using conditions for bias in $\hat{\text{OR}}$ to draw conclusions about bias in $\hat{\text{RP}}$; this issue will be discussed later. Nevertheless, we can derive the following rule about $\hat{\text{RP}}$ bias through simple algebra:

$$
\text{BIAS}(\hat{\text{RP}}, \text{RP}) = 0 \quad \text{if and only if}
$$

$$
\frac{r_E}{r_{\bar{E}}} = \frac{(\mathscr{B} + \mathscr{D})(\mathscr{A}r_E + \mathscr{C})}{(\mathscr{A} + \mathscr{C})(\mathscr{B}r_{\bar{E}} + \mathscr{D})}
$$

(11.4)

It also follows from Expression 11.4 that

$$\text{BIAS}(\hat{RP}, RP) = 0 \qquad \text{if} \qquad r_E = r_{\bar{E}} = 1$$

$$(\text{i.e., } \alpha = \gamma \text{ and } \beta = \delta) \tag{11.5}$$

Rule 11.5 states that there is no selection bias in estimating RP whenever the selection odds for the exposed and unexposed groups (i.e., r_E and $r_{\bar{E}}$, respectively) are both equal to one. This rule gives a sufficient condition for no bias in $\hat{RP}$ but does not provide a necessary condition. Other rules about $\hat{RP}$ bias involving restrictive assumptions on the selection odds (e.g., restricting r_E to be equal to $r_{\bar{E}}$) are stated in the paper by Kleinbaum and colleagues (1981), and these will not be discussed further here.

11.3 EXAMPLES OF SELECTION BIAS

We now provide four examples of selection bias. The first of these considers bias that can result in case-control studies from the choice of comparison groups. The second illustrates Berkson's bias, which is found in case-control studies restricted to hospital populations. The third illustrates how selection bias can result from loss to follow-up in follow-up studies. And the fourth illustrates the problem of selective survival, which concerns bias that may result from the use of prevalence data to draw conclusions about incidence measures.

EXAMPLE 11.1

In this example we look at selection bias resulting from choice of controls. Horwitz and Feinstein (1978) claim that previous case-control findings of a strong association between the use of estrogen (E) and the presence of endometrial cancer (D) are spurious because of selection bias. The bias, which they refer to as "detection bias," results from selective surveillance of estrogen users (in comparison with nonusers) for detection of disease because of vaginal bleeding that is frequently induced by estrogen. In their 1978 study, they propose a method for avoiding such bias by "proper" choice of a control group. Specifically, they recommend that the controls be gynecological patients with benign tumors who are also subject to greater detection among estrogen users than among nonusers. This choice of control group presumably would then compensate for the increased detection of endometrial cancer among estrogen users.

Table 11.1a translates the argument given by Horwitz and Feinstein into our previous notation for selection probabilities. This table also summarizes contradictory arguments offered by Hutchinson and Rothman (1978). Table 11.1b considers a different control group: other gynecological cancer patients. The subscripts used to describe γ and δ correspond to the control group used.

EXAMPLE 11.1 (*continued*)

Table 11.1   Selection Probabilities in Controversy About Estrogen Use (E) and Presence of Endometrial Cancer (D)

a. Controls: Gynecological Patients with Benign Tumors			b. Controls: Other Gynecological Cancer Patients		
	E	$\overline{E}$		E	$\overline{E}$
D	α	β	D	α	β
$\overline{D}$	γ_1	δ_1	$\overline{D}$	γ_2	δ_2

Horwitz and Feinstein (1978):

$\alpha > \beta \qquad \gamma_1 > \delta_1 \qquad \alpha/\beta = \gamma_1/\delta_1$

Hutchinson and Rothman (1978):

$\alpha = \beta \qquad \gamma_1 > \delta_1$

Horwitz and Feinstein (1978):

$\alpha > \beta \qquad \gamma_2 = \delta_2$

Hutchinson and Rothman (1978):

$\alpha = \beta \qquad \gamma_2 = \delta_2$

From Table 11.1a, we see that, because of selective surveillance, Horwitz and Feinstein claim that $\alpha > \beta$; i.e., estrogen users with the disease are more likely to be selected as cases than are nonusers of estrogen with the disease. They also claim that if gynecological patients with benign tumors are chosen for controls, then $\gamma_1 > \delta_1$ and that, moreover, $r_D = \alpha/\beta$ is approximately equal to $r_{\overline{D}} = \gamma_1/\delta_1$. It then follows, from Expression 11.1 for the bias in EÔR, that

$$\text{BIAS(EÔR, EOR)} = (r_D - r_{\overline{D}})/r_{\overline{D}} = 0$$

i.e., there is no selection bias in estimating EOR.

Hutchinson and Rothman (1978), nevertheless, claim that the rationale of Horwitz and Feinstein is erroneous. They argue, instead, that, because nearly all women with invasive endometrial cancer will ultimately have the disease diagnosed, estrogen users (especially long-term users) will be very little overrepresented among a series of women with endometrial cancer. In terms of selection probabilities, then, Hutchinson and Rothman argue that $\alpha = \beta$. Thus, if gynecological patients with benign tumors are chosen to be controls (so that $\gamma_1 > \delta_1$), it follows that

$$r_D = \alpha/\beta = 1 < r_{\overline{D}} = \gamma_1/\delta_1$$

EXAMPLE 11.1 (*continued*)

From Expression 11.3, we then obtain

$$\text{BIAS}(\hat{\text{EOR}}, \text{EOR}) < 0$$

i.e., there is a negative bias, which underestimates the estrogen-cancer association.

To avoid such bias, Hutchinson and Rothman recommend the use of women with other gynecological cancers as controls. This latter group would not be subject to selective screening (because they would have less tendency for vaginal bleeding); moreover, these conditions would nearly always be detected even without screening. As shown in Table 11.1b, using this control group and accepting Hutchinson and Rothman's point of view, we find $\alpha = \beta$ and $\gamma_2 = \delta_2$, so that $\alpha\delta_2/\beta\gamma_2 = 1$. Thus, from Equation 11.1, we have

$$\text{BIAS}(\hat{\text{EOR}}, \text{EOR}) = (\alpha\delta_2/\beta\gamma_2) - 1 = 0$$

i.e., there is no selection bias in estimating EOR. However, using this control group but accepting the arguments of Horwitz and Feinstein, we find $\alpha > \beta$ and $\gamma_2 = \delta_2$, so that

$$r_D = \alpha/\beta > r_{\bar{D}} = \gamma_2/\delta_2 = 1$$

From Expression 11.3, it then follows that

$$\text{BIAS}(\hat{\text{EOR}}, \text{EOR}) > 0$$

i.e., there is a bias (positive), which would lead to overestimation of the estrogen-cancer association, as Horwitz and Feinstein originally claimed.

The discussion in Example 11.1 illustrates how the choice of control group can affect the occurrence of selection bias. The conclusions about such bias must, nevertheless, consider the knowledge and point of view of the investigator regarding specific characteristics of the variables under study as well as the selection process used.

EXAMPLE 11.2

This example of Berkson's bias in a case-control study (from Roberts et al., 1978; Boyd, 1979) uses a prevalence odds ratio (POR) to measure the effect of hypertension (E) as a risk factor for skin cancer (D) in a stable population of 50,000 people. The fourfold table identifying prevalent cases

EXAMPLE 11.2 (*continued*)

of skin cancer for persons with (E) and without ($\bar{E}$) hypertension in this target population is shown in Table 11.2. Since POR = 1, there is no exposure-disease association in the target population.

Table 11.2   Target Population (Prevalent Cases) for a Case-Control Study of Skin Cancer (D) and Hypertension (E)

	E	$\bar{E}$	
D	500	4,500	5,000
$\bar{D}$	4,500	40,500	45,000
	5,000	45,000	50,000

$$POR = \frac{500 \times 40,500}{4,500 \times 4,500} = 1$$

Let us suppose a case-control study is carried out, using samples of cases and noncases drawn from the hospital that serves this community. According to customary procedure, the comparison group is selected from patients admitted to the hospital with a condition believed to be unrelated to the outcome (skin cancer). For the purpose of this illustration, this group will consist of patients with accidental bone fractures (D^*).

By design, the target population has been altered in two ways: it has been restricted to include only those nondiseased who have accidental bone fractures; secondly, only those persons using hospital services have been admitted into the study. Regarding the first alteration, we will further assume that we can describe the distribution of the three clinical conditions being studied (D = skin cancer, D^* = accidental bone fractures, E = hypertension) in the community population of 50,000 by the Venn diagram given in Figure 11.2.

We derived the numbers in the Venn diagram by assuming that the prevalence of each condition is 10% (i.e., there are 5,000 persons with D, 5,000 with E, and 5,000 with D^*) and that the occurrence of one condition in an individual will not affect the likelihood of his or her having one of the other diseases (i.e., probabilities for each condition are independent). For example, the calculation of the 50 persons identified in the figure as having all three conditions involved the following product: 50,000 × .10 × .10 × .10. Also, the calculation of the 4,050 persons identified as

EXAMPLE 11.2 (*continued*)

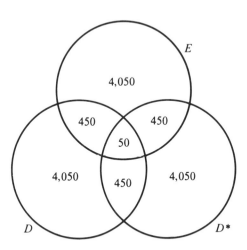

Figure 11.2 Population Distribution of D, D^*, and E

having only D (and neither E nor D^*) was based on the product $50,000 \times .10 \times .90 \times .90$.

Using the Venn diagram, we can obtain the fourfold table to be expected (i.e., the actual population) from the selection of controls (see Table 11.3).

In formulating Table 11.3, we have denoted the actual control group by $\tilde{D}$ and have indicated it to be a subset of the nondiseased (i.e., $\tilde{D} = \overline{D}D^*$). Thus, the $\tilde{D}E$ and $\tilde{D}\overline{E}$ cells exclude persons with disease D. If we had not defined our control group this way, we would have allowed dis-

Table 11.3   Expected (Actual) Population from Choice of Controls

	E	$\overline{E}$
D	500	4,500
$\tilde{D} = \overline{D}D^*$	450	4,050

$$POR^\circ = \frac{500 \times 4,050}{450 \times 4,500} = 1$$

EXAMPLE 11.2 (*continued*)

eased persons to be in the control group. Since the prevalence odds ratio for this table is equal to that of the target population, the choice of controls has not introduced any selection bias into the odds ratio. (Also, the selection probabilities are $\alpha = 1 = \beta$ and $\gamma = .1 = \delta$, so that $\alpha\delta/\beta\gamma = 1$.)

Regarding the second alteration, let us suppose that the probabilities of hospitalization for the community at large are .15 for persons with hypertension (E), .05 for persons with skin cancer (D), and .20 for persons with accidental bone fractures (D^*). If we denote by H_V the event that a person with condition V is hospitalized, then we can write $\mathrm{pr}(H_E) = .15$, $\mathrm{pr}(H_D) = .05$, and $\mathrm{pr}(H_{D^*}) = .20$. We can further argue (see Boyd, 1979) that the probabilities of hospitalization for persons with any two (or all three) conditions are additive; i.e.,

$$\mathrm{pr}(H_{ED}) = \mathrm{pr}(H_E) + \mathrm{pr}(H_D) - \mathrm{pr}(H_E)\mathrm{pr}(H_D)$$

$$\mathrm{pr}(H_{ED^*}) = \mathrm{pr}(H_E) + \mathrm{pr}(H_{D^*}) - \mathrm{pr}(H_E)\mathrm{pr}(H_{D^*})$$

$$\mathrm{pr}(H_{DD^*}) = \mathrm{pr}(H_D) + \mathrm{pr}(H_{D^*}) - \mathrm{pr}(H_D)\mathrm{pr}(H_{D^*})$$

$$\mathrm{pr}(H_{EDD^*}) = \mathrm{pr}(H_E) + \mathrm{pr}(H_D) + \mathrm{pr}(H_{D^*}) - \mathrm{pr}(H_E)\mathrm{pr}(H_D) \\ - \mathrm{pr}(H_E)\mathrm{pr}(H_{D^*}) - \mathrm{pr}(H_D)\mathrm{pr}(H_{D^*}) \\ + \mathrm{pr}(H_E)\mathrm{pr}(H_D)\mathrm{pr}(H_{D^*})$$

Note, e.g., that a person with conditions E and D (but not D^*) may become hospitalized because of E alone, because of D alone, or because of both conditions being present. Hence, $\mathrm{pr}(H_{ED}) = \mathrm{pr}(H_E \text{ or } H_D)$, the latter being the probability of the union of two events.

From the preceding formulas, we can determine the probability of hospitalization and the expected frequency of hospitalized persons for each segment of the Venn diagram, as shown in Figure 11.3. For example, for the 450 people in the population who have both hypertension (E) and bone fractures (D^*) but do not have skin cancer ($\overline{D}$), the probability of being hospitalized is $.15 + .20 - (.15)(.20) = .32$, so that the expected number of hospitalizations is $450 \times .32 = 144$. The remaining percentages and expected numbers are computed as indicated in Table 11.4.

The expected numbers in Table 11.4 can then be grouped to form the fourfold table for the expected hospital population from which the sample will be drawn, as given by Table 11.5. The expected prevalence odds ratio, $\mathrm{POR}^\circ = 1.9$, is nearly twice that of the target population. Thus, we have demonstrated selection bias due to differing rates of hospitalization for the conditions studied. In Table 11.6, this bias is reflected by the selection probabilities α, β, γ, and δ, which yield the following cross product:

EXAMPLE 11.2 (*continued*)

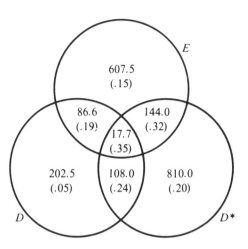

**Figure 11.3 Expected
Hospital Population
and Hospitalization
Probabilities**

Table 11.4   Calculation of Expected Number of Hospitalizations

Segment[a]	Probability of Hospitalization	Expected No. of Hospitalized
$DE \begin{cases} DED* \\ \\ D\bar{E}D* \end{cases}$	.05 + .15 + .20 − (.15)(.05) − (.15)(.20) − (.05)(.20) + (.15)(.05)(.20) = .3540 .05 + .15 − (.05)(.15) = .1925	.3540 × 50 = 17.7 .1925 × 450 = 86.6
$D\bar{E} \begin{cases} D\bar{E}D* \\ D\bar{E}\bar{D}* \end{cases}$	.05 + .20 − (.05)(.20) = .2400 .0500	.2400 × 450 = 108.0 .0500 × 4,050 = 202.5
$\tilde{D}E = \bar{D}ED*$	.15 + .20 − (.15)(.20) = .3200	.3200 × 450 = 144.0
$\tilde{D}\bar{E} = \bar{D}\bar{E}D*$	.2000	.2000 × 4,050 = 810.0
$\bar{D}E\bar{D}*$	.1500	.1500 × 4,050 = 607.5

[a]$\bar{D}$, $\bar{E}$, and $\bar{D}*$ denote the absence of conditions D, E, and $D*$, respectively, and $\tilde{D} = \bar{D}D*$.

EXAMPLE 11.2 (*continued*)

Table 11.5   Expected (Actual) Hospital Population

	E	$\bar{E}$
D	$86.6 + 17.7 = 104.3$	$202.5 + 108.0 = 310.5$
$\bar{D}$	144.0	810.0

$$\text{POR}^\circ = \frac{104.3 \times 810.0}{144.0 \times 310.5} = 1.9$$

$$\alpha\delta/\beta\gamma = (.209 \times .020)/(.032 \times .069) = 1.9 > 1$$

Thus, from Equation 11.3, the bias leads to overestimation of the odds ratio. And from Equation 11.1, we have

$$\text{BIAS}(\hat{\text{POR}}, \text{POR}) = (\text{POR}^\circ - \text{POR})/\text{POR} = (1.9 - 1)/1 = .9$$

In terms of ratios of selection probabilities r_D and $r_{\bar{D}}$, we see that persons with *both* skin cancer and hypertension are about 3 times more likely to be selected into the study than are persons with skin cancer but without hypertension (i.e., $r_D = .209/.069 = 3.03$), whereas persons without skin cancer but with hypertension are only about 1.5 times more likely to be selected than are persons without either skin cancer or hypertension (i.e., $r_{\bar{D}} = .032/.020 = 1.60$). In other words, the selection odds for diseased and nondiseased persons are different:

$$r_D = 3.03 \neq 1.60 = r_{\bar{D}}$$

Moreover, among the four selection probabilities, $\alpha = .209$ is consider-

Table 11.6   Population Selection Probabilities

	E	$\bar{E}$
D	$\alpha = 104.3/500 = .209$	$\beta = 310.5/4{,}500 = .069$
$\bar{D}$	$\gamma = 144.0/4{,}500 = .032$	$\delta = 810.0/40{,}500 = .02$

EXAMPLE 11.2 (*continued*)

ably larger than β, γ, and δ. Thus, in this example, restricting the study to a hospital population is likely to yield a sample that is unrepresentative of the community, because persons with both D and E are much more likely to be selected than persons from any of the other cells of the fourfold table. In other words, persons with both conditions are likely to be overrepresented in the sample in comparison with persons with at most one condition.

A general discussion of the relationship between the size of the (Berkson's) bias and the extent of differences among the three hospitalization rates (for E, D, and D^*) is provided by Boyd (1979). In particular, a general formula for the actual odds ratio in terms of these hospitalization probabilities is as follows:

$$\text{POR}^\circ = \frac{\{1 - [1 - \text{pr}(H_E)][1 - \text{pr}(H_D)][1 - \text{pr}(H_{D^*})\text{pr}(D^*)]\}\text{pr}(H_{D^*})}{\{\text{pr}(H_D) + [1 - \text{pr}(H_D)]\text{pr}(H_{D^*})\text{pr}(D^*)\}}$$
$$\times \{\text{pr}(H_{D^*}) + \text{pr}(H_E) - \text{pr}(H_{D^*})\text{pr}(H_E)\}$$

$$(11.6)$$

where $\text{pr}(D^*)$ denotes the prevalence of condition D^* in the community, and $\text{pr}(H_E)$, $\text{pr}(H_D)$, and $\text{pr}(H_{D^*})$ are the previously defined hospitalization probabilities.

Using this formula, we may derive the following results (see Boyd, 1979):

1. $\text{POR}^\circ = 1$ whenever $\text{pr}(H_E) = 0$; i.e., there is no bias (since $\text{POR} = 1$) if hospitalization due to condition E is not possible.

2. The extent of the bias increases as $\text{pr}(H_E)$ increases.

3. If all three hospitalization probabilities are equal, there may still be selection bias, with the size of the bias increasing as $\text{pr}(D^*)$ increases. However, the size of such bias will be relatively small in comparison to a situation involving markedly different hospitalization probabilities.

4. $\text{POR}^\circ \leq 1$ if $\text{pr}(H_D) > \text{pr}(H_{D^*})$, whereas $\text{POR}^\circ \geq 1$ if $\text{pr}(H_D) < \text{pr}(H_{D^*})$.

As an illustration of the small bias that can result when hospitalization probabilities are all equal, we will consider the same target population and prevalence rates (.10) that we had above, but we will suppose that the hospitalization probabilities are each .05 for E, D, and D^*. Using Equation 11.6, we obtain

$$\text{POR}^\circ = \frac{\{1 - (1 - .05)(1 - .05)[1 - (.05)(.10)]\}(.05)}{[.05 + (1 - .05)(.05)(.10)][.05 + .05 - (.05)(.05)]} = .96$$

EXAMPLE 11.2 (*continued*)

Thus, since POR $= 1$, the bias is insignificant. Note also that the expected hospital population for this example can be described by the fourfold table given in Table 11.7.

Table 11.7   Expected Hospital Population When Hospitalization Probabilities for E, D, and $D*$ Are Each .05

	E	$\bar{E}$
D	51.0	246.4
$\tilde{D}$	43.9	202.5

$$\text{POR}° = \frac{51.0 \times 202.5}{43.9 \times 246.4} = .96$$

EXAMPLE 11.3

This example illustrates selection bias from loss to follow-up. Suppose that the fourfold table describing the five-year incidence of disease D with respect to study factor E for a fixed cohort target population is as shown in Table 11.8a. Here, ROR denotes the risk odds ratio and CIR denotes the cumulative incidence ratio, both of which are measurable in follow-up studies (see Chapter 8).

Let us suppose we conduct a study to follow this population for five years, and let us suppose that subjects who were exposed and later developed the disease were 2.25 times as likely *not to be lost* to follow-up as were subjects who were exposed and later did *not* develop the disease. In addition, suppose that subjects who were not exposed initially, but who later developed the disease, were also 2.25 times as likely not to be lost to follow-up as were unexposed subjects who did not develop the disease. Using our previous notation, we have $\alpha = 2.25\gamma$ and $\beta = 2.25\delta$, from which it follows that

$$r_E = \alpha/\gamma = 2.25 = \beta/\delta = r_{\bar{E}}$$

Thus, from Equation 11.3, BIAS($\hat{\text{ROR}}$, ROR) $= 0$. And from Equation 11.2, we find

EXAMPLE 11.3 (*continued*)

Table 11.8 Selection Bias Caused by Loss to Follow-up

a. Fixed Cohort (Target) Population If No Losses from Five-Year Follow-up		b. Actual Population Based on Expected Losses from Five-Year Follow-up	
E	$\bar{E}$	E	$\bar{E}$

	E	$\bar{E}$		E	$\bar{E}$
D	1,000	500	D	$1,000\alpha = 2,250\gamma$	$500\beta = 1,125\delta$
$\bar{D}$	9,000	9,500	$\bar{D}$	$9,000\gamma$	$9,500\delta$
	10,000	10,000			

$$\text{ROR} = \frac{1,000 \times 9,500}{500 \times 9,000} = 2.11$$

$$\text{CIR} = \frac{1,000/10,000}{500/10,000} = 2.00$$

$$\text{ROR}^\circ = \frac{2,250\gamma \times 9,500\delta}{1,125\delta \times 9,000\gamma} = 2.11$$

$$\text{CIR}^\circ = \frac{2,250\gamma/(2,250\gamma + 9,000\gamma)}{1,125\delta/(1,125\delta + 9,500\delta)} = 1.89$$

$$\text{BIAS}(\hat{\text{CIR}}, \text{CIR}) = \left[\frac{2.25(10,000)(10,625)}{2.25(10,000)(11,250)} - 1 \right]$$
$$= (.94 - 1) = -.06$$

i.e., CIR = 2.0, whereas CIR° = 1.89, as shown in Table 11.8b. You will notice that, although $r_E = r_{\bar{E}}$, there is some bias in estimating CIR, even though the bias is small. However, there is no bias in estimating ROR.

Example 11.3 illustrates that, in follow-up studies, selection bias in estimating CIR may result from loss to follow-up, which concerns the manner in which subjects are selected for analysis after initial selection into the study (Greenland, 1977). The magnitude and direction of the bias in $\hat{\text{CIR}}$ can usually be approximated from Expressions 11.1 and/or 11.3 for the bias in $\hat{\text{OR}}$, although, as we will discuss later, the difference in these biases can be substantial under certain circumstances.

EXAMPLE 11.4

In cross-sectional studies, we obtain *prevalence* data, although we usually are interested in making inferences about *incidence* measures (ROR, CIR, or IDR). This strategy can lead to erroneous conclusions if the probability of death from the disease under study or from other causes is different among the four cells of the target population. To illustrate this problem, which is commonly referred to as *selective survival,* let us suppose that Table 11.9 describes the incidence of disease from time 0 to time 1 for the follow-up of a fixed cohort of 10,000 persons who were disease-free at time 0. We would like to compare the results from this follow-up study with expected results from a cross-sectional study carried out on "survivors" at time 1.

In considering such a cross-sectional study, we will further suppose that the following conditions obtain:

1. No new persons enter the population between time 0 and time 1.
2. Exposed persons who develop the disease are ten times as likely to have died by time 1 as are exposed persons who do not develop the disease.
3. Unexposed persons who develop the disease are twice as likely to have died by time 1 as are unexposed persons who do not develop the disease.
4. The short-term cumulative case fatality for persons who develop the disease between time 0 and time 1 is about 50%, whether exposed or unexposed.

(We recognize that this example is unrealistic, since cross-sectional studies are usually carried out for dynamic populations. However, we find this example convenient pedagogically for illustrating the problem of selective survival.)

Table 11.9 Incidence for Target Population: Time 0 to Time 1

	E	$\bar{E}$		
D	500	800	1,300	ROR = 3
$\bar{D}$	1,500	7,200	8,700	CIR = 2.5
	2,000	8,000	10,000	

EXAMPLE 11.4 (*continued*)

Translating the above information into our previous notation, we find

$$\frac{1-\alpha}{1-\gamma} = 10, \qquad \frac{1-\beta}{1-\delta} = 2, \qquad 1-\alpha = 1-\beta = .50$$

where α, β, γ, and δ represent *selective survival probabilities*. Algebraically, it then follows that $\alpha = .50 = \beta$, $\gamma = .95$, $\delta = .75$, $r_E = \alpha/\gamma = .526$, and $r_{\bar{E}} = .667$. Using Equations 11.1 and 11.2, we can obtain the biases due to selective survival when estimating the incidence measures ROR and CIR with prevalence data–based estimators $\widehat{POR}$ and $\widehat{PR}$, respectively, obtained from a cross-sectional sample at time 1:

$$\text{BIAS}(\widehat{POR}, \text{ROR}) = (.789 - 1) = -.211$$
$$\text{BIAS}(\widehat{PR}, \text{CIR}) = (.866 - 1) = -.134$$

Table 11.10 describes the expected cross-sectional population at time 1 (i.e., the actual population) based on the selective survival probabilities above.

Table 11.10   Expected Cross-Sectional (Actual) Population at Time 1

	E	$\bar{E}$	
D	250	400	$\text{POR}^\circ = 2.368$
$\bar{D}$	1,425	5,400	$\text{PR}^\circ = 2.164$

As a result of selective survival, then, a slightly negative bias occurs when either ROR or CIR is the target parameter. That is, the use of prevalence data at time 1 would lead to an underestimate of incidence measures of association.

11.4 DISCUSSION OF THE EXAMPLES

The numerical examples in the previous section suggest that, when one is considering selection bias in estimating RP, it is sufficient, in practice, to focus on the relatively simple conditions given by Equations 11.1 and 11.3 for the odds ratio. The fact that the odds ratio is frequently a good approximation to the cumulative incidence ratio would appear to lend further support to this practical rule. Nevertheless, this viewpoint is potentially dangerous, as illustrated by the following example.

EXAMPLE 11.5

Consider the same follow-up target population as given in Table 11.8a but with a different set of selection probabilities, namely, $\alpha = 1$, $\beta = 1$, $\gamma = .01$, and $\delta = .01$ (so that $r_E = 100 = r_{\bar{E}}$). Table 11.11 gives the actual population for these probabilities. This table illustrates that, although the disease is rare in the target population, a relatively large selection bias for CIR is encountered, whereas no selection bias is found for OR. The disease is not rare in the actual population, since the overall cumulative incidence is $1,500/1,685 = .89$. In this example, we see that the assessment of selection bias for RP (i.e., CIR or PR), using the conditions for selection bias for OR, must take into account the rare-disease assumption in the altered (i.e., actual) population as well as in the target population. If the disease is rare in both the target and actual populations, then the extent and direction of the bias in estimating RP can be approximately assessed by using Equations 11.1 and 11.3. However, if the rare-disease assumption does not hold in *both* populations, then the bias in $\hat{OR}$ may be quite different from that in $\hat{RP}$.

Table 11.11   Actual Population from Follow-up Loss ($\alpha = 1 = \beta$, $\gamma = .01 = \delta$) in Target Population of Table 11.8a

	E	$\bar{E}$	
D	1,000	500	$ROR° = 2.11 = ROR$
$\bar{D}$	90	95	$CIR° = 1.09 < CIR = 2.00$
	1,090	595	

As these examples have demonstrated, the general mathematical conditions for selection bias in OR and RP given by Expressions 11.1 through 11.5 are applicable to specific measures of effect appropriate for different study designs. Although the underlying mathematical basis is the same, however, it is important to realize that the selection probabilities α, β, γ, and δ take on different interpretations, depending on the study design and the associated type of selection bias under consideration. For example, in follow-up studies (where CIR is customarily the measure of interest), the primary source of bias is loss to follow-up of persons initially selected to be studied. The *initial* selection process from a target (healthy) population to a study population will not contribute to selection bias, because samples of subjects from both the exposed (E) and unexposed ($\bar{E}$) groups in the target population do not have the illness at the beginning of follow-up.

Case-control studies differ considerably from follow-up studies with regard to sources of selection bias. In fact, avoiding or correcting for such biases appears to be much more difficult in case-control studies, and substantial disagreement exists about the merits of such studies (see Ibrahim, 1979). To be specific, the outcome variable (exposure status) in case-control studies has already occurred prior to the time when study subjects (diseased and nondiseased) are selected; consequently, the selection of cases and/or controls may be influenced by exposure status. Some common sources of selection bias in case-control studies involve the initial choice of the control group, the selection of the sampling frame (e.g., a hospital in which there may be differing patterns of service utilization), and exclusions made from the case and control groups. Another source of selection bias in case-control studies, which is tied to the use of prevalent (in contrast to incident) cases, is selective survival. The problem here is that those persons who develop the disease but die prior to the time of the study obviously cannot be included in the study population. If exposure status happens to be over- or underrepresented in the survivors, then the use of prevalence data to estimate incidence-based risk or odds ratios can lead to biased results.

The cross-sectional study contains some of the same sources of selection bias as the case-control study contains (e.g., selection of the sampling frame and selective survival when one is using prevalence data to estimate incidence measures). However, a case-control study can be designed to utilize incident (new) cases, thereby reducing the likelihood of selective survival and possibly other forms of selection bias. However, case-control studies involve sampling from two (or more) populations, whereas cross-sectional studies involve sampling from only one population. Consequently, the case-control study is characterized by additional sources of bias relating to separate selection processes in the choice of comparison groups. For example, unequal diagnostic surveillance, as discussed in the context of studies of endometrial cancer and estrogen use (Horwitz and Feinstein, 1978), is a source of selection bias for a case-control study but can manifest itself in a follow-up study as misclassification.

11.5 WHAT CAN BE DONE ABOUT SELECTION BIAS?

The question of avoiding or correcting for selection bias concerns both what can be done at the design stage (i.e., before data collection has begun) and what can be done at the analysis stage (i.e., after the data have been collected). We discuss both issues below.

Avoiding selection bias through proper design depends on the extent to which the investigator is aware of potential sources of such bias in the anticipated study. If the potential for selection bias can be associated with a possible confounding variable, then such bias may be avoided either by subject restriction with regard to this variable or by accurate measurement of the variable so that it can be controlled in the analysis. For example, in a study of reserpine use as a risk factor for breast cancer (Boston Collaborative Study, 1974), selection bias could have been partially corrected if socioeconomic status had been measured, thus allowing for control at the analysis stage.

11.5.1
Design Aspects

In case-control studies, researchers frequently use two or more control groups, one of which may be a community sample. The primary value of this procedure lies in the detection of selection bias via comparison of estimates of effect from different sets of controls. If the effects do not differ, there is no bias in selection; if they differ, then some selection bias is indicated. However, two effect estimates with the same value may simply be exhibiting the same degree of selection bias. The determination of the most appropriate control group depends largely on the extent of one's a priori knowledge of selection probability ratios. This consideration is the primary issue in the current controversy over choosing the proper controls in studying possible carcinogenic effects of estrogen (Hutchinson and Rothman, 1978), as we previously illustrated.

In follow-up studies, efforts to prevent or to minimize selection bias prior to analysis are primarily involved with ensuring complete follow-up of the initial cohort and obtaining as large a response rate as possible. However, because the presence of selection bias is determined from the selection probabilities *within* the fourfold table, selection bias may occur even with a relatively large overall response rate and/or very little loss to follow-up in each exposure category. Conversely, there may be no selection bias despite small response rates and/or large follow-up losses in each exposure category.

The degree to which selection bias can be corrected after the data have been gathered depends on whether or not reliable estimates of the underlying selection or loss probabilities can be determined. Table 11.12 illustrates how each cell of the fourfold table for the study population can be adjusted if estimates of the selection probabilities $\hat{\alpha}$, $\hat{\beta}$, $\hat{\gamma}$, and $\hat{\delta}$ are available. Corrected estimates of OR and RP can be directly derived from the adjusted study population:

11.5.2
Analysis
Aspects

$$\hat{OR}(\text{corrected}) = \hat{A}\hat{D}/\hat{B}\hat{C} = (\hat{\beta}\hat{\gamma}/\hat{\alpha}\hat{\delta})\,\hat{OR} = (\hat{r}_{\overline{E}}/\hat{r}_E)\hat{OR} = (\hat{r}_{\overline{D}}/\hat{r}_D)\hat{OR}$$

where $\hat{r}_E = \hat{\alpha}/\hat{\gamma}$, $\hat{r}_{\overline{E}} = \hat{\beta}/\hat{\delta}$, $\hat{r}_D = \hat{\alpha}/\hat{\beta}$, $\hat{r}_{\overline{D}} = \hat{\gamma}/\hat{\delta}$, and $\hat{OR} = ad/bc$. Such adjustment is also possible when estimates of only the *ratios* of the unknown selection probabilities are available. (Adjustments are also possible in terms of estimated *loss* probabilities $\hat{\alpha}' = 1 - \hat{\alpha}$, $\hat{\beta}' = 1 - \hat{\beta}$, $\hat{\gamma}' = 1 - \hat{\gamma}$, and $\hat{\delta}' = 1 - \hat{\delta}$.)

Table 11.12   Adjusting the Study Population

STUDY POPULATION						ADJUSTED STUDY POPULATION	
	E	$\overline{E}$		E	$\overline{E}$	E	$\overline{E}$
D	a	b	D	$\hat{\alpha}$	$\hat{\beta}$	$\hat{A} = a/\hat{\alpha}$	$\hat{B} = b/\hat{\beta}$
$\overline{D}$	c	d	$\overline{D}$	$\hat{\gamma}$	$\hat{\delta}$	$\hat{C} = c/\hat{\gamma}$	$\hat{D} = d/\hat{\delta}$

In practice, estimation of the selection or loss probabilities (or even of their ratios) is quite difficult, since it usually requires either information from another study (e.g., a study of those lost to follow-up or of nonrespondents) or knowledge of such selection probabilities for related studies. For these reasons, the investigator must realize that selection bias may exist even though it cannot be precisely determined or adjusted for.

However, if one is able to specify the relative magnitudes of the ratios r_E and $r_{\overline{E}}$ (or r_D and $r_{\overline{D}}$), then one may assess the direction of the bias. For example, if $r_E > r_{\overline{E}}$ (or if $r_D > r_{\overline{D}}$), then any bias found in the odds ratio estimate must be positive.

The potential impact of selection bias may be assessed in terms of "practical" threshold levels for bias, as specified by the investigator, provided that sufficiently narrow ranges for the selection probabilities or their odds can be determined. For instance, if $p*$ denotes the minimum of $\{\alpha, \beta, \gamma, \delta\}$ and if ϵ denotes a threshold level that identifies a "practically insignificant" bias (e.g., $|\theta° - \theta| \leq \epsilon$, where $\theta = $ OR), such a relationship can be derived algebraically (using Expressions 11.1 and 11.2), giving

$$|OR° - OR| \leq \epsilon \quad \text{if and only if} \quad p* \geq 1/\sqrt{1 + \epsilon/OR} \quad (11.7)$$

In Table 11.13, we have used Expression 11.7 to compute values for $p*$ that will ensure that $|OR° - OR| \leq \epsilon$, given ϵ/OR. Thus, if $\epsilon = $ OR/2, then $p*$ must be as large as .82 in order to ensure that no practically important selection bias exists. In contrast, if $\epsilon = $ OR/16, then the corresponding minimum probability is approximately .97.

We note that, for fixed ϵ, the function $1/\sqrt{1 + \epsilon/OR}$ increases toward one as OR increases. In other words, the larger the value of the true odds ratio, the larger the minimum selection probability must be for the investigator to be certain that no meaningful selection bias exists. [Nevertheless, it is not possible to provide convenient guidelines for identifying practical ranges for the selection probabilities (e.g., the value of $p*$) or their odds. Such guidelines would require information about the actual population under study and the specific research design used.]

Table 11.13 Minimum Selection Probabilities,
$p* = 1/\sqrt{1+\epsilon/OR}$, Required for $|OR° - OR| \leq \epsilon$

ϵ/OR	$p*$	ϵ/OR	$p*$
0	1	2	.58
$\vdots$	$\vdots$	4	.45
$\frac{1}{32}$	.98	8	.33
$\frac{1}{16}$	.97	16	.24
$\frac{1}{8}$	.94	32	.17
$\frac{1}{4}$	.89	$\vdots$	$\vdots$
$\frac{1}{2}$	.82	∞	0
1	.71		

In all the deliberations above, we have assumed either that no other sources of bias exist (e.g., information bias or confounding) in the study or that other biases have been sufficiently adjusted for or have canceled one another out. In reality, these assumptions are likely to be untenable; therefore, any corrections for selection bias must be considered in conjunction with corrections for other biases. Clearly, this problem is more complicated than one in which selection bias is the sole consideration.

11.6 CON-CLUDING REMARKS

The following list summarizes the key notation introduced in this chapter.

NOTATION

OR	Odds ratio effect measure (e.g., ROR in follow-up studies, EOR in case-control studies, POR in cross-sectional studies).
RP	Effect measure that is the ratio of two proportions (e.g., RR = CIR in follow-up studies, PR in cross-sectional studies).
OR°	Odds ratio in actual population (which is estimated by $\hat{OR}$).
RP°	Ratio of proportions in actual population (which is estimated by $\hat{RP}$).
$r_D = \alpha/\beta$	Selection odds for diseased subjects.
$r_{\bar{D}} = \gamma/\delta$	Selection odds for nondiseased subjects.
$r_E = \alpha/\gamma$	Selection odds for exposed subjects.
$r_{\bar{E}} = \beta/\delta$	Selection odds for nonexposed subjects.
$\alpha\delta/\beta\gamma$	Selection odds ratio.
$\tilde{D}$	Control group in case-control study (Berkson's bias example), which is a subset of nondiseased ($\bar{D}$) subjects in target population.

$\mathrm{pr}(H_V)$	Probability of being hospitalized because of characteristic V (V may consist of one or more illness conditions).
$\hat{\alpha},\ \hat{\beta},\ \hat{\gamma},\ \hat{\delta}$	Estimated selection probabilities.
$\hat{A},\ \hat{B},\ \hat{C},\ \hat{D}$	Corrected cell counts (e.g., $\hat{A} = a/\hat{\alpha},\ \hat{B} = b/\hat{\beta}$, etc.).
ϵ	Threshold level for a practically insignificant bias—i.e., $\lvert \theta^{\circ} - \theta \rvert \le \epsilon$.
$p*$	Minimum of $\{\alpha,\ \beta,\ \gamma,\ \delta\}$.

PRACTICE EXERCISES

11.1 Determine if the following statements are true or false.

   a. In a case-control study, a primary source of selection bias is loss to follow-up.

   b. In a follow-up study, a primary source of selection bias is selective survival.

   c. If, in a follow-up study, both the exposed (E) and the unexposed ($\bar{E}$) have equal probabilities of loss to follow-up, then there will be no selection bias (due to loss of follow-up) in estimating the CIR.

   d. If, in a case-control study, $r_D = \alpha/\beta = 2.5$ and $r_{\bar{D}} = \gamma/\delta = 1.5$, then there will be selection bias in estimating OR, which will be away from the null (assuming OR ≥ 1).

   e. If, in a follow-up study, $r_E = \alpha/\gamma = 1$ and $r_{\bar{E}} = \beta/\delta = 1$ from loss to follow-up, then there will be no selection bias in estimating the CIR.

   f. If the selection probabilities satisfy $\alpha = \gamma$ and $\beta = 2\delta$, then one may conclude, with regard to estimating the odds ratio, that the true association is likely to be stronger than the observed association. (Hint: Do not assume that OR ≥ 1.)

   g. If it is assumed that OR < 1, that $\alpha = \gamma$, and that $\beta = 2\delta$, then one may conclude that the true association is likely to be stronger than the observed association.

   h. If the bias in the odds ratio is away from the null, then the bias in the risk ratio must also be away from the null.

   i. Suppose that, in a case-control study, the selection probabilities satisfy $\alpha < \beta$ and $\gamma > \delta$. Then, the observed odds ratio is likely to underestimate the true target population odds ratio.

   j. Selective survival concerns the bias that can result when using an estimate of effect based on prevalence data to draw conclusions about an effect based on incidence data.

   k. It is possible to correct a sample estimate of effect for selection bias if reliable estimates of ratios of selection probabilities (e.g., r_E and $r_{\bar{E}}$) can be obtained.

11.2 In Example 11.2 describing Berkson's bias, we have shown, via Expression 11.6, how to determine the bias in the odds ratio that may result from a hospital-based case-control study when there is a risk of hospitalization due to the presence of the exposure conditions (in addition to such a risk for both diseased and nondiseased groups).

   a. For hospitalization probabilities of .05 for each of the E = hypertension,

D = skin cancer, and $D*$ = bone fracture conditions, and for community prevalence rates of .10 for each of these conditions, draw a Venn diagram, analogous to Figure 11.3, that shows the *expected* hospital population and hospitalization probabilities for persons with various combinations of the above three conditions.

b. Use your answer to part a to verify the structure for the expected hospital population given by Table 11.7.

c. Calculate the selection probabilities α, β, γ, and δ for the situation described in part a.

d. For the situation in part a, calculate the bias in the estimated odds ratio, using Expression 11.1. Verify that this result is the same as that obtained by using Expression 11.6.

e. Suppose the hospitalization probability for hypertensives is zero, with the other probabilities in part a remaining unchanged. Verify, using Equation 11.6, that there will be no bias in estimating the odds ratio.

f. Suppose the hospitalization probability for hypertensives is one, with the other probabilities in part a remaining unchanged. What odds ratio will be expected for the hospital population? How does this result compare with the previous results obtained in parts d and e?

g. Suppose the hospitalization probabilities are .15 for E, .20 for D, and .05 for $D*$, with the prevalence rates as before. Compute the expected odds ratio for this situation, and then compare the direction of the bias thus obtained with the direction when the hospitalization probabilities for D and $D*$ are .05 and .20, respectively, as they were in Example 11.2. What general principle about the direction of Berkson's bias has been illustrated here?

11.3 The following questions concern the assessment of selection bias in observational studies where the putative association between salt intake and hypertension is being investigated. It is hypothesized that persons who have a greater intake of salt are at greater risk of developing chronic hypertension. It will be assumed that both variables are dichotomized: *high* and *low* salt intake; *hypertensive* (DBP $\geq$ 95 and/or SBP $\geq$ 160) and *normotensive*. In considering the following questions, you may ignore the possibility of either information bias or confounding. Also, assume that the target CIR, OR, and PR are all greater than one.

Formulate *each* situation below in terms of the selection probabilities $(\alpha, \beta, \gamma, \delta)$, the loss probabilities $(\alpha', \beta', \gamma', \delta')$, or the selection odds $(r_E, r_{\bar{E}}, r_D, r_{\bar{D}})$. Then, answer the following two questions for *each* situation, giving a brief explanation for your answers:

i. Will there be selection bias in estimating the (target population) measure of effect?

ii. Will the selection bias, if it exists, be toward or away from the null value?

a. Consider a *follow-up study* involving an equal number of high- and low-salt consumers who are normotensive at the start of follow-up. It is believed that each group is representative of the population of normotensives with such salt intake patterns. The subjects are followed for five years to monitor the development of hypertension. Suppose that the likelihood of remaining in the study is greater for the exposed than for the unexposed, and that those who become hypertensive and those who remain normotensive within each exposure category are equally likely to remain in the study. What can be said about the bias in estimating ROR and CIR given the above information?

b. Given the same situation as in part a, suppose that 2% of the original cohort becomes hypertensive. If the probability of remaining in the study is greatest for the low-salt normotensives and is lowest for the low-salt hypertensives, while that for high-salt hypertensives and high-salt normotensives is the same, what can be said about the bias in estimating ROR and CIR?

c. Consider a *cross-sectional study* in which a random sample is selected from the population of interest. What would you say about the bias in estimating PR and POR if you had 100% cooperation from those you wished to sample?

d. For the same cross-sectional study described in part c, suppose you knew that low-salt-intake hypertensives, high-salt-intake normotensives, and low-salt-intake normotensives are equally likely to die, but all are 1/5 as likely to die as high-salt-intake hypertensives. You still have 100% cooperation. What can you say about the bias in estimating ROR?

e. Consider a *case-control study,* in which equal numbers of hypertensives (cases) and normotensives (controls) are enrolled. Suppose that hypertensives in the study are gathered from an outpatient clinic designed to screen for hypertensives in the population, using the clinic on a volunteer basis. Normotensives are selected randomly from the surrounding population served by the clinic. Suppose that high-salt-intake hypertensives are four times as likely to be screened as low-salt-intake hypertensives in the clinic and that the sample of normotensives from the surrounding community is indeed a representative sample. What can be said about the bias in estimating EOR?

f. In a type of case-control study similar to that described in part e, suppose that high- and low-salt-intake hypertensives are equally likely to be screened but that high-salt-intake normotensives in the community are more likely to cooperate in the study than are low-salt-intake normotensives in the community. What can be said about the bias in estimating EOR?

REFERENCES   BERKSON, J. 1946. Limitations of the application of fourfold table analysis to hospital data. *Biomet. Bull.* 2: 47–53.

Boston Collaborative Drug Surveillance Program's Report on Reserpine and Breast Cancer. 1974. *Lancet* 2: 669–671.

BOYD, A. V. 1979. Testing for association of diseases. *J. Chronic Dis.* 32: 667–672.

GREENLAND, S. 1977. Response and follow-up bias in cohort studies. *Am. J. Epidemiol.* 106: 184–187.

HORWITZ, R. I., and FEINSTEIN, A. R. 1978. Alternate analytic methods for case-control studies of estrogens and endometrial cancer. *N. Engl. J. Med.* 299: 1089–1094.

HUTCHINSON, G. B., and ROTHMAN, K. J. 1978. Correcting a bias. *N. Engl. J. Med.* 299: 1129–1130.

IBRAHIM, M. A., ed. 1979. The case-control study: Consensus and controversy. *J. Chronic Dis.* 32: 1–144.

KLEINBAUM, D. G.; MORGENSTERN, H.; and KUPPER, L. L. 1981. Selection bias in epidemiologic studies. *Am. J. Epidemiol.* 113: 452–463.

ROBERTS, R. S.; SPITZER, W. O.; DELMORE, T.; and SACKETT, D. L. 1978. An empirical demonstration of Berkson's bias. *J. Chronic Dis.* 31: 119–128.

12

Information Bias

CHAPTER OUTLINE

As introduced in Chapter 10, information bias refers to a distortion in esti- **12.0**
mation of the effect of interest that results when measurement of either the **PREVIEW**
exposure condition (E) or the disease condition (D) is systematically inaccurate. Among the various sources of such error are the use of a measurement device that has a built-in or induced defect; a questionnaire, interview
procedure, or index derived therefrom that does not measure what it pur-
ports to measure; an inaccurate diagnostic procedure (for disease status);
or an incomplete or erroneous data source, e.g., as would occur when subject recall of exposure history is selective. (See Sackett, 1979, for a catalog
of various sources of bias.) Whatever the source of error in the information
obtained, a study subject may, as a result, be misclassified in terms of disease and/or exposure status. In this chapter, we will focus on the potential
consequences of such *misclassification* on the estimated effect measure of
interest, again restricting ourselves to the situation in which both the disease and the exposure variables are dichotomous. We will henceforth use
the term *misclassification bias* (instead of "information bias") to emphasize
our attention here to the consequences of having inaccurate information on
categorically treated factors.

In the discussion to follow, we will demonstrate how the general
framework used in Chapter 11 to describe selection bias also incorporates
misclassification bias: the *target population* is represented here by a fourfold table that assumes no misclassification of any kind, and the *actual
population* is described by a fourfold table reflecting the (expected)
misclassification. In contrast to the fourfold table for the selection bias
situation, the fourfold table for the misclassified actual population represents a *rearrangement* rather than a *subset* of the target population, as
described by Table 12.1. In Table 12.1a, the $\mathcal{A}$ persons who are truly
diseased and exposed (DE) are classified into each of the four cells of
Table 12.1b: $\mathcal{A}_{11}^{\circ}$ are classified as diseased and exposed $(D'E')$; $\mathcal{B}_{11}^{\circ}$ are
classified as diseased and unexposed $(D'\overline{E}')$; $\mathcal{C}_{11}^{\circ}$ as nondiseased and
exposed $(\overline{D}'E')$; and $\mathcal{D}_{11}^{\circ}$ as nondiseased and unexposed $(\overline{D}'\overline{E}')$. In other
words, $\mathcal{A} = \mathcal{A}_{11}^{\circ} + \mathcal{B}_{11}^{\circ} + \mathcal{C}_{11}^{\circ} + \mathcal{D}_{11}^{\circ}$. A similar rearrangement is shown
for the $\mathcal{B}$ persons who are truly $D\overline{E}$, the $\mathcal{C}$ persons who are $\overline{D}E$, and the
$\mathcal{D}$ persons who are $\overline{D}\,\overline{E}$. Consequently, the $\mathcal{A}^{\circ}$ persons (in Table 12.1b)
who are *classified* as diseased and exposed are derived from the four cells
of the target population (Table 12.1a), as expressed by $\mathcal{A}^{\circ} = \mathcal{A}_{11}^{\circ} + \mathcal{A}_{12}^{\circ} + \mathcal{A}_{21}^{\circ} + \mathcal{A}_{22}^{\circ}$; similar statements apply to $\mathcal{B}^{\circ}$, $\mathcal{C}^{\circ}$, and $\mathcal{D}^{\circ}$.

Because we now are considering such a rearrangement, the parame-
ters α, β, γ, and δ, previously defined to relate the target and actual populations for selection bias, can no longer represent probabilities, since
some of these values can exceed one. These parameters can, however, be
expressed as functions of more fundamental sensitivity and specificity parameters, which are probabilities. The *sensitivity* (ϕ) for a given condition
is defined as the probability that a person with the condition will be classified in one's study as having the condition. *Specificity* (ψ) is defined as the
probability that a person without the condition will be classified in one's

Table 12.1   Misclassification Bias: Target Versus Actual Populations

a. Target Population (No Misclassification)

	E	$\overline{E}$
D	$\mathcal{A} = \mathcal{A}^{\circ}_{11} + \mathcal{B}^{\circ}_{11} + \mathcal{C}^{\circ}_{11} + \mathcal{D}^{\circ}_{11}$	$\mathcal{B} = \mathcal{A}^{\circ}_{12} + \mathcal{B}^{\circ}_{12} + \mathcal{C}^{\circ}_{12} + \mathcal{D}^{\circ}_{12}$
$\overline{D}$	$\mathcal{C} = \mathcal{A}^{\circ}_{21} + \mathcal{B}^{\circ}_{21} + \mathcal{C}^{\circ}_{21} + \mathcal{D}^{\circ}_{21}$	$\mathcal{D} = \mathcal{A}^{\circ}_{22} + \mathcal{B}^{\circ}_{22} + \mathcal{C}^{\circ}_{22} + \mathcal{D}^{\circ}_{22}$

$\longrightarrow$

b. Actual (Classified) Population

	E'	$\overline{E}'$
D'	$\mathcal{A}^{\circ} = \mathcal{A}^{\circ}_{11} + \mathcal{A}^{\circ}_{12} + \mathcal{A}^{\circ}_{21} + \mathcal{A}^{\circ}_{22}$	$\mathcal{B}^{\circ} = \mathcal{B}^{\circ}_{11} + \mathcal{B}^{\circ}_{12} + \mathcal{B}^{\circ}_{21} + \mathcal{B}^{\circ}_{22}$
$\overline{D}'$	$\mathcal{C}^{\circ} = \mathcal{C}^{\circ}_{11} + \mathcal{C}^{\circ}_{12} + \mathcal{C}^{\circ}_{21} + \mathcal{C}^{\circ}_{22}$	$\mathcal{D}^{\circ} = \mathcal{D}^{\circ}_{11} + \mathcal{D}^{\circ}_{12} + \mathcal{D}^{\circ}_{21} + \mathcal{D}^{\circ}_{22}$

study as being without the condition. In the ideal study, then, both the sensitivity and specificity should be one. Mathematical expressions for misclassification bias and for possible adjustments to correct for such bias are generally expressible in terms of sensitivity and specificity parameters, as we will show in this chapter.

We will first provide a brief review of the literature; then we will give some simple examples of misclassification bias. Following the examples, we will give a general quantitative formulation of the misclassification problem, including definitions and notation. We will then describe how the bias may be determined in the general situation, which allows for misclassification of *both* the exposure and disease variables. We will also discuss a method for adjusting for such bias with one's study data.

12.1 LITERATURE REVIEW

A classic paper by Bross (1954) considered the effects of misclassification on estimation and hypothesis testing with regard to a single proportion and the difference between two proportions. In comparing two proportions, Bross assumed that the classification system (i.e., the sensitivity and specificity parameters) was the same for each comparison group. We will refer to this assumption as *nondifferential misclassification* in our discussion below. Several other authors (e.g., Fleiss, 1973; Copeland et al., 1977; Greenland, 1980) have (erroneously) attributed to Bross the important result that nondifferential misclassification errors will always tend to deflate the difference between two rates (i.e., the bias is toward the null). This result (Newell, 1962; Keys and Kihlberg, 1963; Gullen et al., 1968) carries over to other effect measures such as the odds and risk ratios (Copeland et al., 1977).

The case of nondifferential and "independent" misclassification of *both* exposure and disease status was examined by Gullen and co-workers (1968), who showed that the bias in estimating the difference between two proportions must, again, be toward the null. However, others (Lilienfeld and Graham, 1958; Fleiss, 1973; Copeland et al., 1977) have pointed out that the assumption of equal sensitivity and specificity rates across populations is not always tenable and that, moreover, the direction of the bias under "differential" misclassification may be either away from or toward the null. Copeland and colleagues (1977) discussed the direction and magnitude of the odds or risk ratio bias for both differential and nondifferential misclassification when only the outcome variable was assumed to be misclassified (i.e., disease status in a follow-up study and exposure status in a case-control study). They also derived formulas for adjusting the risk or the odds ratio from study data to correct for misclassification that is assumed to be nondifferential. Barron (1977) used matrices to extend such adjustment of study data to the case where there is independent nondifferential misclassification of both exposure and disease.

Shy and colleagues (1978) and Gladen and Rogan (1979) examined misclassification bias of risk or odds ratios in the context of environmental studies. In the latter paper, expressions for the bias were derived for nondifferential misclassification involving three or more exposure categories.

Finally, Greenland (1980) has considered the effects of misclassification on both ratio and difference effect measures in the presence of covariates. Greenland demonstrated that misclassification of exposure can spuriously introduce effect modification by a covariate, and that misclassification of a confounder can reintroduce confounding in a summary estimate that controls for confounding by using misclassified data. He also showed that if misclassification of the exposure is nondifferential, then both stratum-specific and adjusted summary measures of effect will be biased toward the null.

The objective of this chapter is to provide a more complete description and clarification of important results contained in the brief literature review above (although Greenland's work on misclassification in the presence of covariates is beyond our scope here). Our discussion will also consider the more general situation of differential and independent misclassification of *both* exposure and disease variables, from which the previous results fall out as special cases. But first we present some examples.

**12.2
EXAMPLES
OF MIS-
CLASSIFI-
CATION IN
ONLY THE
OUTCOME
VARIABLE**

In the first example, we look at a follow-up study with misclassification of disease (from Copeland et al., 1977).

EXAMPLE 12.1

Table 12.2 gives cumulative incidence data (i.e., assuming no measurement error) for hypothetical exposed and unexposed population cohorts.

**Table 12.2   Target Population (No Misclassification)
for Example 12.1**

	E	$\overline{E}$	
D	400	200	$\text{CIR} = \dfrac{400/1{,}000}{200/1{,}000} = 2$
$\overline{D}$	600	800	
	1,000	1,000	

For a follow-up study involving these cohorts, we will assume that disease status will be misclassified with sensitivity of .8 and specificity of .9, as indicated in Table 12.3.

Note that D' = classified as diseased, $\overline{D}'$ = classified as non-diseased, and

$$\text{sensitivity given } E = \text{pr}(D'|DE) = 320/400 = .8$$
$$\text{sensitivity given } \overline{E} = \text{pr}(D'|D\overline{E}) = 160/200 = .8$$
$$\text{specificity given } E = \text{pr}(\overline{D}'|\overline{D}E) = 540/600 = .9$$
$$\text{specificity given } \overline{E} = \text{pr}(\overline{D}'|\overline{D}\,\overline{E}) = 720/800 = .9$$

This information illustrates nondifferential misclassification, which is characterized here by sensitivities and specificities that do not vary with

EXAMPLE 12.1 (*continued*)

Table 12.3   Classification Tables for Example 12.1

	TRUE STATUS (E)				TRUE STATUS ($\bar{E}$)		
	D	$\bar{D}$			D	$\bar{D}$	
CLASSIFIED STATUS D'	320	60	380	CLASSIFIED STATUS D'	160	80	240
$\bar{D}'$	80	540	620	$\bar{D}'$	40	720	760
	400	600	1,000		200	800	1,000

exposure status. (Note that we are assuming no misclassification of exposure status.)

From the row marginals in Table 12.3, we can determine the actual population (that would be expected because of misclassification), as shown in Table 12.4.

Table 12.4   Actual Population (from Misclassification of Disease Status) for Example 12.1

	E	$\bar{E}$
D'	380	240
$\bar{D}'$	620	760
	1,000	1,000

$$CIR° = \frac{380/1,000}{240/1,000} = 1.583$$

Thus, the bias from misclassification is given by

$$BIAS(\hat{CIR}, CIR) = (CIR° - CIR)/CIR = (1.583 - 2)/2 = -.209$$

i.e., the bias is toward the null.

In general, such a bias in the $\hat{CIR}$ will always be toward the null value

EXAMPLE 12.1 (*continued*)

provided the misclassification is *nondifferential*. If the sensitivities or the specificities differ, however, the bias may be either toward or away from the null.

EXAMPLE 12.2

Here, we examine a case-control study with misclassification of exposure (from Copeland et al., 1977). Table 12.5 gives "true" exposure data for prevalent cases and noncases in a hypothetical population.

Table 12.5   Target Population (No Misclassification) for Example 12.2

	E	$\overline{E}$	
D	600	400	1,000
$\overline{D}$	300	700	1,000

$$POR = \frac{600 \times 700}{300 \times 400} = 3.5$$

In a case-control study carried out on this population, we will assume that there is misclassification of exposure with sensitivity of .9 and specificity of .7 for cases, and with sensitivity of .6 and specificity of .9 for controls. (We also assume no misclassification of disease in this example.) Then, the expected classification tables resulting from misclassification will be as given by Table 12.6.

Note that E' = classified as exposed, $\overline{E}'$ = classified as nonexposed, and

$$\text{sensitivity given } D = \text{pr}(E'|DE) = 540/600 = .9$$
$$\text{sensitivity given } \overline{D} = \text{pr}(E'|\overline{D}E) = 180/300 = .6$$
$$\text{specificity given } D = \text{pr}(\overline{E}'|D\overline{E}) = 280/400 = .7$$
$$\text{specificity given } \overline{D} = \text{pr}(\overline{E}'|\overline{D}\,\overline{E}) = 630/700 = .9$$

This example illustrates differential misclassification, characterized here by differing sensitivities and differing specificities over disease categories.

EXAMPLE 12.2 (*continued*)

Table 12.6   Classification Tables for Example 12.2

		TRUE STATUS (D)					TRUE STATUS $(\overline{D})$		
		E	$\overline{E}$				E	$\overline{E}$	
CLASSIFIED STATUS	E'	540	120	660	CLASSIFIED STATUS	E'	180	70	250
	$\overline{E'}$	60	280	340		$\overline{E'}$	120	630	750
		600	400	1,000			300	700	1,000

From the row marginals in Table 12.6, we can then determine the actual population (from misclassification) for this situation, as shown in Table 12.7.

Table 12.7   Actual Population (from Misclassification of Exposure Status) for Example 12.2

	E'	$\overline{E'}$
D	660	340
$\overline{D}$	250	750

$$POR° = \frac{660 \times 750}{250 \times 340} = 5.82$$

Thus, the bias is given by

$$BIAS(P\hat{O}R, POR) = (POR° - POR)/POR = (5.82 - 3.5)/3.5 = .663$$

which is away from the null. In general, such a bias with regard to the odds ratio in a case-control study may be either toward or away from the null if the misclassification is differential over disease categories. However, if only exposure status is misclassified and the misclassification is non-differential, then the bias must be toward the null.

12.3 MISCLASSIFI-CATION BIAS: GENERAL FORMULA-TION

As we have seen in the examples, the nature and extent of bias due to misclassification can be described in the same general framework previously used for consideration of selection bias. Using the general notation given in Table 12.1, we see that misclassification bias with regard to the odds ratio (OR) or to some ratio of proportions (RP = CIR or PR) is again expressible as $(OR° - OR)/OR$ or $(RP° - RP)/RP$, respectively. As suggested by our examples, explicit mathematical expressions for such bias can be obtained in terms of the underlying sensitivity and specificity probabilities that relate the fourfold tables to one another. In this regard, the following notation will be adopted:

D' and $\overline{D}'$ denote classified disease and nondiseased status, respectively.

E' and $\overline{E}'$ denote classified exposure and nonexposure status, respectively.

Then, we define

$$\text{sensitivity for } D \text{ given } E = \phi_{D|E} = \text{pr}(D'|DE)$$

$$\text{specificity for } D \text{ given } E = \psi_{D|E} = \text{pr}(\overline{D}'|\overline{D}E)$$

$$\text{sensitivity for } D \text{ given } \overline{E} = \phi_{D|\overline{E}} = \text{pr}(D'|D\overline{E})$$

$$\text{specificity for } D \text{ given } \overline{E} = \psi_{D|\overline{E}} = \text{pr}(\overline{D}'|\overline{D}\,\overline{E})$$

$$\text{sensitivity for } E \text{ given } D = \phi_{E|D} = \text{pr}(E'|DE)$$

$$\text{specificity for } E \text{ given } D = \psi_{E|D} = \text{pr}(\overline{E}'|D\overline{E})$$

$$\text{sensitivity for } E \text{ given } \overline{D} = \phi_{E|\overline{D}} = \text{pr}(E'|\overline{D}E)$$

$$\text{specificity for } E \text{ given } \overline{D} = \psi_{E|\overline{D}} = \text{pr}(\overline{E}'|\overline{D}\,\overline{E})$$

Table 12.8 describes how these parameters may be identified within appropriate fourfold classification tables that allow for misclassification of exposure and disease. In this context, we define *nondifferential misclassification* to mean that the following four equations

$$\phi_{D|E} = \phi_{D|\overline{E}} = \phi_D, \qquad \psi_{D|E} = \psi_{D|\overline{E}} = \psi_D, \qquad \phi_{E|D} = \phi_{E|\overline{D}} = \phi_E,$$

$$\psi_{E|D} = \psi_{E|\overline{D}} = \psi_E$$

are simultaneously satisfied. In words, this definition means that when one is classifying disease status (D), the sensitivities are the same among both exposed (E) and unexposed ($\overline{E}$) groups, as are the specificities. Similarly, when one is classifying exposure status, the sensitivities are the same among both diseased (D) and nondiseased ($\overline{D}$) groups, as are the specificities.

Finally, we define *independent misclassification* of disease and exposure to mean that the probability of the joint occurrence of any classification outcome concerning disease status (e.g., D') with any classification outcome concerning exposure status (e.g., E'), given the true disease and

Table 12.8   Probabilities of Misclassification for Disease and Exposure

a. Misclassification of Disease

	TRUE (E)				TRUE ($\overline{E}$)	
	D	$\overline{D}$			D	$\overline{D}$
CLASSIFIED D'	$\phi_{D\mid E}$	$1 - \psi_{D\mid E}$		CLASSIFIED D'	$\phi_{D\mid \overline{E}}$	$1 - \psi_{D\mid \overline{E}}$
$\overline{D}'$	$1 - \phi_{D\mid E}$	$\psi_{D\mid E}$		$\overline{D}'$	$1 - \phi_{D\mid \overline{E}}$	$\psi_{D\mid \overline{E}}$

b. Misclassification of Exposure

	TRUE (D)				TRUE ($\overline{D}$)	
	E	$\overline{E}$			E	$\overline{E}$
CLASSIFIED E'	$\phi_{E\mid D}$	$1 - \psi_{E\mid D}$		CLASSIFIED E'	$\phi_{E\mid \overline{D}}$	$1 - \psi_{E\mid \overline{D}}$
$\overline{E}'$	$1 - \phi_{E\mid D}$	$\psi_{E\mid D}$		$\overline{E}'$	$1 - \phi_{E\mid \overline{D}}$	$\psi_{E\mid \overline{D}}$

exposure status, is equal to the product of corresponding classification probabilities for disease and exposure separately. From this definition, it follows, e.g., that

$$\text{pr}(D'E'\mid DE) = \text{pr}(D'\mid DE)\,\text{pr}(E'\mid DE) = \phi_{D\mid E}\,\phi_{E\mid D}$$
$$\text{pr}(\overline{D}'\overline{E}'\mid DE) = \text{pr}(\overline{D}'\mid DE)\,\text{pr}(\overline{E}'\mid DE) = (1 - \phi_{D\mid E})(1 - \phi_{E\mid D})$$
$$\text{pr}(D'E'\mid \overline{D}\,\overline{E}) = \text{pr}(D'\mid \overline{D}\,\overline{E})\,\text{pr}(E'\mid \overline{D}\,\overline{E}) = (1 - \psi_{D\mid \overline{E}})(1 - \psi_{E\mid \overline{D}})$$
$$\text{pr}(\overline{D}'\overline{E}'\mid \overline{D}\,\overline{E}) = \text{pr}(\overline{D}'\mid \overline{D}\,\overline{E})\,\text{pr}(\overline{E}'\mid \overline{D}\,\overline{E}) = \psi_{D\mid \overline{E}}\,\psi_{E\mid \overline{D}}$$

Similar expressions can be obtained for joint (conditional) probabilities involving other combinations of disease and exposure conditions— e.g., $\text{pr}(D'E'\mid D\overline{E})$, etc.

We will next consider the general situation that allows for independent and differential misclassification.

12.4 INDEPEN-DENT MISCLASSIFI-CATION OF BOTH EXPOSURE AND DISEASE

For this general situation, the crucial step for quantifying the bias (when estimating either OR or RP, regardless of study design) involves expressing the *classified* population frequencies $\mathscr{A}°$, $\mathscr{B}°$, $\mathscr{C}°$, and $\mathscr{D}°$ in terms of the *true* population frequencies $\mathscr{A}$, $\mathscr{B}$, $\mathscr{C}$, and $\mathscr{D}$. This can be done through the following four equations, which follow from the definition of independent misclassification given in Section 12.3.

$$\mathscr{A}° = \phi_{D|E}\,\phi_{E|D}\,\mathscr{A} + \phi_{D|\overline{E}}(1 - \psi_{E|D})\,\mathscr{B} + (1 - \psi_{D|E})\,\phi_{E|\overline{D}}\,\mathscr{C}$$
$$+ (1 - \psi_{D|\overline{E}})(1 - \psi_{E|\overline{D}})\,\mathscr{D}$$

$$\mathscr{B}° = \phi_{D|E}(1 - \phi_{E|D})\,\mathscr{A} + \phi_{D|\overline{E}}\,\psi_{E|D}\,\mathscr{B} + (1 - \psi_{D|E})(1 - \phi_{E|\overline{D}})\,\mathscr{C}$$
$$+ (1 - \psi_{D|\overline{E}})\,\psi_{E|\overline{D}}\,\mathscr{D}$$

$$\mathscr{C}° = (1 - \phi_{D|E})\,\phi_{E|D}\,\mathscr{A} + (1 - \phi_{D|\overline{E}})(1 - \psi_{E|D})\,\mathscr{B} + \psi_{D|E}\,\phi_{E|\overline{D}}\,\mathscr{C}$$
$$+ \psi_{D|\overline{E}}(1 - \psi_{E|\overline{D}})\,\mathscr{D}$$

$$\mathscr{D}° = (1 - \phi_{D|E})(1 - \phi_{E|D})\,\mathscr{A} + (1 - \phi_{D|\overline{E}})\,\psi_{E|D}\,\mathscr{B}$$
$$+ \psi_{D|E}(1 - \phi_{E|\overline{D}})\,\mathscr{C} + \psi_{D|\overline{E}}\,\psi_{E|\overline{D}}\,\mathscr{D}$$

(12.1)

Note, e.g., that the first of the equations in Expression 12.1 follows, using the notation in Table 12.1, from applying the independence definition to the relationship:

$$\mathscr{A}° = \mathscr{A}°_{11} + \mathscr{A}°_{12} + \mathscr{A}°_{21} + \mathscr{A}°_{22}$$
$$= (\mathscr{A})\,\mathrm{pr}(D'E'|DE) + (\mathscr{B})\,\mathrm{pr}(D'E'|D\overline{E}) + (\mathscr{C})\,\mathrm{pr}(D'E'|\overline{D}E)$$
$$+ (\mathscr{D})\,\mathrm{pr}(D'E'|\overline{D}\,\overline{E})$$

Formulas for the bias in estimating OR and RP can then be obtained by substituting the expressions on the right from Equation 12.1 into the general expressions for bias given by $(\mathrm{OR}° - \mathrm{OR})/\mathrm{OR}$ and $(\mathrm{RP}° - \mathrm{RP})/\mathrm{RP}$. *These formulas incorporate the misclassification of only one of the two variables as special cases.* In particular, if only disease status is misclassified, then

$$\phi_{E|D} = \phi_{E|\overline{D}} = \psi_{E|D} = \psi_{E|\overline{D}} = 1$$

in Expression 12.1. On the other hand, if only exposure is misclassified, then

$$\phi_{D|E} = \phi_{D|\overline{E}} = \psi_{D|E} = \psi_{D|\overline{E}} = 1$$

in Expression 12.1. One can also demonstrate (e.g., see Gullen et al., 1968) that the bias must be toward the null when there is nondifferential misclassification of both exposure and disease, but that the bias can be in either direction when misclassification is differential.

By solving the above system of equations to obtain expressions for $\mathscr{A}$, $\mathscr{B}$, $\mathscr{C}$, and $\mathscr{D}$ in terms of $\mathscr{A}°$, $\mathscr{B}°$, $\mathscr{C}°$, and $\mathscr{D}°$, we may also derive formulas for adjusting observed estimates of OR and RP to correct for differential misclassification. [Copeland and colleagues (1977) and Barron (1977) give such correction formulas for the nondifferential situation.] The general solution for $\mathcal{A}$, $\mathcal{B}$, $\mathcal{C}$, and $\mathcal{D}$ may be most compactly stated in matrix terms—i.e.,

$$\mathbf{Y} = \mathbf{W}^{-1}\mathbf{Y}^\circ \tag{12.2}$$

where

$$\mathbf{Y} = [\mathcal{A}, \mathcal{B}, \mathcal{C}, \mathcal{D}]' \qquad \mathbf{Y}^\circ = [\mathcal{A}^\circ, \mathcal{B}^\circ, \mathcal{C}^\circ, \mathcal{D}^\circ]'$$

and $\mathbf{W}$ is the matrix of coefficients of $\mathcal{A}$, $\mathcal{B}$, $\mathcal{C}$, and $\mathcal{D}$ given in Expression 12.1, or $\mathbf{W} =$

$$\begin{bmatrix} \phi_{D|E}\phi_{E|D} & \phi_{D|\bar{E}}(1-\psi_{E|D}) & (1-\psi_{D|E})\phi_{E|\bar{D}} & (1-\psi_{D|\bar{E}})(1-\psi_{E|\bar{D}}) \\ \phi_{D|E}(1-\phi_{E|D}) & \phi_{D|\bar{E}}\psi_{E|D} & (1-\psi_{D|E})(1-\phi_{E|\bar{D}}) & (1-\psi_{D|\bar{E}})\psi_{E|\bar{D}} \\ (1-\phi_{D|E})\phi_{E|D} & (1-\phi_{D|\bar{E}})(1-\psi_{E|D}) & \psi_{D|E}\phi_{E|\bar{D}} & \psi_{D|\bar{E}}(1-\psi_{E|\bar{D}}) \\ (1-\phi_{D|E})(1-\phi_{E|D}) & (1-\phi_{D|\bar{E}})\psi_{E|D} & \psi_{D|E}(1-\phi_{E|\bar{D}}) & \psi_{D|\bar{E}}\psi_{E|\bar{D}} \end{bmatrix}$$

Using Equation 12.2, we can correct for misclassification bias in the observed data by correcting each of the sample cell frequencies through the matrix formula

$$\begin{bmatrix} \hat{\mathcal{A}} \\ \hat{\mathcal{B}} \\ \hat{\mathcal{C}} \\ \hat{\mathcal{D}} \end{bmatrix} = \mathbf{W}^{-1} \begin{bmatrix} a \\ b \\ c \\ d \end{bmatrix} \tag{12.3}$$

where a, b, c, and d denote the observed sample frequencies, and $\hat{\mathcal{A}}$, $\hat{\mathcal{B}}$, $\hat{\mathcal{C}}$, and $\hat{\mathcal{D}}$ denote the corresponding corrected frequencies, as shown in Table 12.9. A simplified algebraic formula equivalent to Equation 12.3 when misclassification is nondifferential will be described in the next section.

In using Formula 12.3, we must have accurate estimates for the sensitivity and specificity parameters given in $\mathbf{W}$. If estimates are inaccurate, we may obtain inadmissible (i.e., negative or indeterminate) values for the adjusted cell frequencies $\hat{\mathcal{A}}$, $\hat{\mathcal{B}}$, $\hat{\mathcal{C}}$, and $\hat{\mathcal{D}}$. Moreover, even if good estimates are available, certain values for sensitivity and specificity will yield indeterminate results. The latter situation, in fact, indicates that there are an infinite number of solutions to the system of equations in 12.1. We will illustrate this situation when discussing nondifferential misclassification in the next section.

Accurate estimates of the ϕ's and ψ's must usually be determined from prior studies involving the same or similar populations and the same exposure and/or disease variables. Note, however, that, in a case-control study, the choice of control group can result in sensitivities and specificities for one's study that differ substantially from corresponding

Table 12.9   Correcting for Misclassification in Study Data

	a. Observed Data				b. Corrected Data	

	E'	$\overline{E}'$			E	$\overline{E}$
D'	a	b	n_D	D	$\hat{\mathscr{A}}$	$\hat{\mathscr{B}}$
$\overline{D}'$	c	d	$n_{\overline{D}}$	$\overline{D}$	$\hat{\mathscr{C}}$	$\hat{\mathscr{D}}$
	n_E	$n_{\overline{E}}$	n			n

$$\hat{OR} = \frac{ad}{bc}$$

$$\hat{OR}\,(\text{corrected}) = \frac{\hat{\mathscr{A}}\hat{\mathscr{D}}}{\hat{\mathscr{B}}\hat{\mathscr{C}}}$$

$$\hat{RP} = \frac{a}{b}\left(\frac{n_{\overline{E}}}{n_E}\right)$$

$$\hat{RP}\,(\text{corrected}) = \frac{\hat{\mathscr{A}}}{\hat{\mathscr{B}}}\left[\frac{\hat{\mathscr{B}} + \hat{\mathscr{D}}}{\hat{\mathscr{A}} + \hat{\mathscr{C}}}\right]$$

misclassification probabilities characterizing the population, particularly for nondiseased persons. Similarly, in follow-up studies for which restrictions are imposed in the selection of a comparison group from nonexposed subjects, misclassification probabilities for one's study can differ considerably from those for the population. To properly correct for misclassification in such a situation, one must use, in Formula 12.3, the misclassification probabilities for one's study rather than the population misclassification values.

To illustrate this point, we consider misclassification errors described in Table 12.10. Part a of this table gives the (disease) classification information for a target population. As before, D and D' denote true and classified diseased persons, respectively; $\overline{D}$ and $\overline{D}'$ represent true and classified nondiseased persons, respectively. Part b of this table gives classification information for a study population derived from the target population for a case-control design. The study involves 2,005 controls ($\overline{D}'$), which represents a one-fourth subset of the (8,020) classified nondiseased persons; the entire collection of 2,080 classified diseased persons is also chosen for study. Because of misclassification (using a sensitivity and a specificity of .80 for the target population), it then follows that the study population will contain 85 truly diseased persons (D) and 4,000 truly nondiseased persons among the controls ($\overline{D}$). Consequently, the sensitivity and the specificity for the study population ($\phi_D^* = .94$ and $\psi_D^* = .50$) differ noticeably from corresponding misclassification probabilities in the target population ($\phi_D = .80 = \psi_D$). To properly adjust study data to correct for misclassification in such a study, we must use the misclassification probabilities $\phi_D^* = .94$ and $\psi_D^* = .50$ in Formula 12.3 rather than the target population misclassification probabilities.

Table 12.10   Misclassification Probabilities for Target Population and Study Population in a Case-Control Study

a. Target Population				b. Study Population		
	D	$\bar{D}$			D	$\bar{D}$
D'	80	2,000	2,080	D'	80	2,000	2,080
$\bar{D}'$	20	8,000	8,020	$\bar{D}'$	5	2,000	2,005
	100	10,000	10,100		85	4,000	4,085
	$\phi_D = .80,$	$\psi_D = .80$			$\phi_D^* = .94,$	$\psi_D^* = .50$

For example, suppose that the fourfold table relating exposure to disease in the target population is given by Table 12.11a. Then, for the case-control study design we have described, it follows that the corresponding information for the (actual) study population will be given by Table 12.11b. (These figures assume that there is no misclassification of exposure status and no selection bias from the choice of controls.) If we correct the actual population odds ratio ($OR° = 1.08$) by using Equation 12.3 with the study population misclassification probabilities ($\phi_D^* = .94$, $\psi_D^* = .50$), the corrected odds ratio will turn out to be 3.86, as desired. However, if we use the target population misclassification probabilities in Equation 12.3, the corrected odds ratio becomes 1.14, which is invalid.

Table 12.11   Fourfold Tables for Target and Actual Populations from the Case-Control Study Described by Table 12.10

a. Target Population (No Misclassification)				b. Actual Population (with Misclassification)		
	E	$\bar{E}$			E	$\bar{E}$
D	30	70	100	D'	224	1,856	2,080
$\bar{D}$	1,000	9,000	10,000	$\bar{D}'$	201.5	1,803.5	2,005
	OR = 3.86				$OR° = 1.08$	

**12.5
CORRECT-
ING FOR
NONDIFFER-
ENTIAL
MISCLASSIFI-
CATION**

A straightforward algebraic solution to Equation 12.3 can be derived for nondifferential misclassification—i.e., when $\phi_{D|E} = \phi_{D|\bar{E}} = \phi_D$, $\psi_{D|E} = \psi_{D|\bar{E}} = \psi_D$, $\phi_{E|D} = \phi_{E|\bar{D}} = \phi_E$, and $\psi_{E|D} = \psi_{E|\bar{D}} = \psi_E$. The following formulas for corrected cell frequencies may then be given:

$$\hat{\mathcal{A}} = \frac{\psi_D(n_D\psi_E - b) - (1 - \psi_D)(n_{\bar{D}}\psi_E - d)}{(\phi_D + \psi_D - 1)(\phi_E + \psi_E - 1)}$$

$$\hat{\mathcal{B}} = \frac{\psi_D(n_D\phi_E - a) - (1 - \psi_D)(n_{\bar{D}}\phi_E - c)}{(\phi_D + \psi_D - 1)(\phi_E + \psi_E - 1)}$$

$$\hat{\mathcal{C}} = \frac{\phi_D(n_{\bar{D}}\psi_E - d) - (1 - \phi_D)(n_D\psi_E - b)}{(\phi_D + \psi_D - 1)(\phi_E + \psi_E - 1)}$$

$$\hat{\mathcal{D}} = \frac{\phi_D(n_{\bar{D}}\phi_E - c) - (1 - \phi_D)(n_D\phi_E - a)}{(\phi_D + \psi_D - 1)(\phi_E + \psi_E - 1)}$$

(12.4)

These formulas are indeterminate, however, when the denominator $(\phi_D + \psi_D - 1)(\phi_E + \psi_E - 1)$ equals zero, which can happen if and only if either $\phi_D + \psi_D = 1$ or $\phi_E + \psi_E = 1$. In particular, if $\phi_D = \psi_D = \phi_E = \psi_E = .5$, then the system of equations in 12.1 simplifies to $\mathcal{A}^\circ = \mathcal{B}^\circ = \mathcal{C}^\circ = \mathcal{D}^\circ = (\mathcal{A} + \mathcal{B} + \mathcal{C} + \mathcal{D})/4$. In other words, regardless of the values of $\mathcal{A}$, $\mathcal{B}$, $\mathcal{C}$, and $\mathcal{D}$, each person in the target population has an equal chance of being misclassified into any one of the four cells of the fourfold table. There would, thus, be no point in computing corrected effect estimates for such a situation, since misclassification would have completely invalidated one's study results.

We now consider some examples of the use of these correction formulas.

EXAMPLE 12.3

Suppose we assume we have nondifferential misclassification with $\phi_D = .8$, $\psi_D = .9$, $\phi_E = .9$, and $\psi_E = .7$. Also, suppose we have the observed data given in Table 12.12.

Using Equation 12.4, we can correct for misclassification bias as follows:

$$\text{R}\hat{\text{O}}\text{R(corrected)} = \frac{\begin{array}{l}[.9\{(62)(.7) - 24\} - .1\{(138)(.7) - 76\}] \\ \times [.8\{(138)(.9) - 62\} - .2\{(62)(.9) - 38\}]\end{array}}{\begin{array}{l}[.9\{(62)(.9) - 38\} - .1\{(138)(.9) - 62\}] \\ \times [.8\{(138)(.7) - 76\} - .2\{(62)(.7) - 24\}]\end{array}}$$

EXAMPLE 12.3 (*continued*)

Table 12.12   Follow-up Study Sample Data for Example 12.3

	E'	$\overline{E}'$		
D'	38	24	62	$\hat{ROR} = 1.94$
$\overline{D}'$	62	76	138	$\hat{CIR} = 1.58$
	100	100	200	

$$= \frac{(15.4)(46.2)}{(9.8)(12.6)} = 5.76$$

$$\hat{CIR}\text{(corrected)} = \frac{[.9\{(62)(.7) - 24\} - .1\{(138)(.7) - 76\}]}{[.9\{(62)(.9) - 38\} - .1\{(138)(.9) - 62\}]} \begin{array}{l} \times \, [(200)(.9) - 100] \\ \\ \times \, [(200)(.7) - 100] \end{array}$$

$$= \frac{(15.4)(80)}{(9.8)(40)} = 3.14$$

Note that $(\phi_D + \psi_D - 1)(\phi_E + \psi_E - 1) = .42$, so that $\hat{\mathcal{A}} = 36.7$, $\hat{\mathcal{B}} = 23.3$, $\hat{\mathcal{C}} = 30.0$, and $\hat{\mathcal{D}} = 110.0$.

Notice that despite the relatively high sensitivities and specificities, the adjusted estimates are considerably higher than the unadjusted estimates. Moreover, if we had considered misclassification only in the outcome variable (i.e., disease status, here), the increase in risk and odds ratio estimates from the unadjusted values would be considerably less (e.g., $\hat{CIR}$ changes from 1.58 to 2 when adjusted for disease misclassification only).

EXAMPLE 12.4

We now consider a case-control study yielding the observed data given in Table 12.13. For this study, we will assume that we have misclassification of the outcome (exposure) variable only and that we have the following

EXAMPLE 12.4 (*continued*)

nondifferential estimates of sensitivity and specificity parameters: $\phi_D = \psi_D = 1$, $\phi_E = .9$, and $\psi_E = .7$.

Table 12.13 Case-Control Study Sample Data for Example 12.4

	E'	$\overline{E}'$	
D'	66	34	100
$\overline{D}'$	48	52	100
	114	86	200

$\hat{EOR} = 2.10$

Using Equation 12.4, we can correct $\hat{EOR}$ as follows:

$$\hat{EOR}(\text{corrected}) = \frac{[1.0\{(100)(.7) - 34\} - 0\{(100)(.7) - 52\}] \times [1.0\{(100)(.9) - 48\} - 0\{(100)(.9) - 66\}]}{[1.0\{(100)(.9) - 66\} - 0\{(100)(.9) - 48\}] \times [1.0\{(100)(.7) - 52\} - 0\{(100)(.7) - 34\}]}$$

$$= \frac{(36)(42)}{(24)(18)} = 3.5$$

Here, $(\phi_D + \psi_D - 1)(\phi_E + \psi_E - 1) = .6$, and $\hat{\mathcal{A}} = 60$, $\hat{\mathcal{B}} = 40$, $\hat{\mathcal{C}} = 30$, and $\hat{\mathcal{D}} = 70$.

Thus, as expected, the bias is toward the null, leading to a corrected estimate that exceeds the initial study estimate.

12.6 CONCLUDING REMARKS

We have now seen how errors of misclassification can distort the estimated effect measure and how such distortion can be corrected if reliable estimates of sensitivity and specificity are available. As we did for selection bias, we have considered misclassification bias in isolation from other forms of bias. Further research (e.g., Greenland, 1980) is needed to consider various forms of bias simultaneously. We have also not yet considered distortions in the effect estimate that can result from the presence of variables "extraneous" to the primary association under study. This subject will be discussed in the next chapter on confounding.

The following list summarizes the key notation introduced in this chapter. **NOTATION**

$D, \overline{D}$	True diseased and nondiseased groups, respectively (i.e., no misclassification of disease variable).
$E, \overline{E}$	True exposed and nonexposed groups, respectively (i.e., no misclassification of exposure variable).
$D', \overline{D}'$	Classified diseased and nondiseased groups, respectively (i.e., allowing for possible misclassification of disease variable).
$E', \overline{E}'$	Classified exposed and nonexposed groups, respectively (i.e., allowing for possible misclassification of exposure variable).
$\mathcal{A}_{ij}^{\circ}$	Number of persons classified as exposed and diseased who truly belong to row i and column j of 2×2 table for target population.
$\mathcal{B}_{ij}^{\circ}$	Number of persons classified as nonexposed and diseased who truly belong to row i and column j of 2×2 table for target population.
$\mathcal{C}_{ij}^{\circ}$	Number of persons classified as exposed and nondiseased who truly belong to row i and column j of 2×2 table for target population.
$\mathcal{D}_{ij}^{\circ}$	Number of persons classified as nonexposed and nondiseased who truly belong to row i and column j of 2×2 table for target population.

Note: $\quad \mathcal{A}^{\circ} = \sum_{i=1}^{2} \sum_{j=1}^{2} \mathcal{A}_{ij}^{\circ} \quad \mathcal{B}^{\circ} = \sum_{i=1}^{2} \sum_{j=1}^{2} \mathcal{B}_{ij}^{\circ} \quad \mathcal{C}^{\circ} = \sum_{i=1}^{2} \sum_{j=1}^{2} \mathcal{C}_{ij}^{\circ} \quad \mathcal{D}^{\circ} = \sum_{i=1}^{2} \sum_{j=1}^{2} \mathcal{D}_{ij}^{\circ}$

ϕ	Sensitivity parameter.
ψ	Specificity parameter.
$\phi_{D\mid E}$	Sensitivity for D given $E = \mathrm{pr}(D'\mid DE)$.
$\psi_{D\mid E}$	Specificity for D given $E = \mathrm{pr}(\overline{D}'\mid \overline{D}E)$.
$\phi_{D\mid\overline{E}}$	Sensitivity for D given $\overline{E} = \mathrm{pr}(D'\mid D\overline{E})$.
$\psi_{D\mid\overline{E}}$	Specificity for D given $\overline{E} = \mathrm{pr}(\overline{D}'\mid \overline{D}\,\overline{E})$.
$\phi_{E\mid D}$	Sensitivity for E given $D = \mathrm{pr}(E'\mid DE)$.
$\psi_{E\mid D}$	Specificity for E given $D = \mathrm{pr}(\overline{E}'\mid D\overline{E})$.
$\phi_{E\mid\overline{D}}$	Sensitivity for E given $\overline{D} = \mathrm{pr}(E'\mid \overline{D}E)$.
$\psi_{E\mid\overline{D}}$	Specificity for E given $\overline{D} = \mathrm{pr}(\overline{E}'\mid \overline{D}\,\overline{E})$.

$\mathbf{Y} = [\mathcal{A}, \mathcal{B}, \mathcal{C}, \mathcal{D}]'$ Vector of cell numbers for target 2×2 table when there is no misclassification.

$\mathbf{Y}^\circ = [\mathcal{A}^\circ, \mathcal{B}^\circ, \mathcal{C}^\circ, \mathcal{D}^\circ]'$ Vector of cell numbers for actual 2×2 table that allows for misclassification.

$\mathbf{W}$ Matrix of coefficients involving ϕ and ψ parameters that relate $\mathbf{Y}$ to $\mathbf{Y}^\circ$ in terms of matrix equation $\mathbf{Y} = \mathbf{W}^{-1}\mathbf{Y}^\circ$.

$\hat{\mathcal{A}}, \hat{\mathcal{B}}, \hat{\mathcal{C}}, \hat{\mathcal{D}}$ Cell numbers that have been adjusted by using sample data to correct for misclassification.

$\hat{\mathrm{OR}}$(corrected), $\hat{\mathrm{RP}}$(corrected)   Adjusted sample odds ratio and ratio of proportions, corrected for misclassification.

PRACTICE EXERCISES

12.1 Determine whether the following statements are true or false.

a. Misclassification bias is characterized by an actual population that is a rearrangement of the target population.

b. If there is misclassification of disease status but not of exposure status in a follow-up study, and if the sensitivity probability (ϕ) is the same for exposed and unexposed groups, then whatever bias exists (due to misclassification) must be toward the null.

c. If there is differential misclassification of disease status but not of exposure status in a case-control study, then there may be bias in estimating the odds ratio, which is either away from or toward the null.

d. Suppose there is independent misclassification of both exposure status and disease status. Then $\mathrm{pr}(D'E'|\overline{DE}) = \phi_{D|\overline{E}}\,\psi_{E|D}$.

e. Suppose the observed data are as follows:

	E	$\overline{E}$	
D'	70	30	100
$\overline{D}'$	50	50	100
	120	80	

Also, assume there is nondifferential misclassification of disease, with $\phi_D = .8$ and $\psi_D = .7$, and no misclassification of exposure. Then, the odds ratio may be corrected for misclassification to give the value $\hat{\mathrm{OR}}$(corrected) ≈ 7.4 (to one decimal place).

f. For the same situation described in part e, the bias due to misclassification is away from the null.

g. It is possible to obtain indeterminate results when trying to correct for nondifferential misclassification, even if good estimates of the sensitivity and specificity probabilities are available.

h. If misclassification is nondifferential and independent, with $\phi_D = \psi_D = \phi_E = \psi_E = .5$, then each person in the target population has an equal chance of being misclassified into any one of the four cells of the fourfold table.

i. For the situation described in part h, it is possible to obtain an adjusted estimate of the odds ratio that will correct for misclassification.

j. In a case-control study, one must use misclassification probabilities for one's study rather than use population misclassification values in order to properly correct for misclassification bias.

12.2 The investigators who first studied the type A (coronary-prone) behavior pattern employed a structured personal interview to assess its presence in their subjects. This method, however, was expensive because of the length and complexity of the interview process and the need for rigorously trained interviewers. To reduce the time and cost of such behavior pattern assessment, researchers have constructed a self-administered questionnaire designed to measure the same phenomenon.

Suppose that in 1960 investigators studied 210 white men, free of coronary heart disease (CHD). To test the validity of the questionnaire, the investigators assessed the men's behavior patterns twice, once using the interview and once using the questionnaire. The results were as follows:

		INTERVIEW		
		A	$\overline{A}$	
QUESTIONNAIRE	A'	91	14	105
	$\overline{A}'$	49	56	105
		140	70	210

a. What are the sensitivity (ϕ) and specificity (ψ) of the questionnaire for detecting type A persons, using the interview as the baseline validating criterion?

b. After eight years of follow-up, CHD was detected in 20 subjects (assuming no misclassification of disease), classified in Exercise Table 12.1 by both interview and questionnaire at the start of follow-up. Using the values of ϕ and ψ calculated in part a, and assuming nondifferential misclassification, adjust the $\widehat{CIR}$ calculated from the questionnaire data to correct for misclassification. (Hint: You will need to use the formulas given in Expression 12.4, where *correct* exposure status is assumed to be determined by interview and *classified* exposure status determined by questionnaire.)

c. Why is the result in part b not equal to the $\widehat{CIR}$ for the interview data?

d. Now, consider the additional problem of misclassification of the outcome variable CHD status (in addition to misclassification of behavior type). Assume that the sensitivity for detection of CHD is .8 and the specificity is .9. Also assume that misclassification of disease is independent of misclassification of behavior type. The 2×2 tables relating detected

Exercise Table 12.1

	INTERVIEW				QUESTIONNAIRE		
	A	$\overline{A}$			A'	$\overline{A}'$	
D	16	4	20	D	12	8	20
$\overline{D}$	124	66	190	$\overline{D}$	93	97	190
	140	70	210		105	105	210
	$\hat{\text{CIR}}_{\text{interview}} = 2.0$				$\hat{\text{CIR}}_{\text{questionnaire}} = 1.5$		

CHD to behavior type as determined by interview and by questionnaire (modifying the data to reflect the additional misclassification of CHD) are given in Exercise Table 12.2. Verify the numbers (given in these tables) of *expected* cell counts.

e. Assuming that the correct $\hat{\text{CIR}}$ for assessing the relationship between CHD and behavior type is obtained from the interview data in part b, describe the nature of the bias resulting from misclassification of *both* the exposure and the outcome variables.

Exercise Table 12.2

	INTERVIEW			QUESTIONNAIRE	
	A	$\overline{A}$		A'	$\overline{A}'$
D'	25.2	9.8	D'	18.9	16.1
$\overline{D}'$	114.8	60.2	$\overline{D}'$	86.1	88.9
	$\hat{\text{CIR}}° = 1.29$			$\hat{\text{CIR}}° = 1.17$	

REFERENCES BARRON, B. A. 1977. The effects of misclassification on the estimation of relative risk. *Biometrics* 33: 414–418.

BROSS, I. D. J. 1954. Misclassification in 2 × 2 tables. *Biometrics* 10: 478–486.

COPELAND, K. T.; CHECKOWAY, H.; HOLBROOK, R. H.; and MCMICHAEL, A. J. 1977. Bias due to misclassification in the estimate of relative risk. *Am. J. Epidemiol.* 105(5): 488–495.

FLEISS, J. L. 1973. *Statistical methods for rates and proportions.* New York: Wiley.

GLADEN, B., and ROGAN, W. J. 1979. Misclassification and the design of environmental studies. *Am. J. Epidemiol.* 109(6): 607–616.

GREENLAND, S. 1980. The effect of misclassification in the presence of covariates. *Am. J. Epidemiol.* 112: 564–569.

GULLEN, W. H.; BEARMAN, J. E.; and JOHNSON, E. A. 1968. Effects of misclassification in epidemiologic studies. *Public Health Rep.* 53: 1956–1965.

KEYS, A., and KIHLBERG, J. K. 1963. The effect of misclassification on estimated relative prevalence of a characteristic. *Am. J. Public Health* 53: 1656–1665.

LILIENFELD, A. M., and GRAHAM, S. 1958. Validity of determining circumcision status by questionnaire as related to epidemiological studies of cancer of the cervix. *J. Natl. Cancer Inst.* 21: 713–720.

NEWELL, D. J. 1962. Errors in the interpretation of errors in epidemiology. *Am. J. Public Health* 52: 1925–1928.

SACKETT, D. L. 1979. Bias in analytic research. *J. Chronic Dis.* 32: 51–63.

SHY, C. M.; KLEINBAUM, D. G.; and MORGENSTERN, H. 1978. The effect of misclassification of exposure status in epidemiological studies of air pollution health effects. *Bull. N. Y. Acad. Med.* 54(11): 1155–1165.

13

Confounding

CHAPTER OUTLINE

In most etiologic research, the assessment of an association between two variables must make allowance for certain "extraneous" factors that may affect the relationship studied. The bias in the (crude) estimate that can result when the exposure-disease relationship under study is mixed up with the effects of extraneous variables has traditionally been called *confounding*. The concept of confounding has received considerable attention in epidemiologic literature (Miettinen, 1972, 1974, 1976; Miettinen and Cook, 1981; Dales and Ury, 1979; Fisher and Patil, 1974; Greenland and Neutra, 1980; Kupper et al., 1981). Even so, there still appears to be confusion regarding the definition of confounding, the attributes of a single confounder and of a collection of confounders, and whether such attributes differ because of the type of effect measure chosen, the kind of study design employed (e.g., follow-up versus case-control), and the method of subject selection used (e.g., simple random sampling versus matching). Our purpose in this chapter is to clarify some of these issues, with a minimum of mathematical discussion.

To illustrate the basic principles involved, we will focus, as we did in previous chapters, on the simplistic situation involving a dichotomous disease variable d (with D and $\bar{D}$ denoting the presence and absence of disease, respectively) and a dichotomous exposure variable e (with levels E and $\bar{E}$). Regarding the extraneous variables, we will first consider the characteristics of a confounder in terms of a single dichotomous extraneous factor f (with levels F and $\bar{F}$). Subsequently, we will extend these concepts to allow for several extraneous variables $f_1, f_2, \ldots, f_k$.

The measures of effect we will consider in this chapter are the risk ratio (RR) for follow-up studies and the odds ratio (OR) for case-control and cross-sectional studies. (However, the concepts to be discussed easily carry over to risk difference and incidence density types of measures.) The quantities $\text{c}\hat{\text{R}}\text{R}$ and $\text{c}\hat{\text{O}}\text{R}$ will denote *estimated crude risk and odds ratios* for assessing the e–d relationship; their computation completely ignores the effects of extraneous variables. In contrast, $\text{a}\hat{\text{R}}\text{R}(f_1, f_2, \ldots, f_k)$ and $\text{a}\hat{\text{O}}\text{R}(f_1, f_2, \ldots, f_k)$ will denote *estimated adjusted risk and odds ratios* for quantifying the e–d relationship in a manner that controls for the extraneous factors $f_1, \ldots, f_k$. That is, each of these adjusted estimates either will be some form of weighted average of stratum-specific risk or odds ratios (to be discussed in Chapter 17) or will be describable as an estimated regression coefficient in a mathematical model that relates d and e, taking into account $f_1, \ldots, f_k$ (to be discussed in Chapter 20).

To identify the basic conditions for confounding in terms of the relationships of the extraneous factors with the exposure and disease variables, we need to consider an additional collection of odds ratios. For example, $\hat{\text{OR}}_{ef}$ will denote the sample *unconditional odds ratio* relating the exposure and the extraneous factor f, and $\hat{\text{OR}}_{df|\bar{E}}$ will represent the *conditional odds ratio* relating the disease and the extraneous factor among the sample of unexposed subjects. Also, to distinguish the value of an effect measure in the population from its value in a sample, we will follow the usual convention of placing a "hat" over the effect measure to indicate that it is sample-based rather than population-based.

**13.1
A WORKING
DEFINITION
OF A CON-
FOUNDER**

Without giving a full explanation at this time, we define a *confounder* to be a "risk factor" for the disease under study whose "control" in some appropriate way (either singly or in conjunction with other variables) will reduce or completely correct a bias when estimating the (true) exposure-disease relationship. We will define and discuss the term "risk factor" in Section 13.4. By "control," we refer to an assessment of the $e-d$ relationship at different (combinations of) levels of one or more extraneous variables and, when appropriate, an overall evaluation of the $e-d$ relationship based on a pooling together of information over these various levels. As we will emphasize below, this definition requires us to consider both causal types of relationships, believed to be operating in the target population, and data-based associations.

The data-based criterion for establishing the presence or absence of confounding involves the comparison of a crude effect measure with an "adjusted" effect measure that corrects for distortions due to extraneous variables; confounding is acknowledged to be present when the crude and adjusted measures differ in value. Such a criterion is appropriate only when the adjustment process provides a valid and precise estimate of the parameter of interest (i.e., some adjusted population effect measure). When several extraneous variables are considered simultaneously, the identification of sets of confounders will require the comparison of various adjusted effects. This complex situation will be considered in Chapter 14.

**13.2
SOME EXAM-
PLES WHEN
CONTROL-
LING FOR
ONE EXTRA-
NEOUS
VARIABLE**

We illustrate the above concepts of confounding and related issues with several numerical examples involving the control of a single extraneous variable. We will ignore for now any concern about confounder eligibility requirements (e.g., risk factor status) because of theoretical and/or empirical conditions to be met before data collection and analysis. That is, we will assume in these examples that the variable f being considered for control has already passed the appropriate a priori eligibility tests (e.g., f is a risk factor).

**13.2.1
General
Discussion**

In Table 13.1, we have summarized the essential characteristics of 15 numerical examples. Examples 1–3 are presented in full detail in Table 13.2. (The interested reader may write to the authors for details of the other examples.) The entire collection of examples can be divided into three groups, each of which is associated with one of the following three crude tables of sample data.

Group A: A follow-up study (used in Examples 1, 4, 7, 10, and 13) that yields a crude risk ratio that is moderately large (say greater than 3):

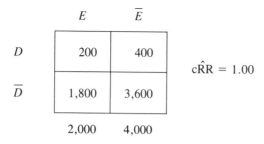

	E	$\overline{E}$
D	200	50
$\overline{D}$	800	950
	1,000	1,000

$c\hat{R}R = 4.00$

Group B: A follow-up study (used in Examples 2, 5, 8, 11, and 14) that yields a crude risk ratio that has the null value 1:

	E	$\overline{E}$
D	200	400
$\overline{D}$	1,800	3,600
	2,000	4,000

$c\hat{R}R = 1.00$

Group C: A case-control study (used in Examples 3, 6, 9, 12, and 15) that yields a crude odds ratio that is moderately different from unity:

	E	$\overline{E}$	
D	550	450	1,000
$\overline{D}$	400	600	1,000

$c\hat{O}R = 1.83$

Each of these 15 examples considers a different stratification of a crude table into two strata, based on some extraneous factor f. You can thus view these results as though a different extraneous factor were being controlled in each example. Also, in discussing these examples, we will assume that the data are obtained by *simple random sampling* rather than by some more restrictive subject selection procedure, like matching. We will briefly mention the implications of matching with regard to confounding later in this chapter; a detailed discussion of such considerations will be given in Chapter 18.

Focusing on Example 1 (in group A), we see from the set of columns labeled "Adjusted vs. Crude" that, although $c\hat{R}R = 4.00$, the two stratum-specific risk ratios are $\hat{R}R_1 = 1.02$ and $\hat{R}R_2 = 1.86$. These results indicate that controlling for the variable f (e.g., by considering the risk ratios at each of the two levels of f) leads to stratum-specific estimated effects that are considerably smaller than the crude estimate of 4.00. Thus, if we do not control for f in these data, we would encounter a bias in the crude estimate of effect, which would manifest itself as a strong $e-d$ association in the crude data. Note that any weighted average of the two stratum-specific values will be no larger than 1.86; we have referred to such an average as an adjusted measure of effect $a\hat{R}R(f)$. Thus, whether we consider the stratum-specific values themselves or some adjusted measure $a\hat{R}R(f)$, the use of $c\hat{R}R$ (equal to 4.00) would yield a (positive) bias *away from the null* (i.e., the estimated crude effect would suggest a stronger relationship than is actually present).

This first example illustrates what is commonly called *confounding*, a phenomenon that is detected in follow-up study data through a comparison of crude and adjusted effects. Mathematically speaking, confounding is said to be present *in the data* because of factor f when

$$c\hat{R}R \neq a\hat{R}R(f) \tag{13.1}$$

Table 13.1   Summary of Examples Showing Confounding and/or Interaction in Randomly Sampled Data

	Example	Study (Effect Measure)	ADJUSTED VS. CRUDE		
			Stratum 1 Estimate	Stratum 2 Estimate	Crude Estimate
Confounding	1	Follow-up (RR)	1.02	1.86	4.00
and Interaction	2	Follow-up (RR)	1.74	3.00	1.00
	3	Case-control (OR)	.96	.45	1.83
No Confounding	4	Follow-up (RR)	4.00	4.00	4.00
and No	5	Follow-up (RR)	1.00	1.00	1.00
Interaction	6	Case-control (OR)	1.83	1.83	1.83
	7	Follow-up (RR)	4.00	4.00	4.00
	8	Follow-up (RR)	1.00	1.00	1.00
	9	Case-control (OR)	1.83	1.83	1.83
Confounding	10	Follow-up (RR)	1.01	1.03	4.00
and No	11	Follow-up (RR)	3.00	3.00	1.00
Interaction	12	Case-control (OR)	.83	.83	1.83
Strong	13	Follow-up (RR)	1.07	9.40	4.00
Interaction,	14	Follow-up (RR)	3.00	.33	1.00
Confounding	15	Case-control (OR)	.36	6.00	1.83
Irrelevant					

Table 13.1 (*continued*)

ASSOCIATION OF e WITH f			ASSOCIATION OF d WITH f			
$\hat{OR}_{ef}$	$\hat{OR}_{ef\mid D}$	$\hat{OR}_{ef\mid \bar{D}}$	$\hat{OR}_{df}$	$\hat{OR}_{df\mid E}$	$\hat{OR}_{df\mid \bar{E}}$	*Type of Bias*
81.00	—	—	(7.56)	4.31	7.98	+ (Confounding)
.11	—	—	(3.54)	4.42	7.11	− (Confounding)
(4.55)	8.67	4.09	(11.71)	21.19	10.00	(Confounding)
1.00	—	—	(7.67)	9.33	6.56	None
1.00	—	—	(12.43)	12.43	12.43	None
(1.11)	1.00	1.00	(2.11)	2.11	2.11	None
16.00	—	—	(2.36)	1.00	1.00	(Other)[a]
9.00	—	—	(1.00)	1.00	1.00	(Other)[a]
(.44)	.44	.44	(.89)	1.00	1.00	(Other)[a]
36.00	—	—	(10.67)	10.35	10.62	+ (Confounding)
.05	—	—	(3.59)	9.60	7.11	− (Confounding)
(4.55)	5.00	5.00	(9.33)	10.00	10.00	(Confounding)
—	—	—	—	—	—	Not relevant
—	—	—	—	—	—	Not relevant
—	—	—	—	—	—	Not relevant

[a]"Other" refers to a bias (e.g., selection or information) that is *not* manifested as (data-based) confounding. For a conclusion that such bias is present, the null value obtained for $\hat{OR}_{df\mid \bar{E}}$ should *not* be possibly due to the vagaries of random sampling.

Expression 13.1 should be taken to mean that the crude effect differs appreciably enough from the adjusted effect (the specific choice of $\hat{aR}R$ being up to the investigator) to produce meaningful distortion in the estimated effect of interest.

Example 1 also illustrates another important phenomenon, which, in general, may or may not accompany the presence of confounding in a set of data. We note that the values 1.02 and 1.86 are sufficiently different from one another to suggest that a different e–d relationship may be operating within each of the two levels of f. This *nonuniformity of stratum-specific estimates of effect* illustrates a form of statistical *interaction*. When such interaction involving a *risk factor f* carries over to the population of interest, its population analog is called *effect modification,* and the risk factor f is called an *effect modifier* (or simply a *modifier*) of the e–d relationship. The term "modifier" means that the e–d association of interest depends on (i.e., is modified by) the factor f. (A more detailed discussion of interaction and effect modification is provided in Chapter 19.)

Table 13.2 Examples Showing Confounding and/or Interaction with Randomly Sampled Data

a. Example 1: Follow-up Data Showing Confounding and Interaction with Positive Bias Away from the Null

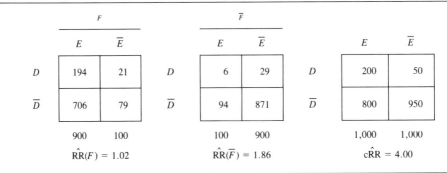

F

	E	$\bar{E}$
D	194	21
$\bar{D}$	706	79
	900	100

$\hat{RR}(F) = 1.02$

$\bar{F}$

	E	$\bar{E}$
D	6	29
$\bar{D}$	94	871
	100	900

$\hat{RR}(\bar{F}) = 1.86$

	E	$\bar{E}$
D	200	50
$\bar{D}$	800	950
	1,000	1,000

$c\hat{RR} = 4.00$

b. Example 1: Additional Tables Showing e–f and d–f Associations

	F	$\bar{F}$
E	900	100
$\bar{E}$	100	900

$\hat{OR}_{ef} = 81.00$

E

	F	$\bar{F}$
D	194	6
$\bar{D}$	706	94

$\hat{OR}_{df|E} = 4.31$

$\bar{E}$

	F	$\bar{F}$
D	21	29
$\bar{D}$	79	871

$\hat{OR}_{df|\bar{E}} = 7.98$

	F	$\bar{F}$
D	215	35
$\bar{D}$	785	966

$\hat{OR}_{df} = 7.56$

c. Example 2: Follow-up Data Showing Confounding and Interaction with Negative Bias Toward the Null

F

	E	$\bar{E}$
D	110	380
$\bar{D}$	390	2,620
	500	3,000

$\hat{RR}(F) = 1.74$

$\bar{F}$

	E	$\bar{E}$
D	90	20
$\bar{D}$	1,410	980
	1,500	1,000

$\hat{RR}(\bar{F}) = 3.00$

	E	$\bar{E}$
D	200	400
$\bar{D}$	1,800	3,600
	2,000	4,000

$c\hat{RR} = 1.00$

Table 13.2 *(continued)*

d. Example 2: Additional Tables Showing *e–f* and *d–f* Associations

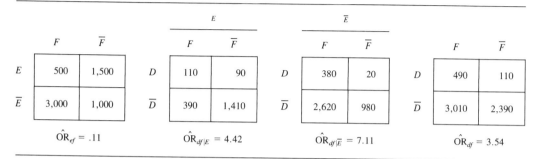

e. Example 3: Case-Control Data Showing Confounding and Interaction with Positive Switchover Bias

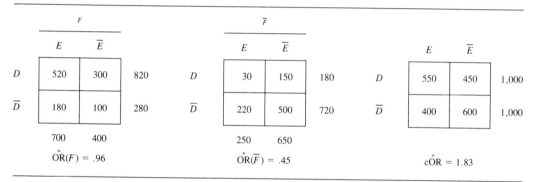

f. Example 3: Additional Tables Showing *e–f* and *d–f* Associations

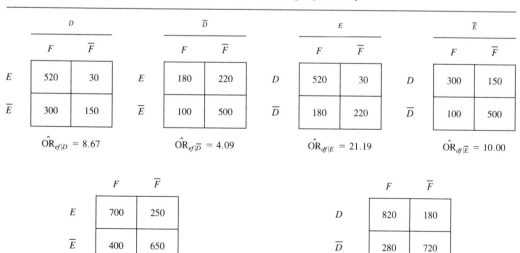

Note that confounding and interaction are different phenomena. In fact, as the remaining examples in Table 13.1 will illustrate, a variable may manifest itself as both a confounder and a modifier, as neither, or as only one of the two. Examples 2 and 3, like Example 1, illustrate *both confounding and interaction*. In Example 2, there is a (negative) bias *toward the null,* since the estimated crude effect indicates that the $e{-}d$ relationship is much weaker (in fact, null) than it is after controlling for f; i.e.,

$$c\hat{R}R = 1.00, \qquad \text{whereas} \qquad \hat{R}R_1 = 1.74 \qquad \text{and} \qquad \hat{R}R_2 = 3.00$$

In contrast to Examples 1 and 2, Example 3 illustrates a situation in which the estimated adjusted effect "switches over" to the side of unity opposite that of the estimated crude effect; in particular,

$$c\hat{O}R = 1.83, \qquad \text{but} \qquad \hat{O}R_1 = .96 \qquad \text{and} \qquad \hat{O}R_2 = .45$$

Proceeding further down Table 13.1, we see that Examples 4–9 illustrate *no confounding and no interaction*; e.g., Example 4 gives

$$c\hat{R}R = \hat{R}R_1 = \hat{R}R_2 = 4.00$$

Examples 10–12, on the other hand, illustrate *confounding without interaction*; e.g., in Example 10, we have

$$c\hat{R}R = 4.00, \qquad \text{but} \qquad \hat{R}R_1 \approx \hat{R}R_2 \approx 1.00$$

Finally, Examples 13–15 illustrate situations in which such strong interaction is encountered that the assessment of confounding becomes irrelevant. For instance, in Example 13, we find

$$\hat{R}R_1 = 1.07 \qquad \text{and} \qquad \hat{R}R_2 = 9.40$$

so that stratum 1 suggests no $e{-}d$ relationship, while evidence of a very strong relationship is reflected in stratum 2. In Examples 14 and 15, the stratum-specific effect estimates are on opposite sides of unity. When situations such as those above are encountered (and the numbers in each stratum are sufficiently large to conclude that f is truly an effect modifier), the confounding effects of f are then of minor importance. Furthermore, as a matter of general analytic strategy (which we will describe in detail in Chapter 20), we recommend that the assessment of interaction should precede any attempt to control for confounding. Indeed, the use of a summary index like $a\hat{R}R(f)$ is recommended only when there is approximate uniformity of estimated effects over the strata (i.e., no "meaningful" interaction). [A word of caution is needed here, since what appears to be interaction may actually be the result of confounding by yet another variable that has not been taken into account. See Lewis (1980) for theoretical and numerical discussions on this point.]

In addition to highlighting the distinction between confounding and interaction, Table 13.1 also illustrates mathematically derived conditions

Table 13.3 Subgroup of Examples Illustrating Conditions for Confounding by Study Design

Example	Study (Effect Measure)	Description	$\hat{OR}_{ef}$	$\hat{OR}_{ef\mid D}$	$\hat{OR}_{ef\mid \bar{D}}$	$\hat{OR}_{df}$	$\hat{OR}_{df\mid E}$	$\hat{OR}_{df\mid \bar{E}}$	Type of Bias
4	Follow-up (RR)	No confounding, no interaction	1.00	—	—	(7.67)	9.33	6.56	None
7		No confounding, no interaction	16.00	—	—	(2.36)	1.00	1.00	(Other)[a]
10		Confounding, no interaction	36.00	—	—	(10.67)	10.35	10.62	+ (Confounding)
6	Case-control (OR)	No confounding, no interaction	(1.11)	1.00	1.00	(2.11)	2.11	2.11	None
9		No confounding, no interaction	(.44)	.44	.44	(0.89)	1.00	1.00	(Other)[a]
12		Confounding, no interaction	(4.55)	5.00	5.00	(9.33)	10.00	10.00	(Confounding)

Note: — denotes an odds ratio value not included in the table because the conditions for confounding in that situation do not involve this odds ratio. ( ) are used to denote odds ratio values that are included for illustrative purposes, although the conditions for confounding in that situation do not involve this odds ratio.

[a]"Other" refers to a bias (e.g., selection or information) that is *not* manifested as (data-based) confounding.

for the presence of confounding (Kupper et al., 1981), conditions that are expressed in terms of unconditional and conditional associations of the risk factor f with the disease (d) and exposure (e) variables. To describe these conditions in detail, we will narrow our focus to a portion of Table 13.1. In particular, Table 13.3 restricts our attention to three of the follow-up study examples (4, 7, 10), and to three of the case-control study examples (6, 9, 12).

**13.2.2.
Follow-up
Studies**

We focus first on the *follow-up study using a risk ratio effect measure*. The conditions necessary for confounding to be present *in the data* (when there is no interaction) are

$$\hat{OR}_{ef} \neq 1 \quad and \quad \hat{OR}_{df|\overline{E}} \neq 1 \tag{13.2}$$

Note that $\hat{OR}_{df|\overline{E}} = \hat{OR}_{df|E}$ under the no-interaction (i.e., uniformity) assumption when f is a dichotomous risk factor.

In Example 4, in which neither confounding nor interaction is present in the data, the first of these conditions is not satisfied. In Example 7, in which there is also no evidence of confounding or interaction in the data, the second condition is not satisfied. However, in Example 10, where confounding is present, both conditions are satisfied; i.e., $\hat{OR}_{ef} = 36.00$, $\hat{OR}_{df|E} = 10.35 \approx \hat{OR}_{df|\overline{E}} = 10.62$. Although we will discuss the implications of these conditions later, in Section 13.5, it is important to note here that the condition $\hat{OR}_{ef} \neq 1$ indicates that the exposure variable is *unconditionally* related to the variable f. In other words, the distribution of f among the exposed is not the same as the distribution of f among the unexposed. As an illustration, Example 4 is contrasted below with Example 10:

		EXAMPLE 4			EXAMPLE 10	
		F	$\overline{F}$		F	$\overline{F}$
E		400	600	E	800	200
$\overline{E}$		400	600	$\overline{E}$	100	900

$$\hat{OR}_{ef} = \frac{400(600)}{600(400)} = 1 \qquad \hat{OR}_{ef} = \frac{800(900)}{200(100)} = 36$$

The second condition in Equation 13.2, $\hat{OR}_{df|\overline{E}} \neq 1$, indicates that the disease variable is *conditionally* (among the unexposed) related to the variable f. We should fully expect this condition to be satisfied *under random sampling* (discounting the possibility of an unrepresentative sample) if we have correctly determined that the variable f is predictive of the disease (i.e., is a risk factor). Consequently, if $\hat{OR}_{df|\bar{E}} = 1$, yet we *know* that f is a risk factor, we can argue, again discounting the vagaries of random sampling, that some form of bias (e.g., selection or information) is present other than data-based confounding. Unfortunately, since $a\hat{RR} = c\hat{RR}$, such bias cannot be corrected at the analysis stage. As an illustration, note that $\hat{OR}_{ef} = 16$ and $\hat{OR}_{df|\bar{E}} = 1.00$ in Example 7. Thus, strictly speaking, there is no evidence of confounding since $c\hat{RR} = a\hat{RR}(f) = 4.00$. However, given that f is truly a risk factor, the fact that the data do not reflect this phenomenon indicates the presence of some sort of bias in $a\hat{RR}(f)$.

If $OR_{ef} \neq 1$ in the population, and f is a risk factor, so that $OR_{df|\bar{E}} \neq 1$, then there is *population-based confounding*; such confounding in the population may be present even when there is no data-based confounding. In Example 7, if $\hat{OR}_{ef} = 16$ reflects the corresponding population value, then there is population-based confounding given that f is a risk factor. However, because of some form of bias, such confounding does *not* manifest itself in the data. Although $a\hat{RR} = c\hat{RR}$ is probably a biased estimate of aRR, no data-based correction can be made. [See Miettinen and Cook (1981) for further discussion on this point.]

We turn now to the *case-control study*, for which the *odds ratio* is the effect measure of interest. The conditions necessary for confounding to be present in the data (when there is no interaction) are

13.2.3
Case-Control
Studies

$$\hat{OR}_{ef|\bar{D}} \neq 1 \quad and \quad \hat{OR}_{df|\bar{E}} \neq 1 \qquad (13.3)$$

Note that $\hat{OR}_{ef|\bar{D}} = \hat{OR}_{ef|D}$ and $\hat{OR}_{df|\bar{E}} = \hat{OR}_{df|E}$ under uniformity. Although the second condition in Expression 13.3 is the same as that in Expression 13.2, the first condition in Expression 13.3 indicates that e must be related to f conditionally (among the nondiseased) when the odds ratio is the effect measure of interest. (This distinction has important implications regarding the use of *matching* in the study design; these will be discussed in Chapter 18).

From Table 13.3, we see that the first condition in Expression 13.3 is not satisfied in Example 6, and the second condition is not satisfied in Example 9. Hence, there is no evidence of confounding in these examples. In Example 12, however, where confounding is present, both conditions in Expression 13.3 are satisfied. As was true for follow-up studies, we would not expect $\hat{OR}_{df|\bar{E}}$ to be unity under random sampling in a case-control study if the extraneous factor f is truly a risk factor (i.e., is predictive of the disease). However, if such is the case (as in Example 9), there is a bias that cannot be corrected by stratifying on f at the analysis stage.

We have now completed a data analysis–oriented discussion of confounding for the single-extraneous-factor case. We will move on to discuss con-

13.2.4
Summary

founding more conceptually. We will first consider the issue of whether or not confounding should be assessed by statistical-testing procedures. Then we will discuss eligibility requirements for the initial selection of extraneous variables, requirements that concern theoretical attributes of such variables over and above characteristics in the data being analyzed. Finally, we will provide a general discussion of confounding involving a single risk factor. Then, in Chapter 14, we will consider problems with confounding involving two or more risk factors.

13.3 SHOULD WE PERFORM A STATISTICAL TEST TO ASSESS CONFOUNDING?

The answer to this question from the epidemiologic literature on confounding (Miettinen, 1974; Fisher and Patil, 1974; Dales and Ury, 1979) has been an unqualified *no*, even though the use of statistical testing to assess confounding is not unheard of in epidemiologic practice. The basic reason for *not* making statistical inferences from tests is that confounding is a *validity* issue that concerns whether or not there is a distortion of the e–d relationship in the data resulting from failure to control for one or more extraneous factors. Even if such a distortion occurs by chance (i.e., the crude and adjusted parameters are equal in the population), it would still have to be corrected in the data in order to obtain a proper estimate of the true e–d association. For example, suppose that the estimated crude and adjusted effects differ greatly [e.g., $c\hat{R}R = 1.3$, but $a\hat{R}R(f) = 5.2$], yet significance testing does not reject the (null) hypothesis that $cRR = aRR(f)$ in the population. The adjusted estimator would still be preferred, because it corrects for the distortion in the data that would remain if the crude estimate were used. The statistical significance of the e–d association is then appropriately assessed by a test (to be described in subsequent chapters) of the null hypothesis H_0: $aRR(f) = 1$. In other words, one should first decide which estimator (crude or adjusted) is more appropriate; *then* one may assess the statistical significance of the chosen estimator.

As a second example, suppose that the crude and adjusted estimates do not differ substantially [e.g., $c\hat{R}R = 2.2$ and $a\hat{R}R(f) = 2.4$], yet testing of the null hypothesis H_0: $cRR = aRR(f)$ indicates that the corresponding population parameters are different. (This situation is likely to occur when the sample size for the study is quite large.) Then, despite the "statistical" difference, no meaningful distortion in the estimate is obtained by using the crude estimate; i.e., it is not necessary to control for f on validity grounds.

In summary, *the use of a statistical test is not appropriate to assess confounding*. Instead, the investigator must make such an evaluation by using data-based comparisons (of crude versus adjusted effects), which address whether a meaningful distortion of the e–d relationship is obtained by using the crude estimate. After the investigator decides which variables need control, he or she can use statistical testing to assess the strength of the e–d association on the basis of the estimator chosen.

Prerequisite to any evaluation of confounding in the data is the consideration of causal relationships that the investigator believes to be operating in the target population. This latter point has not been fully appreciated by many investigators, and, if it is ignored, the result may be unwarranted control of nonconfounders. Such unnecessary adjustment can lower precision and may even introduce bias into the estimate of effect. First, one must permit only *risk factors* (i.e., risk indicators, determinants of disease) to be candidates for control among the entire collection of extraneous variables under consideration. In other words, the definition of a confounder requires that it be a risk factor identified *before* data collection. Second, as we have already described, a confounder must meet a data-based criterion like Equation 13.1.

Broadly speaking, a risk factor is any variable that the investigator determines to be "causally related" (though not necessarily a "direct" cause) and antecedent to illness outcome status (i.e., to the disease) on the basis of substantive knowledge or theory and/or on previous research findings. Age and smoking status, for example, are widely considered to be risk factors for lung cancer, even though the mechanisms by which both variables are determinants of this disease are not well understood. On the other hand, race is not considered to be a risk factor for lung cancer. Also, carrying matches is not a risk factor for lung cancer, although it may be considered as a (poor) surrogate for smoking status. The rationale for restricting potential confounders to risk factors is that primary interest lies in exploring the exposure-disease relationship only after taking into account (i.e., controlling or adjusting for) all other factors known a priori to be causally related to disease development. In other words, if we conclude that there is a strong exposure-disease relationship in our study, we would not want this finding to be explained away by other variables already known to be predictive of the disease.

Admittedly, the decision regarding which extraneous variables to include in the list of risk factors is, in practice, rarely a clear-cut matter. A thorough review of current knowledge and theory about the research question is certainly a necessity. In any case, a cautious approach would entail not being restrictive in the designation of risk factors. After data collection, but prior to the primary data analysis, variables measured for other purposes (e.g., in a broad study designed to evaluate several etiologic questions) may be added to the list of risk factors if they were previously overlooked. Also, a surrogate of a risk factor may have to be used when the latter cannot be readily measured. For example, the number of years spent in a given job in a particular industry is often used as a surrogate measure for the actual amount of exposure to a toxic substance suspected of being an occupationally related carcinogen.

In identifying risk factors, the investigator can be guided by the principle that a variable need not be so identified if it can be considered to be superfluous as a predictor of disease once the risk factors already specified have been taken into account. In other words, in the ideal situation, the investigator need only be concerned about a subset of risk factors that are independent predictors of disease. In practice, this ideal is not easily attainable, nor verifiable, because of the qualitative nature of the process of risk assessment and the theoretical validation criteria that are required at the *population* level (see below). Moreover, the control of confounding does not, as we will later discuss, require us to weed out superfluous risk factors prior to data analysis. Nevertheless, for a proper *understanding* of the characteristics of a confounder, it is useful to consider further this ideal framework.

Quantitatively speaking, the notion of an "independent predictor" of disease suggests a statistical criterion involving *conditional association* between a given risk factor (f_j) and disease status (d). In terms of effect measures we have considered, a reasonable criterion for f_j to be an independent predictor is as follows:

$$\text{OR}_{df_j|\bar{E},\bar{F}_1,\ldots,\bar{F}_k} \neq 1 \quad \text{(excluding } \bar{F}_j) \tag{13.4}$$

This criterion states that the population odds ratio relating the risk factor f_j to d must be different from one, conditional on the absence of all other specified risk factors, including the exposure variable. In a regression context, a related criterion would require a nonzero regression coefficient for each risk factor f_j in a logistic regression model (see Chapter 20), like

$$\mathscr{E}(d) = \left\{1 + \exp\left[-\left(\alpha + \sum_{j=1}^{k} \gamma_j f_j + \beta e\right)\right]\right\}^{-1}$$

where $\mathscr{E}(\cdot)$ denotes statistical expectation and α, γ_j, and β denote regression model parameters.

In the case of a single risk factor, Condition 13.4 reduces to the requirement

$$\text{OR}_{df|\bar{E}} \neq 1 \tag{13.5}$$

which states that the risk indicator status (of f) should obtain even "on the null hypothesis," or, equivalently, among the nonexposed (Miettinen, 1974). The reader will recognize Expression 13.5 as the population analog of the second condition for confounding given in both Expressions 13.2 and 13.3. Thus, if the only risk factor on our list is f, we are presuming that Condition 13.5 holds for our *population*. Assuming that our sample is representative of this population, we would *expect* our data to reflect this association; i.e., we should see $\hat{\text{OR}}_{df|\bar{E}} \neq 1$. The implication with regard to bias for a sample that fails to reflect Condition 13.5 has been illustrated in Section 13.2.

More generally, if a set of independent predictors $f_1, f_2, \ldots, f_k$ can be identified, we would expect Expression 13.4 to be reflected in the data for each f_j (assuming, again, that our sample is representative). If, on the other hand, Expression 13.4 is not supported by the data for a given variable f_j, we can conclude (assuming a representative sample) that f_j is superfluous for control purposes once the other risk factors have been controlled. As we will see in Chapter 14, however, f_j may still be considered to be a confounder if its control, either by itself or in tandem with a subset of other risk factors, will remove confounding.

We wish to point out one other important consideration regarding causal relationships involved in identifying extraneous factors eligible for control. In theory, a list of risk factors should be restricted to variables that cannot be characterized in causal terms as *intervening* in the causal pathway between exposure and disease. A "pure" intervening variable (i.e., a variable g in the causal sequence $e \rightarrow g \rightarrow d$) should not be considered as a potential confounder, since its control can spuriously reduce or eliminate any manifestation in the data of a true association between d and e. Practically speaking, however, it is difficult for the investigator to distinguish intervening variables from risk factors; a cautious approach would retain all risk factors that are not obviously intervening variables.

13.5 SINGLE–RISK FACTOR CONFOUNDING: GENERAL PRINCIPLES

We have already emphasized that confounding (regardless of the number of variables eligible for control) requires consideration both of causal relationships that the investigator believes to be operating in the target population and data-based associations. As we discussed in the previous section, the theoretical eligibility requirement for any extraneous factor is that, on the basis of information external to the study, f be determined to be a non-intervening risk factor for the disease. As we illustrated in Section 13.1, the data-based criterion for confounding involving a single risk factor is that the estimated crude measure of effect (obtained by ignoring the factor f) differ from an adjusted estimate of effect (obtained by controlling for the factor f); i.e., we have

$$\hat{c\theta} \neq \hat{a\theta}(f) \tag{13.6}$$

where θ denotes the effect measure (e.g., θ denotes an odds ratio or risk ratio), $\hat{c\theta}$ denotes the estimated crude effect, and $\hat{a\theta}(f)$ denotes the estimated adjusted effect. [The population analog of Expression 13.6 has been referred to as the "collapsibility" condition by Whittemore (1978). In our terminology, this condition would indicate population-based confounding.] The adjusted measure $\hat{a\theta}(f)$ usually has the form of a weighted sum of stratum-specific measures (based on stratifying on f) and, as such, can be quite misleading when there is nonuniformity of the effect measure across the strata.

13.5.1 Follow-up Study Using the Risk Ratio

When the effect measure is the risk ratio, it follows, from our previous discussion, that *both* $\hat{OR}_{ef}$ and $\hat{OR}_{df|\bar{E}}$ must differ from unity in order for $c\hat{RR}$ to be different from $a\hat{RR}$ (i.e., for data-based confounding to be present). As we have already pointed out, however, the requirement $\hat{OR}_{df|\bar{E}} \neq 1$

may be viewed as corroboration in a representative sample that the variable f is indeed an independent risk factor. Thus, given that f is a risk factor, it may be argued for data representative of the population that the condition $\hat{OR}_{ef} \neq 1$ is the fundamental requirement for data-based confounding in a follow-up study using a risk ratio. The corresponding population-based requirement would be $OR_{ef} \neq 1$.

**13.5.2
Case-Control
Study Using
the Odds Ratio**

When the odds ratio is the effect measure, the conditions for data-based confounding are given by Expression 13.3 in terms of $\hat{OR}_{ef|\overline{D}}$ and $\hat{OR}_{df|\overline{E}}$. The corresponding conditions for population-based confounding are

$$OR_{ef|\overline{D}} \neq 1 \quad \text{and} \quad OR_{df|\overline{E}} \neq 1$$

The risk factor f will therefore be manifest in the data as a confounder (with regard to the odds ratio) when it is differentially distributed between the exposed and unexposed groups in the sample of controls *and* when it reflects its risk factor attribute in the data.

**13.6
CON-
CLUDING
REMARKS**

In this chapter, we have discussed the concept of confounding when only a single potential confounder is under consideration. Clearly, confounding and its proper control continues to be a source of controversy. In particular, the identification of risk factors as potential confounders is not an easy task. Moreover, subjective judgment is often required to decide whether a crude estimate differs enough from an adjusted estimate to warrant control. Finally, various types of bias can yield misleading conclusions from just data-based associations.

These and other problems make the assessment of confounding even more complex when two or more potential confounders require simultaneous consideration. This multi–risk factor situation will be discussed in Chapter 14.

NOTATION

The following list summarizes the key notation introduced in this chapter.

d	Disease variable.
e	Exposure variable.
$f, f_1, \ldots, f_k$	Extraneous variables (risk factors considered for possible control).
$\hat{cRR}$	Estimated crude (i.e., unadjusted) risk ratio measuring e–d association.
$\hat{cOR}$	Estimated crude (i.e., unadjusted) odds ratio measuring e–d association.
$\hat{aRR}(f_1, \ldots, f_k)$	Estimated adjusted risk ratio measuring e–d association after controlling for $f_1, \ldots, f_k$ simultaneously.

$a\hat{\text{OR}}(f_1, \ldots, f_k)$	Estimated adjusted odds ratio measuring e–d association after controlling for $f_1, \ldots, f_k$ simultaneously.
$\hat{\text{OR}}_{ef}$	Estimated unconditional odds ratio measuring e–f association.
$\hat{\text{OR}}_{ef\|D}$	Estimated conditional odds ratio measuring e–f association among diseased subjects.
$\hat{\text{OR}}_{ef\|\overline{D}}$	Estimated conditional odds ratio measuring e–f association among nondiseased subjects.
$\hat{\text{OR}}_{df}$	Estimated unconditional odds ratio measuring d–f association.
$\hat{\text{OR}}_{df\|E}$	Estimated conditional odds ratio measuring d–f association among exposed subjects.
$\hat{\text{OR}}_{df\|\overline{E}}$	Estimated conditional odds ratio measuring d–f association among nonexposed subjects.
$\hat{\text{OR}}_{df_j\|\overline{E},\overline{F}_1, \ldots, \overline{F}_k}$ (excluding $\overline{F}_j$)	Estimated conditional odds ratio measuring d–f_j association among nonexposed subjects who do not have any of the other risk factors being studied.
$\hat{c\theta}$	Crude estimate of parameter θ.
$\hat{a\theta}(f)$	Adjusted estimate of parameter θ after controlling for factor f.

13.1 Let $(D, \overline{D})$ index disease status, $(E, \overline{E})$ exposure status, and (F_1, F_0) the two levels of a potential confounder (gender). Suppose your study results are as shown in Exercise Table 13.1.

PRACTICE EXERCISES

Exercise Table 13.1

	F_1 (MALES)			F_0 (FEMALES)	
	E	$\overline{E}$		E	$\overline{E}$
D	9,100	900	D	900	89,100
$\overline{D}$	990	8,110	$\overline{D}$	10	81,890

a. Calculate $\hat{\text{OR}}$ for males and females separately. Is there evidence of interaction in these data?

b. By combining the E and $\overline{E}$ groups, one obtains the accompanying table involving $(D, \overline{D})$ and (F_1, F_0). Calculate the odds ratio for this table. Is there an unconditional association between gender and disease status?

	F_1 (MALES)	F_0 (FEMALES)
D	10,000	90,000
$\overline{D}$	9,100	81,900

c. The crude table relating disease and exposure (ignoring the potential confounder) is as follows:

	E	$\overline{E}$
D	10,000	90,000
$\overline{D}$	1,000	90,000

Is there evidence of confounding due to gender in this data set?

d. The association between disease status and gender for exposed and non-exposed groups separately can be described by the data in Exercise Table 13.2. Is there an association between gender and disease status *conditional* on exposure status?

Exercise Table 13.2

	E			$\overline{E}$	
	F_1	F_0		F_1	F_0
D	9,100	900	D	900	89,100
$\overline{D}$	990	10	$\overline{D}$	8,110	81,890

e. What is the moral of this exercise with regard to making a decision about confounding based on unconditional associations among the variables being studied?

13.2 Assume that there is no overall association between breast cancer and the use of the drug reserpine in a certain target population of 2 million women. Also, assume that this lack of association carries over to both upper- and lower-socioeconomic-status (SES) groups, each of which contains 1 million women. Let the prevalence of breast cancer (d) and of reserpine use (e) in this population be as given in Exercise Table 13.3.

Exercise Table 13.3

	High SES	Low SES
Breast Cancer Prevalence	20/100,000	20/100,000
Reserpine Use Prevalence	800/10,000	200/10,000

a. From the above information, one can generate Exercise Table 13.4, which relates breast cancer prevalence (D or $\overline{D}$) to reserpine use (E or $\overline{E}$) in this population (you may wish to verify these results). Is there population-based confounding due to SES?

Exercise Table 13.4

	HIGH SES				LOW SES		
	E	$\overline{E}$			E	$\overline{E}$	
D	16	184	200	D	4	196	200
$\overline{D}$	79,984	919,816	999,800	$\overline{D}$	19,996	979,804	999,800
	80,000	920,000	1,000,000		20,000	980,000	1,000,000

	CRUDE		
	E	$\overline{E}$	
D	20	380	400
$\overline{D}$	99,980	1,899,620	1,999,600
	100,000	1,900,000	2,000,000

b. Suppose that the hospitalization probabilities within each SES group are as given in Exercise Table 13.5. From this information, one can generate Exercise Table 13.6, which describes the expected hospital population for a cross-sectional study involving all females in hospitals serving the target population (again, you may wish to verify these results). Calculate the $\widehat{OR}$ for each table. Is there data-based confounding? Interaction?

Exercise Table 13.5

		HIGH SES					LOW SES	
		E	$\overline{E}$				E	$\overline{E}$
D		1	1		D		1	1
$\overline{D}$		.001	.001		$\overline{D}$		.01	.01

Exercise Table 13.6

	HIGH SES			LOW SES			CRUDE	
	E	$\overline{E}$		E	$\overline{E}$		E	$\overline{E}$
D	16	184	D	4	196	D	20	380
$\overline{D}$	80	920	$\overline{D}$	200	9,798	$\overline{D}$	280	10,718

c. On the basis of the data given in part b, what should be the "correct" value of the adjusted odds ratio that controls for confounding? How does this value relate to the corresponding measure of association in the target population?

d. Calculate the selection probabilities α, β, γ, δ for the overall hospital population (both SES groups combined), and then use these values to determine whether there is selection bias due to restricting the study to hospital patients.

e. How is it possible that SES can be a confounder in the hospital population when it is not a confounder in the target population? Support your answer by considering the relevant sample selection probabilities.

13.3 This problem describes a method for quantifying the amount of confounding contributed by a collection of one or more extraneous factors that are simultaneously controlled by stratification (see Miettinen, 1972). The following *background information* is needed.

Suppose that the data are categorized into G strata according to combinations of levels of potential confounders. Let the gth stratum be represented as shown in Exercise Table 13.7. For example, if AGE (old versus young), RACE (black versus white), and GENDER (male versus female) are all potential confounders, we would have $G = 2^3 = 8$ strata: old BM, young BM, old WM, etc.

Exercise Table 13.7

	E	$\overline{E}$	*Total*
D	a_g	b_g	m_{1g}
$\overline{D}$	c_g	d_g	m_{0g}
Total	n_{1g}	n_{0g}	n_g

To measure the amount of confounding by using G strata, we compute an *expected value* for the crude effect under the null hypothesis that the study factor (e) has no independent relationship to the disease (d). For *follow-up studies*, using the risk ratio (RR) as the effect measure, this expected value ($\hat{\mathcal{E}}RR$) is given by the formula

$$\hat{\mathcal{E}}RR = \frac{\sum\limits_{g=1}^{G} \hat{\mathcal{E}}(A_g) \Big/ \sum\limits_{g=1}^{G} n_{1g}}{\sum\limits_{g=1}^{G} b_g \Big/ \sum\limits_{g=1}^{G} n_{0g}}$$

where $\hat{\mathcal{E}}(A_g) = b_g n_{1g}/n_{0g}$ is the expected number of exposed cases under the null hypothesis of no association within the gth stratum. Note that $\hat{\mathcal{E}}(A_g)$ may be obtained by solving the equation

$$\hat{\mathcal{E}}RR_g = \frac{\hat{\mathcal{E}}(A_g)/n_{1g}}{b_g/n_{0g}} = 1$$

for $\hat{\mathcal{E}}(A_g)$, where $\hat{\mathcal{E}}RR_g$ denotes the expected risk ratio for stratum g given no association. Note also that $\hat{\mathcal{E}}RR$ is an "expected crude effect under no association," since it can be written as

$$\hat{\mathcal{E}}RR = \frac{\hat{\mathcal{E}}(A)/n_1}{b/n_0}$$

where $\hat{\mathcal{E}}(A) = \sum_{g=1}^{G} \hat{\mathcal{E}}(A_g)$, $n_1 = \sum_{g=1}^{G} n_{1g}$, $b = \sum_{g=1}^{G} b_g$, $n_0 = \sum_{g=1}^{G} n_{0g}$.

In contrast, the estimated crude effect is given by

$$c\hat{R}R = \frac{a/n_1}{b/n_0}$$

where $a = \Sigma_{g=1}^{G} a_g$.

The magnitude of $\mathscr{E}\hat{R}R$ may be used to measure the amount of confounding in the data. In particular, if $\mathscr{E}\hat{R}R = 1$, then there is no confounding. Also, the more $\mathscr{E}\hat{R}R$ differs from one, the greater is the amount of confounding.

An adjusted estimator of the risk ratio that controls for confounding may be defined (using the above formulation) as the ratio

$$c\hat{R}R/\mathscr{E}\hat{R}R$$

It can be shown that this estimator is equivalent to a *standardized* risk ratio ($s\hat{R}R$), which we will discuss in Chapter 17. This adjusted estimator can alternatively be written in the form of a weighted average of stratum-specific risk ratio estimates. If $\mathscr{E}\hat{R}R = 1$, then it follows that the adjusted estimate ($s\hat{R}R = c\hat{R}R/\mathscr{E}\hat{R}R$) is equal to the crude estimate, which corresponds to our data-based requirement for no confounding, given by Equation 13.1.

For *case-control studies*, where the odds ratio (OR) is the effect measure, the amount of confounding may be quantified by using the expected crude estimate

$$\mathscr{E}\hat{O}R = [\hat{\mathscr{E}}(A)]d/bc$$

Here, $\hat{\mathscr{E}}(A) = \Sigma_{g=1}^{G} \hat{\mathscr{E}}(A_g)$, where $\hat{\mathscr{E}}(A_g) = b_g c_g/d_g$ is the expected number of exposed cases under the null hypothesis that the expected odds ratio is unity in stratum g, and b, c, and d are the respective totals of b_g, c_g, and d_g over all strata. Like the magnitude of $\mathscr{E}\hat{R}R$, the magnitude of $\mathscr{E}\hat{O}R$ can be used to measure the amount of confounding, with $\mathscr{E}\hat{O}R = 1$ indicating no confounding. Also, the ratio

$$s\hat{O}R = c\hat{O}R/\mathscr{E}\hat{O}R$$

represents an adjusted estimate of effect (which we will denote as a standardized odds ratio in Chapter 17).

The questions that follow are intended to illustrate the above procedure for the case-control data (with $G = 2$ strata) given in Exercise Table 13.8.

a. Calculate the stratum-specific odds ratios ($\hat{O}R_g$) and the crude odds ratio. Is gender a confounder in these data?

b. Calculate the expected crude odds ratio ($\mathscr{E}\hat{O}R$) under the null hypothesis of no effect due to E. Is gender a confounder on the basis of the value of $\mathscr{E}\hat{O}R$?

c. Calculate the adjusted odds ratio $c\hat{O}R/\mathscr{E}\hat{O}R$. Is there an association between E and D after adjusting for any gender effect? (Ignore any test for statistical significance.) Compare this adjusted estimate with the stratum-specific estimates ($\hat{O}R_g$).

Exercise Table 13.8

	MEN			WOMEN	
	E	$\overline{E}$		E	$\overline{E}$
D	40	60	D	150	50
$\overline{D}$	50	150	$\overline{D}$	60	40

REFERENCES

DALES, L. G., and URY, H. K. 1979. An improper use of statistical significance testing in studying covariables. *Int. J. Epidemiol.* 7: 373–375.

FISHER, L., and PATIL, K. 1974. Matching and unrelatedness. *Am. J. Epidemiol.* 100: 347–349.

GREENLAND, S., and NEUTRA, R. 1980. Control of confounding in the assessment of medical technology. *Int. J. Epidemiol.* 9(4): 361–367.

KUPPER, L. L.; KARON, J. M.; KLEINBAUM, D. G.; MORGENSTERN, H.; and LEWIS, D. K. 1981. Matching in epidemiologic studies: Validity and efficiency considerations. *Biometrics* 37(2): 271–291.

LEWIS, D. K. 1980. Matching on several variables in epidemiologic studies. Ph.D. dissertation, University of North Carolina at Chapel Hill.

MIETTINEN, O. S. 1972. Components of the crude risk ratio. *Am. J. Epidemiol.* 96: 168–172.

———. 1974. Confounding and effect modification. *Am. J. Epidemiol.* 100(5): 350–353.

———. 1976. Stratification by a multivariate confounder score. *Am. J. Epidemiol.* 104(6): 609–620.

MIETTINEN, O. S., and COOK, E. F. 1981. Confounding: Essence and detection. *Am. J. Epidemiol.* 114(4): 593–603.

WHITTEMORE, A. S. 1978. Collapsibility of multidimensional contingency tables. *J. R. Stat. Soc. B* 40: 328–340.

14

Confounding Involving Several Risk Factors

CHAPTER OUTLINE

Two fundamental principles about the control of confounding need to be considered when, as is the usual situation, two or more risk factors have been identified and measured for possible control:

14.0 PREVIEW

1. *The joint (i.e., simultaneous) control of two or more variables can give different results (i.e., different adjusted estimators) from those obtained by controlling for each variable separately; moreover, the ultimate standard on which all conclusions about confounding and the identification of specific confounders must be based is ideally an adjusted estimate that simultaneously controls for all risk factors under consideration.* The main implication here is that "the need to control a given factor depends ultimately on its characteristics (relatedness to the exposure and the illness), *conditional on whatever other factors are controlled . . .*" (Miettinen, 1974). Failure to consider the combined effects of *all* risk factors measured in a study when assessing confounding may lead to the retention or even the introduction of confounding (see Fisher and Patil, 1974).

2. *Not all the variables in a given list of risk factors may need to be controlled; moreover, depending on the relationships among these risk factors, it is possible that confounding can be corrected by using different subsets of risk factors on the list.* Thus, with regard to bias removal, it is sufficient to use any subset that eliminates such bias (including the one consisting of all the risk factors). Nevertheless, the use of a particular subset for control can be advantageous for other reasons (e.g., to increase precision).

In this chapter, each of the above principles will be considered within the following framework, which is needed to describe the characteristics of confounding when there are several risk factors involved. Letting θ, as before, be any effect measure of interest, we will represent an estimator of θ that simultaneously adjusts for a set of k extraneous factors $f_1, f_2, \ldots, f_k$ by the expression

$$a\hat{\theta}(f_1, f_2, \ldots, f_k)$$

In particular, $a\hat{RR}\ (f_1, f_2, \ldots, f_k)$ and $a\hat{OR}\ (f_1, f_2, \ldots, f_k)$ will denote adjusted risk and odds ratio estimates, respectively. When the f_j are categorical, the adjusted estimate will take the form of a weighted average of stratum-specific estimates of θ. For example, if $k = 3$, $f_1 = $ AGE (two levels), $f_2 = $ RACE (two levels), and $f_3 = $ SEX (two levels), then a given stratum would involve one of the AGE levels (e.g., the younger group), one of the RACE levels (e.g., white), and one of the SEX levels (e.g., male), and there would be $2 \times 2 \times 2 = 8$ strata in all. A general description of the different weighting schemes used to form such adjusted estimates is provided in Chapter 17.

If some of the f_j are continuous variables, the mathematical form of an adjusted estimate is more complex. When mathematical modeling is used to assess the e–d relationship, such an estimate takes the form of an estimated regression coefficient for the exposure variable in the model being used (see Chapter 20).

14.1 DEFINITION OF JOINT CON-FOUNDING

We define *data-based joint confounding due to* $f_1, f_2, \ldots, f_k$ to mean that there is a meaningful difference between the estimated crude effect (which completely ignores all the $f_1, f_2, \ldots, f_k$) and the estimated adjusted effect (which simultaneously controls for all the $f_1, f_2, \ldots, f_k$). Quantitatively, this condition can be stated as

$$\hat{c\theta} \neq \hat{a\theta}(f_1, f_2, \ldots, f_k) \tag{14.1}$$

In contrast, *we define data-based marginal confounding due to* f_j to mean that

$$\hat{c\theta} \neq \hat{a\theta}(f_j) \tag{14.2}$$

[These definitions follow the convention of Lewis (1980).]

As we stated in the first principle given in Section 14.0, the primary criterion for documenting the presence of data-based confounding when all $f_1, f_2, \ldots, f_k$ are eligible for control is given by Expression 14.1. In other words, *confounding is present in the data when there is joint confounding involving all the risk factors*. Thus, ideally, the effect to which all data-based comparisons must be made is $\hat{a\theta}(f_1, f_2, \ldots, f_k)$, the adjusted estimate obtained through the simultaneous control of *all* risk factors. Unfortunately, in practice, there may be so many risk factors in our list relative to the amount of data available that $a\theta(f_1, f_2, \ldots, f_k)$ cannot be estimated with any precision at all. As a result, we may be forced to make decisions by using a proper subset of this large initial set of risk factors. And, if the choice of such a subset becomes difficult, the use of marginal confounding criteria may be the only alternative.

EXAMPLE 14.1

As we now illustrate, incorrect conclusions about joint confounding may result if one considers only the conditions for marginal confounding. In Table 14.1, we present data from a hypothetical follow-up study where two dichotomous variables f and g are eligible for control. From the crude table (part d), it is clear that the crude risk ratio is 2.00. From parts b and c of the table, we see that the separate control of either f or g leads to the same risk ratio estimate of 2.00. In other words,

$$\hat{RR}(F) = \hat{RR}(\overline{F}) = 2.00 = c\hat{RR}$$

and

EXAMPLE 14.1 (*continued*)

Table 14.1   Joint Confounding in the Risk Ratio Without Marginal Confounding (Two Extraneous Variables)

a. Joint Control of f and g

	FG				$F\overline{G}$	
	E	$\overline{E}$			E	$\overline{E}$
D	280	70	D		20	80
$\overline{D}$	120	30	$\overline{D}$		80	320

$\hat{\mathrm{RR}}(FG) = 1.00$ $\hat{\mathrm{RR}}(F\overline{G}) = 1.00$

	$\overline{F}G$				$\overline{F}\,\overline{G}$	
	E	$\overline{E}$			E	$\overline{E}$
D	20	80	D		280	70
$\overline{D}$	80	320	$\overline{D}$		120	30

$\hat{\mathrm{RR}}(\overline{F}G) = 1.00$ $\hat{\mathrm{RR}}(\overline{F}\,\overline{G}) = 1.00$

b. Marginal Control of f Only

	F				$\overline{F}$	
	E	$\overline{E}$			E	$\overline{E}$
D	300	150	D		300	150
$\overline{D}$	200	350	$\overline{D}$		200	350

$\hat{\mathrm{RR}}(F) = 2.00$ $\hat{\mathrm{RR}}(\overline{F}) = 2.00$

EXAMPLE 14.1 (*continued*)

c. Marginal Control of g Only

	G			$\overline{G}$	
	E	$\overline{E}$		E	$\overline{E}$
D	300	150	D	300	150
$\overline{D}$	200	350	$\overline{D}$	200	350

$$\hat{RR}(G) = 2.00 \qquad \hat{RR}(\overline{G}) = 2.00$$

d. Crude Table

	E	$\overline{E}$
D	600	300
$\overline{D}$	400	700

$$c\hat{RR} = 2.00$$

Note: $c\hat{RR} = \hat{RR}(F) = \hat{RR}(\overline{F}) = \hat{RR}(G) = \hat{RR}(\overline{G}) = 2.00$, but $\hat{RR}(FG) = \hat{RR}(F\overline{G}) = \hat{RR}(\overline{F}G) = \hat{RR}(\overline{F}\,\overline{G}) = 1.00$.

$$\hat{RR}(G) = \hat{RR}(\overline{G}) = 2.00 = c\hat{RR}$$

Since there is obviously no interaction when controlling separately for either f or g, it follows that

$$a\hat{RR}(f) = c\hat{RR} \qquad \text{and} \qquad a\hat{RR}(g) = c\hat{RR}$$

That is, from Condition 14.2, there is no data-based marginal confounding due to either f or g. Nevertheless, when we consider the simultaneous control of both variables (see part a of the table), we find that each stratum-specific estimated risk ratio equals 1.00. It thus follows (since there is no interaction when controlling for both f and g) that

$$a\hat{RR}(f, g) = 1.00 \neq 2.00 = c\hat{RR}$$

EXAMPLE 14.1 (*continued*)

Hence, by Expression 14.1, there is data-based joint confounding due to f and g.

Example 14.1 illustrates the importance of using *joint* confounding, whenever possible, as the baseline from which all other confounding issues should be examined. In this regard, we will subsequently address the problem of variable selection as it pertains to the identification of subsets of confounders. It will help us first to specify conditions for no joint confounding in terms of the separate relationships of each f_j to the disease and exposure variables (see Lewis, 1980).

There is no data-based joint confounding with regard to the risk ratio provided that *either*

14.1.1 Follow-up Studies

$$\hat{OR}_{efj}\big|_{\substack{F_1, \ldots, F_k \\ (\text{excluding } F_j)}} = 1 \qquad (14.3)$$

for *each and every f_j, $j = 1, 2, \ldots, k$, or*

$$\hat{OR}_{dfj}\big|_{\substack{\overline{E}, F_1, \ldots, F_k \\ (\text{excluding } F_j)}} = 1 \qquad (14.4)$$

for *each and every f_j, $j = 1, 2, \ldots, k$.* The notation "$F_1, \ldots, F_k$ (excluding F_j)" refers to the consideration of any specified combination of levels of the variables other than f_j. Thus, for Equation 14.3 or 14.4 to be satisfied for a given f_j, the conditional odds ratio being considered must be unity for each and every combination of levels chosen.

There is no data-based joint confounding with regard to the odds ratio provided that *either*

14.1.2 Case-Control Studies

$$\hat{OR}_{efj}\big|_{\substack{\overline{D}, F_1, \ldots, F_k \\ (\text{excluding } F_j)}} = 1 \qquad (14.5)$$

for *each and every f_j, $j = 1, 2, \ldots, k$, or* Equation 14.4 is satisfied. These conditions for *no data-based joint confounding* are direct generalizations, to the multi-risk factor case, of conditions given earlier in Sections 13.5.1 and 13.5.2 for a single risk factor f. Unfortunately, they are *sufficient*, but not necessary, conditions for no joint confounding

(Whittemore, 1978); i.e., it is possible to have no confounding even if such conditions are not satisfied. For the data given in Table 14.1, where there is joint confounding, Equations 14.3 and 14.4 are *not* satisfied for *both f* and *g*, as shown in Table 14.2.

Table 14.2 Conditional Relationships of Risk Factors *f* and *g* with *e* and *d* for the Data in Table 14.1

Exposure Relationships (14.3)	Disease Relationships (14.4)
$\hat{OR}_{ef\|G} = 16.00$	$\hat{OR}_{df\|\bar{E},G} = 9.33$
$\hat{OR}_{ef\|\bar{G}} = .06$	$\hat{OR}_{df\|\bar{E},\bar{G}} = .11$
$\hat{OR}_{eg\|F} = 16.00$	$\hat{OR}_{dg\|\bar{E},F} = 9.33$
$\hat{OR}_{eg\|\bar{F}} = .06$	$\hat{OR}_{dg\|\bar{E},\bar{F}} = .11$

14.2 VARIABLE SELECTION AND CONTROL OF CONFOUNDING

Although Example 14.1 illustrated a situation requiring the simultaneous control of *all* the risk factors under consideration, confounding may be controlled through the use of a proper subset of all the risk factors. Fisher and Patil (1974) have argued that variables requiring control may be identified one at a time by considering the conditional associations with *d* and *e* for each variable, controlling for all other variables. In particular, the criteria suggested by Fisher and Patil for ignoring a given risk factor f_j are Condition 14.3 or 14.4 for follow-up studies and Condition 14.4 or 14.5 for case-control studies. However, a flaw in this strategy relates to the possibility that each and every risk factor may be excluded by using these conditional criteria even when there is joint confounding in the data. We will numerically illustrate, using two risk factors, that it is possible for the control of any one variable to become unnecessary once the other variable has been controlled, even though adjustment for at least one variable is necessary to remove confounding. Moreover, it is possible that the "forward type" of strategy advocated by Fisher and Patil may declare as nonconfounders certain subsets of variables that can also provide for proper (and perhaps more efficient) control of confounding.

Miettinen (1974) has argued, in opposition to Fisher and Patil, that even *unconditional* associations, like those measured by $\hat{OR}_{ef}$ and $\hat{OR}_{df}$, can be used for screening purposes. However, he does advocate the "*selective* use of conditional criteria with the aim of *excluding* from control a factor which superficially would appear to be a confounder." Miettinen's main point is that "to pursue routinely the conditional relationships is a policy whose productiveness is much too low to justify the added efforts and complexities relative to the prevailing approach of first 'screening' on the basis of unconditional criteria." However, the example given in Table 14.1 is precisely of the type that would result in invalid conclusions from such unconditional screening. Whether or not this approach would be appropriate for most practical situations remains to be substantiated through further methodological research.

Underlying the discussion by Fisher and Patil (1974) and by Miettinen (1974) is the philosophy that confounding may be appropriately controlled by adjustment for an "efficient" subset of confounders chosen from the total list of risk factors eligible for control. (As we mentioned earlier, the term "efficient" concerns precision in the effect estimate, a topic to be discussed in later chapters.) Even though the strategies advocated by Fisher and Patil and by Miettinen may both be characterized as "forward selection" approaches for the identification of confounders (analogous, but not equivalent, to forward selection procedures used in regression analysis), a basic conceptual understanding of the conditions that identify an appropriate subset of confounders requires a "backward elimination" viewpoint. In particular, this viewpoint is warranted by the need to consider, as a standard, an adjusted estimator that simultaneously controls for all (or at least the most important) risk factors. We will motivate our discussion concerning the identification of a proper subset of confounders through an example.

EXAMPLE 14.2

The data in Table 14.3 involve two dichotomous risk factors f and g in a follow-up study format. We see from Table 14.3a that there is joint confounding in the data; i.e., $c\hat{R}R = 2.00$, but the control of both f and g yields stratum-specific risk ratios of approximately 1.0. In terms of Criterion 14.1, we have

$$c\hat{R}R = 2.00 \neq 1.0 \approx a\hat{R}R(f, g)$$

where $a\hat{R}R(f, g)$ denotes any weighted average of the four stratum-specific $\hat{R}R$'s.

Focusing now on the control of f and g separately, we see that

$$\hat{R}R(F) = \hat{R}R(\overline{F}) = \hat{R}R(G) = \hat{R}R(\overline{G}) \approx 1.0$$

In terms of adjusted risk ratios, it follows that

$$c\hat{R}R = 2.00 \neq 1.0 \approx a\hat{R}R(f) = a\hat{R}R(g) = a\hat{R}R(f, g)$$

Thus, our example illustrates that we do not need to control for both f and g; it is sufficient to control for either one of these two variables

EXAMPLE 14.2 (*continued*)

separately. In other words, controlling for f is unnecessary once g has been controlled; similarly, g is superfluous after controlling for f.

The manipulation of the data in Table 14.3 will yield the results shown in Table 14.4 concerning the data-based conditional relationships of each risk factor with the exposure and disease variables. From Table 14.4, we see that the conditions for no joint confounding, given by Conditions 14.3 and 14.4 for follow-up studies, are *not* satisfied. In particular, Expression 14.3 is not satisfied for *both* f and g, nor is Expression 14.4. If, on the other hand, either all the odds ratios on the left side of Table 14.4 had been approximately equal to one, or all the odds ratios on the right side had been about one, then there would have been no data-based joint confounding.

From the results in the left-hand column of Table 14.4, it is clear that Condition 14.3 holds approximately for variable f; from the right-hand column, Condition 14.4 is essentially satisfied for variable g. Thus, there is no *residual* confounding due to either f or g. Of course, at least one of these two variables has to be taken into account.

**Table 14.3   Confounding Due to Only One Variable
When There Are Two Risk Factors**

a. Joint Control of f and g

	FG			$F\overline{G}$			$\overline{F}G$			$\overline{F}\,\overline{G}$	
	E	$\overline{E}$		E	$\overline{E}$		E	$\overline{E}$		E	$\overline{E}$
D	555	111	D	5	29	D	15	3	D	25	157
$\overline{D}$	238	48	$\overline{D}$	2	12	$\overline{D}$	62	12	$\overline{D}$	98	628

$\hat{\text{RR}}(FG) = 1.00$ $\hat{\text{RR}}(F\overline{G}) = 1.03$ $\hat{\text{RR}}(\overline{F}G) = .97$ $\hat{\text{RR}}(\overline{F}\,\overline{G}) = 1.02$

EXAMPLE 14.2 (*continued*)

b. Marginal Control of *f* Only

	F			$\overline{F}$	
	E	$\overline{E}$		E	$\overline{E}$
D	560	140	D	40	160
$\overline{D}$	240	60	$\overline{D}$	160	640

$\hat{RR}(F) = 1.00$ $\hat{RR}(\overline{F}) = 1.00$

c. Marginal Control of *g* Only

	G			$\overline{G}$	
	E	$\overline{E}$		E	$\overline{E}$
D	570	114	D	30	186
$\overline{D}$	300	60	$\overline{D}$	100	640

$\hat{RR}(G) = 1.00$ $\hat{RR}(\overline{G}) = 1.03$

d. Crude Table

	E	$\overline{E}$
D	600	300
$\overline{D}$	400	700

$c\hat{RR} = 2.00$

Note: $c\hat{RR} = 2.00$, but all other $\hat{RR}$'s are essentially one. Consequently, control of confounding can be achieved by adjusting for either risk factor alone.

EXAMPLE 14.2 (*continued*)

Table 14.4 Conditional Relationships of the Risk Factors f and g with e and d, Based on Table 14.3

Exposure Relationships (14.3)	Disease Relationships (14.4)
$\hat{OR}_{ef|G} = .97$	$\hat{OR}_{df|\bar{E},G} = 9.25$
$\hat{OR}_{ef|\bar{G}} = 1.23$	$\hat{OR}_{df|\bar{E},\bar{G}} = 9.67$
$\hat{OR}_{eg|F} = 29.21$	$\hat{OR}_{dg|\bar{E},F} = .96$
$\hat{OR}_{eg|\bar{F}} = 36.94$	$\hat{OR}_{dg|\bar{E},\bar{F}} = 1.00$

Example 14.2 clearly illustrates that the proper control of confounding can indeed be achieved by different subsets of the totality of risk factors under consideration. This result leads to the following *general* definitions, which are useful for identifying such subsets.

A *sufficient confounder group* is a *minimal* set of one or more risk factors whose simultaneous control in the analysis will correct for joint confounding in the estimation of the effect of interest. Here, "minimal" refers to the property that, for any such set of variables, *no* variable can be removed from the set without sacrificing validity.

A *confounder* is any risk factor that is a member of a sufficient confounder group.

The use of the term "sufficient" in this context is analogous to its use by Rothman (1976) for the more general philosophical issue of causality.

The following examples are offered to help clarify the use of the above definitions in identifying variables to be controlled in a given analysis.

EXAMPLE 14.3

Assume, as illustrated in Table 14.3, that f and g are the only risk factors eligible for control, and that

$$c\hat{R}R \neq a\hat{R}R(f, g) = a\hat{R}R(f) = a\hat{R}R(g)$$

Then, $\{f\}$ and $\{g\}$ are each sufficient confounder groups, and f and g are each confounders, although both variables do not need to be controlled

EXAMPLE 14.3 (*continued*)

simultaneously. Note that $\{f, g\}$ is not a sufficient confounder group since it is not minimal; i.e., either variable can be removed from the set $\{f, g\}$ without sacrificing validity, as long as the other is retained.

EXAMPLE 14.4

Assume again that f and g are the only risk factors, that

$$c\hat{R}R \neq a\hat{R}R(f, g) = a\hat{R}R(f)$$

but that

$$a\hat{R}R(f, g) \neq a\hat{R}R(g)$$

Then, $\{f\}$ is the only sufficient confounder group, f is the only confounder, and hence f is the only variable requiring control for validity purposes.

EXAMPLE 14.5

Assume that f_1, f_2, and f_3 are the only risk factors in a case-control study, and that

$$c\hat{O}R \neq a\hat{O}R(f_1, f_2, f_3)$$
$$a\hat{O}R(f_1, f_2) = a\hat{O}R(f_2, f_3) = a\hat{O}R(f_1, f_3) = a\hat{O}R(f_1, f_2, f_3)$$
$$a\hat{O}R(f_1) \neq a\hat{O}R(f_1, f_2, f_3)$$
$$a\hat{O}R(f_2) \neq a\hat{O}R(f_1, f_2, f_3)$$
$$a\hat{O}R(f_3) \neq a\hat{O}R(f_1, f_2, f_3)$$

Then, $\{f_1, f_2\}$, $\{f_2, f_3\}$, and $\{f_1, f_3\}$ are the only sufficient confounder groups, and f_1, f_2, and f_3 are confounders (although they do not need to be controlled simultaneously).

EXAMPLE 14.6

Assume that f_1, f_2, f_3, f_4, and f_5 are the only risk factors in a case-control study, that

$$c\hat{O}R \neq a\hat{O}R(f_1, f_2, f_3, f_4, f_5)$$

$$a\hat{O}R(f_1, f_2, f_3, f_4) = a\hat{O}R(f_2, f_5) = a\hat{O}R(f_4) = a\hat{O}R(f_1, f_2, f_3)$$
$$= a\hat{O}R(f_1, f_2, f_3, f_4, f_5)$$

and that $a\hat{O}R$ (any other subset of f's) $\neq a\hat{O}R(f_1, f_2, f_3, f_4, f_5)$. Then, $\{f_2, f_5\}$, $\{f_4\}$, and $\{f_1, f_2, f_3\}$ are the only sufficient confounder groups, and all five variables are confounders (although they do not need to be controlled simultaneously).

14.3 CONCLUDING REMARKS

We reemphasize, after considering the above examples, that the simultaneous control of *all* risk factors makes it unnecessary in the interest of validity to seek out *any* sufficient confounder groups. As we have previously pointed out, however, other criteria may justify the effort in locating certain sufficient confounder groups. In particular, the identification of the sufficient confounder group giving the most precise estimate of effect is important enough to make an examination of such groups worthwhile. Moreover, as we will discuss in Chapter 16, the investigator must frequently consider, in the analysis, the trade-off between controlling for enough risk factors to maintain validity and the possible loss in precision resulting from the control of too many variables.

Finally, we reemphasize our position that the assessment of confounding, including methods for identifying sufficient subsets of confounders, must be predicated on the assumption that there is no meaningful interaction in the data. As we will discuss in later chapters, an appropriate general analysis strategy should first deal with interaction before considering issues of confounding.

NOTATION

The following list summarizes the key notation introduced in this chapter.

$a\hat{\theta}(f_1, f_2, \ldots, f_k)$ — Adjusted estimate of parameter θ after controlling simultaneously for the factors $f_1, f_2, \ldots, f_k$.

$\hat{O}R_{ef_j | F_1, \ldots, F_k \atop (\text{excluding } F_j)}$ — Estimated conditional odds ratio measuring e–f_j association given some combination of levels of $f_1, f_2, \ldots, f_k$ except f_j.

$\hat{\text{OR}}_{df_j|\overline{E},F_1,\ldots,F_k}$
$\quad|_{\text{(excluding } F_j)}$

Estimated conditional odds ratio measuring d–f_j association among nonexposed subjects given some combination of levels of f_1, $f_2, \ldots, f_k$ except f_j.

$\hat{\text{OR}}_{ef_j|\overline{D},F_1,\ldots,F_k}$
$\quad|_{\text{(excluding } F_j)}$

Estimated conditional odds ratio measuring e–f_j association among nondiseased subjects given some combination of levels of f_1, $f_2, \ldots, f_k$ except f_j.

PRACTICE EXERCISES

14.1 Suppose f and g are two distinct risk factors for some disease with dichotomous levels F_1, F_0 and G_1, G_0, respectively. Suppose that the accompanying table gives estimated risk ratios describing the association between the disease and some study factor (exposure) as a function of the various combinations of levels of f and g; the value 1.0 refers to a *marginal* risk ratio, based on collapsing over levels of f or g or over both f and g. Assume that the risk ratio estimates in the cells of the table are of high precision (i.e., are based on large sample sizes).

	G_1	G_0	
F_1	3.0	3.0	1.0
F_0	0.3	3.0	1.0
	1.0	1.0	1.0

Determine whether the following statements are true or false.
a. There is evidence of interaction (i.e., nonuniformity in effect) in the data.
b. There is evidence of confounding in the data.
c. At level G_0, there is no confounding due to factor f.
d. At level F_1, there is no interaction due to factor g.
e. There is evidence that both f and g are effect modifiers.
f. At level F_0, there is no interaction and no confounding.
g. At level G_0, there is confounding but no interaction.
h. It is not necessary to control for either f or g (or both) in order to understand the relationship between d and e.

14.2 Suppose that variables f_1, f_2, and f_3 have been measured in a certain study and that only f_1 and f_2 are considered to be risk factors for some disease (d). Suppose that it is of interest to describe the relationship between this disease and some study factor (e), and that there is no interaction of any kind present in the data. Finally, suppose that the following relationships hold among various odds ratios computed from the data:

$$c\hat{O}R \neq a\hat{O}R(f_1) \qquad a\hat{O}R(f_1, f_2) = a\hat{O}R(f_1)$$

$$c\hat{O}R = a\hat{O}R(f_2) \qquad a\hat{O}R(f_1, f_2) \neq a\hat{O}R(f_2)$$

$$c\hat{O}R = a\hat{O}R(f_3) \qquad a\hat{O}R(f_1, f_3) = a\hat{O}R(f_3)$$

$$c\hat{O}R = a\hat{O}R(f_1, f_2, f_3) \qquad a\hat{O}R(f_1, f_2, f_3) = a\hat{O}R(f_2, f_3)$$

$$c\hat{O}R \neq a\hat{O}R(f_1, f_2)$$

Note: $c\hat{O}R$ denotes the estimated crude odds ratio measuring the e–d association; $a\hat{O}R(f_1, f_2)$ denotes an estimated odds ratio (measuring the e–d association) that "adjusts" for the effects of variables f_1 and f_2 (i.e., it is a weighted average of appropriate stratum-specific effects).

Determine whether the following statements are true or false.
a. There is confounding in the data.
b. Variable f_1 needs to be controlled to avoid confounding.
c. Variable f_2 needs to be controlled to avoid confounding.
d. Variable f_3 needs to be controlled to avoid confounding.
e. Both variables f_1 and f_2 do not need to be controlled simultaneously in order to avoid confounding.
f. $\{f_1, f_2\}$ is a sufficient confounder group.
g. $\{f_1\}$ is a sufficient confounder group.

REFERENCES FISHER, L., and PATIL, K. 1974. Matching and unrelatedness. *Am. J. Epidemiol.* 100: 347–349.

LEWIS, D. K. 1980. Matching on several variables in epidemiologic studies. Ph.D. dissertation, University of North Carolina at Chapel Hill.

MIETTINEN, O. S. 1974. Confounding and effect modification. *Am. J. Epidemiol.* 100(5): 350–353.

ROTHMAN, K. J. 1976. Causes. *Am. J. Epidemiol.* 104(6): 587–592.

WHITTEMORE, A. S. 1978. Collapsibility of multidimensional contingency tables. *J. R. Stat. Soc. B* 40: 328–340.

PART III

Principles and Procedures of Epidemiologic Analysis

15

Statistical Inferences About Effect Measures: Simple Analysis

15.0
PREVIEW

In Chapters 6–9, several absolute and relative measures of epidemiologic import were discussed. In this chapter, we will focus on various statistical inference-making procedures concerning certain of these effect measures. Specifically, we will discuss both statistical hypothesis testing and confidence interval methods.

We will limit our presentation to the so-called simple analysis situation. By "simple," we mean that we will be considering only the relationship between a dichotomous disease variable (with levels D and $\bar{D}$ denoting the presence and absence of disease, respectively) and a dichotomous exposure variable (with levels E and $\bar{E}$). In other words, we will ignore the usually encountered situation where the effects of extraneous variables need to be considered when studying an exposure-disease relationship.

There is no question that a detailed discussion of simple analysis is warranted. First of all, an understanding of this special case is necessary before the general principles of stratified analysis can be appreciated (see Chapter 17). Second, a simple analysis is usually performed even when there are other extraneous variables that must be considered. A simple analysis helps one to decide whether such variables really do affect the exposure-disease relationship by providing a crude measure of effect (obtained by ignoring such variables), which can then be compared with an adjusted effect measure (obtained by controlling or adjusting for such variables), as we saw in the previous chapter.

The phrase "simple analysis" should not be taken to mean that the techniques in this chapter are trivial in their complexity. On the contrary, the hypothesis-testing and confidence interval estimation procedures to be discussed involve important general principles upon which hinge the more complex analysis techniques to be introduced later. Thus, a thorough grasp of the concepts and procedures developed in this chapter is a prerequisite to an understanding of the more general analysis approaches to be presented in later chapters.

In the discussion that follows, we focus first on hypothesis-testing procedures, considering, in turn, the density type of follow-up study, the cumulative type of follow-up study, and the case-control study. In the last part of the chapter, we describe various procedures for the interval estimation of certain epidemiologic effect measures. The general data layouts for the types of studies under consideration have been described in Chapters 6–9. Since we are limiting our discussion to the simple analysis situation, the basic data array for each study will be in the form of a 2×2 table.

15.1
HYPOTHESIS-TESTING PRO-CEDURES

In this section we consider hypothesis tests for three types of studies, density follow-up, cumulative follow-up, and case-control.

The data layout for a density type of follow-up study is shown in Table 15.1 for the simple analysis situation.

From Chapters 6–9, the point estimates of the parameters ID_1, ID_0 (incidence density), IDR (incidence density ratio), and IDD (incidence density difference) are, respectively,

$$\hat{ID}_1 = \frac{a}{L_1} \qquad \hat{ID}_0 = \frac{b}{L_0} \qquad \hat{IDR} = \frac{\hat{ID}_1}{\hat{ID}_0} = \frac{a/L_1}{b/L_0}$$

$$\hat{IDD} = \hat{ID}_1 - \hat{ID}_0 = \frac{a}{L_1} - \frac{b}{L_0}$$

We are interested here in testing the null hypothesis that there is no association between exposure and disease, versus the alternative hypothesis that there is such an association. Statistically speaking, the null hypothesis can be expressed as H_0: $ID_1 = ID_0$ (or, equivalently, IDR $= 1$ or IDD $= 0$), and the appropriate one-sided alternative hypothesis is then H_A: $ID_1 > ID_0$ (or, equivalently, IDR > 1 or IDD > 0). In most applications, one is interested in determining whether the exposure is detrimental to health, and that is why the one-sided alternative is used; unless specifically mentioned otherwise, we will be focusing on this situation.

Since $\hat{ID}_1$ and $\hat{ID}_0$ are not binomial proportions, standard hypothesis-testing methods cannot be used here. One method for testing H_0 versus H_A is to assume that each of the m_1 observed cases represents an independent Bernoulli trial, with "success" and "failure" defined as being in the exposed and unexposed categories, respectively. The probabilities of "success" and "failure" under H_0 are

$$p_0 = L_1/L \qquad \text{and} \qquad q_0 = L_0/L = (1 - p_0)$$

respectively, which are the proportions of the total population time L in (t_0, t) associated with the exposed and unexposed groups. Thus, if A is the random variable denoting the number of cases out of m_1 that are exposed, then, under H_0, it follows from the binomial distribution that

Table 15.1 Data Layout for a Density Follow-up Study

	E	$\overline{E}$	
No. of Cases Developed in (t_0, t)	a	b	$m_1 = (a + b)$
Population-Time of Follow-up in (t_0, t)	L_1	L_0	$L = (L_1 + L_0)$

$$\text{pr}(A \geq a \mid H_0) = \sum_{j=a}^{m_1} C_j^{m_1} p_0^j q_0^{m_1-j} \tag{15.1}$$

where $C_j^{m_1} = m_1! / j! (m_1 - j)!$.

Note that $\text{pr}(A \geq a \mid H_0)$ is the *exact probability* of observing *at least* as many exposed cases as we actually observed (namely, a) if there is no exposure-disease relationship. To put it another way, Expression 15.1 is the probability of observing a result *at least* as rare as the one encountered if H_0 is true. This probability is known as the *P-value*, and it provides a quantification of the *degree of significance* associated with the actual value of the test statistic calculated from the observed data. The P-value is different from the significance level (or α level), since the latter is specified *before* the data are gathered. Clearly, if H_0 is rejected, then the P-value will be less than the significance level.

In our situation, if $\text{pr}(A \geq a \mid H_0)$ is small (say less than .05), then we would probably be willing to reject H_0, with confidence that the risk of doing so incorrectly (i.e., of making a type I error) is fairly small.

A large-sample test of H_0 versus H_A can be constructed by using the normal approximation to the binomial distribution. In particular, since the mean and variance of A under H_0 are $m_1 p_0$ and $m_1 p_0 q_0$, it follows that

$$Z = (A - m_1 p_0) / \sqrt{m_1 p_0 q_0} \tag{15.2}$$

will have (approximately) a standard normal distribution under H_0 if m_1 is sufficiently large and p_0 is not close to zero or one in value. An equivalent testing procedure would involve computing an ordinary "observed versus expected" χ_1^2 statistic from the table below:

	E	$\overline{E}$
Observed	a	b
Expected	$m_1 p_0$	$m_1 q_0$

Of course, this χ_1^2 is mathematically equal to the square of the Z statistic given above, with $A = a$. The large-sample approximation on which this test is based is usually good if $m_1 p_0$ and $m_1 q_0$ both exceed 5; this criterion relates to our earlier comment concerning the sizes of m_1 and p_0.

Before we illustrate the above procedures with a numerical example, we point out that, strictly speaking, the above testing methods are *conditional* testing methods; i.e., the tests perform as described conditional on the assumptions that L_1 and L_0 are fixed constants (i.e., not random variables) and that $m_1 = (a + b)$ is also fixed.

EXAMPLE 15.1

To illustrate the use of the methods we have just described, we will consider the data in Table 15.2. These data pertain to a follow-up study concerning the possible association between obesity and mortality (from all causes) among white women aged 60–75 from a midwestern urban population; a general description of this study was given in Chapter 1.

Table 15.2   Density Type of Data from an Obesity Study

	Obese (E)	Nonobese ($\bar{E}$)	
Deaths During 1960–1967	30	36	$m_1 = 66$
Person-Years of Follow-up, 1960–1967	699	1,399	$L = 2,098$

Here, $a = 30$, $b = 36$, $L_1 = 699$, and $L_0 = 1,399$, so that

$$\hat{\text{IDR}} = \frac{\hat{\text{ID}}_1}{\hat{\text{ID}}_0} = \frac{30/699}{36/1,399} = 1.67$$

To test H_0: IDR $= 1$ versus H_A: IDR > 1, we need the values for p_0 and $q_0 = 1 - p_0$; these are

$$p_0 = L_1/L = 699/2,098 = .333 \quad \text{and} \quad q_0 = .667$$

The random variable A defined earlier has the observed value $a = 30$ for these data. Thus, Expression 15.1 for the exact P-value, namely, $\text{pr}(A \geq a | H_0)$, has the specific form

$$\text{pr}(A \geq 30 | H_0) = \sum_{j=30}^{66} C_j^{66} (.333)^j (.667)^{66-j}$$

This expression is difficult to evaluate without computer assistance. However, an excellent approximation to this exact P-value can be obtained through the use of the large-sample Z test. In fact, using the Z test formula, (15.2), to compute an approximate P-value is the recommended approach

EXAMPLE 15.1 (*continued*)

except in the small-sample situation, where it is then easy to compute the exact value of $\text{pr}(A \geq a|H_0)$.

For the data in Table 15.2, the Z statistic has the value

$$Z = \frac{30 - (66)(.333)}{\sqrt{(66)(.333)(.667)}} = 2.10$$

so that

$$\text{pr}(A \geq 30|H_0) \approx \text{pr}(Z > 2.10|H_0) = (1/2)\,\text{pr}(\chi_1^2 > 4.41|H_0) = .0179$$

The interpretation here is that we have observed an event (namely, the random variable A taking a value greater than or equal to 30) for which the chance is less than 2 in 100 if there really is no relationship between exposure status and disease status (i.e., if IDR = 1). In such a situation, most people would be willing to say that there is strong evidence of a real exposure-disease association just on the basis of the data in Table 15.2.

A word of caution is in order at this point. The analysis in Example 15.1 did not consider the effects of other extraneous factors that may affect the exposure-disease relationship. Such an analysis is generally referred to as a "crude" analysis, and the value 1.67 is called a "crude" estimate of effect, since it is not adjusted for other factors that may need to be controlled (or adjusted for) in the analysis. In fact, it is quite possible that the crude estimate of 1.67, even though it led to the rejection of H_0: IDR = 1 in favor of H_A: IDR > 1 in our simple (i.e., crude) analysis, could be decreased enough after adjustment for other factors so that there would be no postadjustment evidence of an exposure-disease relationship. Of course, the value of $\hat{\text{IDR}}$ after adjustment could also be larger than 1.67. These possibilities will be explored for this particular data set in Chapter 17.

**15.1.2
Cumulative
Type of
Follow-up
Study**

The data layout for a cumulative type of follow-up study is shown in Table 15.3.

To facilitate our discussion, we recast these data into the array shown in Table 15.4. Written in this way, the data layout (with cell entries a, b, c, d) would also be appropriate for displaying the outcome of a case-control or a cross-sectional study.

From Chapters 6–9, the point estimates of the parameters CI_1, CI_0 (cumulative incidence), CIR (cumulative incidence ratio), CID (cumulative incidence difference), and ROR (risk odds ratio) are, respectively,

Table 15.3   Data Layout for a Cumulative Follow-up Study

	E	$\overline{E}$
No. of Cases That Developed in Candidate Population in (t_0, t)	a	b
Size of Candidate Population at Start of Follow-up Period (t_0, t)	n_1	n_0

$$\hat{CI}_1 = \frac{a}{n_1} \qquad \hat{CI}_0 = \frac{b}{n_0}$$

$$\hat{CIR} = \frac{\hat{CI}_1}{\hat{CI}_0} = \frac{a/n_1}{b/n_0}$$

$$\hat{CID} = \hat{CI}_1 - \hat{CI}_0 = \frac{a}{n_1} - \frac{b}{n_0}$$

$$\hat{ROR} = \frac{\hat{CI}_1(1 - \hat{CI}_0)}{\hat{CI}_0(1 - \hat{CI}_1)} = \frac{ad}{bc}$$

The null hypothesis to be tested here is H_0: $CI_1 = CI_0$ (or, equivalently, CIR = ROR = 1 or CID = 0). The one-sided alternative is H_A: $CI_1 > CI_0$ (or, equivalently, CIR > 1, ROR > 1, or CID > 0).

A large-sample test appropriate for this situation is that based on the comparison of two binomial proportions. This test involves a Z statistic of the form

$$Z = \frac{(\hat{CI}_1 - \hat{CI}_0) - 0}{\sqrt{\hat{CI}(1 - \hat{CI})[(1/n_1) + (1/n_0)]}} \tag{15.3}$$

Table 15.4   Revised Data Layout for Table 15.3

	E	$\overline{E}$	
D	a	b	m_1
$\overline{D}$	$c = (n_1 - a)$	$d = (n_0 - b)$	m_0
	n_1	n_0	n

where $\hat{CI} = (a + b)/(n_1 + n_0)$. It can be shown that

$$Z^2 = \chi_1^2 = n(ad - bc)^2/n_1 n_0 m_1 m_0$$

which is the ordinary observed versus expected χ_1^2 statistic calculated from the given 2×2 table. Note that $\chi_1^2 = 0$ when $\hat{ROR} = ad/bc = 1$, and it will be large when ad differs considerably from bc. Statisticians usually agree that this large-sample χ_1^2 test will be reasonably well-behaved when all the expected cell frequencies exceed 5 (although less stringent criteria have also been proposed).

An alternative test for the data above can be developed in the following way. The marginal frequencies in such a 2×2 table (no matter how the sampling was done) provide no information concerning the *strength of association* in the data; they only indicate the amount of information available in the table for quantifying that association. Consequently, then, one would not introduce any bias by regarding all the marginal totals as "fixed" (as opposed to considering one or more marginal totals as "random"). In this case, the statistical concern would be with the distribution of the data in the body of the table, *conditional* on these *fixed* marginal totals.

Since we are dealing specifically with 2×2 tables, the specification of any single cell frequency automatically determines the counts in the other three cells, under the assumption of fixed marginals. Thus, for testing purposes, it suffices to consider a single cell frequency, which is customarily chosen to be the "number of exposed cases," or the "a cell." The observed value (namely, a) is then, under H_0, the realization of a *hypergeometric random variable* (say, A), with probability distribution

$$\text{pr}(A = j|H_0) = C_j^{n_1} C_{m_1-j}^{n_0}/C_{m_1}^n \qquad (15.4)$$

For the realization $A = j$, the data layout is shown in Table 15.5, where

$$\max(0, m_1 - n_0) \leq j \leq \min(n_1, m_1)$$

so as to avoid negative cell entries.

Table 15.5 Data Layout with Fixed Marginal Totals and with $A = j$

	E	$\bar{E}$	
D	j	$m_1 - j$	m_1
$\bar{D}$	$n_1 - j$	$n_0 - m_1 + j$	m_0
	n_1	n_0	

It then follows that the exact P-value for a test of H_0 versus H_A, using 15.4, is

$$\text{pr}(A \geq a|H_0) = \sum_{j=a}^{\min(n_1,m_1)} \text{pr}(A = j|H_0) \qquad (15.5)$$

This testing procedure is known as *Fisher's exact test* (see Ostle, 1963).*

EXAMPLE 15.2

We provide a simple example to illustrate the computations involved in using Equations 15.4 and 15.5 for the data given in the following table:

	E	$\overline{E}$	
D	4	1	$m_1 = 5$
$\overline{D}$	2	6	$m_0 = 8$
	$n_1 = 6$	$n_0 = 7$	

Then we have

$$\text{pr}(A \geq 4|H_0) = \sum_{j=4}^{\min(6,5)} \text{pr}(A = j|H_0) = \sum_{j=4}^{5} \frac{C_j^6 C_{5-j}^7}{C_5^{13}}$$

$$= \frac{C_4^6 C_1^7}{C_5^{13}} + \frac{C_5^6 C_0^7}{C_5^{13}} = \frac{(15)(7)}{1,287} + \frac{(6)(1)}{1,287} = \frac{111}{1,287} \approx .086$$

A large-sample test based on the hypergeometric distribution can also be developed. Under H_0, it can be shown that the mean and variance of A are, respectively, $(n_1 m_1)/n$ and $(n_1 n_0 m_1 m_0)/n^2(n - 1)$. Then, a large-sample test of H_0 versus H_A involves the test statistic

$$Z = \frac{a - [(n_1 m_1)/n]}{\sqrt{(n_1 n_0 m_1 m_0)/n^2(n - 1)}} \qquad (15.6)$$

---

*The term "exact test" is somewhat misleading. We interpret this phrase to mean that it gives the "exact" P-value under the fixed-margins assumption. It does *not* give a test with a type I error rate exactly equal to some prespecified nominal value α, because of the discreteness of the hypergeometric distribution.

or, equivalently,

$$\chi_1^2 = Z^2 = \frac{(n-1)(ad-bc)^2}{n_1 n_0 m_1 m_0} \quad (15.7)$$

This χ_1^2 statistic is known as the *Mantel-Haenszel chi-square statistic* (see Mantel and Haenszel, 1959). It differs from the ordinary χ_1^2 statistic based on squaring Expression 15.3 by the multiplier $(n-1)/n$, which is negligible when n is moderately large.

The "corrected for continuity" version of Equation 15.7 is

$$\chi_1^2 = \left[\frac{|a - (n_1 m_1/n)| - (1/2)}{\sqrt{(n_1 n_0 m_1 m_0)/n^2(n-1)}} \right]^2 = \frac{(n-1)[|ad-bc|-(n/2)]^2}{n_1 n_0 m_1 m_0}$$

$$(15.8)$$

with the numerator never corrected past zero. Expression 15.8 often provides a closer approximation than Equation 15.7 to the exact P-value based on Expressions 15.4 and 15.5. However, the use of a continuity correction has been the subject of considerable debate in the statistical literature (e.g., see Conover, 1974, and comments, directly following his article, by Starmer, Grizzle, and Sen, by Mantel, and by Miettinen). On the basis of our evaluation of this debate and other evidence, we do *not* recommend the use of the continuity correction; thus, it will not appear in formulas given in this book.

The advantages associated with using the Mantel-Haenszel χ_1^2 statistic will become apparent in Chapter 17 (on stratified analysis) and in Chapter 18 (on matching). Briefly, benefits result because the accuracy of the large-sample approximation is dictated by the amount of data accumulated over all strata rather than by the stratum-specific sample sizes. Consequently, the large-sample chi-square approximation will be adequate as long as the total number of subjects is sufficiently large, even though there may be very few subjects in each individual stratum.

EXAMPLE 15.3

We illustrate the procedures for analyzing a cumulative type of follow-up study by using data from the Evans County Heart Disease Study described in Chapter 1. Recall that the purpose of this study was to assess the putative association between endogenous catecholamine level (CAT), which is a fictitious variable constructed for illustrative purposes, and the subsequent seven-year incidence of coronary heart disease (CHD) among a cohort of 609 white males. In our simple (or crude) analysis, we will ignore the effects of other extraneous factors. The data we will consider appear in Table 15.6.

EXAMPLE 15.3 (*continued*)

**Table 15.6   Cumulative Type of Data from the
Evans County Heart Disease Study**

	HI CAT	LO CAT	
CHD	27	44	71
No CHD	95	443	538
	122	487	609

Here, $a = 27$, $b = 44$, $c = 95$, $d = 443$, $n_1 = 122$, $n_0 = 487$, $m_1 = 71$, $m_0 = 538$, and $n = 609$; so,

$$\hat{CIR} = \frac{\hat{CI}_1}{\hat{CI}_0} = \frac{a/n_1}{b/n_0} = \frac{27/122}{44/487} = 2.45$$

The exact P-value for a test of H_0: CIR $= 1$ versus H_A: CIR > 1, based on the hypergeometric distribution, is given by the expression

$$\text{pr}(A \geq 27 | H_0) = \sum_{j=27}^{71} \frac{C_j^{122} C_{71-j}^{487}}{C_{71}^{609}}$$

This equation follows from Expressions 15.4 and 15.5 by noting that $a = 27$ and that $\min(n_1, m_1) = \min(122, 71) = 71$.

Clearly, a computer is needed to evaluate this expression expeditiously. However, an excellent approximation to this exact P-value can be obtained from the Mantel-Haenszel χ_1^2 statistic given by Expression 15.7. Thus, since

$$\frac{(n-1)(ad - bc)^2}{n_1 n_0 m_1 m_0} = \frac{(609 - 1)[(27)(443) - (44)(95)]^2}{(122)(487)(71)(538)} = 16.22$$

it follows that

$$\text{pr}(A \geq a | H_0) \approx (1/2)\,\text{pr}(\chi_1^2 \geq 16.22 | H_0)$$
$$\approx \text{pr}(Z > 4.03 | H_0) < 0.0003$$

EXAMPLE 15.3 (*continued*)

Thus, the crude analysis provides strong evidence of an exposure-disease relationship solely on the basis of the data in Table 15.6.

Note that essentially identical results would have been obtained by using the ordinary χ_1^2 statistic, as given by the square of Expression 15.3, since the correction factor $(n - 1)/n = (608/609) = .9984 \approx 1$. In Example 15.3, the sample sizes are large enough to ensure that the χ_1^2 tests are accurate, so that the use of Fisher's exact test is unnecessary to obtain a valid P-value. However, in small-sample situations, it is mandatory to assess the significance of the findings via procedures like Fisher's exact test, which is valid regardless of the size of the data set.

**15.1.3
Case-Control
Study**

All the different types of case-control studies discussed in Chapter 5 lead to data that can be put into the tabular format of Table 15.7.

Table 15.7   Data Layout for a Case-Control Study

	E	$\overline{E}$	
D	a	b	m_1
$\overline{D}$	c	d	m_0
	n_1	n_0	n

The sample odds ratio ad/bc is the key statistic here, and the interpretation given to this estimate depends on the type of study under consideration. In density types of studies, for example, it is used to estimate IDR. In cumulative types of studies, it estimates the risk odds ratio ROR, which approximates CIR when the risks are small. And in cross-sectional studies, it estimates the prevalence odds ratio POR, which is essentially equal to the prevalence ratio PR for diseases with low prevalence.

A direct way to test whether ad/bc is significantly greater than one is to use the hypergeometric distribution procedures discussed in Section 15.1.2.

EXAMPLE 15.4

To illustrate the approach, we consider the data in Table 15.8, which represent the results of a hypothetical case-control study involving random samples of 10 cases and 50 controls.

Table 15.8 Results from a Hypothetical Case-Control Study Using Randomly Sampled Cases and Controls

	E	$\bar{E}$	
D	8	2	10
$\bar{D}$	30	20	50
	38	22	60

For these data, the estimated exposure odds ratio is $\widehat{\text{EOR}} = ad/bc = (8)(20)/(2)(30) = 2.67$.

To assess whether the observed value of 2.67 is significantly greater than 1, we can calculate an exact P-value associated with the test of H_0: EOR $= 1$ versus H_A: EOR > 1, using the hypergeometric distribution results given earlier. The exact P-value for these data, based on Expressions 15.4 and 15.5, is

$$\text{pr}(A \geq 8 | H_0) = \sum_{j=8}^{10} \frac{C_j^{38} C_{10-j}^{22}}{C_{10}^{60}} = .150 + .048 + .006 = .204$$

which means that there is not sufficient evidence to reject the null hypothesis of no association.

The large-sample Mantel-Haenszel χ_1^2 statistic given by Expression 15.7 has the value

$$\chi_1^2 = \frac{(60 - 1)[(8)(20) - (2)(30)]^2}{(38)(22)(10)(50)} = 1.41$$

which is associated with a one-sided P-value between .10 and .15. This result roughly approximates that found by using the exact P-value for-

---

EXAMPLE 15.4 (*continued*)

mula. Our conclusion from these analyses is that there is no evidence of an exposure-disease relationship for the data in Table 15.8, although we caution that this simple treatment of the data has not involved the consideration of other extraneous factors.

This concludes our discussion of simple analysis procedures from an hypothesis-testing perspective. We next turn to a consideration of interval estimation techniques, which are related to the hypothesis-testing methods just presented.

15.2 CONFIDENCE INTERVAL PROCEDURES

The purpose of this section is to provide a discussion of some general methods for constructing confidence intervals for certain epidemiologic effect measures. Our presentation will focus mainly on large-sample interval estimation techniques, since most such procedures are computationally easy to use and provide reasonably valid results. However, we will briefly discuss the construction of exact types of confidence intervals in Section 15.2.3.

A considerable amount of statistical research has been devoted to developing both exact and approximate interval estimation techniques for the risk ratio and the odds ratio. For an excellent discussion of several of these procedures, see Fleiss (1979) and Breslow and Day (1981). It is not our purpose here to describe and compare all these different approaches. Rather, we will be content to illustrate the use of some of the more popular procedures. The approximate confidence interval techniques we will discuss in the following two sections have been shown numerically to provide valid answers when based on moderate to large sample sizes. In such circumstances, these answers agree reasonably well with those obtained by using more esoteric procedures (e.g., certain exact types of methods as discussed by Breslow and Day, 1981). We will continue to focus on the simple analysis situation, and we will illustrate the use of the confidence interval formulas with some of the data sets presented earlier.

The general setting for our discussion is as follows. Suppose that θ denotes the parameter of interest and that $\hat{\theta}$ is our point estimator of θ. For example, θ could be the CID, so that $\hat{\theta}$ would be $\hat{\text{CID}} = \hat{\text{CI}}_1 - \hat{\text{CI}}_0$; or θ could be ln EOR, so that $\hat{\theta}$ would be ln $\hat{\text{EOR}}$. One form of a $100(1 - \alpha)\%$ large-sample confidence interval for θ has the general structure

$$\hat{\theta} \pm Z_{1-\alpha/2} \sqrt{\hat{\text{Var}}(\hat{\theta})}$$

where $Z_{1-\alpha/2}$ is that value of a standard normal variate Z such that $\text{pr}(Z > Z_{1-\alpha/2}) = \alpha/2$, and where $\hat{\text{Var}}(\hat{\theta})$ is an estimate of the variance of

$\hat{\theta}$. The basic assumption involved in the construction of this confidence interval is that the quantity

$$(\hat{\theta} - \theta)/\sqrt{\hat{\text{Var}}(\hat{\theta})}$$

has an approximate standard normal distribution for moderate to large samples.

To utilize this form of confidence interval, we obviously must have a value for $\hat{\text{Var}}(\hat{\theta})$. The complexity involved in coming up with that value will depend on the form of the estimator $\hat{\theta}$. For example, when $\hat{\theta}$ is a linear function (e.g., a difference as opposed to a ratio) of independent random variables whose variances are easy to obtain, then the expression for $\hat{\text{Var}}(\hat{\theta})$ can be derived directly. As an illustration, from well-known properties of the binomial distribution, it follows that

$$\hat{\text{Var}}(\hat{\text{CID}}) = \hat{\text{Var}}(\hat{\text{CI}}_1 - \hat{\text{CI}}_0) = \hat{\text{Var}}(\hat{\text{CI}}_1) + \hat{\text{Var}}(\hat{\text{CI}}_0)$$

$$= \frac{\hat{\text{CI}}_1(1 - \hat{\text{CI}}_1)}{n_1} + \frac{\hat{\text{CI}}_0(1 - \hat{\text{CI}}_0)}{n_0}$$

Thus, a $100(1 - \alpha)\%$ large-sample confidence interval for CID (i.e., the risk difference RD) is

$$\hat{\text{CID}} \pm Z_{1-\alpha/2} \sqrt{\frac{\hat{\text{CI}}_1(1 - \hat{\text{CI}}_1)}{n_1} + \frac{\hat{\text{CI}}_0(1 - \hat{\text{CI}}_0)}{n_0}}$$

However, many epidemiologic effect measure estimators are ratios of random variables, which greatly complicates the task of finding an expression for $\hat{\text{Var}}(\hat{\theta})$. In fact, the differences in behavior of confidence intervals for effect measures like risk ratios and odds ratios essentially depend on what technique is employed to estimate $\text{Var}(\hat{\theta})$. We will now discuss two such techniques in detail, namely, the first-order Taylor series approximation method and Miettinen's test-based method (Miettinen, 1976).

To illustrate how Taylor series confidence intervals are constructed, let us focus on a particular application. Suppose we wish to find a $100(1 - \alpha)\%$ confidence interval for the CIR (i.e., for the risk ratio RR). The point estimator of CIR is $\hat{\text{CIR}} = \hat{\text{CI}}_1/\hat{\text{CI}}_0$, and we are thus inclined initially to consider the interval

15.2.1 Taylor Series Confidence Intervals

$$\hat{\text{CIR}} \pm Z_{1-\alpha/2} \sqrt{\hat{\text{Var}}(\hat{\text{CIR}})}$$

Although it is possible to derive an approximate expression for $\hat{\text{Var}}(\hat{\text{CIR}})$ by using a Taylor series, this form of interval is *not* recommended. The main reason for not using this particular interval is that there is asymmetry in the distribution of possible values for the risk ratio, which leads to a distortion in the nominal confidence coefficient. That is, the interval will not cover the true parameter value the purported $100(1 - \alpha)\%$ of the time. Similar criticism has been leveled at an analogous interval for the odds ratio (see Fleiss, 1979).

One recommended approach for alleviating this asymmetry problem is to work with the estimator ln CÎR rather than with CÎR; the *natural logarithmic transformation* is often used by statisticians to transform a highly skewed distribution to one that is more (approximately) normal in appearance. The use of this transformation means that a two-step procedure must be employed to derive the desired confidence interval for CIR. First, a $100(1 - \alpha)\%$ large-sample confidence interval for ln CIR is obtained; this interval is of the form

$$\ln \text{CÎR} \pm Z_{1-\alpha/2} \sqrt{\hat{\text{Var}}(\ln \text{CÎR})}$$

Then, since $\text{CIR} = \exp(\ln \text{CIR})$, the desired upper and lower endpoints of the $100(1 - \alpha)\%$ large-sample confidence interval for CIR are found by taking antilogarithms of the corresponding endpoints of the interval for ln CIR. The resulting large-sample $100(1 - \alpha)\%$ confidence interval for CIR, based on the use of this natural logarithmic transformation, takes the general form

$$(\text{CÎR}) \exp[\pm Z_{1-\alpha/2} \sqrt{\hat{\text{Var}}(\ln \text{CÎR})}]$$

We now need to find an expression for $\hat{\text{Var}}(\ln \text{CÎR})$. Although an exact expression for this variance cannot readily be found, we can obtain a good approximation to it by employing the following general result. For two random variables X and Y such that $Y = f(X)$, then

$$\hat{\text{Var}}(Y) \approx [df(\hat{\mu}_X)/dX]^2 \; \hat{\text{Var}}(X)$$

where $df(\hat{\mu}_X)/dX$ is the derivative of $f(X)$ with respect to X evaluated at the estimate $\hat{\mu}_X$ of the mean μ_X of X. This result is based on a first-order (or linear) Taylor series approximation to Y of the form

$$Y = f(\mu_X) + [df(\mu_X)/dX] \; (X - \mu_X)$$

Confidence intervals based on this variance approximation method are generally referred to as *Taylor series confidence intervals*. The behavior of such confidence intervals is very much dependent on the accuracy of this linear approximation, which tends to be good for large samples.

To illustrate the use of this variance approximation formula, we let $Y = \ln \hat{\text{CI}}_1$ and $X = \hat{\text{CI}}_1$, so that $Y = f(X) = \ln X$ is the functional relationship between Y and X. Then, $d(\ln X)/dX = 1/X$, so that

$$\hat{\text{Var}}(\ln \hat{\text{CI}}_1) \approx \left(\frac{1}{\hat{\text{CI}}_1}\right)^2 \hat{\text{Var}}(\hat{\text{CI}}_1) = \frac{1}{(\hat{\text{CI}}_1)^2} \cdot \frac{\hat{\text{CI}}_1(1 - \hat{\text{CI}}_1)}{n_1} = \frac{1 - \hat{\text{CI}}_1}{n_1 \hat{\text{CI}}_1}$$

Similarly,

$$\hat{\text{Var}}(\ln \hat{\text{CI}}_0) \approx (1 - \hat{\text{CI}}_0)/n_0 \hat{\text{CI}}_0$$

Then, since $\ln \hat{\text{CIR}} = \ln \hat{\text{CI}}_1 - \ln \hat{\text{CI}}_0$ and $\hat{\text{CI}}_1$ and $\hat{\text{CI}}_0$ are independent, it follows that

$$\hat{\text{Var}}(\ln \hat{\text{CIR}}) = \hat{\text{Var}}(\ln \hat{\text{CI}}_1) + \hat{\text{Var}}(\ln \hat{\text{CI}}_0) \approx \frac{1 - \hat{\text{CI}}_1}{n_1 \hat{\text{CI}}_1} + \frac{1 - \hat{\text{CI}}_0}{n_0 \hat{\text{CI}}_0}$$

Thus, the $100(1 - \alpha)\%$ Taylor series confidence interval for the CIR is

$$(\hat{\text{CIR}}) \exp\left[\pm Z_{1-\alpha/2} \sqrt{\frac{1 - \hat{\text{CI}}_1}{n_1 \hat{\text{CI}}_1} + \frac{1 - \hat{\text{CI}}_0}{n_0 \hat{\text{CI}}_0}}\right] \qquad (15.9)$$

This form of interval has been recommended by Katz and colleagues (1978) on the basis of results of extensive simulation studies.

EXAMPLE 15.5

To illustrate the use of Expression 15.9, we will construct a 95% interval for the CIR, using the data in Table 15.6. With these data, Expression 15.9 becomes

$$(2.45) \exp\left[\pm 1.96 \sqrt{\frac{1 - (27/122)}{122(27/122)} + \frac{1 - (44/487)}{487(44/487)}}\right] = (2.45)e^{\pm .436}$$

which leads to the interval $(1.584, 3.789)$. Note that this Taylor series interval does *not* include one; this result agrees with the result from our χ_1^2 test, which favored the rejection of H_0: CIR $= 1$. In this regard, we feel it is generally good practice to construct confidence intervals in combination with testing hypotheses, since the confidence interval lengths provide a direct measure of the precision in the effect estimation procedure.

One can use an argument analogous to that above to develop a confidence interval for the odds ratio. We simply state the final result, which is

$$\left(\frac{ad}{bc}\right) \exp\left(\pm Z_{1-\alpha/2} \sqrt{\frac{1}{a} + \frac{1}{b} + \frac{1}{c} + \frac{1}{d}}\right) \qquad (15.10)$$

EXAMPLE 15.6

For the data in Table 15.8, the 95% Taylor series confidence interval for EOR, based on Expression 15.10, is

EXAMPLE 15.6 (*continued*)

$$(2.67)\exp\left(\pm\ 1.96\ \sqrt{\frac{1}{8} + \frac{1}{2} + \frac{1}{30} + \frac{1}{20}} \right) = (2.67)e^{\pm 1.650}$$

or (.513, 13.903). This interval includes the null value one, which is in agreement with the large *P*-value of .204 and the insignificant χ_1^2 value obtained earlier. Because of the small values of *a* and *b* in Table 15.8, this large-sample interval is quite wide. The wide interval is indicative of poor precision in the estimation of the odds ratio. This result emphasizes the fact that large-sample intervals can be very insensitive and should not be used unless moderate to large numbers are present in each of the cells of the tables under consideration.

15.2.2
Test-based
Confidence
Intervals

As an alternative to the somewhat complex Taylor series method, Miettinen (1976) has suggested a "quick and dirty" way to calculate a *test-based confidence interval*, the motivation being to avoid determining an expression for $\text{Var}(\hat{\theta})$ directly. The statistical properties of his suggested procedure have not as yet received sufficient study; Halperin (1977) and Miettinen (1977) have discussed some of the pros and cons of the technique, as have Fleiss (1979) and Gart (1979). It has been our experience that the test-based intervals give about the same results as the Taylor series intervals for large samples and that neither approach is very good for small samples.

The rationale behind Miettinen's test-based confidence interval approach is as follows. If we want to test $H_0: \theta = \theta_0$ versus some alternative hypothesis, the appropriate large-sample test statistic is

$$Z = (\hat{\theta} - \theta_0)/\sqrt{\text{Var}_0(\hat{\theta})}$$

or, equivalently,

$$\chi_1^2 = (\hat{\theta} - \theta_0)^2/\text{Var}_0(\hat{\theta})$$

where $\text{Var}_0(\hat{\theta})$ is the variance of $\hat{\theta}$ under H_0. If we could calculate the appropriate χ_1^2 value *independently* of the above formula, which necessitates obtaining $\text{Var}_0(\hat{\theta})$ *directly*, then we could solve the above expression to obtain the value of $\text{Var}_0(\hat{\theta})$ *indirectly*, as

$$\text{Var}_0(\hat{\theta}) = (\hat{\theta} - \theta_0)^2/\chi_1^2$$

The χ_1^2 value in the denominator of this expression is generally taken to be the Mantel-Haenszel χ_1^2 statistic value.

Usually one can arrange matters so that θ_0 or a function of θ_0 is equal to zero. For example, if θ is the CID or the EF (etiologic fraction), then

$\theta_0 = 0$; and ln $\theta_0 = 0$ for those parameters like the risk ratio and the odds ratio whose null value is one. In the former case, the resulting test-based confidence interval has the general structure

$$\hat{\theta} \pm Z_{1-\alpha/2} \sqrt{\hat{\theta}^2/\chi_1^2}$$

In the second case, the test-based interval is

$$(\hat{\theta})\exp[\pm Z_{1-\alpha/2} \sqrt{(\ln \hat{\theta})^2/\chi_1^2}]$$

A comparison of the structure of these intervals with the corresponding Taylor series intervals in Section 15.2.1 highlights the basic difference, namely, that $\hat{\theta}^2/\chi_1^2$ or $(\ln \hat{\theta})^2/\chi_1^2$ is employed as a crude estimate of Var($\hat{\theta}$) or Var(ln $\hat{\theta}$) instead of a more rigorously developed estimate (as is used in the Taylor series intervals). One major criticism leveled at the test-based interval is that, strictly speaking, the quantity $\hat{\theta}^2/\chi_1^2$ or $(\ln \hat{\theta})^2/\chi_1^2$ is an estimate of the (null) variance of $\hat{\theta}$ or ln $\hat{\theta}$ under H_0, which is really only appropriate when H_0 is true. This is the reason that the test-based intervals tend, on the average, to be a little narrower than the Taylor series intervals. This discrepancy does not disappear for large samples, but it is usually negligible when the parameter of interest is not far away from its null value (e.g., $.2 \leq OR \leq 4$).

For computational purposes, the two forms of the test-based interval just given are best written, respectively, as

$$\hat{\theta}(1 \pm Z_{1-\alpha/2}/\sqrt{\chi_1^2}) \qquad (15.11)$$

and

$$\hat{\theta}^{(1 \pm Z_{1-\alpha/2}/\sqrt{\chi_1^2})} \qquad (15.12)$$

EXAMPLE 15.7

We will demonstrate how to use these formulas with the data sets in Tables 15.2, 15.6, and 15.8. The data in Table 15.2 illustrate why the test-based interval approach is sometimes quite appealing. The fact that these data involve person-years information means that we are dealing with rates rather than proportions, and the statistical properties of estimators of rates are not the same as those of estimators of proportions. As a result, Taylor series intervals are difficult (although not impossible) to develop in such situations; so, it is much easier to use the test-based intervals, since χ^2 tests for such data are readily available.

For the data in Table 15.2, the χ_1^2 statistic has the value $(2.10)^2 = 4.41$. This χ_1^2 value is used to find test-based intervals for both IDD and IDR, since this value is employed to test H_0: $ID_1 = ID_0$, a null hypothesis that is equivalent to both IDD = 0 and IDR = 1. So, using Expressions

EXAMPLE 15.7 (*continued*)

15.11 and 15.12, we find 95% test-based confidence intervals for IDD and IDR to be, respectively,

$$[(30/699) - (36/1,399)](1 \pm 1.96/\sqrt{4.41}) \qquad \text{or} \qquad (.001, .033)$$

and

$$\left(\frac{30/699}{36/1,399}\right)^{(1 \pm 1.96/\sqrt{4.41})} \qquad \text{or} \qquad (1.035, 2.695)$$

These intervals do not contain the null values of the effect measures. This consistency with the result of the χ_1^2 test is one of the desirable properties of the test-based interval estimation procedure. That is, the $100(1 - \alpha)\%$ test-based confidence interval does or does not contain the null value of the effect measure according to whether the associated χ_1^2 test does not or does reject the null hypothesis of no effect at the α level of significance.

A 95% test-based confidence interval for the CIR, using the data in Table 15.6, is, from Expression 15.12,

$$(2.45)^{(1 \pm 1.96/\sqrt{16.22})} \qquad \text{or} \qquad (1.584, 3.789)$$

Note that this interval is the same as the one obtained by using the Taylor series approach; of course, this is generally not the case.

Finally, a 95% test-based confidence interval for EOR, using the data in Table 15.8, is

$$(2.67)^{(1 \pm 1.96/\sqrt{1.41})} \qquad \text{or} \qquad (.528, 13.506)$$

This interval is slightly narrower than the corresponding Taylor series interval, (.513, 13.903). Both intervals are quite wide and indicate no evidence of an exposure-disease relationship.

**15.2.3
Exact Types of
Confidence
Intervals for
the OR**

In this section we will discuss briefly the construction of exact types of confidence intervals for the odds ratio. Use of these intervals would be recommended when dealing with small to moderate cell sample sizes. The computations involved in the construction of the intervals require computer assistance; however, there are algorithms available (e.g., see Thomas, 1971).

The statistical theory on which exact types of intervals are based uses the data layout shown in Table 15.9. This layout was previously considered in Table 15.5. For this table, the random variable A, assuming fixed margins and under H_0: OR $= 1$, had the hypergeometric distribution given

**Table 15.9 Data Layout for Exact Confidence Intervals
for the OR**

	E	$\overline{E}$	
D	j	$m_1 - j$	m_1
$\overline{D}$	$n_1 - j$	$n_0 - m_1 + j$	m_0
	n_1	n_0	

by Expression 15.4. More generally, if the OR is not restricted to be equal to one, then A has the *noncentral* hypergeometric distribution

$$\text{pr}(A = j|\text{OR}) = C_j^{n_1} C_{m_1-j}^{n_0}(\text{OR})^j \Big/ \sum_u C_u^{n_1} C_{m_1-u}^{n_0}(\text{OR})^u \quad (15.13)$$

where $\sum\limits_u$ is the sum over all values of u for which

$$\max(0, m_1 - n_0) \le u \le \min(n_1, m_1)$$

It can be shown that Expression 15.13 reduces to 15.4 when the OR is equal to one.

Exact confidence intervals for the OR are obtained, via Expression 15.13, by using an argument tied to hypothesis testing. In particular, to construct an exact $100(1 - \alpha)\%$ confidence interval for the OR by using Expression 15.13, we need to determine all values of OR that are "consistent with the observed data" (i.e., consistent with observing $A = a$) in the sense that the two-sided exact test of H_0: OR $= 1$ versus H_A: OR $\ne 1$, with critical region (i.e., type I error rate) of size α, would not lead to the rejection of H_0. That is, we wish to determine values $\hat{\text{OR}}_L$ and $\hat{\text{OR}}_U$ satisfying the following criteria:

$\hat{\text{OR}}_L$ is the *smallest value* of OR for which Expression 15.13 satisfies

$$\sum_{\text{all } j \ge a} \text{pr}(A = j|\hat{\text{OR}}_L) \ge \frac{\alpha}{2} \quad (15.14)$$

$\hat{\text{OR}}_U$ is the *largest value* of OR for which Expression 15.13 satisfies

$$\sum_{\text{all } j \le a} \text{pr}(A = j|\hat{\text{OR}}_U) \ge \frac{\alpha}{2} \quad (15.15)$$

These values of OR yield the confidence interval statement

$$\text{pr}(\hat{\text{OR}}_L \le \text{OR} \le \hat{\text{OR}}_U) = (1 - \alpha)$$

The determination of $\hat{OR}_L$ and $\hat{OR}_U$, using Expressions 15.14 and 15.15, generally requires computer assistance (Thomas, 1971), and even this aid is of questionable value for moderate to large data sets. Fortunately, with data sets of at least moderate size, it is possible to approximate the probabilities in 15.14 and 15.15 and hence to obtain approximate values for $\hat{OR}_L$ and $\hat{OR}_U$.

The best-known approximation procedure is that of Cornfield (1956). Cornfield's confidence limits (say $\hat{OR}_L^*$ and $\hat{OR}_U^*$) generally offer the closest approximations to $\hat{OR}_L$ and $\hat{OR}_U$, and they come nearest to preserving the nominal confidence coefficient (e.g., 95%) of any of the intervals we have previously considered (see Gart and Thomas, 1972).

To determine $\hat{OR}_L^*$ for a $100(1 - \alpha)\%$ confidence interval, Cornfield first finds a_L^* as the *smallest* real root of the quartic equation in a_L of the form

$$\left(a - a_L - \frac{1}{2}\right)^2\left(\frac{1}{a_L} + \frac{1}{m_1 - a_L} + \frac{1}{n_1 - a_L} + \frac{1}{n_0 - m_1 + a_L}\right) = Z_{1-\alpha/2}^2$$

subject to the condition

$$\max(0, m_1 - n_0) \le a_L^* \le \min(n_1, m_1)$$

Then he calculates $\hat{OR}_L^*$ from the equation

$$\hat{OR}_L^* = a_L^*(n_0 - m_1 + a_L^*)/(m_1 - a_L^*)(n_1 - a_L^*) \qquad (15.16)$$

Similarly,

$$\hat{OR}_U^* = a_U^*(n_0 - m_1 + a_U^*)/(m_1 - a_U^*)(n_1 - a_U^*) \qquad (15.17)$$

where a_U^* is the *largest* real root of the quartic equation in a_U of the form

$$\left(a - a_U + \frac{1}{2}\right)^2\left(\frac{1}{a_U} + \frac{1}{m_1 - a_U} + \frac{1}{n_1 - a_U} + \frac{1}{n_0 - m_1 + a_U}\right) = Z_{1-\alpha/2}^2$$

subject to the condition

$$\max(0, m_1 - n_0) \le a_U^* \le \min(n_1, m_1)$$

EXAMPLE 15.8

As a numerical illustration, we will consider, as did Cornfield (1956), a subset of the case-control data on smoking and lung cancer given by Wynder and Cornfield (1953). These data appear in Table 15.10. Note that $\hat{EOR} = (60)(11)/(3)(32) = 6.875$.

EXAMPLE 15.8 (*continued*)

Table 15.10   Case-Control Data

	E (*Smoker*)	$\overline{E}$ (*Nonsmoker*)	
D (*Lung Cancer Patient*)	60	3	$m_1 = 63$
$\overset{.}{D}$ (*Control*)	32	11	$m_0 = 43$
	$n_1 = 92$	$n_0 = 14$	

For these data, it can be shown (with computer assistance) that $a_L^* = 56.0956$, so that, from Expression 15.16,

$$\hat{OR}_L^* = \frac{(56.0956)(14 - 63 + 56.0956)}{(63 - 56.0956)(92 - 56.0956)} = 1.606$$

Also, $a_U^* = 62.1852$, so that Expression 15.17 becomes

$$\hat{OR}_U^* = \frac{(62.1852)(14 - 63 + 62.1852)}{(63 - 62.1852)(92 - 62.1852)} = 33.751$$

The Cornfield interval is, then, (1.606, 33.751).

Mantel and Fleiss (1980) have described a simple check to see whether Cornfield's approximate interval $(\hat{OR}_L^*, \hat{OR}_U^*)$ is a reasonable one to use instead of the more tedious-to-calculate exact interval $(\hat{OR}_L, \hat{OR}_U)$ based on Expressions 15.14 and 15.15. For 95% confidence limits, one simply checks whether the intervals

$$a_L^* \pm 1.96 \left(\frac{1}{a_L^*} + \frac{1}{m_1 - a_L^*} + \frac{1}{n_1 - a_L^*} + \frac{1}{n_0 - m_1 + a_L^*} \right)^{-1/2} \quad (15.18)$$

and

$$a_U^* \pm 1.96 \left(\frac{1}{a_U^*} + \frac{1}{m_1 - a_U^*} + \frac{1}{n_1 - a_U^*} + \frac{1}{n_0 - m_1 + a_U^*} \right)^{-1/2} \quad (15.19)$$

are both contained within the range of possible values for a under the fixed-margins assumption, namely,

$$\max(0, m_1 - n_0) \leq a \leq \min(n_1, m_1)$$

EXAMPLE 15.9

For the data in Table 15.10, the intervals 15.18 and 15.19 are, respectively,

$$(52.36, 59.83) \quad \text{and} \quad (59.15, 65.22)$$

Since $\max(0, m_1 - n_0) = 49$ and $\min(n_1, m_1) = 63$, interval 15.19 does not meet the desired condition for these data, but it is close enough to say that the Cornfield approximation is permissible to use.

For comparison purposes, the 95% Taylor series confidence interval for EOR for these data is, from Expression 15.10,

$$(\hat{EOR}) \exp\left(\pm 1.96 \sqrt{\frac{1}{a} + \frac{1}{b} + \frac{1}{c} + \frac{1}{d}} \right)$$

or

$$(6.875) \exp\left(\pm 1.96 \sqrt{\frac{1}{60} + \frac{1}{3} + \frac{1}{32} + \frac{1}{11}} \right)$$

or

$$(6.875)e^{\pm 1.347} \quad \text{or} \quad (1.788, 26.440)$$

The 95% test-based confidence interval for EOR, based on Expression 15.12, is

$$\hat{EOR}^{(1 \pm 1.96/\sqrt{x_1^2})}$$

where, from Expression 15.7,

$$\chi_1^2 = \frac{(106 - 1)[(60)(11) - (3)(32)]^2}{(92)(14)(63)(43)} = 9.572$$

Thus, we have

$$(6.875)^{(1 \pm 1.96/\sqrt{9.572})} \quad \text{or} \quad (6.875)^{(1 \pm .6335)}$$

or

$$(2.027, 23.318)$$

EXAMPLE 15.9 (*continued*)

The Taylor series interval is somewhat unreliable because of the small frequency (namely, 3) in the $\overline{DE}$ cell, and the test-based interval is too narrow since $\hat{EOR}$ is quite far away from one.

This concludes our discussion on hypothesis testing and confidence interval estimation in the simple analysis situation. Extensions of these concepts to more complex situations will be presented in later chapters. Also, we point out that the preceding discussion was not designed to cover all the various interval estimation procedures that are available. For example, we did not discuss some of the confidence interval methods for estimating parameters like the attributable risk (e.g., see Walter, 1976, and Leung and Kupper, 1981a, 1981b). The interested reader can consult the appropriate references for further details.

15.3 CONCLUDING REMARKS

The following list summarizes the key notation introduced in this chapter.

NOTATION

A	Random variable denoting the number of exposed cases.
a	Sample realization of A.
$pr(A = j\vert H_0)$	Probability that A takes the particular value j under some null hypothesis H_0.

Density Type of Follow-up Study

$\hat{ID}_1 = a/L_1$	Estimated incidence density for exposed subjects.
$\hat{ID}_0 = b/L_0$	Estimated incidence density for nonexposed subjects.
$\hat{IDR} = \hat{ID}_1/\hat{ID}_0$	Estimated incidence density ratio.
$\hat{IDD} = \hat{ID}_1 - \hat{ID}_0$	Estimated incidence density difference.
$p_0 = L_1/L$	Proportion of L associated with exposed subjects.
$q_0 = L_0/L = 1 - p_0$	Proportion of L associated with nonexposed subjects.

Cumulative Type of Follow-up Study, Case-Control Study, or Cross-sectional Study

$\hat{CI}_1 = a/n_1$	Estimated cumulative incidence for exposed subjects.

$$\hat{CI}_0 = b/n_0$$ Estimated cumulative incidence for nonexposed subjects.

$$\hat{CIR} = \hat{CI}_1/\hat{CI}_0(= \hat{RR})$$ Estimated cumulative incidence ratio (risk ratio).

$$\hat{CID} = \hat{CI}_1 - \hat{CI}_0$$
$$(= \hat{RD})$$ Estimated cumulative incidence difference (risk difference).

$$\hat{ROR} = \frac{\hat{CI}_1(1 - \hat{CI}_0)}{\hat{CI}_0(1 - \hat{CI}_1)}$$ Estimated risk odds ratio.

$$= \frac{ad}{bc}$$

$$\hat{EOR} = ad/bc$$ Estimated exposure odds ratio.

PRACTICE EXERCISES

15.1 A case-control study was carried out to investigate the theory that a certain study factor e is a determinant of some rare disease d. A representative group of new (incident) cases of the disease arising in a given population over a five-year period was identified. These cases were then compared to a random sample of an equal number of noncases from that same population regarding previous exposure to the study factor (with E denoting some previous exposure and $\overline{E}$ denoting no previous exposure). Exercise Table 15.1 gives the frequency of previous exposure to the study factor for cases (D) and noncases $(\overline{D})$.

Exercise Table 15.1

	E	$\overline{E}$	Total
D	28	22	50
$\overline{D}$	20	30	50
Total	48	52	100

a. Estimate the exposure odds ratio (EOR) for the data. Can we say (using this point estimate alone) that there is statistical evidence of an association between the study factor and the disease? Explain.

b. Assess the statistical significance of the observed $\hat{EOR}$ value, using a Mantel-Haenszel χ^2 test. Determine the one-sided P-value and interpret this result.

c. Calculate a 95% large-sample confidence interval for EOR. Assume that $\hat{EOR}$ is lognormally distributed and that the standard error (SE) of ln $\hat{EOR}$ can be estimated as

$$\hat{SE}(\ln \hat{EOR}) \approx \sqrt{\frac{1}{a} + \frac{1}{b} + \frac{1}{c} + \frac{1}{d}}$$

where a, b, c, and d are the numbers of exposed cases, unexposed cases, exposed noncases, and unexposed noncases, respectively.

d. Calculate a 95% test-based interval, using the information obtained in part b. Again, assume that EÔR is lognormally distributed. Compare this interval with the one calculated in part c. Which interval is more "conservative" (i.e., wider)?

15.2 A small clinical trial was conducted to test the effectiveness of vitamin C in preventing the common cold. In May 1968, 30 white male assembly workers from a small urban community were randomized into two groups: those who were to receive 30-day supplies of vitamin C each month of the study, to be taken daily in prescribed doses (the *treatment group*); and those who were to receive 30-day supplies of a placebo each month (the *control group*). At the start of the study, the subjects ranged in age from 20 to 49 and were free of any diagnosed infections or chronic diseases known to be related to individual susceptibility to the common cold. The subjects were asked to report monthly to the company physician (who was also the principal investigator) to receive their monthly allotment of vitamin C or placebo, to be examined or questioned regarding new occurrences of the illness under study as well as other conditions, and to be questioned about drug compliance for the previous month. The subjects were not aware of their group (treatment) status, nor was the investigator (i.e., this study was a double-blind study).

The study was terminated in November 1968, six months after the initial exam. Several subjects were not followed for the entire follow-up period for either of two reasons: failure to report to the physician as scheduled, or failure to comply with the allotted regimen (as prescribed by the investigator). Exercise Table 15.2 summarizes the data for each subject. There were 15

Exercise Table 15.2

Subject Number	Age	Assigned Group	No. of Months Observed	No. of Occurrences of Common Cold
1	34	T	6	0
2	49	C	5	2
3	36	T	6	0
4	26	C	2	0
5	25	T	6	0
6	42	C	6	1
7	27	T	5	1
8	30	C	6	0
9	33	T	6	1
10	47	C	3	1
11	28	T	3	0
12	41	C	6	2
13	42	T	5	1
14	33	C	4	1
15	20	T	6	0
16	34	C	3	0
17	27	T	5	0

Exercise Table 15.2 (*continued*)

Subject Number	Age	Assigned Group	No. of Months Observed	No. of Occurrences of Common Cold
18	43	C	5	0
19	48	T	3	1
20	35	C	6	2
21	39	T	6	0
22	24	C	4	0
23	45	T	6	0
24	46	C	5	0
25	38	T	6	1
26	29	C	5	1
27	46	T	4	0
28	37	C	5	0
29	24	T	6	0
30	22	C	4	0

treatment (T) and 15 control (C) subjects who were followed for between two and six months. Multiple occurrences of the common cold were observed in 3 subjects. Assume that each cold lasted one-third of a month and that all colds started one-third of a month prior to the end of the observation period, or earlier.

a. Estimate the average incidence density for the treatment group (i.e., $\hat{ID}_1$) and for the control group (i.e., $\hat{ID}_0$), using the data given. Calculate the estimated incidence density ratio ($\hat{IDR}$).

b. Is the observed $\hat{IDR}$ significantly less than one? Use two methods to test H_0: IDR = 1 versus H_A: IDR < 1: (i) a large-sample Z test and (ii) an exact test.

c. Calculate a 95% test-based confidence interval for IDR, using the large-sample Z test result obtained in part b.

d. What would your suggestions be for improving the analysis of these data?

REFERENCES   BRESLOW, N. E., and DAY, N. E. 1981. *Statistical methods in cancer research. Vol. I: The analysis of case-control studies*. Lyon, France: IARC Scientific Publications No. 32; Chap. IV.

CONOVER, W. J. 1974. Some reasons for not using the Yates continuity correction on 2 × 2 contingency tables. *J. Am. Stat. Assoc.* 69(346): 374–382.

CORNFIELD, J. 1956. A statistical problem arising from retrospective studies. In *Proceedings of the 3rd Berkeley symposium on mathematical statistics and probability*, edited by J. Newman, pp. 135–148. Berkeley: University of California Press.

FLEISS, J. L. 1979. Confidence intervals for the odds ratio in case-control studies: The state of the art. *J. Chronic Dis.* 32(1/2): 69–77.

GART, J. J. 1979. Statistical analyses of the relative risk. *Environ. Health Perspec.* 32: 157–167.

GART, J. J., and THOMAS, D. G. 1972. Numerical results on appropriate confidence limits for the odds ratio. *J. R. Stat. Soc. B* 34: 441–447.

HALPERIN, M. 1977. Estimability and estimation in case-referent studies (letter to the editor). *Am. J. Epidemiol.* 105: 496–498.

KATZ, D.; BAPTISTA, J.; AZEN, S. P.; and PIKE, M. C. 1978. Obtaining confidence intervals for the risk ratio in cohort studies. *Biometrics* 34(3): 469–474.

LEUNG, H. M., and KUPPER, L. L. 1981a. Comparisons of confidence intervals for attributable risk. *Biometrics* 37(2): 293–302.

———. 1981b. Interval estimation using the folded logarithmic transformation. *Commun. Stat.* A10(10): 997–1015.

MANTEL, N., and FLEISS, J. L. 1980. Minimum expected cell size requirements for the Mantel-Haenszel one-degree-of-freedom chi-square test and a related rapid procedure. *Am. J. Epidemiol.* 112(1): 129–134.

MANTEL, N., and HAENSZEL, W. 1959. Statistical aspects of the analysis of data from retrospective studies of disease. *J. Nat. Cancer Inst.* 22(4): 719–748.

MIETTINEN, O. S. 1976. Estimability and estimation in case-referent studies. *Am. J. Epidemiol.* 103(2): 226–235.

———. 1977. Author's reply to letter by M. Halperin. *Am. J. Epidemiol.* 105: 498–502.

OSTLE, B. 1963. *Statistics in research.* Ames: Iowa State University Press.

THOMAS, D. G. 1971. Exact confidence limits for an odds ratio in a 2 × 2 table. *Appl. Stat.* 20: 105–110.

WALTER, S. D. 1976. The estimation and interpretation of attributable risk in health research. *Biometrics* 32: 829–849.

WYNDER, E. L., and CORNFIELD, J. 1953. Cancer of the lung in physicians. *N. Eng. J. Med.* 248: 441–444.

16

Overview of Options for Control of Extraneous Factors

CHAPTER OUTLINE

Having discussed and illustrated in earlier chapters several important general concepts regarding the control of extraneous variables, we now wish to review these concepts. Then we will describe several options for the process of control, options that are available both at the design and at the analysis stages of a study.

16.0 PREVIEW

The term "control" has had many different usages in the statistical and applied research literature (see Feinstein, 1977). Our definition of the term is motivated by the desire to make an appropriate comparison of study factor (i.e., exposure) groups. In particular, by "control of extraneous variables," we mean the assessment of the effect of the exposure E on the disease D at different combinations of levels of the extraneous variables, in conjunction with an overall (i.e., summary) evaluation, when appropriate, of the E–D relationship, based on pooling together information over these various levels. This definition, while suggestive of stratified analyses, also conceptually incorporates mathematical modeling approaches, which address essentially the same goals.

16.1 DEFINITION OF CONTROL

We have previously mentioned three reasons for the control of extraneous factors: (1) to make internally valid statistical estimates of and tests about the parameters of interest (e.g., to eliminate or minimize confounding); (2) to improve the precision of estimates and the power of tests; and (3) to shed light on any possible causal mechanisms regarding disease etiology (e.g., to assess effect modification or to decide whether a variable is intervening).

16.2 REASONS FOR CONTROL

The concept of *internal validity*, as it is used here, is essentially concerned with the presence or absence of systematic error in data. Such error results from methodological aspects of the design and/or analysis other than sampling variability—e.g., the selection of subjects, the quality of information obtained, and the extraneous variables taken into account in the analysis.

As we previously discussed, confounding refers to the distortion (or bias) in the point estimator of the effect that is due to the mixing of the "true" effect with the effects of other factors (i.e., confounders). In most observational studies, the investigator must wait until the analysis stage to control or adjust for confounders, requiring that data be collected on variables that are likely to be confounding (i.e., *potential* confounders). In practice, variables identified as potential confounders are generally determinants of the disease (i.e., risk factors), with such identification being based on current knowledge of disease etiology and previous empirical findings. However, variables that are intervening in the causal path between exposure and disease should not be treated as potential confounders, since their control could spuriously mask a nonnull E–D association.

Operationally, a potential confounder is considered an actual confounder if adjustment for this variable in the data results in a "meaningful" change in the estimate of the exposure effect on disease, conditional on all other potential confounders. One important implication of this definition is that a factor will not appear to be confounding unless it is "associated with" both the exposure and the disease in the data (Miettinen, 1974). (The phrase "associated with" was clarified in Chapter 13, on confounding.) Thus, "stepwise" mathematical-modeling procedures using a pool of potential confounders and the exposure as the set of candidate independent variables can give misleading results, because they rely solely on the adjusted association between potential confounders and the disease for purposes of variable selection (without simultaneously considering the relationship of these potential confounders to the exposure). In other words, improving precision in the estimation of the response via regression analysis does not ensure that confounding is adequately controlled.

The concept of *precision* is essentially concerned with the amount of random error in the estimate of effect. One approach to quantification of precision involves calculating the reciprocal of the estimated variance of the estimator of effect. An approximately equivalent alternative is to look at confidence interval width. Precision considerations should *not* take precedence over concerns for validity. The investigator must, in any case, consider the trade-offs involved in trying both to increase precision and to maintain validity. Such trade-offs apply to the use of stratified analysis as well as to mathematical-modeling approaches for control.

Over and above issues of confounding and precision, it is of paramount importance to assess the degree to which risk factors *modify* the effect of the exposure on the disease. We have questioned the value of efforts to control for confounding when effect modification, as manifested in the data as statistical interaction, is present. In such circumstances, the most logical strategy for analysis would be to evaluate the E–D association, including considerations of confounding and precision, within combinations of the various levels of the modifier(s).

16.3 OPTIONS FOR CONTROL

Once the collection of extraneous variables to be considered for control is identified, procedures for control may be implemented either at the design (i.e., sampling) stage or at the analysis stage. Four general options are usually available (Miettinen, 1975), and the use of a combination of these options may be worthwhile. Another option, which is characteristic of experimental studies (e.g., clinical trials), is the use of *randomization* in the allocation of the study factor (e.g., exposure status) to study subjects. The purpose of randomization is to evenly distribute the presence of extraneous factors among exposure groups in order to make these groups comparable. Nevertheless, as Rothman (1977) has pointed out, randomization in experiments does not preclude the presence of confounding, with the degree of confounding expected being inversely related to the size of the comparison groups. Since our primary focus in this text concerns observational (rather than experimental) studies, we will not discuss further the properties of randomization.

The four options for control are restriction, matching followed by stratification, stratification without matching, and mathematical modeling. Each of these will be discussed in detail in subsequent chapters. Here, we provide a brief overview.

1. *Restriction in the study design.* This approach to control simply involves specifying narrow ranges of values for one or more extraneous variables as criteria for admissibility into the study (e.g., restriction to white males only or to ages between 40 and 50). Note that restriction applies to both index and comparison subjects (i.e., to both exposed and unexposed in a follow-up study or to both cases and controls in a case-control study).

2. *Matching in the study design and sampling procedure, followed by stratification in the analysis, based on the matching.* Matching involves the use of constraints in the selection of the comparison group, the goal being to make the distribution of the extraneous variable(s) within the comparison group similar (or identical) to the corresponding distribution in the index group. Note that matching can be viewed as imposing a "partial restriction" on the values of the extraneous variables, since only the comparison group values are restricted. The analysis of matched data requires stratification, with each matched group considered as a separate stratum. Matching will be discussed in detail in Chapter 18.

3. *Stratification in the analysis without matching.* We have illustrated this approach in earlier chapters. This option essentially involves restriction of the analysis (rather than the sampling scheme) to narrow ranges (i.e., strata) of the extraneous variable(s), with pooling of the information over all strata if appropriate (i.e., if there is no interaction).

4. *Mathematical modeling in the analysis.* This approach involves the use of some form of multivariable regression analysis based on a mathematical model relating exposure, extraneous variables, and illness outcome. In follow-up studies, the dependent variable is generally a measure of illness outcome; in case-control studies, the dependent variable may be either exposure status or illness outcome (see Chapter 20). When the dependent variable is binary, the most popular multivariable-modeling approach involves the use of a logistic model, with estimation of model parameters based on maximum likelihood or least squares techniques. Among other approaches for binary outcomes, Miettinen's (1976) confounder summarization method can be considered to be a combination of model fitting followed by stratification. When the dependent variable is continuous (which is not our focus in this text), the most widely used modeling approach is analysis of covariance (Kleinbaum and Kupper, 1978).

At this point, we provide a brief review of regression-modeling concepts. A regression model can be expressed in the general form

$$\mathcal{E}(Y|x_1, x_2, \ldots, x_k) = f(x_1, x_2, \ldots, x_k)$$

where $\mathcal{E}$ denotes expected value, f denotes a function, Y is the dependent variable, and the x's are the independent variables. A function that is linear in the regression coefficients is often written as

$$\mathcal{E}(Y|x_1, x_2, \ldots, x_k) = \alpha + \sum_{j=1}^{k} \beta_j x_j$$

A popular regression model, which we discuss in detail in Chapter 20, is the *logistic model,* given by

$$\mathcal{E}(Y|x_1, x_2, \ldots, x_k) = \left\{ 1 + \exp\left[-\left(\alpha + \sum_{j=1}^{k} \beta_j x_j \right) \right] \right\}^{-1}$$

The logistic model is "inherently linear" in the sense that it can be made linear in the regression coefficients by employing the *logit transformation* (see Chapter 20).

If the dependent variable is binary, the expected value expression simplifies to a probability statement:

$$\mathcal{E}(Y|x_1, x_2, \ldots, x_k) = \mathrm{pr}(Y = 1|x_1, x_2, \ldots, x_k)$$

Consequently, when we later focus on the logistic model for binary disease variables, we can write this general model in the form

$$\mathrm{pr}(Y = 1|x_1, x_2, \ldots, x_k) = \left\{ 1 + \exp\left[-\left(\alpha + \sum_{j=1}^{k} \beta_j x_j \right) \right] \right\}^{-1}$$

16.4 GUIDELINES CONCERNING THE CHOICE OF CONTROL OPTION

The first opportunity to choose a control option arises during the development of the study design or sampling procedure. See Table 16.1, which summarizes the pros and cons of the various options. Here, the investigator must make a decision, for each risk factor, about restricting the range of permissible values, matching in the selection of the comparison series, or waiting until the analysis stage to control (i.e., by stratified analysis or by some form of mathematical modeling or by both).

The main argument for restriction is that it provides efficient control (i.e., no confounding or effect modification, and high precision) within the range of admissibility, if that range is sufficiently narrow. Moreover, restriction is convenient and inexpensive, it simplifies the analysis and interpretation, and it allows one to use alternative control procedures for other extraneous variables. On the negative side, restriction means that statistical inferences cannot be made outside the range of admissibility.

Once study design restriction requirements have been specified, the next step involves the choice of either matching in the study design (fol-

Table 16.1 Options for Control of Extraneous Variables

Study Stage Initiated	Option	Advantages	Disadvantages
Design	Restriction	Complete control Convenient Inexpensive Easy analysis	Can't make (general) inferences beyond restricted categories May have "residual confounding" if restrictions are not fine enough
	Matching	Efficiency (i.e., precision) Feasibility: good way to control for certain factors (see Chapter 18)	Cost Flexibility Feasibility: depends on size of control pool available
Analysis	Stratification	Minimum assumptions required Direct, logical strategy Straightforward computational procedure	Run out of numbers in many strata Lose information by categorizing Various ways to form strata Interpretation is difficult with several extraneous variables
	Mathematical modeling	Feasible with small numbers Provides "smoothing" Provides individual "prediction" of risk Allows continuous variables Allows several exposure variables	Restrictive assumptions Choice of model may be difficult Choice of variables to evaluate may be difficult Variable selection from initial variables is difficult Interpretation is difficult Standard computer algorithms may give misleading results

lowed by an analysis that considers the matching) or controlling in the analysis after selecting unmatched samples. Four factors must be considered when making this choice: *sensitivity* (i.e., precision, statistical power), *cost, feasibility,* and *flexibility*. The reader is referred to more detailed discussions of these factors in the biostatistical and epidemiologic literature (e.g., see Miettinen, 1970; McKinlay, 1977; Kupper et al., 1981).

In the field of epidemiology, there is probably no technique that is more misunderstood and hence misused than that of matching, particularly with regard to the purpose that matching serves in controlling confounding and the circumstances in which matching is likely to be worthwhile. Specifically, it is not often appreciated (cost, feasibility, and flexibility issues aside) that the choice of matching or not matching primarily relates to efficiency considerations (i.e., precision in estimation of effect and power in hypothesis testing) rather than to validity issues (i.e., the control of confounding). A properly analyzed unmatched sample generally preserves validity as well as a correctly handled matched sample does.

In general, it is usually less expensive to choose a random sample of the comparison group than to select matched controls, although matching might be justifiable on cost grounds if the acquisition cost per subject is low. Matching is quite feasible when there is a large group of comparison subjects from which to form appropriate matches. With regard to flexibility, since the distribution of the matching factor will be about the same in each group, matching usually precludes analysis of the matching factor's relationship to the group designation variable (i.e., disease status for case-control studies and exposure status for follow-up studies).

Once the study design and sampling requirements have been specified, any further efforts at control must take place at the analysis stage. Of the two general approaches available, stratification is often preferred to modeling because it is easy to carry out, understand, and describe (via contingency tables), and because it requires minimal statistical assumptions for inference-making purposes. Nevertheless, simultaneous control through stratification of even a moderate number of potential confounders usually results in insufficient information (i.e., small cell frequencies) in many strata, thus making inferences and interpretations of the data quite unreliable. Moreover, even if adequate numbers are present in all cells, the use of stratified analyses to pinpoint sources of confounding and/or effect modification becomes strategically complex. Additional drawbacks include loss of information associated with the categorization process itself (which can be particularly severe for continuous variables), the possibility that "residual" confounding may remain if stratum boundaries are too broad, and variability in interpretations resulting from the way variables are categorized.

The primary reasons we use multivariable mathematical-modeling techniques to control simultaneously for several extraneous variables are to help with the insufficient-numbers problem, often encountered when using stratified analyses, and to provide "smoothing." By the latter term, we mean that modeling may lead to a simplified, parsimonious description of the effects, which "smoothes out" (i.e., dampens) variation contributed by unimportant variables.

Like stratified analysis, modeling is used to address issues concerning effect modification and confounding and to obtain, when appropriate, a test of overall association and an estimate of overall effect. In certain circumstances, the results from modeling may provide more insight than the results from simple stratified analysis (e.g., when an easily interpretable "best model" becomes clear-cut upon data analysis). Also, modeling can sometimes be used to "predict" individual risk. However, in our experience, the results from modeling are sometimes difficult to interpret. Specific problems associated with mathematical modeling would include difficulties in choosing the "correct" model and the appropriate estimation procedure, and difficulties in verifying the reasonableness of the assumptions required for valid significance testing. Also, the several alternative modeling approaches available have yet to be sufficiently scrutinized and compared in terms of performance. As we will describe and illustrate in Chapters 20–24, Miettinen's confounder summarization method represents an attempt to combine the advantages of mathematical modeling and stratification while avoiding their disadvantages; however, this method has problems of its own.

It is our opinion that no single method of analysis can be singled out as optimal. We generally recommend, whether or not there are sufficient numbers, that stratified analysis be used to some extent prior to and in conjunction with mathematical modeling. Even when the sample size is small, one may gain valuable qualitative insight into the nature of confounding and interaction by stratification on one, two, or three factors at a time. Also, by using mathematical modeling, one may identify an efficient subset of confounders and/or modifiers for subsequent consideration via stratified analysis. We will discuss strategies for analysis in more detail in Chapters 20 and 21.

16.5 CONCLUDING REMARKS

REFERENCES

FEINSTEIN, A. R. 1977. *Clinical biostatistics*. St. Louis: Mosby.

KLEINBAUM, D. G., and KUPPER, L. L. 1978. *Applied regression analysis and other multivariable methods*. Boston: Duxbury Press.

KUPPER, L. L.; KARON, J. M.; KLEINBAUM, D. G.; MORGENSTERN, H.; and LEWIS, D. K. 1981. Matching in epidemiologic studies: Validity and efficiency considerations. *Biometrics* 37(2): 271–291.

MCKINLAY, S. M. 1977. Pair-matching—A reappraisal of a popular technique. *Biometrics* 33: 725–735.

MIETTINEN, O. S. 1970. Matching and design efficiency in retrospective studies. *Am. J. Epidemiol.* 91: 111–118.

———. 1974. Confounding and effect modification. *Am. J. Epidemiol.* 100: 350–353.

———. 1975. *Principles of epidemiologic research*. Unpublished manuscript. Cambridge, Mass.: Harvard University.

———. 1976. Stratification by a multivariate confounder score. *Am. J. Epidemiol.* 104(6): 609–620.

ROTHMAN, K. J. 1977. Epidemiologic methods in clinical trials. *Cancer* 39: 1771–1775.

17

Stratified Analysis

CHAPTER OUTLINE

Stratified analysis is one of two general approaches commonly used for control of extraneous variables at the analysis stage, the other approach being some form of mathematical modeling. The appeal of stratification is the straightforward manner by which control is achieved, the easy-to-follow-and-understand computations required, and the relatively small number of statistical assumptions necessary for inference making. However, these characteristics pertain more to the procedure itself than to the broad objective of achieving simultaneous control of several variables. With the latter objective in mind, then, stratification becomes worthwhile under the three following conditions:

17.0 PREVIEW

1. There are sufficient numbers in all strata.
2. An appropriate choice of control variables can be made.
3. An appropriate categorization scheme for each variable can be identified (i.e., categories are meaningful and there is no residual confounding).

This chapter describes the details and problem areas associated with the *procedure* involved in stratified analysis; for the most part, therefore, we will assume that conditions 1–3 above are met. However, using data from the previously described (Chapter 1) study of the relationship of cate-cholamine level to incidence of coronary heart disease in Evans County, Georgia, we will also illustrate problems in interpretation that typically arise when simultaneously considering several control variables.

Given a specified set of control variables, we may describe the procedure of stratified analysis through the following five steps.

17.1 OVERVIEW OF THE PROCEDURE

Step 1. Categorize each of the variables to be controlled.

Step 2. For the categories defined in step 1, organize the study subjects into combinations of categories of each control variable; these combinations are called *strata*. For dichotomous disease and exposure variables, the data in the gth stratum can be described by one of two formats, as shown in Table 17.1; the format depends on the study design used.

Table 17.1   Data Layout for the *g*th Stratum ($g = 1, 2, \ldots, G$)

a. **Cumulative Follow-up, Case-Control, or Cross-sectional Studies**   b. **Density Follow-up Studies**

	E	$\bar{E}$	
D	a_g	b_g	m_{1g}
$\bar{D}$	c_g	d_g	m_{0g}
	n_{1g}	n_{0g}	n_g

	E	$\bar{E}$	
No. of Cases Developed in (t_0, t)	a_g	b_g	$m_{1g} = a_g + b_g$
Population-Time of Follow-up in (t_0, t)	L_{1g}	L_{0g}	$L_g = L_{1g} + L_{0g}$

Step 3.   Carry out simple analyses (as described in Chapter 15) within each stratum, using a Mantel-Haenszel χ^2 test for association and an estimate of effect (e.g., risk ratio, odds ratio, risk difference, incidence density ratio, or incidence density difference) appropriate for the design used.

Step 4.   If considered appropriate, carry out and interpret an overall test for association between exposure and disease that accumulates the information contained in each stratum in such a way as to control for confounding. The test statistic most commonly recommended is a Mantel-Haenszel statistic extended for stratified data.

Step 5.   If considered appropriate, accumulate information over the strata to obtain point and/or interval (summary) estimates of overall effect. The point estimates are typically in the form of weighted averages of stratum-specific estimates. The interval estimates may be those using either Taylor series or test-based approximations of variance (described in Chapter 15 for the simple analysis case), although other (more exact) procedures are available also.

In addition to the above steps, the analysis may include a step to assess the functional (e.g., linear) relationship among estimates of effect over the strata, provided the strata are defined on an ordinal scale. For example, if three age strata distinguish among old, middle-aged, and young subjects, it may be of interest to evaluate whether stratum-specific estimates of, say, the risk ratio increase as age increases.

As indicated above, there are two decision points in the analysis procedure, steps 4 and 5, which involve a certain amount of subjectivity. Either one or both of these steps may be considered inappropriate if there is considerable evidence of statistical *interaction,* as indicated by nonuniformity of the estimates of effect over the strata.

Subjectivity enters for two reasons. First, as we will discuss in detail later (in Chapter 19 on interaction, effect modification, and synergism), the assessment of interaction depends on the statistical model chosen to define the state of no interaction. [For example, the homogeneity of several risk ratios is equivalent to no interaction on a "multiplicative" scale (Kupper and Hogan, 1978).] The choice of model, in turn, requires the subjective judgment of the investigator regarding the underlying scale for measuring interaction, which must consider the purpose of one's study and current knowledge of the relationships among the variables of interest. Second, once a model (i.e., scale) is specified, the assessment of homogeneity of effect should not rely exclusively on the results of a statistical test. The investigator's judgment is required to interpret the clinical importance of differences that are obtained among stratum-specific point estimates. [Testing for interaction is typically accomplished through mathematical-modeling procedures, as discussed and illustrated in Chapters 19–24. A suitable test for stratified data (Breslow and Day, 1980) is described in Practice Exercise 17.6 at the end of this chapter.]

EXAMPLE 17.1

To illustrate the subjective decision problem arising from comparison of stratum-specific estimates of effect, we consider the three situations identified in Table 17.2, which concerns estimation of a risk ratio, using two strata. In considering each stratum, we will assume that there are sufficient numbers in each stratum, so that the risk ratio estimates are reasonably precise.

For situation 1, the estimates provided show *opposite effects* in each stratum; i.e., in stratum 1, the risk ratio is less than one, whereas in stra-

Table 17.2 Examples Pertaining to Decisions About Interaction in Stratified Analysis

	$\hat{\text{RR}}$		*Overall Test?*	*Overall Summary Estimate?*
Situation	*Stratum 1*	*Stratum 2*		
1 (Opposite direction)	.7	3.5	No	No
2 (Same direction)	1.5	4.8	Maybe	Maybe
3 (Uniform effect)	2.3	2.9	Yes	Yes

EXAMPLE 17.1 *(continued)*

tum 2 the risk ratio is greater than one. For such a situation, it is possible that opposite effects may cancel each other when using either an overall test or summary estimate, thus giving a misleading impression of no overall association. For this reason, we do not recommend the use of either an overall test or a summary estimate when the direction of effect differs among the strata.

When stratum-specific effects are all in the same direction, as illustrated by situation 2, a spurious appearance of no association cannot arise from cancellation of opposite effects. For situation 2, then, it may be worthwhile to perform an overall test or use a summary estimate or both, depending on the investigator's judgment of how large the difference is between stratum-specific effects and/or how stable these estimates are.

Finally, situation 3 shows stratum-specific effects of approximately the same magnitude, so that summarization over the strata would not mask important stratum-specific results.

We emphasize that, in considering any of the situations in Table 17.2 (vis-à-vis the appropriateness of steps 4 and 5 of a stratified analysis), the investigator must exercise some judgment as to the clinical importance of the observed differences among stratum-specific estimates as well as to the stability of these estimates.

**17.2
A GENERAL
EXAMPLE**

We illustrate the results of stratified analysis by using the previously discussed data set from the Evans County heart disease study (see Chapter 1). Recall that the study concerned the putative association between endogenous catecholamine level (CAT) and the subsequent seven-year incidence of coronary heart disease (CHD) among a cohort of 609 white males. The variable CAT, which was fabricated for illustrative purposes, has been dichotomized into categories "high" (the top quintile of cohort values) and "low." Other factors, considered as potential confounders, include the following variables, which were measured at the onset of follow-up (1960–1962): AGE, serum cholesterol (CHL), diastolic blood pressure (DBP), Quetelet's index (QTI; weight, in pounds, times 100, divided by height, in inches squared), smoking status (SMK; smoker/nonsmoker), any electrocardiogram abnormality (ECG; yes/no), socioeconomic status (SES; an index ranging from 12 for highest level to 84 for lowest level), and type of occupation (OCC; farm/nonfarm). Also, a dichotomous hypertension variable (HPT) was considered, the two levels being "high" (systolic blood pressure at least 160 and/or diastolic blood pressure at least 95) and "low."

Table 17.3   Crude Analysis of CAT–CHD Data

	HI CAT	LO CAT	
CHD	27	44	71
$\overline{CHD}$	95	443	538
	122	487	609

$$c\hat{R}R = \frac{27/122}{44/487} = 2.45$$

$$\chi^2_{MH} = \frac{608[(27)(443) - (44)(95)]^2}{(122)(487)(71)(538)}$$

$$= 16.22 \quad (P < .001)$$

For this data set, a simplified crude analysis, which would provide a first step in evaluating the nature and extent of the CAT–CHD relationship, would involve consideration of the CAT–CHD information given in Table 17.3.

17.2.1 Crude Analysis

In the table, the term $c\hat{R}R$ denotes the crude risk ratio estimate, and χ^2_{MH} denotes the Mantel-Haenszel chi-square statistic for the simple test of H_0: no CAT–CHD association. On the basis of the χ^2_{MH} value, the true risk ratio relating CAT to CHD appears to be greater than one; moreover, the strength of the relationship, on the basis of the crude risk ratio point estimate of 2.45, is moderately high. Nevertheless, these results certainly ignore consideration of various sources of bias that may have occurred either from inappropriate selection of subjects into the study or from misclassification of subjects into CAT or CHD categories (problems we have discussed in Chapters 11 and 12). Moreover, even assuming that such biases are nonexistent, have been corrected, or are considered to be of a nature that will not seriously alter the measure of association, these results do not take into account the effects (i.e., confounding or interaction) that other known risk factors might have on the CAT–CHD relationship.

An initial approach commonly used for dealing with a multivariable control problem is to carry out stratified analyses for various combinations of risk factors that have been measured. A summary of such analyses for evaluating the CAT–CHD relationship is presented in Table 17.4. In this table, we have provided overall Mantel-Haenszel χ^2 test statistics and corresponding P-values, plus three different summary (adjusted) risk ratio measures ($a\hat{R}R$, $s\hat{R}R$, and $s'\hat{R}R$, which will be described later in this chapter) for each collection of control variables specified. The degree of confounding can be estimated from a comparison of these summary indices with the crude risk ratio ($c\hat{R}R$), which is also provided (in the last column of the table).

17.2.2 Stratified Analyses

Table 17.4   Summary of Stratified Analyses for CAT–CHD Association

Control Variables Involved	Number of Strata	MH TEST OF SIGNIFICANCE, CAT–CHD ASSOCIATION		ESTIMATED SUMMARY EFFECT MEASURES			
		χ^2_{MHS} Value	P-Value (One-sided)	a$\hat{\text{R}}$R	s$\hat{\text{R}}$R	s'$\hat{\text{R}}$R	c$\hat{\text{R}}$R
1. None	1	16.22	.000	—	—	—	2.45
2. AGE	7[a]	5.29	.011	1.79[†]	1.65	1.74	2.45
3. AGE	2	6.99	.004	1.91	1.88	2.04	2.45
4. SMK	2	16.45	.000	2.44	2.46	2.45	2.45
5. ECG	2	9.31	.001	2.15	1.98	2.38	2.45
6. OCC	2	17.51	.000	2.51	2.54	2.51	2.45
7. CHL	2	17.48	.000	3.28	2.37	3.48	2.45
8. HPT	2	7.26	.004	2.19	1.64	3.19	2.45
9. QTI	2	16.09	.000	2.54	2.45	2.42	2.45
10. SES	2	16.85	.000	2.75	2.38	2.71	2.45
11. AGE, SMK	4	5.76	.008	1.83	1.72	1.94	2.45
12. AGE, ECG	4	4.15	.021	1.71	1.65	1.83	2.45
13. AGE, OCC	4	6.93	.004	1.93	1.85	2.03	2.45
14. AGE, CHL	4	7.39	.003	2.97[†]	1.69	3.14	2.45
15. AGE, HPT	4	2.94	.043	1.68[†]	1.14	1.77	2.45
16. AGE, QTI	4	6.52	.005	1.86	1.85	2.00	2.45
17. AGE, SES	4	8.28	.002	2.12	1.83	2.26	2.45
18. SMK, CHL	4	18.02	.000	3.40[†]	2.40	3.54	2.45
19. CHL, HPT	4	8.34[†]	.002[†]	2.45[†]	1.45[†]	3.92[†]	2.45
20. SMK, ECG, AGE	8	2.24[†]	.067[†]	1.51[†]	1.49[†]	2.45[†]	2.45
21. SMK, AGE, HPT	8	2.07	.075	1.85[†]	1.07	2.40	2.45
22. CHL, AGE, HPT	8	3.55[†]	.030[†]	1.83[†]	.93[†]	2.70[†]	2.45
23. SMK, CHL, AGE	8	6.26	.006	2.77[†]	1.54	3.15	2.45
24. ECG, AGE, QTI	8	3.68	.028	3.23[†]	1.63	2.48	2.45
25. AGE, OCC, HPT	8	2.66[†]	.051[†]	1.62[†]	1.09[†]	1.73[†]	2.45
26. SMK, CHL, ECG	8	7.89	.003	2.87[†]	1.64	3.11	2.45
27. AGE at LO CHL and LO HPT	2	13.14	.000	6.08[†]	4.97	2.31	5.77
28. AGE at LO CHL and HI HPT	2	4.40	.018	.49	.45	.67	.72
29. AGE at HI CHL and HI HPT	2	22.99	.000	13.70[†]	13.52	13.78	12.83
30. AGE, SMK, ECG at LO CHL	8	.36[†]	.275[†]	.91[†]	.82[†]	1.61[†]	1.85

Note: The continuous variables are dichotomized as follows: AGE ($\geq$55, <55); CHL ($\geq$250, <250); QTI ($\geq$3.57, <3.57); SES ($\geq$57, <57).

[a]The seven age strata are 40–44, 45–49, 50–54, 55–59, 60–64, 65–69, and 70+.

[†]The dagger denotes that .50 was added to all cell entries of any stratum containing at least one zero cell.

Unfortunately, the need to consider a variety of analyses for different subsets of variables—e.g., AGE alone, AGE and CHL, etc.—makes an interpretation of the results somewhat complicated. The basic question is, again, whether there is a significant CAT–CHD relationship and, if so, what is its magnitude. An inspection of Table 17.4 indicates that the answer may vary, depending on which subset of variables is actually considered. This problem is complicated by our inability to stratify on many variables at once, since this procedure can result in insufficient numbers in the strata. Furthermore, we must consider the possibility that nonuniformity of the effect measure over the strata (i.e., statistical interaction) may preclude the use of an overall χ^2 test or summary statistic. In fact, the information in Table 17.4 is not detailed enough to permit adequate discussion of interaction or precision issues, which require consideration of the data in individual strata.

Some interpretation of the results in this table is possible, nevertheless. First of all, it appears that if AGE alone is controlled, whether using two or seven strata, then the CAT–CHD relationship is somewhat weaker than originally indicated from the crude results—i.e., there is some confounding by AGE. Notice, for example, that all the summary risk ratio estimates presented in either rows 2 or 3 of the table are closer to one than is the crude estimate and that, moreover, the chi-square value is considerably reduced from the chi-square of 16.22 for the crude table. Similar interpretations are appropriate for ECG and HPT, treated separately, although there is somewhat more variability among summary estimates for each of these factors. Also, when considered separately, the remaining variables provide little indication of confounding, with the exception of CHL, for which two of the three summary estimates are higher than the crude estimate. From these results for variables stratified singly, therefore, it would appear that AGE, ECG, HPT, and CHL should be the primary candidate variables to be considered for the control of confounding.

This interpretation, though reasonable, must be considered tentative on several grounds. First of all, sample sizes are small in many strata, and estimates are somewhat arbitrary when there are zero cells in some strata (as indicated by the † in the table). Second, consideration of interaction (i.e., identifying the modifiers) may indicate additional variables to be controlled or may eliminate the need to consider confounding except within specific levels of such modifiers. Third, as illustrated in Chapter 14, consideration of variables two or more at a time may indicate confounding that might not be manifested when variables are treated singly. Or, alternatively, confounding might not be indicated when variables are controlled together, even though it is suggested when variables are treated individually. Finally, when variables such as AGE, ECG, HPT, and CHL, which are initially identified as possible confounders, are controlled together, some of them may appear to be superfluous with regard to confounding. For example, when AGE and ECG are controlled together (row 12 in the table), the adjusted estimate (a$\hat{\text{R}}$R = 1.71) does not appear to be meaningfully different from the adjusted estimate for AGE alone ($a\hat{R}R = 1.91$ in row 3).

**17.2.3
Interaction**

Regarding the assessment of interaction, an initial approach using stratified analysis would involve comparing risk ratio estimates in different strata for variables taken one at a time. For example, Table 17.5 provides results obtained when separately stratifying on CHL, HPT, and AGE.

From inspection of the risk ratio estimates in Table 17.5, it appears that both CHL and HPT are modifiers, since these estimates are noticeably different in the two strata for each variable, whereas there is no clear evidence of interaction involving AGE. Notice, however, that the evidence for nonuniformity of risk ratios by CHL level is clouded by the imprecision of the estimate for high-CHL persons.

Like the assessment of confounding, the assessment of interaction must consider the simultaneous control of risk factors of interest. For example, Table 17.6 presents stratum-specific risk ratios when CHL, AGE, and HPT are controlled simultaneously.

Examination of this table provides insights not apparent from previous information. There is certainly evidence of interaction, since there is considerable variation in the stratum-specific risk ratios. Nevertheless, specific identification of either confounders or modifiers is somewhat clouded by the lack of sufficient numbers in several strata (particularly those left blank in the table), a situation that typically occurs when two or more variables are controlled. However, it appears that the relationship is different for low versus high CHL, since both risk ratios at high CHL are very large, whereas those at low CHL and high HPT are small. Moreover, at low CHL, high HPT, and AGE above 55, the risk ratio is less than one, suggesting a possible protective effect of CAT on CHD, which may therefore require special consideration. There is also interaction involving AGE at low CHL and high HPT, whereas there appears to be no such interaction at high CHL and HPT. In other words, the use of an overall chi-square and summary estimate (steps 4 and 5 of stratified analysis) seems appropriate within high CHL and HPT, but it is questionable otherwise.

**17.2.4
Conclusions**

In light of the previous comments about interaction, we must view with caution the test statistic and adjusted estimates given in row 22 of Table 17.4 for the simultaneous control of CHL, AGE, and HPT. Although some confounding involving these variables is evident (i.e., $c\hat{R}R = 2.45$, whereas $a\hat{R}R = 1.83$ and $s\hat{R}R = .93$ when all three variables are controlled), the nature of interaction identified from Table 17.6 is a more important finding. Furthermore, these results suggest that control of confounding should be carried out separately within combinations of categories of CHL and HPT, as illustrated by rows 27–29 of Table 17.4, which use AGE as the only control variable. From these rows, we find a high CAT–CHD

Table 17.5 Stratifying on CHL, HPT, and AGE Separately

---

a. CHL Alone

	LOW			HIGH	
	CAT	$\overline{CAT}$		CAT	$\overline{CAT}$
CHD	20	37	CHD	7	7
$\overline{CHD}$	94	353	$\overline{CHD}$	1	90

$\hat{RR} = 1.85$ $\hat{RR} = 12.13$

$\chi^2 = 5.70$ $(P = .009)$ $\chi^2 = 40.83$ $(P < .001)$

---

b. HPT Alone

	LOW			HIGH	
	CAT	$\overline{CAT}$		CAT	$\overline{CAT}$
CHD	8	20	CHD	19	24
$\overline{CHD}$	16	310	$\overline{CHD}$	79	133

$\hat{RR} = 5.50$ $\hat{RR} = 1.27$

$\chi^2 = 22.78$ $(P < .001)$ $\chi^2 = .72$ $(P = .20)$

---

c. AGE Alone

	<55			≥55	
	CAT	$\overline{CAT}$		CAT	$\overline{CAT}$
CHD	4	24	CHD	23	20
$\overline{CHD}$	21	309	$\overline{CHD}$	74	134

$\hat{RR} = 2.22$ $\hat{RR} = 1.83$

$\chi^2 = 2.49$ $(P = .06)$ $\chi^2 = 4.80$ $(P = .01)$

risk ratio (between 13 and 14) when CHL is high; in contrast, we find indication of a possible protective effect of CAT when CHL is low and HPT is high.

The simultaneous control of the other risk factors—i.e., SMK, ECG, OCC, QTI, and SES—might alter such conclusions, though, particularly regarding the assessment of interaction. However, when considered two or

Table 17.6   Risk Ratios from Stratifying on CHL, AGE, and HPT Simultaneously

	AGE < 55	AGE 55+
	n = 200	n = 101
LO CHL, *LO HPT*	$1.33^{\dagger}$ (P = .28)	6.15 (P < .001)
	n = 95	n = 108
LO CHL, *HI HPT*	1.02 (P = .49)	.40 (P = .007)
	n = 33	n = 20
HI CHL, *LO HPT*	—[a]	—[a]
	n = 30	n = 22
HI CHL, *HI HPT*	$14.00^{\dagger\dagger}$ (P < .001)	13.33 (P < .001)

[a]Zero on margin of table.

[†]Zero cell; all cells adjusted by adding .5 to compute risk ratio estimate.

[††]Zero cell; no adjustment needed to calculate risk ratio estimate.

three at a time (e.g., rows 11–13, 16–18 of Table 17.4), these variables do not appear to contribute to confounding over and above that contributed by AGE, CHL, and HPT. Moreover, the additional consideration of more than three risk factors through stratified analysis is precluded by the small numbers that would result.

Thus, as we have seen, the control of several risk factors by way of stratified analysis can be quite complicated because of problems of insufficient numbers, which result when too many variables are controlled, and because of difficulties in assessing the nature of interaction. For these reasons, mathematical modeling approaches are usually considered in addition to or in lieu of stratified analysis (although modeling has problems of its own).

We turn now to some of the specific details of the procedure involved in a stratified analysis. We will first describe the Mantel-Haenszel test for overall association; then we will discuss methods for both point and interval estimation of effect.

17.3 TESTING FOR OVERALL ASSOCIATION

The *Mantel-Haenszel (MH) test* (1959) is the most widely used and recommended method of testing for overall association in a stratified analysis. This test, as we will show below, is a straightforward generalization of the χ^2 test for simple analysis (i.e., when there is only one stratum) described in Chapter 15. The test is applicable to the analysis of both matched and unmatched data (we will leave the matched analysis for Chapter 18).

The MH test statistic for stratified analysis is based on a hypergeometric model for cumulative follow-up, case-control (density or cumulative), and cross-sectional studies. For density follow-up studies, a binomial model is utilized. In all cases, regardless of the study design, the procedure (for dichotomous disease and exposure variables) is a large-sample test using a *one-degree-of-freedom chi-square statistic,* whose basic structure is of the general form

$$\chi^2_{\text{MHS}} = [a - \mathcal{E}_0(A)]^2 / \text{Var}_0(A) \qquad (17.1)$$

where
a = total number of exposed cases (summed over all strata)
A = random variable for which a is the realization in the sample under consideration
$\mathcal{E}_0(A)$ = expected total number of exposed cases under the null hypothesis of no association between exposure and disease
$\text{Var}_0(A)$ = variance of the total number of exposed cases under the same null hypothesis

The specific form that $\mathcal{E}_0(A)$ and $\text{Var}_0(A)$ take depends on the study design used, as we now describe.

**17.3.1
Case-Control,
Cumulative
Follow-up, and
Cross-sectional
Studies**

The data configuration for stratum g in each of these studies was shown in Table 17.1a. As we argued for the simple analysis case, no matter how the sampling was carried out, the marginal frequencies n_{1g}, n_{0g}, m_{1g}, and m_{0g} convey no information about the degree (i.e., strength) of association within a given stratum but, rather, indicate only the amount of information (i.e., precision) in the stratum. Consequently, the marginal frequencies within each stratum may be assumed to be "fixed," so that only the distribution of the numbers in the body of the table need be considered random. It follows that the specification of any single cell frequency automatically determines the counts in the other three cells in the table. Thus, for testing purposes, it is sufficient to focus entirely on the a cell, i.e., the number of exposed cases. The test statistic to be used, therefore, is based on the distribution of the quantity

$$A = \sum_{g=1}^{G} A_g$$

where A_g is the random variable indicating the number of exposed cases in the gth stratum (for which a_g is its sample realization), and where G denotes the total number of strata.

The expected value and variance of A can be obtained by summing over all strata expected values and variances, respectively, derived from the separate distributions of the stratum-specific A_g. [Summation of variances requires the assumption that data from different strata are independent.] Since, under H_0 and assuming fixed marginals, A_g is a hypergeometric random variable, it then follows (in a manner analogous to the simple analysis situation of Chapter 15) that

$$\mathcal{E}_0(A) = \sum_{g=1}^{G} \mathcal{E}_0(A_g) = \sum_{g=1}^{G} \frac{n_{1g} m_{1g}}{n_g}$$

and

$$\mathrm{Var}_0(A) = \sum_{g=1}^{G} \frac{n_{1g} n_{0g} m_{1g} m_{0g}}{(n_g - 1)n_g^2}$$

For purposes of calculation, the quantity inside the brackets of the numerator of Expression 17.1 simplifies to $\sum_g (a_g d_g - b_g c_g)/n_g$. Thus, the usual χ^2_{MHS} *computing formula* (without the continuity correction) *for case-control, cumulative follow-up, and cross-sectional studies* is given by

$$\chi^2_{\mathrm{MHS}} = \left(\sum_{g=1}^{G} \frac{a_g d_g - b_g c_g}{n_g} \right)^2 \bigg/ \sum_{g=1}^{G} \frac{n_{1g} n_{0g} m_{1g} m_{0g}}{(n_g - 1)n_g^2} \qquad (17.2)$$

which should be compared to a tabled value of the chi-square distribution with one degree of freedom.

Note that the large-sample assumptions for this test pertain to the pooled information over all strata rather than stratum-specific numbers.

Consequently, in the use of the test, it is permissible to have relatively little information in specific strata as long as the total number of subjects on the margins over all strata is sufficiently large. Specific criteria for appropriate sample size have been suggested by Mantel and Fleiss (1980). They recommend using χ^2_{MHS} provided both

$$\mathscr{E}_0(A) - \left[\sum_{g=1}^{G} \max(0, m_{1g} - n_{0g})\right] \quad \text{and} \quad \left[\sum_{g=1}^{G} \min(n_{1g}, m_{1g})\right] - \mathscr{E}_0(A)$$

exceed five.

Note also that the test statistic given by Equation 17.2 does not include a correction for continuity. There has been considerable debate in the statistical literature over the value of the continuity correction; e.g., see Conover (1974), Starmer and colleagues (1974), and Mantel (1974). For a more recent discussion of this question with regard to the Mantel-Haenszel test above, see Li and colleagues (1979).

EXAMPLE 17.2

As an example of the use of the Mantel-Haenszel procedure, we consider the control of AGE and ECG in evaluating the CAT–CHD association from the Evans County data described earlier (see Table 17.4, row 12). The four strata resulting from using dichotomous categories of both AGE and ECG are presented in Table 17.7. Notice that the stratum-specific risk ratios in this table are all in the same direction (greater than one) and are not noticeably different from one another (i.e., there is little interaction), so that use of an overall test is appropriate. Notice, also, that three of the four stratum-specific $\hat{RR}$'s are nonsignificant and that the $\hat{RR}$ in the other stratum is of borderline significance, which is not surprising since each stratum contains at least one small cell entry. The total margin sizes (in the crude table) are large, nevertheless, justifying use of the MH test. Using Formula 17.2, we make the following calculations:

$$\chi^2_{MHS} = \frac{\left[\dfrac{(1)(257) - (17)(7)}{282} + \dfrac{(3)(52) - (7)(14)}{76} + \dfrac{(9)(107) - (15)(30)}{161} \right. }{\left[\dfrac{(8)(274)(18)(264)}{(281)(282)^2} + \dfrac{(17)(59)(10)(66)}{(75)(76)^2} + \dfrac{(39)(122)(24)(137)}{(160)(161)^2} \right.}$$

$$\left. + \dfrac{(14)(27) - (5)(44)}{90}\right]^2$$

$$\left. + \dfrac{(58)(32)(19)(71)}{(89)(90)^2}\right]$$

Table 17.7 Stratifying on AGE and ECG to Assess CAT–CHD Association in a Follow-up Study

a. $g = 1$, AGE < 55, ECG $= 0$

	CAT	$\overline{CAT}$	
CHD	1	17	18
$\overline{CHD}$	7	257	264
	8	274	

$\hat{RR}_1 = 2.01$ (N.S.)

b. $g = 2$, AGE < 55, ECG $= 1$

	CAT	$\overline{CAT}$	
CHD	3	7	10
$\overline{CHD}$	14	52	66
	17	59	76

$\hat{RR}_2 = 1.49$ (N.S.)

c. $g = 3$, AGE 55+, ECG $= 0$

	CAT	$\overline{CAT}$	
CHD	9	15	24
$\overline{CHD}$	30	107	137
	39	122	161

$\hat{RR}_3 = 1.88$ ($P = .05$)

d. $g = 4$, AGE 55+, ECG $= 1$

	CAT	$\overline{CAT}$	
CHD	14	5	19
$\overline{CHD}$	44	27	71
	58	32	90

$\hat{RR}_4 = 1.54$ (N.S.)

e. Crude Table

	CAT	$\overline{CAT}$	
CHD	27	44	
$\overline{CHD}$	95	443	487
	122		

$c\hat{RR} = 2.45$ ($P < .001$)

Note: N.S. denotes nonsignificant stratum-specific χ^2_{MH} test.

EXAMPLE 17.2   (*continued*)

$$= \frac{(.4894 + .7632 + 3.1863 + 1.7556)^2}{.4661 + 1.5281 + 3.7721 + 3.4731}$$

$$= 4.15 \quad (P = .02, \text{ one-sided})$$

Thus, on the basis of the overall χ^2_{MHS} test, we would conclude that there is a (borderline) significant CAT–CHD association, controlling for both AGE and ECG. Quantifying the strength of this association would require an appropriate choice of point and/or interval estimate, which we discuss in later sections. Note, however, that the use of this test (or any test) alone is not sufficient to indicate which, if any, variable, AGE or ECG, is a confounder. To evaluate such confounding, we would have to compare various adjusted estimates controlling for AGE and ECG simultaneously with the crude estimate 2.45 and with adjusted estimates controlling separately for AGE and ECG.

EXAMPLE 17.3

To illustrate why the utility of the MH test is questionable when stratum-specific risk ratios are in the opposite direction, consider the appropriateness of this test for the data given in Table 17.8.

Table 17.8   Example of Inappropriate Use of MH Test (Follow-up Study)

	a. Stratum 1			**b. Stratum 2**			**c. Crude Table**	
	E	$\overline{E}$		E	$\overline{E}$		E	$\overline{E}$
D	15	5	D	5	15	D	20	20
$\overline{D}$	85	95	$\overline{D}$	95	85	$\overline{D}$	180	180

$\hat{RR}_1 = 3.00 \quad (P = .01)$ $\hat{RR}_2 = .33 \quad (P = .01)$ $c\hat{RR} = 1.00$

EXAMPLE 17.3 (*continued*)

From Table 17.8, we see that there is a moderately large, positive (e.g., deleterious) effect in stratum 1 ($\hat{RR}_1 = 3$), whereas there is a moderately large but negative (e.g., protective) effect in stratum 2 ($\hat{RR}_2 = .33$). That is, the two effects are both strong and significant, but they are in the opposite direction. However, the use of a Mantel-Haenszel test in such a case would yield a χ^2_{MHS} of zero:

$$\chi^2_{MHS} = \frac{\left[\dfrac{(15)(95) - (5)(85)}{200} + \dfrac{(5)(85) - (15)(95)}{200}\right]^2}{\dfrac{(100)(100)(20)(180)}{(199)(200)^2} + \dfrac{(100)(100)(20)(180)}{(199)(200)^2}} = 0$$

Thus, an MH test can misleadingly indicate no association when there are strong but opposite effects in different strata that cancel each other in the computation of the test statistic.

**17.3.2
Density
Follow-up
Studies**

The general data configuration for the gth stratum of density follow-up studies was previously given in Table 17.1b. Under the null hypothesis of no exposure-disease association, it may be assumed, as was previously done for a simple analysis, that A_g is a binomial variable with probabilities of success and failure, respectively, given by

$$p_{0g} = L_{1g}/L_g \qquad \text{and} \qquad q_{0g} = 1 - p_{0g} = L_{0g}/L_g$$

and with the number of trials given by $m_{1g} = a_g + b_g$.

It follows, then, that the null mean and variance of $A = \Sigma^G_{g=1} A_g$ are given by

$$\mathcal{E}_0(A) = \sum_{g=1}^{G} \mathcal{E}_0(A_g) = \sum_{g=1}^{G} m_{1g}p_{0g} = \sum_{g=1}^{G} \frac{m_{1g}L_{1g}}{L_g} \tag{17.3}$$

$$\text{Var}_0(A) = \sum_{g=1}^{G} \text{Var}_0(A_g) = \sum_{g=1}^{G} m_{1g}p_{0g}q_{0g} = \sum_{g=1}^{G} \frac{m_{1g}L_{1g}L_{0g}}{L_g^2} \tag{17.4}$$

where the variance calculation assumes that the data from different strata are independent. Thus, in large samples (i.e., $\Sigma_g m_{1g}$ large), we can use the test statistic

$$\chi^2_{MHD} = \frac{[a - \mathcal{E}_0(A)]^2}{\text{Var}_0(A)} \tag{17.5}$$

which can be compared with a tabled value of the chi-square distribution with one degree of freedom, where χ^2_{MHD} denotes the *Mantel-Haenszel test statistic for density follow-up studies* and $\mathcal{E}_0(A)$ and $\text{Var}_0(A)$ are given by Expressions 17.3 and 17.4, respectively.

EXAMPLE 17.4

As an application of the MH test to density studies, consider the data in Table 17.9, which concerns a follow-up investigation of the possible association between obesity and mortality (from all causes) among white women of ages 60–75 from a midwestern urban population. A detailed description of this study was previously given in Chapter 1.

Table 17.9 gives stratum-specific information based on categories of ages "attained" by each subject (see the footnote in the table). The analysis given below may be criticized on the grounds that data in different strata are not independent, since the same person may be counted in more than one stratum. This point is debatable, however, since the person-years in different strata represent nonoverlapping periods of follow-up.

For this stratification, the statistic given in Equation 17.5 for testing an overall association, which controls for (attained) age, is calculated as follows. Using Equation 17.3, we obtain

$$\mathcal{E}_0(A) = \frac{16(234.5)}{799} + \frac{22(264.5)}{709} + \frac{28(200)}{610} = 22.2040$$

Using Equation 17.4, we obtain

$$\text{Var}_0(A) = \frac{16(234.5)(544.5)}{(779)^2} + \frac{22(264.5)(444.5)}{(709)^2} + \frac{28(200)(410)}{(610)^2}$$

$$= 14.6825$$

Thus,

$$\chi^2_{\text{MHD}} = \frac{[a - \mathcal{E}_0(A)]^2}{\text{Var}_0(A)} = \frac{(30 - 22.2040)^2}{14.6825} = 4.14 \quad (P = .02)$$

These test results provide some (i.e., borderline significant) evidence of an overall association of obesity with death in older women after controlling for age. Note, however, that inspection of the stratum-specific IDRs indicates that the extent of the association is somewhat weak (i.e., all IDRs are below 2). Methods for determining summary point estimates that accumulate such information over several strata are described in Section 17.4.

Table 17.9 Density Data from Obesity Study Stratified by Attained Age

a. Ages 60–64

	Obese	Nonobese	
Deaths During 1960–1967	7	9	16
Person-Years During 1960–1967	234.5	544.5	779

$I\hat{D}R_1 = 1.81$ (N.S.)

b. Ages 65–69

	Obese	Nonobese	
Deaths During 1960–1967	11	11	22
Person-Years During 1960–1967	264.5	444.5	709

$I\hat{D}R_2 = 1.68$ (N.S.)

c. Ages 70–74

	Obese	Nonobese	
Deaths During 1960–1967	12	16	28
Person-Years During 1960–1967	200	410	610

$I\hat{D}R_3 = 1.54$ (N.S.)

d. Crude Table

	Obese	Nonobese	
Deaths During 1960–1967	30	36	66
Person-Years During 1960–1967	699	1,399	2,098

$c I\hat{D}R = 1.67$ $(P \approx .02)$

Note: The experience of a given subject may contribute data to one or more strata, depending on the ages attained by that subject during the study period. For example, a woman who enters the study (on January 1) at age 62 and dies (on July 1) at age 68 will contribute 3 person-years and no deaths to age category 60–64 plus 4.5 person-years and 1 death (on July 1) to age category 65–69. N.S. denotes nonsignificant test.

The Mantel-Haenszel test based on Equation 17.2 has been shown to have optimal statistical properties ("uniformly most powerful") in the case where stratum-specific odds ratios are uniform over the strata (Radhakrishna, 1965). Nevertheless, the statistical literature contains other test procedures proposed for the same problem. Several of these, though based on a different rationale, give approximately the same numerical chi-square values when the stratum-specific sample sizes are at least moderate. All these alternatives have the same theoretical rationale, discussed below.

**17.3.3
Alternative
Test
Procedures**

Let θ denote the effect measure, $\hat{\theta}_g$ its estimate from the gth stratum, and W_g a weight applied to this stratum. Then, depending on the type of estimate being used, an overall (weighted) estimate of effect can be given by either

$$\hat{\theta} = \sum_{g=1}^{G} W_g \hat{\theta}_g \Big/ \sum_{g=1}^{G} W_g \qquad (17.6)$$

or

$$\hat{\theta} = \exp\left(\sum_{g=1}^{G} W_g \ln \hat{\theta}_g \Big/ \sum_{g=1}^{G} W_g\right) \qquad (17.7)$$

Formula 17.6 is appropriate when $\hat{\theta}_g$ is either a *difference measure* (e.g., risk difference) or a *certain type of ratio measure* (e.g., "standardized" risk or odds ratios, to be described later). Formula 17.7 is appropriate only when $\hat{\theta}_g$ is a *ratio measure weighted according to precision*, i.e., in terms of $\mathrm{Var}(\ln \hat{\theta}_g)$.

Using the quantity $\hat{\theta}$, we can generally formulate the null hypothesis to be tested as

$$H_0: \mu_{\hat{\theta}} = \theta_0$$

where $\theta_0 = 0$ for difference measures and $\theta_0 = 1$ for ratio measures. The test statistic will then have one of the following forms:

$$\chi^2 = (\hat{\theta} - \theta_0)^2 / \hat{\mathrm{Var}}_0(\hat{\theta})$$

which is used when $\hat{\theta}$ is expressible in terms of Equation 17.6, or

$$\chi^2 = (\ln \hat{\theta})^2 / \hat{\mathrm{Var}}_0(\ln \hat{\theta})$$

when $\hat{\theta}$ is expressible in terms of Equation 17.7.

For the notation previously given in Table 17.1a, some specific choices of $\hat{\theta}_g$ and W_g that have been proposed for cumulative follow-up, case-control, or cross-sectional studies are as follows:

Follow-up studies: $\hat{\theta}$ expressible as Equation 17.6, where

$$\hat{\theta}_g = (a_g/n_{1g}) - (b_g/n_{0g}) \qquad \text{(Cochran's ordinary difference;}$$
$$\text{Cochran, 1954)}$$

$$W_g = n_{1g} n_{0g} / n_g$$

$\hat{\theta}$ expressible as Equation 17.6, where

$$\hat{\theta}_g = \frac{(a_g/n_{1g}) - (b_g/n_{0g})}{m_{1g} m_{0g} / n_g^2} \qquad \text{(Cochran's standardized difference;}$$
$$\text{Cochran, 1954)}$$
$$W_g = m_{1g} m_{0g} n_{1g} n_{0g} / n_g^3 \approx 1/\hat{\text{Var}}_0(\hat{\theta}_g)$$

$\hat{\theta}$ expressible as Equation 17.7, where

$$\hat{\theta}_g = a_g n_{0g} / b_g n_{1g} \qquad (= \hat{\text{RR}}_g)$$
$$W_g = m_{1g} n_{1g} n_{0g} / m_{0g} n_g \approx 1/\hat{\text{Var}}_0(\ln \hat{\theta}_g)$$

Case-control or cross-sectional studies: $\hat{\theta}$ expressible as Equation 17.7, where

$$\hat{\theta}_g = a_g d_g / b_g c_g \qquad (= \hat{\text{OR}}_g) \qquad \text{(logit; Woolf, 1955)}$$

$$W_g = \frac{1}{\dfrac{1}{a_g} + \dfrac{1}{b_g} + \dfrac{1}{c_g} + \dfrac{1}{d_g}} \approx \frac{1}{\hat{\text{Var}}(\ln \hat{\theta}_g)}$$

All the above alternatives give approximately the same computational value as the Mantel-Haenszel statistic of Equation 17.2 when stratum-specific sample sizes are at least moderate, but they have inferior statistical credentials otherwise. Thus, use of the MH test is preferable. Note, in particular, that the test statistic using Cochran's standardized difference will give a value twice as large as χ^2_{MHS} if the strata represent individual matched pairs (i.e., $n_g = 2$ for all g). The test based on the logit (Woolf, 1955) can also give results highly discrepant from those of the MH test when there are small stratum-specific sample sizes, even when modified, as suggested by Haldane (1955), with the addition of .5 to each cell of the fourfold table.

17.4 POINT ESTIMATION OF OVERALL EFFECT

Overall (i.e., summary) estimators of effect, which accumulate information over several strata, may take the form of *weighted averages*, as given by Expressions 17.6 and 17.7, or *maximum likelihood (ML) estimators*, the latter being asymptotically optimal (in terms of having minimum variance in very large samples). Asymptotic ML estimators may be conveniently obtained by fitting mathematical models for stratified data, a technique we will describe in Chapter 20. Exact ML estimators (see Gart, 1979), which make use of the exact hypergeometric distributions of the A_g under the (conditional) fixed-marginals assumption, will not be addressed here. Such estimators can be closely approximated by other estimators (Gart, 1970; Dayal, 1978), even in small samples. Also, they are somewhat inconvenient computationally, requiring special computer programs (e.g., see Thomas, 1975) not widely available in packaged form.

We thus focus in this section on the various types and properties of weighted averages of the form given by Expression 17.6 or 17.7. In choosing the weights W_g, we usually adopt one of three general approaches: the weights may be chosen (1) to achieve optimal precision in the estimate, (2) to reflect what we consider to be the relative importance of the various strata, or (3) to achieve standardization of results relative to a standard population (see Miettinen, 1972). Of these, the precision-based approach is usually preferable, because the others require some subjectivity on the part of the investigator and also because a precision-based approach is logically called for to provide optimally narrow interval estimates (i.e., of minimum width) when there is approximate uniformity of effect over the strata. Adjusted point estimates based on different weighting schemes will all have approximately the same value if there is approximate uniformity of effect over the strata. However, if there is considerable nonuniformity of effect, the utility of any summary measure is questionable.

For adjusted estimates of the form

$$\hat{\theta} = \sum_{g=1}^{G} W_g \hat{\theta}_g / \sum_{g=1}^{G} W_g$$

17.4.1 Weighting for Precision: General Formulation

it may be shown (we omit the proof) that the choice of W_g that minimizes the unconditional variance $\mathrm{Var}(\hat{\theta})$ is given by

$$W_g = 1/\mathrm{Var}(\hat{\theta}_g)$$

If the adjusted estimate is of the form

$$\hat{\theta} = \exp\left(\sum_{g=1}^{G} W_g \ln \hat{\theta}_g / \sum_{g=1}^{G} W_g\right)$$

then the choice of W_g that minimizes $\mathrm{Var}(\ln \hat{\theta})$ is given by

$$W_g = 1/\mathrm{Var}(\ln \hat{\theta}_g)$$

Thus, on precision grounds, the *optimal weights* are given by the reciprocals (i.e., inverses) of the variances of the stratum-specific estimators or their natural logarithms. These optimal weights are, however, unknown parameter values. Consequently, only approximate optimality can be achieved by replacing these weights with their corresponding sample estimates

$$W_g = 1/\hat{\mathrm{Var}}(\hat{\theta}_g) \tag{17.8}$$

or

$$W_g = 1/\hat{\mathrm{Var}}(\ln \hat{\theta}_g) \tag{17.9}$$

in the above two weighted average formulas, respectively.

The use of natural logarithms in Equations 17.7 and 17.9 is generally restricted to ratio effect measures, primarily because, for moderate to large samples, $\ln \hat{\theta}_g$ tends to be more normally distributed than does $\hat{\theta}_g$. Further justification for the use of logarithms based on extensive simulation work has been provided by Katz and colleagues (1978).

17.4.2 Formulas for Weighted Averages by Study Design

Table 17.16, which is presented for the reader's convenience at the end of this chapter, provides formulas for a variety of weighted average estimators that may be computed for different study designs. This table also contains formulas for interval estimators, which we will discuss in Section 17.5.

The estimators given in the table can be categorized into three broad classes:

1. *Precision-based weighted averages,* which use weights given by Equation 17.8 or 17.9. These estimators are denoted in the table by $a\hat{R}R$, $a\hat{R}D$, $a\hat{O}R$, $a\hat{I}DR$, and $a\hat{I}DD$ for the respective parameters indicated. The variances used in determining the weights for $a\hat{R}R$, $a\hat{O}R$, etc. often involve Taylor series approximations (similar to those described for the simple analysis situation). Also, where indicated, both null and nonnull variances are used for stratum-specific weighting.

2. *Mantel-Haenszel weighted averages,* which we describe in the next subsection. These estimators are denoted in the table by $m\hat{O}R$, $m\hat{R}R$, and $m\hat{I}DR$. The $m\hat{O}R$ is well known (Mantel and Haenszel, 1959; Dayal, 1978), whereas the other two are ad hoc estimators that have not been studied.

3. *Standardized weighted averages,* which use weights derived from a standard population with frequencies s_g, $g = 1, 2, \ldots, G$, for the different strata. These estimators are generally denoted by $S\hat{R}R$, $S\hat{R}D$, $S\hat{O}R$, $S\hat{I}DR$, and $S\hat{I}DD$ for the respective parameters. In addition, we earlier used (in Table 17.4) the estimators $s\hat{R}R$ and $s'\hat{R}R$ to represent *special cases* of $S\hat{R}R$ resulting from particular choices for the standard. The estimator $s\hat{R}R$, which Miettinen (1972) called the *internally standardized risk ratio,* uses weights based on the marginal frequencies for exposed subjects (i.e., $s_g = n_{1g}$). The estimator $s'\hat{R}R$, which Miettinen called the *externally standardized risk ratio,* uses weights based on the marginal frequencies for unexposed subjects (i.e., $s_g = n_{0g}$). Analogous special cases can be defined (Miettinen, 1972) from $S\hat{O}R$, where $s\hat{O}R$ uses the exposed noncases (i.e., $s_g = c_g$) and $s'\hat{O}R$ uses the nonexposed noncases (i.e., $s_g = d_g$).

Although standardized estimators are not preferable on precision grounds to the two other types of weighted averages, standardization is appropriate for providing unconfounded summary comparisons with a known standard population. Also, standardization may be used to estimate excess case occurrence due to exposure in a specified population (Miettinen, 1974).

Mantel and Haenszel, in their classic paper (1959), proposed several sum- **17.4.3**
mary estimators for use in "retrospective" (i.e., case-control) studies. The **Mantel-**
most notable of these is the $m\hat{OR}$, which is defined as follows: **Haenszel**

Estimators

$$m\hat{OR} = \sum_{g=1}^{G} \frac{a_g d_g}{n_g} \bigg/ \sum_{g=1}^{G} \frac{b_g c_g}{n_g} \qquad (17.10)$$

Note that if $b_g c_g \neq 0$ for all g, this estimator may be expressed as a
weighted average of stratum-specific odds ratios, as follows:

$$m\hat{OR} = \sum_{g=1}^{G} W_g \hat{OR}_g \bigg/ \sum_{g=1}^{G} W_g$$

where $W_g = b_g c_g / n_g$.

As Mantel and Haenszel point out, an interesting property of the $m\hat{OR}$
is that it equals unity only when the Mantel-Haenszel chi-square statistic,
given by Equation 17.2, is zero. Thus, there is a direct mathematical connection between the $m\hat{OR}$ and the χ^2_{MHS} test, which is not characteristic of
the other summary estimators.

Another advantage of the $m\hat{OR}$ over other summary odds ratio estimators is that it may be used without modification when there are zero frequencies within the body of some of the stratum-specific tables.

EXAMPLE 17.5

Consider the problem of obtaining a summary odds ratio estimate that
involves the two strata given in Table 17.10. The zero cell frequency obtained in stratum 1 of the data precludes the use of either the precision-
based $a\hat{OR}$ or any standardized $S\hat{OR}$ given in Table 17.16. A modified
precision-based estimate is available, though, using the Woolf-Haldane
adjustment (Haldane, 1955; Anscombe, 1956), which adds the quantity .5
to each cell frequency. The adjusted $a\hat{OR}$ then becomes

$$a\hat{OR} = \exp\left\{\left[\frac{1}{\frac{1}{7.5} + \frac{1}{3.5} + \frac{1}{.5} + \frac{1}{10.5}} \ln\frac{(7.5)(10.5)}{(3.5)(.5)}\right.\right.$$

$$\left.\left. + \frac{1}{\frac{1}{5} + \frac{1}{5} + \frac{1}{1} + \frac{1}{9}} \ln\frac{(5)(9)}{(5)(1)}\right] \bigg/ \left[\frac{1}{\frac{1}{7.5} + \frac{1}{3.5} + \frac{1}{.5} + \frac{1}{10.5}}\right.\right.$$

EXAMPLE 17.5   (*continued*)

$$+ \cfrac{1}{\cfrac{1}{5}+\cfrac{1}{5}+\cfrac{1}{1}+\cfrac{1}{9}}\Big]\Big\}$$

$$= \exp(.3754 \ln 45 + .6246 \ln 9) = 16.47$$

Nevertheless, Gart (1970) has indicated that the Woolf-Haldane estimate does not, in general, perform as well as the $m\hat{OR}$ when stratum-specific sample sizes are small. (In particular, the $m\hat{OR}$ is a statistically consistent estimator of an underlying common odds ratio over the strata, and it yields values close to those obtained when using exact ML estimation.) Moreover, even on intuitive grounds, the use of an arbitrary adjustment (such as adding .5 to each cell within the table) is undesirable and can be avoided entirely with the $m\hat{OR}$, which yields the following estimate:

$$m\hat{OR} = \frac{[(7)(10)/20] + [(5)(9)/20]}{[(3)(0)/20] + [(5)(1)/20]} = \frac{3.50 + 2.25}{0 + .25} = 23.00$$

Table 17.10   Stratified Data Involving a Zero Cell Frequency

	a. Stratum 1				**b. Stratum 2**		
	E	$\bar{E}$			E	$\bar{E}$	
D	7	3	10	D	5	5	10
$\bar{D}$	0	10	10	$\bar{D}$	1	9	10
	7	13			6	14	
	$\hat{OR}_1$ indeterminate				$\hat{OR}_2 = 9$		

One final property of the $m\hat{OR}$ worth mentioning here is that, in the special case when pair matching is performed as part of the study design, the $m\hat{OR}$ is the conditional (i.e., assuming fixed margins) ML estimator of the odds ratio (Miettinen, 1968, 1969). In general, however, the $m\hat{OR}$ and both conditional and unconditional ML estimators of common odds ratios differ. (See Hauck, 1979, for a comparison of the variance of the $m\hat{O}R$ with that of the unconditional ML estimator.)

Although the $m\hat{O}R$ was initially recommended in the context of retrospective studies, it may be used to approximate the risk ratio in a follow-up study (under the usual rare disease assumption). Alternatively, an ad hoc risk ratio analog, which we call $m\hat{R}R$, may be defined as follows:

$$m\hat{R}R = \sum_{g=1}^{G} \frac{a_g n_{0g}}{n_g} \bigg/ \sum_{g=1}^{G} \frac{b_g n_{1g}}{n_g} \qquad (17.11)$$

This estimator, like $m\hat{O}R$, can be equivalently expressed as a weighted average of stratum-specific risk ratios:

$$m\hat{R}R = \sum_{g=1}^{G} W_g \hat{R}R_g \bigg/ \sum_{g=1}^{G} W_g$$

where $W_g = b_g n_{1g}/n_g$ (provided that all $b_g n_{1g} \neq 0$).

An analogous ad hoc estimator can also be defined for incidence density studies (Rothman and Boice, 1979), as follows:

$$m\hat{I}D R = \sum_{g=1}^{G} \frac{a_g L_{0g}}{L_g} \bigg/ \sum_{g=1}^{G} \frac{b_g L_{1g}}{L_g} \qquad (17.12)$$

where L_{0g}, L_{1g}, and L_g denote population-time experience for the exposed, unexposed, and total groups, respectively.

17.4.4 Examples of Summary Point Estimation

In this section, we provide some numerical examples to illustrate and compare the various formulas described above (Table 17.16) for summary estimation of effect.

EXAMPLE 17.6

Here we will examine cumulative incidence follow-up data. We consider again the control of AGE and ECG in evaluating the CAT–CHD association from the Evans County data described earlier (see Table 17.4, row 12). The four strata resulting from dichotomous categorization of both AGE and ECG were presented in Table 17.7. As we previously described, very little interaction was indicated from comparison of the stratum-specific risk ratio estimates, and the χ^2_{MHS} test yielded a computed test statistic of 4.15, with a corresponding (one-sided) P-value of $P = .02$. We may conclude, therefore, that there is a significant overall CAT–CHD ef-

EXAMPLE 17.6   (*continued*)

fect at the .05 level (though not at the .01 level) after controlling for AGE and ECG.

We now illustrate quantification of the strength of this effect through computation of $a\hat{R}R$, $s\hat{R}R$, $s'\hat{R}R$, $m\hat{R}R$, and $m\hat{O}R$ (using formulas given in Table 17.16). For $a\hat{R}R$, the stratum-specific weights are given, in general, by

$$W_g = \frac{1}{\hat{\text{Var}}(\ln \hat{R}R_g)} = \frac{1}{(c_g/n_{1g}a_g) + (d_g/n_{0g}b_g)}$$

From the data (Table 17.7), we then obtain

$$W_1 = \frac{1}{[7/(8)(1)] + [257/(274)(17)]} = 1.0751$$

$$W_2 = \frac{1}{[14/(17)(3)] + [52/(59)(7)]} = 2.4974$$

$$W_3 = \frac{1}{[30/(39)(9)] + [107/(122)(15)]} = 6.9473$$

$$W_4 = \frac{1}{[44/(58)(14)] + [27/(32)(5)]} = 4.4856$$

Thus

$$a\hat{R}R = \exp\left(\frac{\begin{array}{r}1.0751 \ln 2.01 + 2.4974 \ln 1.49 + 6.9473 \ln 1.88 \\ + 4.4856 \ln 1.54\end{array}}{1.0751 + 2.4974 + 6.9473 + 4.4856}\right)$$

$$= \exp(.5377) = 1.71$$

We now compute standardized risk ratios, as follows:

$$s\hat{R}R = \frac{s_1(a_1/n_{11}) + s_2(a_2/n_{12}) + s_3(a_3/n_{13}) + s_4(a_4/n_{14})}{s_1(b_1/n_{01}) + s_2(b_2/n_{02}) + s_3(b_3/n_{03}) + s_4(b_4/n_{04})}$$

$$= \frac{s_1(1/8) + s_2(3/17) + s_3(9/39) + s_4(14/58)}{s_1(17/274) + s_2(7/59) + s_3(15/122) + s_4(5/32)}$$

Note that the weights W_g for $s\hat{R}R$ are given, in general, by $W_g = s_g\hat{\text{CI}}_{0g}$, so that

$$W_1 = s_1(17/274) \qquad W_2 = s_2(7/59) \qquad W_3 = s_3(15/122)$$

$$W_4 = s_4(5/32)$$

EXAMPLE 17.6 (*continued*)

For computation of the internally standardized risk ratio, $s\hat{R}R$, the standard population is $s_g = n_{1g}$, so that $s_1 = 8$, $s_2 = 17$, $s_3 = 39$, and $s_4 = 58$. The weights for $s\hat{R}R$ are, therefore, $W_1 = .50$, $W_2 = 2.02$, $W_3 = 4.80$, and $W_4 = 9.07$. Thus

$$s\hat{R}R = \frac{8(1/8) + 17(3/17) + 39(9/39) + 58(14/58)}{8(17/274) + 17(7/59) + 39(15/122) + 58(5/32)}$$

$$= \frac{27}{16.3709} \quad \left(= \frac{\text{observed cases among exposed}}{\text{expected cases among exposed}} \right)$$

$$= 1.65$$

For computation of the externally standardized risk ratio, $s'\hat{R}R$, the standard population is $s_g = n_{0g}$, so that $s_1 = 274$, $s_2 = 59$, $s_3 = 122$, and $s_4 = 32$. The weights for $s'\hat{R}R$ are, therefore, $W_1 = 17.00$, $W_2 = 7.00$, $W_3 = 15.00$, and $W_4 = 5.00$. Notice that, in a comparison of the weights for $s\hat{R}R$ and $s'\hat{R}R$, the former gives most weight to stratum 4 and least weight to stratum 1, whereas the latter, $s'\hat{R}R$, gives the most weight to stratum 1 and least to stratum 4. Thus

$$s'RR = \frac{274(1/8) + 59(3/17) + 122(9/39) + 32(14/58)}{274(17/274) + 59(7/59) + 122(15/122) + 32(5/32)}$$

$$= \frac{80.5397}{44} \quad \left(= \frac{\text{expected cases among nonexposed}}{\text{observed cases among nonexposed}} \right)$$

$$= 1.83$$

Finally, the $m\hat{R}R$ and $m\hat{O}R$ are computed as follows:

$$m\hat{R}R = \frac{1(274/282) + 3(59/76) + 9(122/161) + 14(32/90)}{17(8/282) + 7(17/76) + 15(39/161) + 5(58/90)} = 1.70$$

$$m\hat{O}R = \frac{1(257/282) + 3(52/76) + 9(107/161) + 14(27/90)}{17(7/282) + 7(14/76) + 15(30/161) + 5(44/90)} = 1.89$$

Note that the weights for $m\hat{R}R$ are $W_1 = .48$, $W_2 = 1.57$, $W_3 = 3.63$, and $W_4 = 3.22$, which are in the same relative order as the weights for $a\hat{R}R$. This feature accounts for the similarity between the $a\hat{R}R$ and $m\hat{R}R$ values. The weights for $m\hat{O}R$ are $W_1 = .42$, $W_2 = 1.29$, $W_3 = 2.80$, and $W_4 = 2.44$, which also correspond to those for $a\hat{R}R$. However, because $m\hat{O}R$ estimates the odds ratio, it is somewhat different from $m\hat{R}R$.

The five summary estimates are, thus, not all identical. Nevertheless, each gives roughly the same information about the strength of the CAT–

EXAMPLE 17.6 (*continued*)

CHD association. Except for the mÔR, the differences among these estimates can be attributed to different relative weighting schemes, as summarized in Table 17.11.

Table 17.11   Relative Weights for Adjusted Risk and Odds Ratios for the Data of Table 17.7

Adjusted Estimator	$W_1 / \sum_{g=1}^{4} W_g$	$W_2 / \sum_{g=1}^{4} W_g$	$W_3 / \sum_{g=1}^{4} W_g$	$W_4 / \sum_{g=1}^{4} W_g$
aR̂R = 1.71	.07	.17	.46	.30
sR̂R = 1.65	.03	.12	.30	.55
s'R̂R = 1.83	.39	.16	.34	.11
mR̂R = 1.70	.05	.18	.41	.36
mÔR = 1.89	.06	.19	.40	.35

EXAMPLE 17.7

Consider the information presented in Table 17.12, which gives hypothetical data stratified by age for a case-control study of the smoking habits of male patients with lung cancer.

Table 17.12   Hypothetical Case-Control Data on Smoking (SMK) and Lung Cancer (LC), Stratified by Age

	a. Ages 40–49		**b. Ages 50–59**	
	SMK	$\overline{SMK}$	*SMK*	$\overline{SMK}$
LC	160	3	100	1
$\overline{LC}$	125	9	98	5

$$\hat{OR}_1 = 3.84 \quad (P = .02) \qquad \hat{OR}_2 = 5.10 \quad (P = .05)$$

EXAMPLE 17.7 (*continued*)

Table 17.12 (*continued*)

	c. Ages 60+			d. Crude Table	
	SMK	$\overline{SMK}$		*SMK*	$\overline{SMK}$
LC	40	0	*LC*	300	4
$\overline{LC}$	45	4	$\overline{LC}$	268	18

$\hat{OR}_3 = 8.01^{\dagger}$ (*P* = .03) $\quad$ $c\hat{OR} = 5.04$ (*P* < .001)

$^{\dagger}\hat{OR}_3$ was computed after adding .5 to each cell within the fourfold table for stratum 3.

For the data in Table 17.12, the Mantel-Haenszel chi-square test statistic that controls for age is $\chi^2_{MHS} = 10.24$ (one-sided *P* < .001). To quantify the strength of this association, we can compute (using formulas in Table 17.16) adjusted odds ratios, as summarized in Table 17.13. These estimates are all slightly different; nevertheless, they give roughly the same information about the extent of the association. Note that for $s\hat{OR}$ and

Table 17.13 Adjusted Odds Ratios and Their Relative Weights for the Data of Table 17.12

Adjusted Estimator	$W_1 \Big/ \sum\limits_{g=1}^{3} W_g$	$W_2 \Big/ \sum\limits_{g=1}^{3} W_g$	$W_3 \Big/ \sum\limits_{g=1}^{3} W_g$
$a\hat{OR} = 4.51^{\dagger}$	.63	.24	.13
$s\hat{OR} = 4.90$	.68	.32	.00
$s'\hat{OR} = 5.04$	.75	.25	.00
$m\hat{OR} = 5.22^{a}$	—	—	—

†The weight for stratum 3 in the computation for $a\hat{OR}$ was obtained after adding .5 to each cell frequency for that stratum.
^{a}The $m\hat{OR}$ is not a weighted average of odds ratios in this example because $b_3 c_3 / n_3 = 0$ in stratum 3.

EXAMPLE 17.7 (*continued*)

s'ÔR, no weight is given to the estimated odds ratio for stratum 3. Also, because of the zero cell frequency in stratum 3, the mÔR cannot be computed as a weighted average of odds ratios. In fact, if the weights $W_g = b_g c_g / n_g$ were used, the resulting weighted average would be 4.19 and not 5.22.

EXAMPLE 17.8

To illustrate point estimation for density studies, we continue with the data given in Table 17.9, which concerns the follow-up investigation of a possible association between obesity and mortality among white women, aged 60–75, from a midwestern urban population. For these data, we previously found that the overall Mantel-Haenszel chi-square statistic for density data, which controls for (attained) age, was significant at the .05 level ($P = .02$), even though each stratum-specific χ^2 was not individually significant.

Results for the quantification of the strength of the overall association are presented in Table 17.14 (using the formulas of Table 17.16). The four summary estimates obtained are identical when rounded to two decimal places. This result can be seen to follow from the use of almost identical relative weights for each estimator.

Table 17.14 Adjusted Incidence Density Ratios for the Data of Table 17.9

Adjusted Estimator	$W_1 \Big/ \sum\limits_{g=1}^{3} W_g$	$W_2 \Big/ \sum\limits_{g=1}^{3} W_g$	$W_3 \Big/ \sum\limits_{g=1}^{3} W_g$
aID̂R = 1.65	.23	.35	.42
sID̂R = 1.65	.21	.36	.43
s'ID̂R = 1.65	.25	.31	.44
mID̂R = 1.65	.22	.34	.44

In concluding this section, we reemphasize our recommendation to use precision-based estimates except in certain special cases calling for Mantel-Haenszel or standardized estimators. As we have previously pointed out, the use of an overall summary estimate is usually inappropriate if there is considerable interaction in the data, as represented by nonuniformity of stratum-specific estimates of effect. If there is little evidence of interaction, then all forms of summary estimation will yield roughly the same numerical results, and the logical choice of estimator is the one that is most precise (i.e., has the smallest variance). As we have seen in the case-control example (Example 17.5), however, when some stratum-specific cell frequencies are zero, use of precision-based estimates such as a$\hat{\text{OR}}$ will usually require adjustments for avoiding an indeterminate result. Since the value of the summary estimate can vary markedly with the specific form of adjustment (e.g., adding .5 to each cell versus adding .1 to each cell), the use of such estimates may be criticized as being arbitrary and possibly misleading. Alternatively, therefore, when there are zero frequencies, the use of Mantel-Haenszel estimates (m$\hat{\text{OR}}$, m$\hat{\text{RR}}$, or m$\hat{\text{IDR}}$) should be preferred, since they can usually be calculated without adjustment. Also, even if there are no zeros, precision-based estimators have poor performance compared to Mantel-Haenszel estimators whenever the majority of nonnull cell expectations fall below four or so.

Interval estimates of weighted averages from stratified data take one of the following two forms:

$$\hat{\theta} \pm Z_{1-\alpha/2}\sqrt{\hat{\text{V}}\text{ar}(\hat{\theta})} \qquad (17.13)$$

when $\hat{\theta}$ is a *difference measure*, or

$$\hat{\theta} \exp[\pm Z_{1-\alpha/2}\sqrt{\hat{\text{V}}\text{ar}(\ln \hat{\theta})}] \qquad (17.14)$$

17.5 INTERVAL ESTIMATION OF EFFECT

when $\hat{\theta}$ is a *ratio measure*. (These forms are identical to those previously described for the simple analysis situation in Chapter 15.)

The specific expression for the general interval estimate given by Expression 17.13 or 17.14 will depend on the manner in which the variance estimates are calculated (and, of course, on the study design and corresponding effect measure used). As was true for the simple analysis case, there are two approaches for determining the variance: *direct approximation* (which may involve use of a Taylor series approximation) and *test-based approximation*. [As we mentioned in Chapter 15, the test-based approach has been criticized by Halperin (1977), who showed that confidence limits for ratio measures will tend to be too narrow. Although this problem does not become severe unless the association is very strong, it is not remedied by large sample sizes. Gart (1979) also criticized the test-based procedure as being "not correct in principle, in asymptotic theory, nor in exact evaluation" in certain cases.]

Two other procedures for interval estimation are based on the exact and large-sample conditional distributions of the A_g. Formulas are analogous to those previously described for simple analysis and, though quite complicated computationally, have been programmed by Thomas (1975). For further discussion see Gart (1971), who warns that exact estimates become important when the data are thin in many strata.

**17.5.1
Formulas for
Direct and
Test-based
Interval
Estimates**

Specific formulas, listed separately by effect measure within a given study design, are provided in Table 17.16 (last column), at the end of the chapter, for both direct and test-based interval estimates. For certain measures in this table, we have presented only the test-based interval because a convenient directly derivable variance formula was not available. In fact, the primary value of the test-based interval is that it can be used whenever a direct expression for the variance of a summary effect measure cannot be readily derived. Also, it is easy to compute once a Mantel-Haenszel chi-square statistic has been obtained.

For stratified data, *test-based intervals for difference measures* of any type (e.g., $\hat{\theta} = $ a$\hat{R}$D, s$\hat{R}$D, aI$\hat{D}$D, or sI$\hat{D}$D) have the following form:

$$\hat{\theta}(1 \pm Z_{1-\alpha/2}/\chi_{MHS}) \qquad (17.15)$$

where χ_{MHS} is the square root of the general chi-square test statistic (17.1) for testing for overall association in a stratified analysis.

Test-based intervals for ratio estimators of any type ($\hat{\theta} = $ a$\hat{R}$R, a$\hat{O}$R, aI$\hat{D}$R, etc.) have the following form:

$$\hat{\theta}^{(1 \pm Z_{1-\alpha/2}/\chi_{MHS})} \qquad (17.16)$$

For interval estimates where weights are *precision-based*, it can be shown that, for *difference measures* (i.e., a$\hat{R}$D, aI$\hat{D}$D), Expression 17.13 reduces (assuming the W_g are nonrandom) to the form

$$\hat{\theta} \pm Z_{1-\alpha/2} \Big/ \sqrt{\sum_{g=1}^{G} W_g} \qquad (17.17)$$

where $\hat{\theta} = \Sigma_g W_g \hat{\theta}_g / \Sigma_g W_g$ and $W_g = 1/\hat{V}ar(\hat{\theta}_g)$.

For *ratio measures* (i.e., a$\hat{R}$R, a$\hat{O}$R, and aI$\hat{D}$R), Expression 17.14 reduces (assuming, again, that the W_g are nonrandom) to

$$\hat{\theta} \exp\left(\pm Z_{1-\alpha/2} \Big/ \sqrt{\sum_{g=1}^{G} W_g}\right) \qquad (17.18)$$

where $\hat{\theta} = \exp(\Sigma_g W_g \ln \hat{\theta}_g / \Sigma_g W_g)$ and $W_g = 1/\hat{V}ar(\ln \hat{\theta}_g)$.

**17.5.2
Examples**

We now provide numerical examples to illustrate the computation of the interval estimates and to compare results from direct and test-based approaches.

EXAMPLE 17.9

We first consider a cumulative incidence follow-up study. When we controlled for AGE and ECG in evaluating the CAT–CHD association for the

EXAMPLE 17.9 (*continued*)

Evans County data described earlier (Tables 17.4 and 17.7), we found, for precision-based weighting, that

$$a\hat{R}R = 1.71 \qquad \sum_{g=1}^{4} W_g = 15.01 \qquad \chi_{MHS} = \sqrt{4.15} = 2.04$$

With these results, we can obtain 95% direct and test-based interval estimates for aRR by using Expressions 17.18 and 17.16, respectively.

The 95% direct precision-based confidence interval is

$$a\hat{R}R \exp\left(\pm Z_{1-\alpha/2} \Big/ \sqrt{\sum_{g=1}^{4} W_g} \right) = 1.71 \exp[\pm 1.96/\sqrt{15.01}]$$

which gives the interval estimate (1.03, 2.84).

A 95% test-based confidence interval is

$$a\hat{R}R^{(1 \pm Z_{1-\alpha/2}/\chi_{MHS})} = 1.71^{(1 \pm 1.96/2.04)}$$

which gives the interval estimate (1.02, 2.86).

Using Expression 17.16 again, we can also obtain the following 95% test-based intervals for other summary indices.

$$
\begin{aligned}
s\hat{R}R &= 1.65: & (1.02, 2.67) \\
s'\hat{R}R &= 1.83: & (1.02, 3.27) \\
m\hat{R}R &= 1.70: & (1.02, 2.83) \\
m\hat{O}R &= 1.89: & (1.03, 3.48)
\end{aligned}
$$

EXAMPLE 17.10

Consider again the case-control data in Table 17.12, which concern an assessment of the SMK–LC relationship, controlling for AGE. For these data, we found that

$$a\hat{O}R = 4.51 \qquad \sum_{g=1}^{3} W_g = 3.44 \qquad \chi_{MHS} = \sqrt{10.24} = 3.20$$

With these results, we can obtain 95% precision-based and test-based interval estimates for aOR by using Expressions 17.18 and 17.16 again.

EXAMPLE 17.10   (*continued*)

The 95% precision-based confidence interval is

$$a\hat{O}R \ exp\left(\pm Z_{1-\alpha/2} \Big/ \sqrt{\sum_{g=1}^{3} W_g}\right) = 4.51 \ exp(\pm 1.96/\sqrt{3.44})$$

which yields the interval estimate (1.57, 12.98).
A 95% test-based confidence interval is

$$a\hat{O}R^{(1\pm Z_{1-\alpha/2}/\chi_{MHS})} = 4.51^{(1\pm 1.96/3.20)}$$

which yields the interval estimate (1.79, 11.35).
Other 95% test-based intervals are as follows:

$$s\hat{O}R = 4.90: \quad (1.85, \ 12.97)$$
$$s'\hat{O}R = 5.04: \quad (1.87, \ 13.57)$$
$$m\hat{O}R = 5.22: \quad (1.90, \ 14.36)$$

EXAMPLE 17.11

Now, we turn to the previous density study described in Table 17.9, which concerns the putative association between obesity and mortality, controlling for attained age. For these data, we previously found, for precision-based weighting, that

$$a\hat{ID}R = 1.65 \qquad \sum W_g = 14.68 \qquad \chi_{MHD} = \sqrt{4.14} = 2.03$$

With these results and using Expressions 17.18 and 17.16, we can obtain 95% precision-based and test-based intervals, respectively.
The 95% precision-based confidence interval is

$$a\hat{ID}R \ exp\left(\pm Z_{1-\alpha/2} \Big/ \sqrt{\sum W_g}\right) = 1.65 \ exp(\pm 1.96/\sqrt{14.68})$$

which gives the interval (.99, 2.75).
A 95% test-based interval is

$$a\hat{ID}R^{(1\pm Z_{1-\alpha/2}/\chi_{MH})} = 1.65^{(1\pm 1.96/2.03)}$$

which gives the interval (1.02, 2.68).
Notice that the test-based interval is consistent with the results of the Mantel-Haenszel test, since the 95% interval does not contain one, and,

> **EXAMPLE 17.11** (*continued*)
>
> correspondingly, $P = .02 < .05$. This is not the case for the precision-based interval obtained for aIDR. In general, a $100(1 - \alpha)\%$ precision-based interval may include the null value (one, in this case) even if the χ^2_{MH} test rejects the null hypothesis at the α level.

In this section, we provide an overview of methods for carrying out stratified analyses when there are more than two exposure categories. Research contributions in this area, which we will refer to below, have included work by Mantel and Haenszel (1959), Mantel (1963), Clayton (1974), and Karon (1978). The general data layout considered is a collection of 2 by c contingency tables representing the various strata. Table 17.15 gives the notation for the data for the gth stratum.

17.6 EXTENSIONS TO SEVERAL EXPOSURE CATEGORIES

Table 17.15 Data Layout for Stratum g in a Stratified Analysis Involving c Exposure Categories

		E_1	E_2	$\cdots$	E_{c-1}	E_c	
Disease Factor	D	a_{1g}	a_{2g}	$\cdots$	$a_{c-1,g}$	a_{cg}	m_{1g}
	$\bar{D}$	$n_{1g} - a_{1g}$	$n_{2g} - a_{2g}$	$\cdots$	$n_{c-1,g} - a_{c-1,g}$	$n_{cg} - a_{cg}$	m_{0g}
		n_{1g}	n_{2g}	$\cdots$	$n_{c-1,g}$	n_{cg}	n_g

EXPOSURE FACTOR

It is typical to consider one of the exposure levels in the Table 17.15 as a referent category with which the other categories may be compared. In such a case, it is convenient, for ease of interpretation, to designate category E_c as the referent.

As is true for the case of dichotomous disease and exposure categories, it is of primary interest to test for overall association, controlling for the potential confounding of those variables used to form strata, and to arrive at overall (adjusted) summary measures of effect over all the strata. Proposed procedures for testing hypotheses involve chi-square statistics that represent extensions of the Mantel-Haenszel chi-square (χ^2_{MHS}) given by Equation 17.2 for the dichotomous case. Two different testing situations have been distinguished; one assumes the exposure variable to be *nominal* (Mantel and Haenszel, 1959) and the other assumes the exposure variable to be *ordinal* (Mantel, 1963). The test statistics for these two cases, which we will describe below, can be most compactly expressed in matrix terms (Clayton, 1974).

In estimating overall effect or any stratum-specific effects, investigators have traditionally preferred to compute several (i.e., $c - 1$) effect measures, each of which incorporates a common referent category. For example, $(c - 1)$ odds ratios, $\hat{OR}_{1g}, \hat{OR}_{2g}, \ldots, \hat{OR}_{c-1,g}$, might be used for the gth stratum and $a\hat{OR}_1, a\hat{OR}_2, \ldots, a\hat{OR}_{c-1}$ might be used as $(c - 1)$ precision-based summary measures, with each estimator having exposure category E_c for a referent group. Alternatively, however, one could use a single overall measure in the form of a correlation coefficient or weighted average of correlation coefficients (Mantel, 1963). We prefer the use of several relative effect measures to the use of a single measure for reasons of interpretability, particularly when the exposure variable is ordinal, so that a dose-response type of relationship can be assessed.

Since the above orientation to estimation requires no additional formulas, we focus the remaining discussion on an abbreviated description of the test procedures (which apply to cumulative follow-up, case-control, and cross-sectional studies).

17.6.1 ($c - 1$) Nominal Levels of Exposure

Mantel and Haenszel (1959) have described the test procedure for this case as involving the sum of $(c - 1)$ chi-square statistics, which is approximately distributed as a chi-square variable with $(c - 1)$ degrees of freedom under the null hypothesis of no association. The conceptual basis of their test, which is similar to that of the dichotomous exposure situation, assumes that all stratum-specific marginals are fixed. Thus, the test statistic considers only the variation attributable to $(c - 1)$ of the random variables A_{ig}, whose sample realizations are the a_{ig}'s in Table 17.15. Thus, for example, if $c = 3$, then the test involves the sum of a chi-square statistic based on A_{1g} and a chi-square statistic based on A_{2g}, with the latter being adjusted in some fashion to account for the correlation between A_{2g} and A_{1g}. Although a simple algebraic formula for the test statistic is not possible, a convenient matrix formula has been provided by Clayton (1974), which is as follows:

$$\chi^2_{MHN} = \mathbf{H}'[\hat{V}ar_0(\mathbf{H})]^{-1}\mathbf{H} \tag{17.19}$$

which should be compared to a tabled value of the chi-square distribution with $(c - 1)$ degrees of freedom. In the formula, χ^2_{MHN} denotes the Mantel-Haenszel statistic for *nominal* exposure categories, $\mathbf{H}$ denotes the vector of total observed minus expected values for the first $(c - 1)$ categories of diseased subjects, and $\hat{V}ar_0(\mathbf{H})$ denotes the estimated null variance-covariance matrix of the vector $\mathbf{H}$.

The test procedure proposed by Mantel (1963) for this case uses a one-degree-of-freedom chi-square statistic based on a sum of scores that are assigned to the levels of exposure. We denote the score for the ith ordinal category in the gth stratum by y_{ig}; then the random variable for the sum of scores (A_g^*) for all individuals in row 1 of Table 17.15 (i.e., the diseased group D) is given by

$$A_g^* = \sum_{i=1}^{c} A_{ig} y_{ig}$$

The test statistic then has the following form:

$$\chi_{\mathrm{MHO}}^2 = \left[\sum_{g=1}^{G} a_g^* - \sum_{g=1}^{G} \mathscr{E}_0(A_g^*) \right]^2 \Big/ \sum_{g=1}^{G} \hat{\mathrm{Var}}_0(A_g^*) \qquad (17.20)$$

In this formula, χ_{MHO}^2 denotes the Mantel-Haenszel statistic for *ordinal* exposure categories,

$$a_g^* = \text{sample realization of } A_g^*$$

$$\mathscr{E}_0(A_g^*) = \left(\frac{m_{1g}}{n_g} \right) \sum_{i=1}^{c} n_{ig} y_{ig}$$

$$\hat{\mathrm{Var}}_0(A_g^*) = (m_{1g} m_{0g} / n_g) \hat{\sigma}_g^2$$

with

$$\hat{\sigma}_g^2 = \left(\frac{1}{n_g - 1} \right) \left[\sum_{i=1}^{c} n_{ig} y_{ig}^2 - \left(\sum_{i=1}^{c} n_{ig} y_{ig} \right)^2 \Big/ n_g \right]$$

the latter denoting the sample variance of the scores for the column marginals.

In using this test statistic, Karon (1978) has pointed out that monotone scores (e.g., $y_{1g} = c$, $y_{2g} = c - 1$, . . . , $y_{c-1,g} = 1$, $y_{cg} = 0$) have yielded a relatively powerful test in most situations, but it can give poor power (in terms of low χ^2 values) in certain circumstances. In particular, the maximum value of χ_{MHO}^2 for all possible choices of scoring systems is χ_{MHN}^2, given by Expression 17.19. However, if the exposure variable is considered to be nominal, the use of χ_{MHN}^2 will require $(c - 1)$ degrees of freedom, whereas χ_{MHO}^2 requires only one degree of freedom. Also, the expression given by Equation 17.20 is invariant under a linear transformation of the scores (i.e., the same chi-square value will be obtained if the scoring goes from c to 1 or from $c - 1$ to 0). Other scoring procedures that may be considered include "natural" scores (e.g., midpoints of the dosage levels comprising a given exposure category) and ridit-type or other rank scores (see Karon, 1978, for further discussion on the choice of scores).

**17.7
CON-
CLUDING
REMARKS**

Stratified analysis is an extremely useful and direct approach for providing control of confounding. Nevertheless, as we have illustrated by our general example (Section 17.2), interpretation of stratified analyses becomes more and more difficult as the number of variables to be controlled increases, even though the procedure itself is fairly straightforward. In addition, the procedure requires a certain amount of subjective evaluation on the part of the investigator, particularly with regard to the usefulness of carrying out either an overall test for association or computing summary point and interval estimates.

For completeness, we describe several different types of summary effect measures in Table 17.16. All the measures considered are used in practice to varying degrees, but, in general, we prefer the use of precision-based estimators in the case when there is relatively little interaction, and we note that the usefulness of any summary estimator is limited when there is considerable interaction.

In the next chapter, we will see how the analysis of matched data may be viewed as a special case of stratified analysis. We will also compare the design characteristics of matching vis-à-vis the use of stratification after unmatched sampling, giving the advantages and disadvantages of each. Mathematical-modeling approaches, which may be used as alternatives to stratified analysis, will be discussed in Chapters 20–24, following a somewhat philosophical discussion of the concepts of interaction, effect modification, and synergism (Chapter 19).

NOTATION

The following list summarizes the key notation introduced in this chapter. (Also see Table 17.16.)

g	Indicator of the gth stratum (group).
G	Number of strata (i.e., $g = 1, 2, \ldots, G$).
$a = \sum_{g=1}^{G} a_g$	Observed total number of exposed cases.
χ^2_{MHS}	Mantel-Haenszel chi-square statistic for cumulative follow-up, case-control, or cross-sectional studies.
χ^2_{MHD}	Mantel-Haenszel chi-square statistic for density follow-up studies.
$\hat{\theta}_g$	Stratum-specific estimator of θ using the data in stratum g.
W_g	Weight assigned to stratum g (used in calculating a weighted average of stratum-specific estimates).

Table 17.16 Formulas for Point and Interval Estimation of Overall Effect in Stratified Analysis

a. Cumulative Incidence Follow-up Studies (Risk Difference and Risk Ratio)[a]

STRATUM g

	E	$\overline{E}$	
D	a_g	b_g	m_{1g}
$\overline{D}$	c_g	d_g	m_{0g}
	n_{1g}	n_{0g}	n_g

Description	$\hat{\theta}$	$\hat{\theta}_g$	W_g	$100(1-\alpha)\%$ Interval Estimate
Risk difference using inverse variance weights derived from binomial variance estimates	$\widehat{\mathrm{aRD}} = \dfrac{\sum W_g \widehat{\mathrm{RD}}_g}{\sum W_g}$	$\widehat{\mathrm{RD}}_g = \dfrac{a_g}{n_{1g}} - \dfrac{b_g}{n_{0g}}$	$\dfrac{1}{\widehat{\mathrm{Var}}(\widehat{\mathrm{RD}}_g)} = \dfrac{1}{\left(\dfrac{a_g c_g}{n_{1g}^3} + \dfrac{b_g d_g}{n_{0g}^3}\right)}$	$\widehat{\mathrm{aRD}} \pm \dfrac{Z_{1-\alpha/2}}{\sqrt{\sum W_g}}$ $\qquad$ $\widehat{\mathrm{aRD}}\left(1 \pm \dfrac{Z_{1-\alpha/2}}{\chi_{\mathrm{MH}}}\right)$
Standardized risk difference	$\widehat{\mathrm{SRD}} = \dfrac{\sum s_g a_g/n_{1g} - \sum s_g b_g/n_{0g}}{}$ $\left(= \dfrac{\sum W_g \widehat{\mathrm{RD}}_g}{\sum W_g}\right)$	$\widehat{\mathrm{RD}}_g = \dfrac{a_g}{n_{1g}} - \dfrac{b_g}{n_{0g}}$	$\dfrac{1}{\widehat{\mathrm{Var}}_0(\widehat{\mathrm{RD}}_g)} = \dfrac{n_g n_{1g} n_{0g}}{m_{1g} m_{0g}}$ s_g, a standard population frequency	$\widehat{\mathrm{SRD}} \pm Z_{1-\alpha2} \sqrt{\dfrac{\sum s_g^2 \left(\dfrac{a_g c_g}{n_{1g}^2} + \dfrac{b_g d_g}{n_{0g}^2}\right)\left(\dfrac{1}{n_{1g}} + \dfrac{1}{n_{0g}}\right)}{(\sum s_g)^2}}$ $\qquad$ $\widehat{\mathrm{SRD}}\left(1 \pm \dfrac{Z_{1-\alpha/2}}{\chi_{\mathrm{MH}}}\right)$
Risk ratio using inverse variance weights derived from Taylor series approximation for variance	$\widehat{\mathrm{aRR}} = \exp\left(\dfrac{\sum W_g \ln \widehat{\mathrm{RR}}_g}{\sum W_g}\right)$	$\widehat{\mathrm{RR}}_g = \dfrac{a_g n_{0g}}{b_g n_{1g}}$	$\dfrac{1}{\widehat{\mathrm{Var}}(\ln \widehat{\mathrm{RR}}_g)} = \dfrac{1}{\left(\dfrac{c_g}{n_{1g} a_g} + \dfrac{d_g}{n_{0g} b_g}\right)}$	$\widehat{\mathrm{aRR}} \exp\left(\pm \dfrac{Z_{1-\alpha/2}}{\sqrt{\sum W_g}}\right)$ $\qquad$ $\widehat{\mathrm{aRR}}^{(1 \pm Z_{1-\alpha/2}/\chi_{\mathrm{MH}})}$
Standardized risk ratio	$\widehat{\mathrm{SRR}} = \dfrac{\sum s_g a_g/n_{1g}}{\sum s_g b_g/n_{0g}}$ $\left(= \dfrac{\sum W_g \widehat{\mathrm{RR}}_g}{\sum W_g}\right)$	$\widehat{\mathrm{RR}}_g = \dfrac{a_g n_{0g}}{b_g n_{1g}}$	$\dfrac{1}{\widehat{\mathrm{Var}}_0(\ln \widehat{\mathrm{RR}}_g)} = \dfrac{m_{1g} n_{1g} n_{0g}}{m_{0g} n_g}$ $s_g b_g/n_{0g}$, where s_g denotes a standard population frequency	$\widehat{\mathrm{SRR}} \exp\left[\pm Z_{1-\alpha2} \sqrt{\dfrac{\sum s_g^2 a_g c_g/n_{1g}^3}{(\sum s_g a_g/n_{1g})^2} + \dfrac{\sum s_g^2 b_g d_g/n_{0g}^3}{(\sum s_g b_g/n_{0g})^2}}\right]$ $\qquad$ $\widehat{\mathrm{SRR}}^{(1 \pm Z_{1-\alpha/2}/\chi_{\mathrm{MH}})}$
MH risk ratio (MH odds ratio described in part b)	$\widehat{\mathrm{mRR}} = \dfrac{\sum a_g n_{0g}/n_g}{\sum b_g n_{1g}/n_g}$ $\left(= \dfrac{\sum W_g \widehat{\mathrm{RR}}_g}{\sum W_g}\right)$, provided all $b_g n_{1g} \neq 0$	$\widehat{\mathrm{RR}}_g = \dfrac{a_g n_{0g}}{b_g n_{1g}}$	$\dfrac{b_g n_{1g}}{n_g}$	$\widehat{\mathrm{mRR}}^{(1 \pm Z_{1-\alpha/2}/\chi_{\mathrm{MH}})}$

Table 17.16 (continued)

Table 17.16   (*continued*)

Table 17.16   Formulas for Point and Interval Estimation of Overall Effect in Stratified Analysis

STRATUM g

	E	$\bar{E}$	
D	a_g	b_g	m_{1g}
$\bar{D}$	c_g	d_g	m_{0g}
	n_{1g}	n_{0g}	n_g

b. Case-Control and Cross-sectional Studies (Odds Ratio)

Description	$\hat{\theta}$	$\hat{\theta}_g$	W_g	$100(1-\alpha)\%$ Interval Estimate
Odds ratio using inverse variance weights derived from Taylor series approximations	$\hat{a\text{OR}} = \exp\left(\dfrac{\sum W_g \ln \hat{\text{OR}}_g}{\sum W_g}\right)$	$\hat{\text{OR}}_g = \dfrac{a_g d_g}{b_g c_g}$	$\dfrac{1}{\hat{\text{Var}}(\ln \text{OR}_g)} = \dfrac{1}{\dfrac{1}{a_g}+\dfrac{1}{b_g}+\dfrac{1}{c_g}+\dfrac{1}{d_g}}$	$\hat{a\text{OR}} \exp\left(\pm Z_{1-\alpha/2} \Big/ \sqrt{\sum W_g}\right)$
Standardized odds ratio	$\hat{\text{SOR}} = \dfrac{\sum s_g a_g / c_g}{\sum s_g b_g / d_g}$ $\left(= \dfrac{\sum W_g \hat{\text{OR}}_g}{\sum W_g}\right)$	$\hat{\text{OR}}_g = \dfrac{a_g d_g}{b_g c_g}$	$s_g b_g / d_g$, where s_g denotes a standard population frequency	$\hat{\text{SOR}}^{(1\pm Z_{1-\alpha/2}/\chi_{\text{MH}})}$
MH odds ratio	$\hat{\text{mOR}} = \dfrac{\sum a_g d_g / n_g}{\sum b_g c_g / n_g}$ $\left(= \dfrac{\sum W_g \hat{\text{OR}}_g}{\sum W_g}\right)$, provided all $b_g c_g \neq 0$	$\hat{\text{OR}}_g = \dfrac{a_g d_g}{b_g c_g}$	$\dfrac{b_g c_g}{n_g}$	$\hat{\text{mOR}}^{(1\pm Z_{1-\alpha/2}/\chi_{\text{MH}})}$

c. Density Studies (Density Difference and Density Ratio)

	E	$\bar{E}$	
No. of New Cases in (t_0, t)	a_g	b_g	m_g
Population-Time	L_{1g}	L_{0g}	L_g

Table 17.16   (*continued*)

Description	$\hat{\theta}$	$\hat{\theta}_g$	W_g	$100(1-\alpha)\%$ Interval Estimate
Incidence density difference using inverse variance weights	$a\hat{\mathrm{I}}\mathrm{DD} = \dfrac{\sum W_g \mathrm{I}\hat{\mathrm{D}}\mathrm{D}_g}{\sum W_g}$	$\mathrm{I}\hat{\mathrm{D}}\mathrm{D}_g = \dfrac{a_g}{L_{1g}} - \dfrac{b_g}{L_{0g}}$	$\dfrac{1}{\hat{\mathrm{V}}\mathrm{ar}_0(\mathrm{I}\hat{\mathrm{D}}\mathrm{D}_g)} = \dfrac{L_{1g}L_{0g}}{m_{1g}}$	$a\hat{\mathrm{I}}\mathrm{DD} \pm \dfrac{Z_{1-\alpha/2}}{\sqrt{\sum W_g}}$ $a\hat{\mathrm{I}}\mathrm{DD}\left(1 \pm \dfrac{Z_{1-\alpha/2}}{\chi_{\mathrm{MH}}}\right)$
Standardized incidence density difference	$S\hat{\mathrm{I}}\mathrm{DD} = \dfrac{\sum s_g a_g}{L_{1g}} - \dfrac{\sum s_g b_g}{L_{0g}}$ $\left(= \dfrac{\sum W_g \mathrm{I}\hat{\mathrm{D}}\mathrm{D}_g}{\sum W_g}\right)$	$\mathrm{I}\hat{\mathrm{D}}\mathrm{D}_g = \dfrac{a_g}{L_{1g}} - \dfrac{b_g}{L_{0g}}$	s_g, a standard population frequency	$S\hat{\mathrm{I}}\mathrm{DD} \pm Z_{1-\alpha/2}\sqrt{\dfrac{\sum s_g^2 m_{1g}}{L_{1g}L_{0g}}}\left(\sum s_g\right)^2$ $S\hat{\mathrm{I}}\mathrm{DD}\left(1 \pm \dfrac{Z_{1-\alpha/2}}{\chi_{\mathrm{MH}}}\right)$
Incidence density ratio using inverse variance weights	$a\hat{\mathrm{I}}\mathrm{DR} = \exp\left(\dfrac{\sum W_g \ln \mathrm{I}\hat{\mathrm{D}}\mathrm{R}_g}{\sum W_g}\right)$	$\mathrm{I}\hat{\mathrm{D}}\mathrm{R}_g = \dfrac{a_g L_{0g}}{b_g L_{1g}}$	$\dfrac{1}{\hat{\mathrm{V}}\mathrm{ar}_0(\mathrm{I}\hat{\mathrm{D}}\mathrm{R}_g)} = \dfrac{m_{1g}L_{1g}L_{0g}}{L_g^2}$	$a\hat{\mathrm{I}}\mathrm{DR} \exp\left(\pm \dfrac{Z_{1-\alpha/2}}{\sqrt{\sum W_g}}\right)$ $a\hat{\mathrm{I}}\mathrm{DR}^{(1\pm Z_{1-\alpha/2}/\chi_{\mathrm{MH}})}$
Standardized incidence density ratio	$S\hat{\mathrm{I}}\mathrm{DR} = \dfrac{\sum s_g a_g / L_{1g}}{\sum s_g b_g / L_{0g}}$ $\left(= \dfrac{\sum W_g \mathrm{I}\hat{\mathrm{D}}\mathrm{R}_g}{\sum W_g}\right)$	$\mathrm{I}\hat{\mathrm{D}}\mathrm{R}_g = \dfrac{a_g L_{0g}}{b_g L_{1g}}$	$\dfrac{s_g b_g}{L_{0g}}$, where s_g denotes a standard population frequency	$S\hat{\mathrm{I}}\mathrm{DR}^{(1\pm Z_{1-\alpha/2}/\chi_{\mathrm{MH}})}$
MH incidence density ratio	$m\hat{\mathrm{I}}\mathrm{DR} = \dfrac{\sum a_g L_{0g}/L_g}{\sum b_g L_{1g}/L_g}$ $\left(= \dfrac{\sum W_g \mathrm{I}\hat{\mathrm{D}}\mathrm{R}_g}{\sum W_g},\right.$ $\left.\text{provided all } b_g L_{1g} \neq 0\right)$	$\mathrm{I}\hat{\mathrm{D}}\mathrm{R}_g = \dfrac{a_g L_{0g}}{b_g L_{1g}}$	$\dfrac{b_g L_{1g}}{L_g}$	$m\hat{\mathrm{I}}\mathrm{DR}^{(1\pm Z_{1-\alpha/2}/\chi_{\mathrm{MH}})}$

Note: For strata with zero cell frequencies, regardless of study design, an indeterminate value for $\hat{\theta}_g$ or W_g may be avoided by modifying each cell frequency in such strata with the addition of .5; i.e., replace a_g, b_g, c_g, and d_g with $a_g + .5$, $b_g + .5$, $c_g + .5$, and $d_g + .5$, respectively. Such adjustment is not usually necessary for mRR, mOR, and mIDR.

[a]Analogous formulas for estimating adjusted prevalence differences and prevalence ratios in cross-sectional studies may be obtained by substituting $\hat{\mathrm{PD}}$ and $\hat{\mathrm{PR}}$ for $\hat{\mathrm{RD}}$ and $\hat{\mathrm{RR}}$, respectively, throughout. Also, $\chi_{\mathrm{MH}} = \sqrt{\chi_{\mathrm{MHS}}^2}$.

$$\hat{\theta} = \begin{cases} \dfrac{\displaystyle\sum_{g=1}^{G} W_g \hat{\theta}_g}{\displaystyle\sum_{g=1}^{G} W_g} & \text{Weighted average of stratum-specific esti-} \\[2em] & \text{mates } \hat{\theta}_g. \\[2em] \exp\left(\dfrac{\displaystyle\sum_{g=1}^{G} W_g \ln \hat{\theta}_g}{\displaystyle\sum_{g=1}^{G} W_g}\right) & \text{Exponentiated weighted average of natural lo-} \\ & \text{garithms of stratum-specific estimates } \hat{\theta}_g. \end{cases}$$

$\hat{aRD}$	Estimated adjusted risk difference using precision-based weights for $\hat{RD}_g$, $g = 1$, $2, \ldots, G$.
$\hat{aRR}$	Estimated adjusted risk ratio using precision-based weights for $\ln \hat{RR}_g$.
$\hat{aOR}$	Estimated adjusted odds ratio using precision-based weights for $\ln \hat{OR}_g$.
$\hat{aIDD}$	Estimated adjusted incidence density difference using precision-based weights for $\hat{IDD}_g$.
$\hat{aIDR}$	Estimated adjusted incidence density ratio using precision-based weights for $\hat{IDR}_g$.
$\hat{mOR}$	Mantel-Haenszel adjusted odds ratio estimate.
$\hat{mRR}$	Mantel-Haenszel adjusted risk ratio estimate.
$\hat{mIDR}$	Adjusted incidence density ratio estimate.
$s_1, \ldots, s_G$	Frequency distribution over the G strata for the standard population.
$\hat{SRR}$	Estimated standardized risk (cumulative incidence) ratio.
$\hat{SRD}$	Estimated standardized risk (cumulative incidence) difference.
$\hat{sRR}$	Internally standardized risk ratio estimate (based on using the exposed group distribution as the standard).
$s'\hat{RR}$	Externally standardized risk ratio estimate (based on using the nonexposed group distribution as the standard).
$\hat{SOR}$	Estimated standardized odds ratio.
$\hat{sOR}$	Internally standardized odds ratio estimate (based on using exposed noncases as the standard).

s'$\hat{\text{OR}}$	Externally standardized odds ratio estimate (based on using nonexposed noncases as the standard).
SI$\hat{\text{D}}$R	Estimated standardized incidence density ratio.
SI$\hat{\text{D}}$D	Estimated standardized incidence density difference.
χ^2_{MHN}	Mantel-Haenszel chi-square statistic when exposure categories are treated nominally.
χ^2_{MHO}	Mantel-Haenszel chi-square statistic when exposure categories are treated ordinally.
y_{ig}	Score for the ith ordinal category in stratum g.
$a_g^* = \sum_{i=1}^{c} a_{ig} y_{ig}$	Observed weighted sum of scores for all persons in the diseased group sample in stratum g.

Each of the problems below concerns stratified analyses of *hypothetical* study data. We provide summaries of computer results for Exercises 17.1– 17.3 and 17.5 to reduce the amount of hand computation required. You may, nevertheless, wish to carry out some calculations directly to gain familiarity with the formulas being used (see Table 17.16).

PRACTICE EXERCISES

17.1 A researcher conducted a follow-up study on the utilization of swine flu vaccine at a large southern university during the fall of 1976. The investigator devised a detailed questionnaire to measure what she termed the "perception of swine flu." The instrument consisted of items measuring such things as perceived likelihood of getting the disease, perceived severity of the disease, perceived transmission of the disease, and perceived costs and benefits of vaccination. A single score was calculated for each subject on the basis of the entire response pattern. The scores were then dichotomized into two categories: receptive perception (R) and nonreceptive perception ($\bar{R}$). "Receptive" indicates that the person is aware of the disease, feels that the chance of getting it is worthy of concern, considers the consequences of getting the disease to be severe, and believes that getting the vaccine will help. "Nonreceptive" implies the opposite set of attitudes. The conjecture under investigation is that a person with a receptive perception of the disease will be more likely to opt for vaccination than will a person with a nonreceptive perception.

    A random sample of 600 sophomores was selected from those students who were enrolled in the university at the beginning of the fall semester in 1976. The questionnaire was administered to each subject during the last two weeks of September. Since each person receiving the vaccine was registered with the student health service, the investigator was able to check the records between October and December to determine whether each subject in the sample had been vaccinated. Exercise Table 17.1 summarizes the study population by type of perception (R versus $\bar{R}$), vaccination behavior (V versus $\bar{V}$), race (W versus B), and gender (M versus F).

Exercise Table 17.1

	VACCINATED (V)		NOT VACCINATED ($\bar{V}$)		
Race-Gender	R	$\bar{R}$	R	$\bar{R}$	Total
WM	68	17	172	43	300
WF	8	12	52	78	150
BM	1	4	9	36	50
BF	81	9	9	1	100
Total	158	42	242	158	600

The computer summary results are as follows:

ANALYSIS=V BY R, BY GENDER

	a	b	c	d	n	$\hat{R}R$	χ^2_{MH}	P-VALUE
MALE	69	21	181	79	350	1.31	1.62	.101
FEMALE	89	21	61	79	250	2.83	35.64	.000
:OVERALL	158	42	242	158	600	1.88	20.50	.000

a$\hat{R}R$	s$\hat{R}R$	s'$\hat{R}R$	m$\hat{R}R$	χ^2_{MH}	P-VALUE
1.98	1.88	2.07	2.00	26.92	.000

ANALYSIS=V BY R, BY RACE

	a	b	c	d	n	$\hat{R}R$	χ^2_{MH}	P-VALUE
WHITE	76	29	224	121	450	1.31	2.01	.078
BLACK	82	13	18	37	150	3.15	44.71	.000
:OVERALL	158	42	242	158	600	1.88	20.50	.000

a$\hat{R}R$	s$\hat{R}R$	s'$\hat{R}R$	m$\hat{R}R$	χ^2_{MH}	P-VALUE
1.84	1.88	1.88	1.88	23.66	.000

ANALYSIS=V BY R, BY RACE AND GENDER

	a	b	c	d	n	$\hat{R}R$	χ^2_{MH}	P-VALUE
WM	68	17	172	43	300	1.00	.00	.500
WF	8	12	52	78	150	1.00	.00	.500
BM	1	4	9	36	50	1.00	.00	.500

	a	b	c	d	n	$\hat{RR}$	χ^2_{MH}	P-VALUE
BF	81	9	9	1	100	1.00	.00	.500
:OVERALL	158	42	242	158	600	1.88	20.50	.000

a$\hat{RR}$	s$\hat{RR}$	s'$\hat{RR}$	m$\hat{RR}$	χ^2_{MH}	P-VALUE
1.00	1.00	1.00	1.00	.00	.500

a. What can you conclude about the association between perception of disease and vaccine acceptance on the basis of the estimated crude risk ratio comparing the proportion vaccinated among receptive perceivers (R) with the corresponding proportion among nonreceptive perceivers ($\bar{R}$)?

b. Why are the adjusted estimates a$\hat{RR}$, s$\hat{RR}$, and s'$\hat{RR}$ (see the summarized computer results), based on controlling just for gender (i.e., ignoring race), not all equal?

c. Ignoring race, does gender appear to be confounding the association between perception of disease and vaccine acceptance? Explain.

d. Ignoring gender, does race appear to be confounding the association between perception of disease and vaccine acceptance? Explain.

e. Stratify on both race and gender simultaneously. How do the resulting four stratum-specific risk ratio estimates compare with the crude risk ratio estimate and the adjusted estimates based on controlling for gender and race separately?

f. What conclusion can you draw about the effect of sex and race on the observed relationship between perception of swine flu and vaccine acceptance?

g. Based on the study described, is perception of swine flu a *determinant* of vaccination acceptance? Explain.

17.2 Researchers conducted a case-control study of bladder cancer to test its putative association with dietary consumption of substance E. Cases and noncases were selected randomly from white male hospital patients between 50 and 60 years of age residing in a large metropolitan area. Exercise Table 17.2 summarizes the data by history of cigarette smoking. From previous investigations, it is known that smoking is a risk factor for bladder cancer. Note that consumption of substance E has been dichotomized into consumers (E) and nonconsumers ($\bar{E}$).

Exercise Table 17.2

	SMOKERS			NONSMOKERS	
	E	$\bar{E}$		E	$\bar{E}$
D	35	5	D	10	15
$\bar{D}$	30	10	$\bar{D}$	10	30

The computer results are summarized below.

ANALYSIS=D BY E, BY SMK STATUS

	a	b	c	d	n	OR̂	V̂ar(ln OR̂)	OR̂$_L$	OR̂$_U$	χ^2_{MH}	P-VALUE
									←95% CI→		
SMK	35	5	30	10	80	2.33	.361905	.72	7.59	2.03	.077
NONSMK	10	15	10	30	65	2.00	.300000	.68	5.85	1.60	.103
:OVERALL	45	20	40	40	145	2.25	.122222	1.13	4.46	5.43	.010

aOR̂	aOR̂$_L$	aOR̂$_U$	sOR̂	s'OR̂	mOR̂	χ^2_{MH}	P-VALUE
	|←95% CI→|					
2.14	.97	4.74	2.25	2.08	2.15	3.60	.029

In answering the following questions, assume that the potential confounding effects of age have been appropriately controlled by restriction.

a. What is the estimated crude odds ratio comparing cases and noncases with regard to previous consumption of substance E? Is this odds ratio significantly greater than one (use $\alpha = .01$)?

b. Compare the two estimated smoking-specific odds ratios to each other and to the crude odds ratio estimate. Also, compare corresponding P-values. What do these results indicate with regard to confounding, interaction, and precision?

c. On the basis of an examination of one or more (appropriate) adjusted estimates of overall effect, does smoking status appear to be a confounding variable in these data?

d. Test for the significance of the association of E with bladder cancer by using a two-strata Mantel-Haenszel statistic. Compare the resulting P-value with those obtained in parts a and b.

e. On the basis of the above results, would you recommend controlling for smoking status? Explain.

f. Calculate Taylor series–based and test-based 95% interval estimates for the adjusted odds ratio (aOR). Compare the intervals obtained.

g. Do the data support the theory that consumption of substance E is related to the occurrence of bladder cancer? Explain.

17.3 Investigators conducted a cross-sectional study of a rural community in the southern United States to test the putative association between educational background and hypertension. In 1960, a random sample of 720 adults was selected from a biracial community. Hypertension was defined as SPB $\geq$ 160 mmHg and/or DBP $\geq$ 95 mmHg. No one in the community was known to be on antihypertensive therapy in 1960. Education was also dichotomized into two categories: those with more than a ninth-grade education (>9) and those with a ninth-grade education or less ($\leq$9). Exercise Table 17.3 summarizes the frequency of hypertension (H) and normotension (N) by level of education, race, and gender.

Exercise Table 17.3

Race-Gender	EDUCATION > 9		EDUCATION ≤ 9		Total
	H	N	H	N	
WM	8	64	19	89	180
WF	11	109	14	66	200
BM	17	15	43	85	160
BF	21	33	34	92	180
Total	57	221	110	332	720

The computer results are summarized below.

ANALYSIS=HYP BY EDUC, BY RACE AND GENDER

	a	b	c	d	n	$\hat{OR}$	$\hat{Var}(\ln \hat{OR})$	$\hat{OR}_L$	$\hat{OR}_U$	χ^2_{MH}	P-VALUE
								|←95% CI→|			
WM	8	19	64	89	180	.59	.204493	.24	1.42	1.42	.117
WF	11	14	109	66	200	.48	.186663	.20	1.11	3.03	.041
BM	17	43	15	85	160	2.24	.160511	1.02	4.91	4.14	.021
BF	21	34	33	92	180	1.72	.118203	.88	3.38	2.51	.057
:OVERALL	57	110	221	332	720	.78	.034172	.54	1.12	1.84	.088

a$\hat{OR}$	a$\hat{OR}_L$	a$\hat{OR}_U$	s$\hat{OR}$	s'$\hat{OR}$	m$\hat{OR}$	χ^2_{MH}	P-VALUE
	|←95% CI→|						
1.13	.76	1.67	1.01	1.57	1.11	.29	.294

ANALYSIS=HYP BY EDUC, BY GENDER FOR WHITES

	a	b	c	d	n	$\hat{OR}$	$\hat{Var}(\ln \hat{OR})$	$\hat{OR}_L$	$\hat{OR}_U$	χ^2_{MH}	P-VALUE
								|←95% CI→|			
WM	8	19	64	89	180	.59	.204493	.24	1.42	1.42	.117
WF	11	14	109	66	200	.48	.186663	.20	1.11	3.03	.041
:OVERALL	19	33	173	155	380	.52	.095167	.28	.94	4.70	.015

a$\hat{OR}$	a$\hat{OR}_L$	a$\hat{OR}_U$	s$\hat{OR}$	s'$\hat{OR}$	m$\hat{OR}$	χ^2_{MH}	P-VALUE
	|←95% CI→|						
.53	.28	.97	.52	.54	.53	4.28	.019

ANALYSIS=HYP BY EDUC, BY GENDER FOR BLACKS

	a	b	c	d	n	$\hat{OR}$	$\hat{Var}(\ln \hat{OR})$	$\hat{OR}_L$	$\hat{OR}_U$	χ^2_{MH}	P-VALUE
								|←95% CI→|		
BM	17	43	15	85	160	2.24	.160511	1.02	4.91	4.14	.021
BF	21	34	33	92	180	1.72	.118203	.88	3.38	2.51	.057
:OVERALL	38	77	48	177	340	1.82	.065786	1.10	3.01	5.51	.009

$a\hat{OR}$	$a\hat{OR}_L$	$a\hat{OR}_U$	$s\hat{OR}$	$s'\hat{OR}$	$m\hat{OR}$	χ^2_{MH}	P-VALUE
	←95% CI→						
1.93	1.15	3.21	1.92	2.01	1.93	6.40	.006

a. On the basis of the crude data (i.e., ignoring the variables race and gender), does there appear to be an association between education and hypertension in the data?

b. If you consider the four stratum-specific prevalence odds ratios ($\hat{OR}_g$), should you alter the conclusion you made in part a? Explain.

c. Using a precision-based estimated adjusted odds ratio, a Taylor series–based 95% interval estimate, and a Mantel-Haenszel test statistic in each case, describe the association between educational background and hypertension for each race separately, controlling for gender.

d. For each race separately, is there confounding by gender? Explain.

e. Suppose that the investigator also wished to control, in the analysis, for other known risk factors of hypertension, such as age, obesity, salt intake, physical exercise, and smoking. What problem would be expected to occur if stratified analyses were used for such control purposes?

17.4 Consider again the data for the vitamin C trial described in Exercise 15.2. Several subjects were not followed for the entire follow-up period for one of two reasons: failure to report to the physician as scheduled or failure to comply with the regimen. Exercise Table 17.4 summarizes the data. It should be noted that multiple occurrences of the common cold were observed in three subjects. Assume that each cold lasted a third of a month, and that all colds occurred more than a third of a month prior to the end of the observation period for each individual. In the table, T = treatment and C = control.

a. Stratifying the data into three age groups (20–29, 30–39, and 40–49), estimate the crude incidence density ratio (cIDR) and the three age-specific incidence density ratios (IDR$_g$), comparing treatment to control subjects.

b. Calculate the precision-based adjusted estimate of the incidence density ratio (a$\hat{I}$DR), adjusting for the three categories of age. Is age a confounding factor? That is, did the randomization procedure eliminate the confounding effect of age in these data?

c. Appropriately test the significance of the association of interest by using Miettinen's modification of the stratified Mantel-Haenszel statistic. You will need to assume that cold occurrences are independent events, even when there is more than one occurrence in the same subject. Do these data support the hypothesis that vitamin C helps to prevent the common cold?

d. Compute a 95% test-based confidence interval for the aIDR, assuming that aI$\hat{D}$R is lognormally distributed.

Exercise Table 17.4

Subject	Age	Assigned Group	No. of Months Observed	No. of Occurrences of Common Cold	Person-Months
1	34	T	6	0	6
2	49	C	5	2	4.33
3	36	T	6	0	6
4	26	C	2	0	2
5	25	T	6	0	6
6	42	C	6	1	5.67
7	27	T	5	1	4.67
8	30	C	6	0	6
9	33	T	6	1	5.67
10	47	C	3	1	2.67
11	28	T	3	0	3
12	41	C	6	2	5.33
13	42	T	5	1	4.67
14	33	C	4	1	3.67
15	20	T	6	0	6
16	34	C	3	0	3
17	27	T	5	0	5
18	43	C	5	0	5
19	48	T	3	1	2.67
20	35	C	6	2	5.33
21	39	T	6	0	6
22	24	C	4	0	4
23	45	T	6	0	6
24	46	C	5	0	5
25	38	T	6	1	5.67
26	29	C	5	1	4.67
27	46	T	4	0	4
28	37	C	5	0	5
29	24	T	6	0	6
30	22	C	4	0	4

e. Calculate a point estimate of the prevented fraction (aPF) adjusting for age, and also compute a 95% test-based confidence interval for the aPF. Assume that $(1 - \hat{\text{aPF}})$ is lognormally distributed. Use the computational formula

$$\hat{\text{aPF}} = \frac{a[1 - (\text{aI}\hat{\text{D}}\text{R})]}{a + b(\text{aI}\hat{\text{D}}\text{R})}$$

where

   a = total number of occurrences of the common cold in the treatment group

b = total number of occurrences of the common cold in the placebo group

17.5 A researcher conducted a case-control study to investigate the possible association between cigarette smoking and myocardial infarction (MI). One hundred hospitalized cases with a first (recently diagnosed) acute MI were compared to 110 noncases who were hospitalized for noncardiovascular conditions and who had no history or symptoms of coronary heart disease. All subjects were white males between the ages of 50 and 54; they were categorized as having "high" or "low" social status (SS) according to their occupation, education, and income. Current cigarette smoking practice was divided into three categories: nonsmokers (NS), light smokers (LS), who smoke a pack or less each day, and heavy smokers (HS), who smoke more than a pack per day. Exercise Table 17.5 describes the disease status (D) of the study population as a function of smoking status and social status.

Exercise Table 17.5

	HIGH SS			LOW SS		
	HS	LS	NS	HS	LS	NS
D	9	6	5	29	36	15
$\bar{D}$	10	20	20	15	30	15
Total	19	26	25	44	66	30

The computer results are summarized below.

ANALYSIS=D BY HSMK, BY SS

	a	b	c	d	n	$\hat{OR}$	$\hat{Var}(\ln \hat{OR})$	$\hat{OR}_L$	$\hat{OR}_U$	χ^2_{MH}	P-VALUE
								$\mid\leftarrow$ 95% CI $\rightarrow\mid$			
HI SS	9	5	10	20	44	3.60	.461111	.95	13.62	3.64	.028
LO SS	29	15	15	15	74	1.93	.234483	.75	4.99	1.85	.087
:OVERALL	38	20	25	35	118	2.66	.144887	1.26	5.61	6.68	.005

a$\hat{OR}$	a$\hat{OR}_L$	a$\hat{OR}_U$	s$\hat{OR}$	s'$\hat{OR}$	m$\hat{OR}$	χ^2_{MH}	P-VALUE
$\mid\leftarrow$ 95% CI $\rightarrow\mid$							
2.38	1.10	5.16	2.17	2.35	2.39	4.97	.013

ANALYSIS=D BY LSMK, BY SS

	a	b	c	d	n	$\hat{OR}$	$\hat{Var}(\ln \hat{OR})$	$\hat{OR}_L$	$\hat{OR}_U$	χ^2_{MH}	P-VALUE
								$\mid\leftarrow$ 95% CI $\rightarrow\mid$			
HI SS	6	5	20	20	51	1.20	.466667	.31	4.58	.07	.396

| LO SS | 36 | 15 | 30 | 15 | 96 | 1.20 | .194444 | .51 | 2.85 | .17 | .340 |
| :OVERALL | 42 | 20 | 50 | 35 | 147 | 1.47 | .122381 | .74 | 2.92 | 1.21 | .136 |

		|←95% CI→|				
$a\hat{O}R$	$a\hat{O}R_L$	$a\hat{O}R_U$	$s\hat{O}R$	$s'\hat{O}R$	$m\hat{O}R$	χ^2_{MH}	P-VALUE
1.20	.58	2.48	1.20	1.20	1.20	.24	.312

ANALYSIS=D BY COMBINED SMK, BY SS

								←95% CI→			
	a	b	c	d	n	$\hat{O}R$	$\hat{Var}(\ln \hat{O}R)$	$\hat{O}R_L$	$\hat{O}R_U$	χ^2_{MH}	P-VALUE
HI SS	15	5	30	20	70	2.00	.350000	.63	6.38	1.38	.120
LO SS	65	15	45	15	140	1.44	.170940	.64	3.25	.79	.187
:OVERALL	80	20	75	35	210	1.87	.104405	.99	3.52	3.77	.026

		|←95% CI→|				
$a\hat{O}R$	$a\hat{O}R_L$	$a\hat{O}R_U$	$s\hat{O}R$	$s'\hat{O}R$	$m\hat{O}R$	χ^2_{MH}	P-VALUE
1.61	.83	3.12	1.52	1.58	1.62	2.01	.078

a. Calculate and interpret the two estimated crude odds ratios ($c\hat{O}R$) and the four SS-specific estimated odds ratios ($\hat{O}R_g$), comparing heavy and light smokers to nonsmokers.

b. Calculate the $m\hat{O}R$ for each smoking category compared to nonsmokers, adjusting for SS. Is SS a confounding factor?

c. How can the use of the $m\hat{O}R$ be criticized (in terms of the weights being used) when assessing a possible dose-response effect of smoking? What advantage, if any, does the use of $s'\hat{O}R$ have in this regard?

d. Test for a significant dose-response effect due to smoking by using the Mantel extension of the Mantel-Haenszel test (which allows for several ordinal exposure categories). Use scores of 0, 1, and 2 for nonsmokers, light smokers, and heavy smokers, respectively.

e. Reanalyze the data after combining the higher two smoking categories (i.e., LS and HS). Calculate $c\hat{O}R$ and $m\hat{O}R$. Also, test the association by using a Mantel-Haenszel statistic. Compare these results to the findings in parts a–d.

f. What proportion of acute MIs in the study population is due to cigarette smoking? Note: You should compute an adjusted etiologic fraction ($m\hat{E}F$) based on controlling for SS; use the formula

$$m\hat{E}F = \frac{a}{m_1}\left(\frac{m\hat{O}R - 1}{m\hat{O}R}\right)$$

where a/m_1 is the proportion of the total number of cases who smoke, and $m\hat{O}R$ is the value computed in part e.

g. Compute a 95% test-based confidence interval for mEF, using the results of part e. Assume that $(1 - m\hat{E}F)$ is lognormally distributed; use the Mantel statistic from part d, not the Mantel-Haenszel statistic from part e.

17.6 This problem considers various methods for testing for interaction, using stratified data. The two examples in Exercise Table 17.6 (from Mantel et al., 1977) will be used to illustrate each method.

Exercise Table 17.6

a. Example 1

	STRATUM 1				STRATUM 2		
	E	$\overline{E}$			E	$\overline{E}$	
D	100	15	115	D	5	15	20
$\overline{D}$	5	20	25	$\overline{D}$	5	400	405
	105	35	140		10	415	425
	$\hat{OR}_1 = 26.67$				$\hat{OR}_2 = 26.67$		

b. Example 2

	STRATUM 1				STRATUM 2		
	E	$\overline{E}$			E	$\overline{E}$	
D	95	405	500	D	375	125	500
$\overline{D}$	5	495	500	$\overline{D}$	125	375	500
	100	900	1,000		500	500	1,000
	$\hat{OR}_1 = 23.22$				$\hat{OR}_2 = 9.00$		

From a visual comparison of the estimated stratum-specific odds ratios, there is apparently no interaction in the data of Example 1 but considerable interaction in the Example 2 data.

a. Zelen (1971) suggested a procedure for testing the null hypothesis of uniformity of stratum-specific odds ratios. His test statistic is given by the formula

$$\chi^2_{\text{Zelen}} = \sum_{g=1}^{G} \chi^2_{\text{MH},g} - \chi^2_{\text{MHS}}$$

where $\chi^2_{MH,g}$ is the Mantel-Haenszel chi-square for the gth stratum and χ^2_{MHS} is the Mantel-Haenszel chi-square for stratified data (as given by Equation 17.2). Under the null hypothesis of uniformity in stratum-specific odds ratios, Zelen claims that this test statistic has approximately a chi-square distribution with $(G - 1)$ degrees of freedom.

   Using the following information (you may wish to verify these numbers), calculate Zelen's test statistic for each example and comment on the results.

Example 1: $\chi^2_{MH,1} = 48.75$ $\chi^2_{MH,2} = 46.74$ $\chi^2_{MHS} = 77.40$

Example 2: $\chi^2_{MH,1} = 89.91$ $\chi^2_{MH,2} = 249.75$ $\chi^2_{MHS} = 339.67$

b. Fleiss (1973) suggested an alternative procedure for testing uniformity of effect (which he attributes to Yates). His test statistic is based on the use of the "standardized difference" (instead of the odds ratio) as the effect measure. With the usual data layout for the gth stratum (Table 17.1a), the stratum-specific standardized difference ($\hat{\Delta}_g$) is defined as follows:

$$\hat{\Delta}_g = (a_g d_g - b_g c_g) n_g^2 / n_{1g} n_{0g} m_{1g} m_{0g}$$

The test statistic is then

$$\chi^2_{Fleiss} = \sum_{g=1}^{G} W_g \hat{\Delta}_g^2 - \left(\sum_{g=1}^{G} W_g \hat{\Delta}_g\right)^2 \Big/ \sum_{g=1}^{G} W_g$$

where $W_g = n_{1g} n_{0g} m_{1g} m_{0g} / n_g^3$. Under the null hypothesis, this statistic may also be compared to a tabulated value of the chi-square distribution with $(G - 1)$ degrees of freedom.

   From the above information, the standardized differences and Fleiss's chi-square statistic for each of the two examples are as given in Exercise Table 17.7. How do these results compare with the results from Zelen's procedure? What would you conclude about the appropriateness of Zelen's test?

Exercise Table 17.7

	Example 1	Example 2
$\hat{\Delta}_1$	3.57	2.0
$\hat{\Delta}_2$	10.34	2.0
χ^2_{Fleiss}	18.30	0

c. In Section 17.1, another procedure for testing for uniformity of effect was mentioned (Breslow and Day, 1980). The computational form of this test statistic is given by

$$\chi_I^2 = \sum_{g=1}^{G} \frac{(a_g - a_g')^2}{\hat{\text{Var}}_0(A_g)}$$

The subscript I in χ_I^2 denotes an "interaction" test statistic, A_g is the random variable denoting the number of exposed cases in the gth stratum, and a_g is the observed value (i.e., sample realization) of A_g. Here, the fitted values a_g' satisfy the equation

$$\frac{a_g'(m_{0g} - n_{1g} + a_g')}{(m_{1g} - a_g')(n_{1g} - a_g')} = \hat{\psi}$$

$\hat{\psi}$ denotes any (adjusted) estimator of a common odds ratio, and

$$\hat{\text{Var}}_0(A_g) = \left(\frac{1}{a_g'} + \frac{1}{m_{1g} - a_g'} + \frac{1}{n_{1g} - a_g'} + \frac{1}{m_{0g} - n_{1g} + a_g'}\right)^{-1}$$

As is done with the other two test statistics, the calculated value of χ_I^2 is compared with a tabulated value of the chi-square distribution with $(G - 1)$ degrees of freedom.

Using $\hat{\psi} = \text{a}\hat{\text{OR}}$, we have computed the values in Exercise Table 17.8 for a_g' and $\hat{\text{Var}}_0(A_g)$, $g = 1, 2$ (you may wish to verify these results). On the basis of the above information, carry out the test procedure, using χ_I^2 for *each* example, and compare your results with those obtained from the other test procedures.

Exercise Table 17.8

	aÔR	a_1'	a_2'	$\hat{\text{Var}}_0(A_1)$	$\hat{\text{Var}}_0(A_2)$
Example 1	26.67	100	5	3.0612	2.1314
Example 2	9.80	89.17	378.95	9.2568	45.8719

REFERENCES

ANSCOMBE, F. J. 1956. On estimating binomial response relations. *Biometrika* 43: 461–464.

BRESLOW, N. E., and DAY, N. E. 1980. *Statistical methods in cancer research.* Lyon, France: IARC Publications; Chap. 4.

CLAYTON, D. G. 1974. Some odds ratio statistics for the analysis of ordered categorical data. *Biometrika* 61: 525–531.

COCHRAN, W. G. 1954. Some methods for strengthening the common χ^2 tests. *Biometrics* 10: 417–451.

CONOVER, W. J. 1974. Some reasons for not using the Yates continuity correction on 2 × 2 contingency tables. *J. Am. Stat. Assoc.* 69(346): 374–382.

DAYAL, H. H. 1978. On the desirability of the Mantel-Haenszel summary measure in case-control studies of multifactor etiology of disease. *Am. J. Epidemiol.* 108: 506–511.

FLEISS, J. L. 1973. *Statistical methods for rates and proportions*. New York: Wiley.

GART, J. J. 1970. Point and interval estimation of the common odds ratio in the combination of 2×2 tables with fixed margins. *Biometrika* 57: 471–475.

———. 1971. The comparison of proportions: A review of significance tests, confidence intervals and adjustments for stratification. *Rev. Int. Stat. Inst.* 39: 148–169.

———. 1979. Statistical analyses of the relative risk. *Environ. Health Perspect.* 32: 157–167.

HALDANE, J. B. S. 1955. The estimation and significance of the logarithm of a ratio of frequencies. *Ann. Hum. Genet.* 20: 309–314.

HALPERIN, M. 1977. Estimability and estimation in case-referent studies (letter to the editor). *Am. J. Epidemiol.* 105: 496–498.

HAUCK, W. W. 1979. The large sample variance of the Mantel-Haenszel estimator of a common odds ratio. *Biometrics* 35: 817–819.

KARON, J. M. 1978. The effect of scoring methods on the chi-square for contingency tables with ordinal classes. Paper presented at the annual meeting of the American Statistical Association, San Diego, Calif., August.

KATZ, D.; BAPTISTA, J.; AZEN, S. P.; and PIKE, M. C. 1978. Obtaining confidence intervals for the risk ratio in cohort studies. *Biometrics* 34(3): 469–474.

KUPPER, L. L., and HOGAN, M. D. 1978. Interaction in epidemiologic studies. *Am. J. Epidemiol.* 108(6): 447–453.

LI, S.; SIMON, R. M.; and GART, J. J. 1979. Small sample properties of the Mantel-Haenszel test. *Biometrika* 66: 181–183.

MANTEL, N. 1963. Chi-square tests with one degree of freedom: Extensions of the Mantel-Haenszel procedure. *J. Am. Stat. Assoc.* 58: 690–700.

———. 1974. Comment and a suggestion. *J. Am. Stat. Assoc.* 69: 378–380.

MANTEL, N.; BROWN, C.; and BYAR, D. P. 1977. Tests for homogeneity of effect in an epidemiologic investigation. *Am. J. Epidemiol.* 106(2): 125–129.

MANTEL, N., and FLEISS, J. L. 1980. Minimum expected cell size requirements for the Mantel-Haenszel one-degree of freedom chi-square test and a related rapid procedure. *Am. J. Epidemiol.* 112(1): 129–134.

MANTEL, N., and HAENSZEL, W. 1959. Statistical aspects of the analysis of data from retrospective studies of disease. *J. Nat. Cancer Inst.* 22(4): 719–748.

MIETTINEN, O. S. 1968. The matched pairs design in the case of all-or-none responses. *Biometrics* 24: 339–352.

———. 1969. Individual matching with multiple controls in the case of all-or-none responses. *Biometrics* 22: 339–355.

———. 1972. Standardization of risk ratios. *Am. J. Epidemiol.* 96(6): 383–388.

———. 1974. Confounding and effect modification. *Am. J. Epidemiol.* 100: 350–353.

RADHAKRISHNA, S. 1965. Combination of results from several 2×2 contingency tables. *Biometrics* 21: 86–98.

ROTHMAN, K. J., and BOICE, J. D. 1979. *Epidemiologic analysis with a programmable calculator*. NIH Publ. No. 79–1649. Washington, D.C.: Government Printing Office.

STARMER, C. F.; GRIZZLE, J. E.; and SEN, P. K. 1974. Comment. *J. Am. Stat. Assoc.* 69: 376.

THOMAS, D. G. 1975. Exact and asymptotic methods for the combination of 2×2 tables. *Comput. Biomed. Res.* 8: 423–446.

WOOLF, B. 1955. On estimating the relation between blood group and disease. *Ann. Hum. Genet.* 19: 251–253.

ZELEN, M. 1971. The analyses of several 2×2 contingency tables. *Biometrika* 58: 129–137.

18

Matching in
Epidemiologic Studies

**18.0
PREVIEW**

In Chapter 16, when discussing options for the control of extraneous factors, we pointed out that efforts to control confounding could be made both at the design stage of a study (e.g., by employing some type of subject selection procedure like restriction) and at the analysis stage (e.g., by using stratification or multivariable-modeling techniques). In this chapter we discuss a popular method of subject selection called *matching,* which has often been used by epidemiologists for the express purpose of controlling confounding.

The widely held belief that matching is a panacea for confounding has resulted in its misuse in many epidemiologic research studies, especially case-control studies. In the discussion to follow, we will explain what purpose matching serves with regard to the control of confounding, and we will point out, with some carefully chosen numerical examples, the advantages and disadvantages of matching with respect to statistical efficiency (e.g., as reflected in precision in effect estimation and power in hypothesis testing). In considering these numerical examples, we will also illustrate the appropriate methods for analyzing certain types of matched data.

**18.1
DEFINITION
OF
MATCHING**

Matching involves the employment of constraints in the selection of the *referent* (or *comparison*) *group,* which is the unexposed ($\overline{E}$) group in a follow-up study or the control ($\overline{D}$) group in a case-control study. These constraints are aimed at making this referent group similar to the *index group* (i.e., the E group in a follow-up study or the D group in a case-control study) with respect to the distributions of one or more *potentially confounding factors.* [Note: By a "potential confounder," we mean a risk factor (see Chapter 13) that a priori can be expected to manifest itself as a confounder in data representative of the population (e.g., in data chosen by random sampling).]

Thus, matching is a type of *partial restriction* on subject selection, partial in the sense that only the referent group is chosen in accord with certain constraints. In particular, the usual data-gathering approach is, first, to select a group of index subjects (e.g., by randomly sampling the population of candidate index subjects) and then to restrict the choice of referents in order to ensure that the two groups are similar with respect to the observed distributions, in the index group, of certain important extraneous factors. Clearly, then, a matched referent group will be more similar to the observed index group than to the original population of candidate referent subjects. We use the word "similar" rather than "identical" because the index and matched referent groups will generally not be identically distributed after matching—nor do they need to be. The degree of similarity will depend on the type and the extent of matching employed.

**18.2
TYPES OF
MATCHING
SCHEMES**

To discuss types of matching schemes, we must distinguish between matching on *continuous variables* (e.g., age, weight, blood pressure) and matching on *categorical variables* (e.g., gender, race). (Of course, any continuous variable can be categorized and treated as such.)

Matching on some continuous variable (say X) necessitates the specification of a rule for deciding when an index subject's value (say X_1) and a referent subject's value (say X_0) for this variable are "close enough" to declare the two subjects to be matched. One recommended procedure is known as *caliper matching;* one specifies a caliper (or tolerance) c and then declares the index and referent subjects to be matched if $|X_1 - X_0| \le c$. If c is very small (i.e., quite close to zero), the tighter the match will be on X—but, correspondingly, the more difficult it will be to find pairs of subjects to satisfy the stringent matching criterion. An analytical investigation of the properties of this procedure and others (e.g., nearest-neighbor matching) for matching on continuous variables is discussed in Raynor and Kupper (1977); other related discussions are given by Billewicz (1965) and Rubin (1973).

We will not pursue further the issues associated with matching on continuous variables, since, in standard epidemiologic practice, variables are often categorized for purposes of matching. (But note that caliper matching defines categories for X of width c, with each such category possibly containing only one pair of subjects if c is small enough.)

For the remainder of this chapter, we will focus on *category matching*. Under this procedure, variables to be matched on are either inherently categorical (e.g., race, gender) or are made to be categorical (e.g., age in five-year groupings). Index and referent subjects are said to be matched on a variable if they are in the same category of that variable. (Note that the properties of the matching process are affected by the way the categories are defined, as is true for any type of stratification-based procedure.) When, as is often the case, category matching is done on several variables at once, index and referent subjects are said to be matched when they are in the same category for each and every one of the matching variables under consideration. For example, a subset of all subjects matched on age, race, and gender might consist of black females between the ages of 40 and 44. For stratified analysis purposes, this subset would be considered as a single stratum, even though it involves a combination of categories for three distinct matching variables.

The popular technique of *pair matching* refers to the special situation when each stratum is assumed, for analysis purposes, to contain exactly one index subject and one referent subject. However, this assumption will generally lead to an inefficient stratified analysis when the pairing is artificial and thus unnecessary. For example, it is common practice to associate each index subject with a *single* referent subject of the same age (category), race, and sex. However, within each stratum, as defined by combinations of categories of these factors (e.g., black females, ages 40–44), any member of the index group could be paired up with any member of the referent group without altering the basic within-stratum structure. Retaining such "random" pairing in the analysis is clearly unwarranted and leads to a chi-square statistic value that is slightly smaller than the appropriate one involving fewer strata (see Lewis, 1980). We will illustrate, with some numerical examples, the loss in efficiency due to such overmatching. McKinlay (1977) and Kupper and colleagues (1981) also provide discussions regarding the advantages and disadvantages of pair matching.

Performing a matched pairs analysis is justifiable only when the number of matching variables is large enough (or the categorization is refined enough) so that most, or all, of the individual strata will contain only one index subject and one referent subject. In some instances, statistical efficiency can be slightly improved by discarding referent subjects until each stratum contains only a single pair, especially when the number of referents per stratum varies considerably among those strata containing more than one referent.

One final comment on pair matching: The pairs referred to in the above discussion need to be distinguished from so-called naturally occurring pairs (e.g., twins, halves of the same material, etc.). For naturally occurring pairs, there is an inherent relationship (or dependency) over and above that artificially introduced by simply comparing, through stratified analysis, pairs of individuals who are similar with respect to the values of certain extraneous factors.

A generalized form of pair matching is a procedure known as R-to-1 matching, where each stratum is considered to contain one index subject and exactly R referent subjects; the special case $R = 1$ is, of course, pair matching. We will have more to say about R-to-1 matching later on in this chapter, especially with regard to the proper choice for R.

In the most general category-matching situation, a particular stratum (say the gth) may contain R_g referent subjects and S_g index subjects, giving a *matching ratio* of R_g/S_g (which is not necessarily an integer). If this matching ratio varies with g, then we have a *variable–matching ratio plan*. If the matching ratio does not vary over the strata (e.g., R-to-1 matching), then we have a *fixed–matching ratio plan*. With either plan, the appropriate stratified analysis would still accumulate intrastratum information; in terms of statistical efficiency, however, a fixed–matching ratio plan is usually more desirable.

18.3 ADVANTAGES AND DISADVANTAGES OF CATEGORY MATCHING

In this section, we discuss, in a general way, some of the pros and cons associated with the use of category matching as a method of subject selection in epidemiologic research studies. We will defer our quantitative discussion of statistical validity and efficiency until Section 18.4.

Some of the *benefits* associated with category matching can accrue in the following situations:

1. Matching on variables like sibship or neighborhood of residence can lead to efficient adjustment for the potentially confounding effects of a wide range of social and economic factors that would be difficult, if not impossible, to measure and hence to control. Matching on such surrogates, even when unnecessary, often promotes a feeling of security and so has something to recommend it on political grounds. (Of course, the indiscrim-

inate use of such matching is to be avoided, because it is possible to "match out" an important association of interest, like one involving an economic, environmental, or social risk factor correlated with such surrogates.) Matching on multiple-valued factors such as sibship or area of residence— or, indeed, on any variable whose values constitute a complex nominal scale—would reduce the variability over strata with regard to the ratio of the number of comparison subjects to the number of index subjects. This reduction would be particularly true when dealing with small sample sizes. As we have pointed out, such variability in the matching ratio can lead to inefficient analyses and even to completely uninformative strata.

2. Matching is sometimes the obvious sampling method of choice with regard to savings in time and money. For example, when the cases in a case-control study are chosen from medical records in different hospitals or in different companies within some industry, it is preferable, for reasons of simplicity and convenience in data collection (and also possibly on validity and efficiency grounds), to choose controls for each case from that same set of hospital or company records. One can then check, at the analysis stage, whether hospital-to-hospital or company-to-company differences need to be taken into account statistically (i.e., whether the grouping of cases and controls by hospital or by company must be retained in the analysis).

3. Matching in the selection of the referent group with respect to a given set of potential confounders does not preclude controlling for other confounding factors that show up during data analysis. In other words, one can match on risk factors considered a priori to be highly likely to manifest themselves as strong confounders in the data, and still retain the flexibility to adjust (if necessary) for other factors at the analysis stage. This feature will be illustrated by example in Chapter 24.

4. Category matching a set of referent subjects to a sample of index subjects (e.g., obtained by random sampling) can often lead to a more statistically efficient analysis than will choosing the same number of referents by random sampling. This would be the case when the matching variables are risk factors expected to be differentially distributed between the exposed and unexposed groups in the data under random sampling (i.e., are expected to be actual confounders). For dichotomous disease and exposure variables, the expected gain in efficiency over random sampling arising from matching on a *single* dichotomous potential confounder has been demonstrated analytically by Kupper and colleagues (1981). The advantages in category matching on two possibly correlated dichotomous potential confounders have been documented by Lewis (1980). We will illustrate how this expected gain arises via a numerical example in Section 18.4. We point out (again, see Kupper and colleagues, 1981) that the magnitude of the expected gain in efficiency is more pronounced in follow-up studies than in case-control studies. Also, the size of the gain varies directly with the strength of the relationship between the potential con-

founder and disease status (i.e., the "stronger" the risk factor being matched on, the "larger" will be the gain in efficiency over random sampling). See Samuels (1981) for further theoretical discussion on matching and design efficiency.

Some of the *negative aspects* of category matching in epidemiologic research studies are the following:

1. Matching can be a costly enterprise, both with regard to the *direct* costs of time and labor required to find the appropriate matches and the *indirect* costs (in terms of information loss) due to the discarding of available referents not able to satisfy the matching criteria. In fact, when the category-matching constraints are so demanding that they result in a 50% or more reduction in the size of the matched referent group relative to that available under random sampling [which, according to McKinlay (1977) is not an unrealistic possibility], then random sampling can become the more statistically efficient method of subject selection (e.g., see Kupper et al., 1981; Lewis, 1980).

2. The referent group chosen by matching ends up being more like the index group than like the underlying population of referents being sampled, whereas a randomly sampled referent group would tend to reflect the characteristics of the underlying referent population. In particular, matching generally precludes the evaluation of the underlying population relationships between the matching variables and exposure status in a follow-up study or between the matching factors and disease status in a case-control study.

3. Category matching in case-control studies can sometimes lead to a loss in efficiency relative to random sampling. The extent of the loss depends on the strength of certain population-based associations of the matching factor with disease status and with exposure status. In particular, matching on a nonrisk factor in a case-control study invariably results in some loss in efficiency, although the magnitude of the loss is not always of importance. In any event, unnecessary matching is usually more detrimental to statistical efficiency in case-control studies than it is in follow-up studies.

The implication to be derived from this list of pros and cons is that matching can be a fruitful activity in both follow-up and case-control studies if prior knowledge about important relationships among the disease, exposure, and all potentially confounding variables is available and is used properly. When in doubt, the safest strategy is to match only on strong risk factors expected to be differentially distributed between the exposed and unexposed study subjects. Cost and logistic considerations also need to be taken into account when entertaining the idea of matching on one or more extraneous factors.

In this section, we will provide a numerical example to illustrate how category matching can lead to a gain in statistical efficiency over random sampling when matching on a potential confounder in follow-up or case-control studies. We will focus on the special situation involving a dichotomous disease variable (with D and $\bar{D}$ denoting the presence and absence of disease, respectively), a dichotomous exposure variable (with levels E and $\bar{E}$), and a *single* dichotomous matching factor f (with levels F_0 and F_1). In addition, we will ignore cost considerations.

**18.4
CATEGORY
MATCHING:
VALIDITY
AND
EFFICIENCY**

Although this setting is, admittedly, the simplest one we can consider, it will nevertheless be sufficient to illustrate the salient points regarding validity and efficiency we wish to make. Furthermore, it is not so naive a setting as to rule out generalizing many of the principles to more complex situations involving several matching factors, and the simplicity has the obvious advantage of making the discussion easier to understand.

Our numerical illustration will involve comparing Mantel-Haenszel χ_1^2 test statistics and various confidence intervals, computed by using sample 2×2 tables *expected* from random sampling and category matching. The data from the hypothetical population is presented in Table 18.1.

This artificial population has been constructed so that f is *not* an effect modifier for either the risk ratio (RR) or the odds ratio (OR) but *is* a confounder in the population. In particular, the population crude RR is 5.14, which is substantially different from the value of 4.00 in both the F_0 and F_1 strata. Also, the crude OR value is 5.46, whereas the stratum-specific OR values are 4.125 and 4.26.

Note that f is related to disease, both unconditionally and conditionally on exposure status, and to exposure, both unconditionally and

Table 18.1 Hypothetical Population

Disease	STRATUM F_0 Exposure E	$\bar{E}$	Total	STRATUM F_1 Exposure E	$\bar{E}$	Total	TOTAL POPULATION Exposure E	$\bar{E}$	Total
D	160	480	640	1,280	640	1,920	1,440	1,120	2,560
$\bar{D}$	3,840	47,520	51,360	14,720	31,360	46,080	18,560	78,880	97,440
Total	4,000	48,000	52,000	16,000	32,000	48,000	20,000	80,000	100,000
RR	4.00			4.00			5.14		
OR	4.125			4.26			5.46		

conditionally on disease status, as shown by the following set of odds ratios:

$$OR_{df|\bar{E}} = 2.02 \qquad OR_{df|E} = 2.09 \qquad OR_{df} = 3.34$$

$$OR_{ef|\bar{D}} = 5.81 \qquad OR_{ef|D} = 6.00 \qquad OR_{ef} = 6.00$$

Here, for example, $OR_{df|\bar{E}}$ is the odds ratio quantifying the association between disease status and the factor f among the unexposed, and this odds ratio gives an indication of the strength of f as a risk factor. According to our criteria for confounding, given in Chapter 13, f is a potential confounder. If there is no effect modification with respect to RR and OR in this population, then it follows, for purely mathematical reasons, that $OR_{df|\bar{E}} = OR_{df|E}$ and that $OR_{ef|\bar{D}} = OR_{ef|D} = OR_{ef}$. Since the stratum-specific odds ratios are *not exactly* equal, these equalities hold only approximately. These equalities should be kept in mind throughout our later discussions about confounding in the data, the conditions for which involve the sample analogs of these population-based odds ratios.

In the efficiency comparisons to follow, we will assume that the index subjects are chosen through random sampling. Subjects will be selected from the referent population either by random sampling or by category matching on the factor f. We will consider the follow-up and case-control study situations separately.

18.4.1
Follow-up
Study

Consider a follow-up study to estimate RR by using 1,000 exposed and 1,000 unexposed subjects selected from the population in Table 18.1. As shown in Table 18.2, a random sample of 1,000 exposed subjects would, on expectation, yield 200 and 800 persons in strata F_0 and F_1, respectively, whereas a random sample of 1,000 unexposed subjects would (on the average) have 600 in stratum F_0 and 400 in stratum F_1. In contrast, a category matching of the unexposed group to the exposed group would necessitate selecting random samples of 200 and 800 persons from the unexposed F_0 and F_1 groups, respectively. For both random sampling and category matching, the expected numbers of subjects in the 2×2 tables showing the relation between exposure and disease in each stratum are given in Table 18.2. The expected data from random sampling will, of course, exactly mimic the population structure given in Table 18.1.

Category Matching Versus Random Sampling Results

Table 18.3 gives the risk ratio estimates, associated Mantel-Haenszel χ_1^2 statistic values, and the 95% large-sample precision-based (with Taylor series–computed weights) confidence intervals.

As we mentioned earlier in this chapter, the stratified analysis methods discussed in Chapter 17 are appropriate for category-matched data as

Table 18.2   Follow-up Study to Estimate Risk Ratio; Expected Cell Counts

a. Unexposed Chosen by Random Sampling

	STRATUM F_0			STRATUM F_1			TOTAL		
	Exposure			Exposure			Exposure		
Disease	E	$\overline{E}$	Total	E	$\overline{E}$	Total	E	$\overline{E}$	Total
D	8	6	14	64	8	72	72	14	86
$\overline{D}$	192	594	786	736	392	1,128	928	986	1,914
Total	200	600	800	800	400	1,200	1,000	1,000	2,000

b. Unexposed Chosen by Category Matching on f

	STRATUM F_0			STRATUM F_1			TOTAL		
	Exposure			Exposure			Exposure		
Disease	E	$\overline{E}$	Total	E	$\overline{E}$	Total	E	$\overline{E}$	Total
D	8	2	10	64	16	80	72	18	90
$\overline{D}$	192	198	390	736	784	1,520	928	982	1,910
Total	200	200	400	800	800	1,600	1,000	1,000	2,000

Table 18.3   Statistics Related to the Estimation of Risk Ratio

Choice of Unexposed	RISK RATIO ESTIMATES				95% Confidence Intervals for aRR	χ_1^2 Values
	Crude	For F_0	For F_1	$a\hat{R}R$		
Random sampling	5.14	4.00	4.00	4.00	(2.20, 7.26)	23.83
Category matching	4.00	4.00	4.00	4.00	(2.41, 6.65)	33.98

well as for data obtained via random sampling, with the strata defined a priori (i.e., before sampling) by the various combinations of categories of the matching factors. In our particular example, we have two strata, and the use of Formula 17.2 for the matched data in Table 18.2 yields

$$
\chi^2_{MHS} = \frac{\left\{\left[\dfrac{8(198) - 2(192)}{400}\right] + \left[\dfrac{64(784) - 16(736)}{1,600}\right]\right\}^2}{\dfrac{(200)(200)(10)(390)}{(400 - 1)(400)^2} + \dfrac{(800)(800)(80)(1,520)}{(1,600 - 1)(1,600)^2}} = 33.98
$$

With regard to the interval estimation of RR, it is reasonable to compute the precision-based estimator $a\hat{R}R$ since there is uniformity of effect across strata. In particular, if $\hat{R}R_g$ denotes the estimator of RR in stratum F_g, then

$$
\ln(a\hat{R}R) = (W_0 \ln \hat{R}R_0 + W_1 \ln \hat{R}R_1)/(W_0 + W_1)
$$

where W_g is an estimator of $[\text{Var}(\ln \hat{R}R_g)]^{-1}$, the reciprocal of the variance of $\ln \hat{R}R_g$. From Expression 17.18 and Table 17.16, the corresponding large-sample 95% confidence interval for RR (using Taylor series–based weights) is of the general form

$$
(a\hat{R}R) \exp(\pm 1.96/\sqrt{W_0 + W_1})
$$

where

$$
W_g = \left(\frac{c_g}{n_{1g}a_g} + \frac{d_g}{n_{0g}b_g}\right)^{-1}
$$

For the matched data in Table 18.2, we have

$$
W_0 = \left[\frac{(192)}{(200)(8)} + \frac{(198)}{(200)(2)}\right]^{-1} = 1.626
$$

$$
W_1 = \left[\frac{(736)}{(800)(64)} + \frac{(784)}{(800)(16)}\right]^{-1} = 13.223
$$

So the 95% confidence interval is

$$
(4.00) \exp(\pm 1.96/\sqrt{1.626 + 13.223})
$$

or $(2.405, 6.652)$. For comparison, the test-based interval is

$$
(4.00)^{(1 \pm 1.96/\sqrt{33.98})} \qquad \text{or} \qquad (2.510, 6.375)
$$

Observations and Interpretations

From Table 18.3, a comparison of the appropriate Mantel-Haenszel χ^2_1 statistic and confidence interval for random sampling (whose computation requires stratification because of the confounding present) with the corresponding values computed above for the matched data clearly indicates that category matching leads to a more precise estimate of the population RR than does random sampling. More detailed studies we have made (see Kupper et al., 1981) show that category matching on potential confounders generally results in an increase in precision relative to random sampling in follow-up studies, provided that the matching requirements are not so stringent as to result in a severe reduction (say 50% or more) in the size of the unexposed group relative to that for random sampling. It is worth pointing out here that the decision to match or not match in both follow-up and case-control studies is one that should be motivated mainly by efficiency considerations, since a proper analysis (e.g., stratification) ensures validity regardless of whether category matching or random sampling is the method of subject selection. (Of course, this statement assumes that other types of bias, as described in Chapters 10–12, are not present.)

Another important observation to be made here is that the crude risk ratio for the matched data is 4.00, which means that there is no confounding in these data with regard to estimating the risk ratio. This result is not surprising, since category matching on f has ensured that the *sample* unconditional odds ratio relating f and exposure, namely, $\widehat{OR}_{ef}$, will have the value one in the matched data (see Table 18.2). And, as we know (see Chapter 13), this is one of the conditions for no confounding when the risk ratio is the effect measure. Note that category matching on f in a follow-up study precludes examining the true exposure-factor f relationship in the underlying population; e.g., $OR_{ef} = 6.00$ for the population in Table 18.1, but $\widehat{OR}_{ef} = 1$ in the matched sample. On the other hand, the matched sample odds ratios relating disease and the factor f, *conditionally* on exposure status, will still reflect (on the average) the corresponding population values, since the E and $\bar{E}$ groups (and *not* the D and $\bar{D}$ groups) are being matched. As one might anticipate, the opposite is true for case-control studies, since the D and $\bar{D}$ groups are involved in the matching process.

Rationale for Performing a Stratified Analysis

The reader may be wondering why we bothered to perform a stratified analysis after a category matching of the unexposed group to the exposed group with respect to the risk factor f had been done. The matching process itself has ensured that the crude risk ratio for the matched data will provide the correct *point estimate* of the population RR (given the no effect modification assumption). Nevertheless, a stratified analysis is required for both precision and validity reasons.

With regard to precision, a stratified analysis (which takes the matching into account) can be shown to be slightly more statistically efficient than the crude analysis (which ignores the matching). This result occurs because the risk factor f, even though not a confounder in the data, is still predictive of the disease. For our example, the 95% confidence interval for RR, based on the combined table after matching, is (2.404, 6.654), which is just a shade wider than the stratified analysis–based interval. In addition, the matched sample crude χ_1^2 value of 33.91 is slightly less than the stratified analysis–based value of 33.98.

The argument for preferring the stratified analysis on validity grounds, although somewhat subtle, goes as follows. As we pointed out in Chapter 15, the crude Mantel-Haenszel χ_1^2 value is directly proportional to the quantity $(ad - bc)^2$, so that the closer the crude odds ratio is to one, the smaller will be the crude χ_1^2 value. Furthermore, since the crude odds ratio calculated from the combined table after matching can be shown to be slightly biased toward the null value of one when $\hat{OR}_{ef|\bar{D}} \neq 1$, it follows that the crude χ_1^2 value will be slightly lower than the value based on stratification when $\hat{OR}_{ef|\bar{D}} \neq 1$. Fortunately, this bias in follow-up studies is generally small. In particular, for the special case of a single dichotomous factor f, $\hat{OR}_{ef|\bar{D}} = \hat{OR}_{ef|D} = \hat{OR}_{ef}$ under uniformity in the odds ratio, and matching ensures that $\hat{OR}_{ef} = 1$. (Again, see Table 18.2 for a numerical illustration.)

Thus, even though both the loss in precision and the amount of bias are usually very small when using the crude analysis, the stratified analysis is still to be preferred. As we will see in Section 18.4.2, the bias in the crude exposure odds ratio after matching in case-control studies is somewhat more pronounced, because $\hat{OR}_{ef|\bar{D}}$ reflects (on the average) the population-based odds ratio $OR_{ef|\bar{D}}$, which could be large.

Matched Pairs Analysis Results

To complete our discussion of the follow-up study, let us suppose that a matched pairs analysis is employed (see the discussion in Section 18.2). The distribution of the expected numbers of pairs is given in Table 18.4. Here, u_{11} is the number of exposed-unexposed pairs in which both members develop the disease, u_{10} is the number of such pairs in which the

Table 18.4 Follow-up Study Using Pair Matching; Expected Numbers of Pairs (Rounded to Integers)

Disease Status, Exposed	DISEASE STATUS, UNEXPOSED		*Total*
	D	*$\bar{D}$*	
D	$u_{11} = 1$	$u_{10} = 71$	72
$\bar{D}$	$u_{01} = 17$	$u_{00} = 911$	928
Total	18	982	1,000

exposed member develops the disease but the unexposed member does not, etc.

The *maximum likelihood estimator* of the population risk ratio (assuming uniformity) is $(u_{11} + u_{10})/(u_{11} + u_{01})$, which, in this example, has the value $72/18 = 4.00$. The McNemar χ_1^2 test statistic (e.g., see Fleiss, 1973), which can be shown to be a special case of the Mantel-Haenszel statistic when there is one index subject and one referent subject in each stratum, has the value

$$\frac{(u_{10} - u_{01})^2}{(u_{10} + u_{01})} = \frac{(71 - 17)^2}{(71 + 17)} = 33.14$$

Note that this value is slightly smaller than the stratified χ_1^2 value of 33.98 based on two strata, reflecting the slight loss in power resulting from unnecessary stratification.

Miettinen's test-based confidence interval method yields a 95% confidence interval of (2.50, 6.41). For comparison, the corresponding test-based intervals for samples in which the unexposed are selected by using random sampling and category matching are (2.29, 6.98) and (2.51, 6.38), respectively. Note that category matching is slightly more efficient than pair matching (as expected), and that random sampling of the unexposed is clearly the least efficient of the three procedures.

18.4.2 Case-Control Study

We will now consider a case-control study designed to estimate the exposure odds ratio. We will assume that a random sample of 256 diseased persons from the population in Table 18.1 is to be selected, and that an equal number of controls is to be chosen either by random sampling or by category matching on the factor f. Table 18.5 gives the expected numbers of persons in the stratum-specific 2×2 tables relating exposure and disease for these two methods of sampling the referent population.

Category Matching Versus Random Sampling Results

Estimates of the exposure odds ratio and associated statistics are presented in Table 18.6.

In contrast to the follow-up study situation, note from Table 18.6 that the category-matching process has *not* controlled confounding. The crude exposure odds ratio calculated from the matched sample is 3.70, which is substantially smaller than the precision-based aEÔR value of 4.24. This numerical result illustrates the general point that category matching in a case-control study does *not* in and of itself eliminate confounding, meaning that some sort of control of confounding (e.g., stratification) is still necessary at the analysis stage.

As we mentioned in Section 18.4.1, the reason for the discrepancy between the crude exposure odds ratio after matching and aEÔR in our

**Table 18.5   Case-Control Study to Estimate Exposure Odds Ratio;
Expected Cell Counts (Rounded to Integers)**

a. Nondiseased Chosen by Random Sampling

Disease	STRATUM F_0 Exposure			STRATUM F_1 Exposure			TOTAL Exposure		
	E	$\overline{E}$	Total	E	$\overline{E}$	Total	E	$\overline{E}$	Total
D	16	48	64	128	64	192	144	112	256
$\overline{D}$	10	125	135	39	82	121	49	207	256
Total	26	173	199	167	146	313	193	319	512

b. Nondiseased Chosen by Category Matching on f

Disease	STRATUM F_0 Exposure			STRATUM F_1 Exposure			TOTAL Exposure		
	E	$\overline{E}$	Total	E	$\overline{E}$	Total	E	$\overline{E}$	Total
D	16	48	64	128	64	192	144	122	256
$\overline{D}$	5	59	64	61	131	192	66	190	256
Total	21	107	128	189	195	384	210	302	512

Table 18.6   Statistics Related to the Estimation of Exposure Odds Ratio

Choice of Nondiseased	EXPOSURE ODDS RATIO ESTIMATES				95% Confidence Intervals for aEOR	χ_1^2 Values
	Crude	For F_0	For F_1	$a\hat{E}OR$		
Random sampling	5.43	4.17	4.20	4.20	(2.75, 6.40)	46.92
Category matching	3.70	3.93	4.30	4.24	(2.85, 6.31)	53.41

example is that $\hat{OR}_{ef|\overline{D}}$ is decidedly different from one, reflecting a similarly strong association in the population. In this regard, it is important to remember that category matching on f in a case-control study does *not* affect the *conditional* odds ratio relating exposure and f in the sense that these sample values will (on the average) reflect the corresponding population values. It should also be clear that such matching does make $\hat{OR}_{df} = 1$ and alters $\hat{OR}_{df|E}$ from the corresponding population value, thus making it impossible to validly assess the disease-factor f population relationship. Although unlikely, $\hat{OR}_{df|E}$ could be close to one after matching even when $OR_{df|E}$ is large (e.g., when f is a "strong" risk factor). Even so, the crude exposure odds ratio after matching would still be biased toward one when $\hat{OR}_{ef|\overline{D}} \neq 1$, thus necessitating a stratified analysis.

Observations and Interpretations

An inspection of Table 18.6 clearly indicates the presence of confounding in both the randomly sampled data and the category-matched data. A comparison of the appropriate stratified analyses for the two data sets in Table 18.5 indicates that a category-matched sample leads to a slightly more efficient analysis than does a random sample of the controls. This numerical result supports our earlier general statements that, from an efficiency standpoint, it is best to match on strong risk factors that are expected to be differentially distributed between the exposed and unexposed groups when representative (e.g., random) samples are chosen. Such a situation was illustrated for the population described in Table 18.1.

However, while category matching would certainly be recommended on efficiency grounds for this particular population, category matching in a case-control study is generally not as beneficial, in terms of statistical efficiency, as it is in a follow-up study. Even when one is matching on a risk factor in a case-control study, it is possible to lose efficiency relative to random sampling, with the size of the loss depending on the strength of the associations of the matching factor with disease and with exposure in the underlying population. In the extreme case when f is not a risk factor, so that $OR_{df|E} = 1$, category matching in a case-control study invariably results in some loss in efficiency, although the magnitude of the loss is often small. In contrast, no gain or loss in efficiency will result when matching on a nonrisk factor in a follow-up study.

In summary, the safest strategy in case-control studies is to match only on potential confounders that are known to be *strong* risk factors, since unnecessary matching is more likely to yield a loss in efficiency relative to random sampling in case-control studies than it is in follow-up studies. Of course, this statement assumes that there will be sufficient data available to control efficiently at the analysis stage for other confounders not matched on at the design stage; such analyses will be illustrated in Chapter 24. Also, it is important to remember that cost considerations have been ignored, and any conclusions regarding the relative efficiency of category matching to random sampling will be altered when, for example, matching constraints result in a reduction in the number of available referents relative to random sampling (see Kupper et al., 1981).

Matched Pairs Analysis Results

To complete our discussion of case-control studies, let us suppose that a matched pairs analysis is performed. The distribution of the expected numbers of pairs is given in Table 18.7.

Table 18.7   Case-Control Study Using Pair Matching; Expected Numbers of Pairs (Rounded to Integers)

Exposure Status, Diseased	EXPOSURE STATUS, NONDISEASED		*Total*
	E	*$\bar{E}$*	
E	$v_{11} = 42$	$v_{10} = 102$	144
$\bar{E}$	$v_{01} = 24$	$v_{00} = 88$	112
Total	66	190	256

The maximum likelihood estimator of the exposure odds ratio is given as the ratio of the off-diagonal elements, namely, v_{10}/v_{01}, which has the value $102/24 = 4.25$. The McNemar χ_1^2 statistic, which is the Mantel-Haenszel χ_1^2 when each stratum contains exactly one case and one control, has the general form $(v_{10} - v_{01})^2/(v_{10} + v_{01})$. Its value for the data in Table 18.7 is $(102 - 24)^2/(102 + 24) = 48.28$, which (as expected) is smaller than the Mantel-Haenszel two-strata value of 53.41.

A 95% test-based confidence interval for EOR is (2.82, 6.39). For comparison, the corresponding intervals (based on *not* rounding the expected cell counts to whole numbers) for random sampling and category matching are (2.79, 6.41) and (2.88, 6.25), respectively. Thus, a stratified analysis using two strata after matching is slightly better than a matched pairs analysis, and both of these are, in turn, just slightly more efficient than stratification after a random sampling of the controls.

**18.4.3
Summary of
Results**

Kupper and colleagues (1981) have conducted a theoretical and numerical evaluation of the relative efficiency of category matching to random sampling, taking into account the possible loss in efficiency from a reduction in the size of the available matched referent group due to matching constraints. The analysis comparisons that were made are summarized in Table 18.8. For each sampling method and study design, the type of analysis required to obtain a valid and most precise estimate of the effect measure is given.

Our conclusions concerning the preferred sampling strategy for choosing the referent group, based solely on statistical considerations and assuming no relationship between the method of sampling and the size of the referent group, are summarized in Table 18.9.

In contrast to some of the conclusions in Table 18.9, choosing the referent group by random sampling may be advantageous when matching results in a substantial loss in the available number of referents. This situation may occur when a matched referent group is no more than 40% to 50% of the size of a randomly sampled referent group when estimating the risk ratio in a follow-up study, or is less than 50% to 65% of the size when estimating the exposure odds ratio in a case-control study.

Table 18.8   Recommendations for Analysis Based on Validity and Precision, by Study Design, Population Associations, and Method of Sampling

		SELECTION OF THE COMPARISON GROUP	
Study Design	*Presence of Confounding and Population Associations*	*Category Matching*	*Random Sampling*
Follow-up (using RR)	No: $OR_{ef} = 1$, $OR_{df|\bar{E}} \neq 1$	Stratified[a]	Stratified[a]
	No: $OR_{df|\bar{E}} = 1$	Unstratified[b]	Unstratified
	Yes: $OR_{ef} \neq 1$, $OR_{df|\bar{E}} \neq 1$	Stratified[a]	Stratified
Case-control (using OR)	No: $OR_{ef|\bar{D}} = 1$	Unstratified[b]	Unstratified
	No: $OR_{ef|\bar{D}} \neq 1$, $OR_{df|\bar{E}} = 1$	Stratified	Unstratified
	Yes: $OR_{ef|\bar{D}} \neq 1$, $OR_{df|\bar{E}} \neq 1$	Stratified	Stratified

[a]The unstratified data provide a valid point estimate of the RR. A stratified analysis can be more efficient.
[b]The unstratified and stratified data yield the same estimate for $Var(\ln \hat{R}R)$ or $Var(\ln \hat{O}R)$. However, the Mantel-Haenszel chi-square for the stratified data is slightly smaller than that for the unstratified data.

Table 18.9   Summary of Conclusions About Efficiency Based on Comparisons in Table 18.8 (Cost Considerations Ignored)

Study Type	*No Population Confounding*	*Population Confounding*
Follow-up	$OR_{ef} = 1$ or $OR_{df|\bar{E}} = 1$; no expected gain or loss from matching	$OR_{ef} \neq 1$ and $OR_{df|\bar{E}} \neq 1$; expected gain from matching
Case-control	$OR_{ef|\bar{D}} = 1$; no expected gain or loss from matching	$OR_{ef|\bar{D}} \neq 1$ and $OR_{df|\bar{E}} \neq 1$; expected gain from matching when EOR and exposure rates are small to moderate; expected loss from matching when EOR and exposure rates are large
	$OR_{ef|\bar{D}} \neq 1$ and $OR_{df|\bar{E}} = 1$; expected loss from matching when EOR and exposure rates are large	

18.5
***R*-TO-1**
MATCHING

As we discussed in Section 18.2, R-to-1 matching refers to the situation where each stratum, for analysis purposes, contains one index subject and exactly R referent subjects. Since R-to-1 matching is used quite often by epidemiologists, we devote some time to discussing the typical analysis of such data, which is a straightforward special case of the general Mantel-Haenszel stratified analysis methodology.

18.5.1
Analysis
Methods

In the general R-to-1 matched data layout, we have G strata, each of which consists of R members of the referent group and one member of the index group. For the gth stratum based on, say, a case-referent study with dichotomous disease and exposure factors, the 2×2 table would appear as follows:

	E	$\bar{E}$	
D	Y_g	$(1 - Y_g)$	1
$\bar{D}$	X_g	$(R - X_g)$	R
			$(1 + R)$

Here, Y_g equals one if the case has the attribute E and equals zero if not; X_g is the number of referents out of R with the attribute E.

Given this layout, the Mantel-Haenszel statistic can be shown to have the special structure

$$\chi^2_{\text{MHS}} = \left(R \sum_{g=1}^{G} Y_g - \sum_{g=1}^{G} X_g \right)^2 \Bigg/$$
$$\left[(1 + R) \sum_{g=1}^{G} (X_g + Y_g) - \sum_{g=1}^{G} (X_g + Y_g)^2 \right] \qquad (18.1)$$

Note that $\sum_{g=1}^{G} Y_g$ and $\sum_{g=1}^{G} X_g$ are, respectively, the total number of cases and referents *over all G strata* possessing the attribute E, and $(X_g + Y_g)$ is the total number of subjects in the gth stratum with the attribute E.

The Mantel-Haenszel estimator of the population odds ratio is

$$\text{m}\hat{\text{OR}} = \sum_{g=1}^{G} Y_g (R - X_g) \Bigg/ \sum_{g=1}^{G} X_g (1 - Y_g) \qquad (18.2)$$

which is a special case of the general formula given in Table 17.16. For $R = 1$, m$\hat{\text{OR}}$ reduces to the matched pairs estimator of EOR given in Section 18.4.2.

EXAMPLE 18.1

As an example of the use of these formulas, we will consider data from a study by Trichopoulos and colleagues (1969), which has also been used by Miettinen (1969, 1970). The data come from a case-control study involving 18 cases with ectopic pregnancy following at least one earlier pregnancy; there were $R = 4$ controls matched to each case on the following variables: order of pregnancy, age, and husband's age. The history of induced abortions terminating any of the preceding pregnancies was recorded for the case and the referents. The data appear in Table 18.10.

For these data, $G = 18$, $R = 4$, $\sum_{g=1}^{18} Y_g = 12$, $\sum_{g=1}^{18} X_g = 16$, and $\sum_{g=1}^{18} (X_g + Y_g)^2 = 76$. Thus, using Expression 18.1, we obtain

Table 18.10   Previous History of Induced Abortion in Cases with Tubal Pregnancy and in Matched Controls

| | | CONTROL NO. | | | | | | |
Case No.	Case	1	2	3	4	Y_g	X_g	$(X_g + Y_g)^2$
1	−	−	−	−	−	0	0	0
2	+	−	+	−	−	1	1	4
3	+	−	−	−	−	1	0	1
4	−	−	−	−	−	0	0	0
5	−	+	−	−	−	0	1	1
6	+	−	−	−	−	1	0	1
7	+	−	−	−	−	1	0	1
8	−	−	−	−	−	0	0	0
9	+	+	−	−	+	1	2	9
10	+	−	+	−	−	1	1	4
11	+	−	+	+	−	1	2	9
12	−	−	−	−	−	0	0	0
13	+	+	+	+	+	1	4	25
14	+	−	−	+	−	1	1	4
15	+	−	−	+	−	1	1	4
16	+	+	−	−	−	1	1	4
17	−	−	−	−	−	0	0	0
18	+	+	−	−	+	1	2	9
Total						12	16	76

Source: Trichopoulos et al., 1969.

EXAMPLE 18.1 (*continued*)

$$\chi^2_{\text{MHS}} = \frac{[(4)(12) - (16)]^2}{[(1 + 4)(16 + 12) - (76)]} = 16$$

The value of mÔR for these data is most easily calculated after recasting the data in Table 18.10 into the following array:

NUMBER OF CONTROLS WITH ATTRIBUTE E

	$X_g = 4$	$X_g = 3$	$X_g = 2$	$X_g = 1$	$X_g = 0$
$E:Y_g = 1$	1	0	3	5	3
$\overline{E}:Y_g = 0$	0	0	0	1	5

D (to the left of the table)

It then follows (ignoring zero cells) that Formula 18.2 gives

$$\text{mÔR} = \frac{(1)(1)(4 - 4) + (3)(1)(4 - 2) + (5)(1)(4 - 1) + (3)(1)(4 - 0)}{(1)(1)(1 - 0) + (5)(0)(1 - 0)}$$

$$= 33$$

On the basis of a complex iterative method of Miettinen (1970), the conditional maximum likelihood estimate of the population odds ratio is 22.57, and his 90% confidence interval is (3.93, 210.60).

The data in Table 18.10 will be considered again in Chapter 24.

**18.5.2
What Size
Should R Be?**

Miettinen (1969) and others have shown that there is little to gain by using $R > 4$. Ury (1975) has calculated the Pitman efficiency (which is like the reciprocal of an asymptotic variance ratio) of the Mantel-Haenszel test, using R controls per case, to McNemar's test (i.e., $R = 1$), obtaining the value $2R/(R + 1)$. The table below, which gives values of $2R/(R + 1)$ as a function of R, demonstrates the "diminishing returns" phenomenon once R exceeds 4.

R	1	2	3	4	5	6	$+\infty$
$2R/(R + 1)$	1.000	1.333	1.500	1.600	1.667	1.714	2

In summary, we are in favor of category matching on potential confound-ers in both follow-up and case-control studies when reliable information, based on knowledge of the disease process and on previous research stud-ies, indicates that such factors are well-established and strong disease de-terminants (i.e., they are acknowledged to be strong risk factors). In such situations, matching will increase efficiency relative to random sampling of the referent population, with the increase being a direct function of the extent to which the matching factors are expected to be differentially dis-tributed between the exposed and unexposed subjects in the data after rep-resentative sampling.

As we pointed out earlier, a gain in efficiency from category matching is expected to be less substantial in case-control studies than in follow-up studies. In addition, matching on variables that are either weak risk factors or are not risk factors at all (i.e., overmatching) is more detrimental in terms of efficiency in case-control studies. Also, cost and logistical consid-erations cannot be ignored when decisions regarding matching are being made at the design stage of an epidemiologic investigation.

Finally, as we mentioned in Section 18.3, in a matched design, one may control or adjust at the analysis stage for factors not matched on at the design stage. In Chapter 24, we will illustrate this feature by using multi-variable analysis procedures for matched data based on the logistic model.

18.6 CONCLUDING REMARKS

The following list summarizes the key notation introduced in this chapter.   **NOTATION**

R	Number of referent subjects per matched group under a fixed matching ratio plan (e.g., $R = 1$ for pair matching).
S	Number of index subjects per matched group under a fixed matching ratio plan (e.g., $S = 1$ for pair matching).
R_i	Number of referent subjects in the ith matched group under a variable matching ratio plan.
S_i	Number of index subjects in the ith matched group under a variable matching ratio plan.

The 2×2 table data layouts for matched pairs analysis are shown on the following page.

Follow-up Study

UNEXPOSED

	D	$\overline{D}$
D	u_{11}	u_{10}
$\overline{D}$	u_{01}	u_{00}

EXPOSED

Case-Control Study

NONDISEASED

	E	$\overline{E}$
E	v_{11}	v_{10}
$\overline{E}$	v_{01}	v_{00}

DISEASED

The 2×2 table data layout for an R-to-1 matched analysis (stratum g) is as follows:

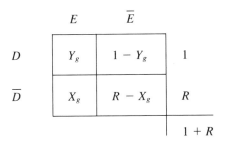

	E	$\overline{E}$	
D	Y_g	$1 - Y_g$	1
$\overline{D}$	X_g	$R - X_g$	R
			$1 + R$

$$Y_g = \begin{cases} 1 \text{ if case has attribute } E \\ 0 \text{ otherwise} \end{cases}$$

X_g = number of referents out of R who have attribute E

PRACTICE EXERCISES

18.1 Consider a hypothetical case-control study carried out to assess the association between a dichotomous study factor (with levels E and $\overline{E}$) and a particular disease. Let the gth stratum (based on stratification on one or more control variables) be represented as shown in Exercise Table 18.1.

Exercise Table 18.1

	E	$\overline{E}$	Total
D	a_g	b_g	m_{1g}
$\overline{D}$	c_g	d_g	m_{0g}
Total	n_{1g}	n_{0g}	n_g

As we described in Chapter 17, Mantel and Haenszel (1959) developed both an estimate of the population odds ratio (mOR̂) and a chi-square test of significance (with one degree of freedom). The purpose of this exercise is to develop the corresponding estimates and test statistics for certain types of matched analyses of case-control study data. It is important to realize that each matched set (e.g., one case and one control, as in pair matching) is actually a stratum. That is, matched analysis refers to a special type of stratified analysis.

a. Derive the specific form of the Mantel-Haenszel estimate of the population odds ratio (mOR̂) for a one-to-one matched data set (i.e., for pair matching). Let the data layout be represented as shown in Exercise Table 18.2. For example, there are v_{11} pairs (or strata) for which both the case and control are exposed.

Exercise Table 18.2

		$\overline{D}$		
D	E	$\overline{E}$	Total
E	v_{11}	v_{10}	$v_{1.}$
$\overline{E}$	v_{01}	v_{00}	$v_{0.}$
Total	$v_{.1}$	$v_{.0}$	$v_{..}$

b. The conditional maximum likelihood estimator of the odds ratio is v_{10}/v_{01}. Is this measure equal to the one derived in part a?

c. Derive the specific form of the mOR̂ for a two-to-one matched data set. Let the data layout be represented as shown in Exercise Table 18.3. Here, v_{ij} = the number of matched sets with i exposed cases and j exposed non-cases, $i = 0, 1$ and $j = 0, 1, 2$.

Exercise Table 18.3

		$\overline{D}$		
D	$2E$	$E/\overline{E}$	$2\overline{E}$	Total
E	v_{12}	v_{11}	v_{10}	$v_{1.}$
$\overline{E}$	v_{02}	v_{01}	v_{00}	$v_{0.}$
Total	$v_{.2}$	$v_{.1}$	$v_{.0}$	$v_{..}$

d. The maximum likelihood estimator of the odds ratio for two-to-one matching is

$$A + \sqrt{A^2 + [(v_{10} + v_{11})/(v_{01} + v_{02})]}$$

where

$$A = (4v_{10} + v_{11} - 4v_{02} - v_{01})/4(v_{01} + v_{02})$$

Is this maximum likelihood estimator equal to the estimator found in part c? (Hint: A numerical example may provide the answer.)

e. Derive the specific form of the Mantel-Haenszel chi-square statistic for a pair-matched case-control study, using the data layout given in Exercise Table 18.2. You should end up with McNemar's test statistic involving only the discordant pairs.

18.2 An investigator plans to conduct a case-control study in a county hospital in order to examine the relationship between social status (SS) and birth weight (BW), controlling for the potential confounding effect of maternal age at birth. Exercise Table 18.4 describes the *total population* of live births, giving the numbers of infants with normal birth weight (NBW) and low birth weight (LBW) (i.e., $<2,500$ gm) in 1970 by maternal age (<21 or ≥ 21) and the social status (LSS or HSS) of that parent with the greater income. Suppose the investigator identifies *all* LBW infants in 1970 and compares them to an equal number of NBW infants (with a birthweight of 2,500 gm or more) from the same hospital.

To answer the following questions, you will have to compute the expected frequencies for appropriate 2×2 tables.

Exercise Table 18.4

Weight	MATERNAL AGE < 21		MATERNAL AGE ≥ 21	
	LSS	HSS	LSS	HSS
LBW	60	20	20	20
NBW	540	540	180	540
Total	600	560	200	560

a. Assume that the NBW infants are sampled randomly from the source population (i.e., no matching). Calculate the crude odds ratio (cÔR) comparing LSS and HSS births, and compute the internally standardized odds ratio (sÔR) adjusting for maternal age. Test the statistical significance of the SS–BW association with a Mantel-Haenszel chi-square, both ignoring and controlling for maternal age. Comment.

b. Now, assume that the investigator individually matches on maternal age. Each LBW infant is paired with a randomly selected NBW infant (≥2,500 gm). Calculate the maximum likelihood estimator of the population odds ratio, using a paired analysis, and test the statistical significance of this association. Compare these results to the findings in part a. [Hint: First determine the expected cell frequencies of infants (not pairs) for each stratum of maternal age; the sums of these cell frequencies over the strata are equal to the marginals of the table involving paired observations.]

c. Suppose that the investigator uses category matching (as in part b) but then fails to stratify by maternal age in the analysis. Estimate the population odds ratio by using the unstratified data after matching. Is this estimate a valid one? Explain.

d. Compare the benefits and limitations of pairwise matching in case-control studies.

18.3 A researcher conducted a retrospective follow-up study on a group of male, blue-collar workers to assess the possible association between rotating shifts and the reporting of lower back pain (LBP). Between 1950 and 1960, 80 males were hired (by a factory in Ohio) to rotate shifts irregularly for a salary 15% more than that paid to workers of regular, steady shifts. The company utilized the rotating workers to meet the need for personnel during the three regular eight-hour shifts. Because this group was believed to be highly self-selected, the investigator felt that several potential confounders could best be controlled via a matched design. Thus, each worker on a rotating shift (R) was paired with a nonrotating worker ($\bar{R}$) on the following variables: year of birth (± 2 years), year of hire (± 2 years), age at hire (± 2 years), continuous duration of employment (ensuring that each regular worker could be followed on the job for the same number of years as the rotating worker), type of job, race, and marital status. Using company records of mandatory biannual medical exams, the investigator was able to determine which workers reported LBP during subsequent years of employment (until 1975). Exercise Table 18.5 summarizes the number of matched pairs by type of shift (R versus $\bar{R}$) and the subsequent development of LBP.

Exercise Table 18.5

		$\bar{R}$		
		LBP	$\overline{LBP}$	*Total*
R	*LBP*	20	20	40
	$\overline{LBP}$	10	30	40
	Total	30	50	80

a. Calculate the maximum likelihood estimate of the risk ratio comparing rotating shift workers to regular shift workers. Test the statistical significance of the observed association.

b. Suppose that the investigator also wished to study the relationship between one of the matched variables (e.g., type of job) and the incidence of LBP. Can this be done?

c. The statistical advantages of matching (in terms of efficiency) can more easily be realized in a follow-up design than in a case-control design. Nevertheless, matching in a case-control study is very common, while matching in a follow-up study is less common. Why?

REFERENCES   BILLEWICZ, W. Z. 1965. The efficiency of matched samples: An empirical investigation. *Biometrics* 21: 623–643.

FLEISS, J. L. 1973. *Statistical methods for rates and proportions*. New York: Wiley.

KUPPER, L. L.; KARON, J. M.; KLEINBAUM, D. G.; MORGENSTERN, H.; and LEWIS, D. K. 1981. Matching in epidemiologic studies: Validity and efficiency considerations. *Biometrics* 37(2): 271–292.

LEWIS, D. K. 1980. Matching on several variables in epidemiologic studies. Ph.D. dissertation, University of North Carolina at Chapel Hill.

MCKINLAY, S. M. 1977. Pair-matching—A reappraisal of a popular technique. *Biometrics* 33: 725–735.

MANTEL, N., and HAENSZEL, W. 1959. Statistical aspects of the analysis of data from retrospective studies of disease. *J. Natl. Cancer Inst.* 22(4): 719–748.

MIETTINEN, O. S. 1969. Individual matching with multiple controls in the case of all-or-none responses. *Biometrics* 22: 339–355.

———. 1970. Estimation of relative risk from individually matched series. *Biometrics* 23: 75–86.

RAYNOR, W. J., and KUPPER, L. L. 1977. Matching on a continuous variable in case-control studies. University of North Carolina, Institute of Statistics Mimeo Series No. 1127.

RUBIN, D. R. 1973. Matching to remove bias in observational studies. *Biometrics* 29: 159–183.

SAMUELS, M. L. 1981. Matching and design efficiency in epidemiologic studies. *Biometrika* 68: 577–588.

TRICHOPOULOS, D.; MIETTINEN, O. S.; and POLYCHRONOPOULOU, A. 1969. Induced abortions and ectopic pregnancy. Unpublished manuscript.

URY, H. K. 1975. Efficiency of case-control studies with multiple controls per case: Continuous or dichotomous data. *Biometrics* 31: 643–649.

19

Interaction, Effect Modification, and Synergism

CHAPTER OUTLINE

**19.0
PREVIEW**

The purpose of this chapter is to clarify the concepts underlying the terms interaction, effect modification, and synergism. The confusion surrounding the exact meaning and interpretation of each of these terms is evident to anyone who has been reading the current epidemiologic literature, especially the continuing discourse in the *American Journal of Epidemiology*.

Most standard dictionaries define *synergism* as "the action of separate substances that in combination produce an effect *greater* than that of any component taken alone." (*Antagonism*, the antithesis of synergism, refers to the situation when the combined effect is *less* than that of any individual effect.) An often-cited example of a supposed synergistic effect in epidemiology concerns smokers who also inhale asbestos fibers as a result of their occupation. Several epidemiologic studies (e.g., see Hammond and Selikoff, 1973) have found that such individuals apparently have a much higher risk of developing lung cancer than do individuals who are exposed to one, but not both, of these harmful agents. Epidemiologic research studies, such as those carried out to assess the combined smoking-asbestos exposure effect, provide extremely relevant data, since human beings are invariably exposed to several deleterious substances during their lifetimes.

It is no wonder, then, that epidemiologists and statisticians alike have been actively involved in developing methods for interpreting the results from epidemiologic research studies designed to provide information regarding the "synergistic" potential of different types of exposures. More specifically, a good deal of attention has been devoted to quantifying the "amount of synergism" present in data and to developing associated statistical inference-making procedures. Unfortunately, much of the work has been done without keeping in mind the subtle distinction between synergism and statistical interaction.

The term "synergism" is most appropriately reserved to the description of biologic mechanisms of action (e.g., the characterization of the mode of action of two drugs on the nervous system of mice when administered simultaneously), and information regarding such basic biologic processes is generally obtainable only through carefully designed and well-controlled laboratory experiments. In contrast, statistical interaction, which is the phenomenon that epidemiologists and statisticians have been measuring with their epidemiologic study results, concerns quantitative relationships not necessarily related to basic biologic mechanisms.

The above remarks should not be taken to mean that the assessment of interaction in such circumstances is unimportant. On the contrary, such an effect can have meaningful public health implications and can contribute to an understanding of disease etiology. The point we make here is that statistical interaction and synergism are distinctly different phenomena. Also, the statistical assessment of interaction between two different exposures, based on epidemiologic study data, can be very misleading without an awareness of certain basic mathematical facts about interaction quantification.

In the next section, we provide a brief literature review, the purpose being to give a chronological overview of the progress in conceptualizing interaction and synergy. Section 19.2 discusses the concept of synergism, and Section 19.3 presents statistical interaction and effect modification.

19.1 LITERATURE REVIEW

As early as 1974, Rothman proposed that "synergism" be defined as a deviation from a particular null state in which the joint effect of two or more (discrete) causes of disease is equal to the *sum* of the separate effects, with the effect being defined as excess risk above background. (This definition does not, in fact, pertain to synergism; it suggests an *additive model* for the state of "no interaction," as will be discussed in Section 19.3.) Rothman (1976) also proposed a ratio type of index to quantify such a deviation, and he developed associated confidence interval estimation procedures.

Hogan and colleagues (1978) reexamined and provided further insight into the rationale underlying Rothman's conceptualization (1974) and quantification (1976) of "synergism" (really, interaction). They derived simpler and more appropriate hypothesis-testing and confidence interval methods for cohort studies. Kupper and Hogan (1978) followed with a theoretical discussion on the connection between case-control and cohort study models for the assessment of interaction. They emphasized that the quantification of interaction is very much model-dependent, as was also pointed out by Miettinen (1974) and Mantel and colleagues (1977). This model dependency attribute will be illustrated dramatically in Section 19.3.

Walter and Holford (1978) further elaborated on the Kupper-Hogan discussion of additive and multiplicative models for assessing interaction, and they advocated that the choice of model should involve consideration of the causal relationships under investigation. Blot and Day (1979) argued that departure from additivity is the type of interaction effect with the most public health import. Rothman and co-workers (1980) supported this position in their paper, in which they discussed interaction from four conceptual perspectives, biological, statistical, public health, and individual decision making. Saracci (1980) has also commented on the first three of these perspectives.

This brief and qualitative review of the literature should be sufficient to convince the reader that there has been both confusion and disagreement among researchers about the meaning and interpretation of the concepts of synergism (or antagonism) and interaction. In the next few sections, we will attempt to synthesize the various ideas presented in the articles just discussed into a logical presentation of what we believe are the key principles.

19.2 SYNERGISM

We have defined synergism to be a biological response produced by simultaneous exposure to two or more agents that exceeds the combined actions of the agents when working in an "independent" manner. Although the word "independent" is admittedly vague in this context, the understanding is that synergistic agents work together mechanistically (e.g., at the cellular level) to produce an effect greater than that expected by their separate actions. It is our contention that the term "synergism" [or, as Rothman and colleagues (1980) call it, "biologic interaction"] can be characterized only in terms of experimentally verifiable biologic models describing modes of action of substances at the cellular level. In fact, we prefer *not* to involve the word "interaction" at all when describing this type of basic mechanistic phenomenon, mainly because of the confusion that has resulted from its use in this context in the past.

To reinforce our position, we cite a paper by Hamilton (1982), who has demonstrated that, under a plausible multifactor model for carcinogenesis, a 2^2 factorial experiment analyzed by using popular statistical measures of interaction (see Section 19.3) may yield little information about mechanistic synergism. In particular, a deviation from additivity in effects can occur even when the agents under study independently influence cancer initiation, on the basis of multistage theory. Another example comes from the field of molecular pharmacology (see Ashford and Cobby, 1974), where synergism has been characterized as requiring a synthesis of information from both theoretical biologic principles and basic experimental evidence. Such basic mechanistic information is not obtainable from the standard epidemiologic research study.

The goal in the statistical analysis of an epidemiologic study is to describe the relationships present in the observed data, with risk prediction often as a companion objective. As we have emphasized, this goal does not relate to the assessment of mechanistic synergism, or of causality in general, but it *need not* do so for the purpose of providing valuable information regarding both etiologic and public health concerns. As Rothman and colleagues (1980) point out by example, a multivariable risk function might be very useful for the early identification of persons at high risk for developing a certain type of cancer, even though such a function would generally not provide any information regarding mechanisms of action at the biologic level (e.g., *basic* etiology). Indeed, most or all of the important variables in such a screening function may at best be correlates of the true causes of the disease, but the model can still perform well.

In building multivariable functions for analyzing epidemiologic data, we wish to find a regression model that is as simple as possible in structure and yet is consistent with the observed data. The quantification of statistical interaction (e.g., by introducing cross-product terms into such regression models) is an important step in finding a useful statistical model, and such quantification need not be tied to specific biologic models in order to be worthwhile. However, there are numerous difficulties involved in the interpretation of statistical interaction. The next section clarifies some of the issues involved.

The main point we make in this section is as follows: *An assessment regarding the presence or absence of interaction from a set of data depends on how one defines the state of no interaction.*

The above statement has the following implications. First, the statistical quantification of interaction is very much model-dependent, since any such quantification would be expressed as a deviation from the statistical (*not* biologic) model assumed to represent the state of no interaction. Common statistical models suggested for such purposes are often *not* motivated by basic biologic considerations, and, as such, they do not aid in quantifying mechanistic synergism. Second, interaction is a characteristic of the observed data, and it should be looked upon as a manifestation of the interaction present in the population from which the data came. Such "population interaction," when involving two risk factors, has been called *effect modification* (see Miettinen, 1974). Thus, a measure of interaction for a set of data (e.g., a calculated index or a sample regression coefficient) would be used to estimate the corresponding population measure of effect modification, which is equally model-dependent. To be consistent with standard terminology, we will use the term "interaction," regardless of whether it is population-based or sample-based.

19.3 STATISTICAL INTERACTION AND EFFECT MODIFICATION

To illustrate why the assessment of interaction is model-dependent, we will focus on a simple situation. Consider two factors, A and B. Let A_1 and A_0 denote the presence and absence of A, respectively, and let B_1 and B_0 be defined similarly. We define the following probabilities (i.e., risks for developing disease):

19.3.1 Additive and Multiplicative Models

$$R_{11} = \mathrm{pr}(D|A_1B_1) \qquad R_{10} = \mathrm{pr}(D|A_1B_0)$$

$$R_{01} = \mathrm{pr}(D|A_0B_1) \qquad R_{00} = \mathrm{pr}(D|A_0B_0) = \text{background risk}$$

For example, then, R_{11} is the probability of developing disease (over some specified time period) given exposure to both factors A and B; R_{10} is the probability of developing disease given exposure to A but not to B; etc. Next, we define the corresponding risk ratios:

$$\mathrm{RR}_{11} = R_{11}/R_{00} \qquad \mathrm{RR}_{10} = R_{10}/R_{00} \qquad \mathrm{RR}_{01} = R_{01}/R_{00}$$

We can now specify, in terms of mathematical relationships among these risk ratios, the two states of no interaction that are invariably considered when analyzing epidemiologic data. The first state is "no interaction on an *additive* scale" (in terms of excesses over one), or

$$(\mathrm{RR}_{11} - 1) = (\mathrm{RR}_{10} - 1) + (\mathrm{RR}_{01} - 1) \qquad (19.1)$$

Expression 19.1 is equivalent to additivity in the attributable risks (see

Cole and MacMahon, 1971):

$$(R_{11} - R_{00}) = (R_{10} - R_{00}) + (R_{01} - R_{00}) \qquad (19.2)$$

Writing Expression 19.2 as

$$T = R_{11} - R_{10} - R_{01} + R_{00} = 0$$

we can see that considering Conditions 19.1 and 19.2 is equivalent to considering the standard analysis of variance contrast for assessing interaction in the following 2×2 table:

	B_0	B_1
A_0	R_{00}	R_{01}
A_1	R_{10}	R_{11}

Rothman's (1976) index S is

$$S = \frac{(R_{11} - R_{00})}{(R_{10} - R_{00}) + (R_{01} - R_{00})}$$

and it should be clear that S is greater than, equal to, or less than one whenever T is greater than, equal to, or less than zero. Hogan and colleagues (1978) have documented some of the statistical advantages in using the index T instead of S to assess deviations from additivity in cohort studies.

The second state is referred to as "no interaction on a *multiplicative scale*":

$$RR_{11} = RR_{10} \cdot RR_{01} \qquad (19.3)$$

Expression 19.3 can be written equivalently as

$$\ln RR_{11} = \ln RR_{10} + \ln RR_{01} \qquad (19.4)$$

which represents additivity in the natural logarithms of the risk ratios. Walter (1976) has provided motivation for considering this multiplicative formulation when quantifying interaction effects in terms of the proportions of diseased persons *attributable* to exposure to both A and B, to A but not B, and to B but not A. Bishop and colleagues (1975) have strongly advocated the use of loglinear models like (19.4) to test for interaction effects using maximum likelihood methods.

The following numerical example dramatically illustrates how one's conclusion concerning the presence or absence of interaction in a data set depends on the statistical model chosen to represent the state of no interaction.

EXAMPLE 19.1

Consider the hypothetical data in Table 19.1, which is based on a cohort follow-up study of 100 individuals in each of four exposure categories. For these data, the estimated risks (i.e., the $\hat{CI}$ values) are

$$\hat{R}_{11} = 40/100 = .40 \qquad \hat{R}_{10} = \hat{R}_{01} = 20/100 = .20$$
$$\hat{R}_{00} = 10/100 = .10$$

So, the estimated risk ratios (or cumulative incidence ratios) are

$$\hat{RR}_{11} = .40/.10 = 4 \quad \text{and} \quad \hat{RR}_{10} = \hat{RR}_{01} = .20/.10 = 2$$

Thus, since $\hat{RR}_{11} = \hat{RR}_{10} \cdot \hat{RR}_{01}$, there is no evidence of interaction on a multiplicative scale.

Table 19.1 Hypothetical Data

	A_1B_1	A_1B_0	A_0B_1	A_0B_0
D	40	20	20	10
$\bar{D}$	60	80	80	90
	100	100	100	100

However, since

$$\hat{T} = \hat{R}_{11} - \hat{R}_{10} - \hat{R}_{01} + \hat{R}_{00}$$
$$= .40 - .20 - .20 + .10 = .10$$

which is greater than zero, there is evidence of a possible interaction effect as reflected in a deviation from additivity. Methods for testing whether $\hat{T}$ is *significantly* different from zero and for finding a confidence interval for T are discussed by Hogan and colleagues (1978).

EXAMPLE 19.1 (*continued*)

In summary, these data agree exactly with Equations 19.3 and 19.4, but they deviate from the conditions specified by Expressions 19.1 and 19.2. In other words, there is no evidence of interaction under a multiplicative no-interaction model, but there is some evidence of interaction when additivity is taken as the state of no interaction. Actually, these seemingly conflicting results are to be expected. In fact, we can show mathematically that if one of the conditions 19.1 or 19.3 holds, then the other condition will not hold unless either RR_{10} or RR_{01} is equal to one. (Of course, it is possible for *neither* condition to hold in a given application.) Thus, it should be clear that an investigator must be cognizant of the definition employed for the state of no interaction before he or she can validly interpret an observed interaction effect.

The results in Example 19.1 can be related to discussions by Mantel and colleagues (1977) on testing for homogeneity of effect and by Miettinen (1974) on effect modification. Their concept of the presence or the absence of interaction pertains to whether or not a particular effect measure (e.g., a risk ratio or an odds ratio) varies in value over categories or strata based on the levels of some factor. As an illustration using our example, suppose we form the tables given in Table 19.2, which enable us to quantify (in terms of a risk ratio) the relationship between disease and exposure factor A for each of the strata defined by the two levels of factor B.

Table 19.2   Relationship Between Disease and Factor A at Different Levels of Factor B

	a. Stratum 1 (B_1)			b. Stratum 0 (B_0)	
	A_1	A_0		A_1	A_0
D	40	20	D	20	10
$\overline{D}$	60	80	$\overline{D}$	80	90
	100	100		100	100
	$\hat{RR}_{B_1} = 2$			$\hat{RR}_{B_0} = 2$	

Since $\hat{RR}_{B_1} = \hat{RR}_{B_0}$, there is uniformity in the effect measure over strata, although we have demonstrated the presence of interaction when measured as a deviation from additivity. What this result means is that an assessment regarding nonuniformity of risk ratios over strata is equivalent to an assessment regarding interaction based on a multiplicative no-interaction model. In contrast, note that the risk difference (RD) estimates are $\hat{RD}_1 = .20$ and $\hat{RD}_0 = .10$, which reflects the observed deviation from additivity.

The above discussion has focused on cohort follow-up studies, where the risk ratio RR is the effect measure. However, everything that has been said up to now is equally true for the case-control study, the only modification being that the odds ratio OR replaces the risk ratio RR in all the formulas and related conclusions. In particular, the odds ratio corresponding to

$$RR_{ij} = R_{ij}/R_{00} = \text{pr}(D|A_iB_j)/\text{pr}(D|A_0B_0)$$

is

$$OR_{ij} = \frac{R_{ij}(1 - R_{00})}{R_{00}(1 - R_{ij})} = \frac{\text{pr}(A_iB_j|D)\ \text{pr}(A_0B_0|\overline{D})}{\text{pr}(A_0B_0|D)\ \text{pr}(A_iB_j|\overline{D})}$$

for $i = 0, 1$ and $j = 0, 1$. For further details, the interested reader is encouraged to consult Kupper and Hogan (1978), who have provided a detailed discussion linking case-control and cohort follow-up study models for the assessment of interaction.

Which of the above two no-interaction conditions, additive or multiplicative, should be considered when analyzing epidemiologic data to check for the presence or absence of interaction? *For addressing public health concerns regarding disease frequency reduction, deviations from additivity appear to have the most relevance.* This opinion has also been given by Blot and Day (1979), Rothman and colleagues (1980), and Saracci (1980). On the other hand, analysis of multiplicative models often contributes to the understanding of disease etiology, as will be illustrated by example in Chapters 22–24. Also, multiplicative relationships are anticipated from a variety of basic biologic models (e.g., see Peto, 1977; Whittemore and Keller, 1978). Nevertheless, with regard to epidemiologic data, deviations from additivity can arise that have public health import, even when such data perfectly agree with a multiplicative no-interaction model.

As an example, consider the results of several published studies (see Saracci, 1977), which have suggested that the risk ratio for lung cancer following joint exposure to cigarette smoking and asbestos can be approximated by the product of the risk ratios for smoking exposure alone and asbestos exposure alone. Yet, these same sets of data reflect large positive deviations from additivity. (This result is to be expected, since

$\hat{RR}_{11} - \hat{RR}_{10} - \hat{RR}_{01} + 1$ will be greater than zero if $\hat{RR}_{11} \geq \hat{RR}_{10} \cdot \hat{RR}_{01}$ and if both $\hat{RR}_{10}$ and $\hat{RR}_{01}$ exceed one.) Thus, if the model of 19.3 is considered to represent the no-interaction state, then one would say that there is no evidence of an asbestos-smoking interaction effect. However, it is known that the excess number of people who develop lung cancer if exposed to both asbestos and cigarette smoking is much greater than the sum of excess numbers resulting from exposure to either agent alone. In such a situation, the additive model, 19.1, is obviously more appropriate than the multiplicative model, 19.3, for documenting the excess case load due to combined exposure to asbestos and cigarette smoking. It is important to note here that consideration of basic biologic modes of action is not necessary for the success of this type of epidemiologic evaluation of interaction. Departures from additivity of risk differences (or, equivalently, of excess risk ratios) should be the focus whenever public health issues are involved, no matter what the underlying biologic mechanisms might be.

19.3.2
Interaction
Assessment via
Regression
Analysis

The usual statistical approach for assessing interaction when analyzing complex epidemiologic data sets is to fit regression models that contain one or more cross-product terms (e.g., terms of the form X_1X_2, $X_1X_2X_3$, etc.). One then concludes that there is evidence of interaction if one or more of the estimated regression coefficients associated with these product terms is significantly different from zero.

Unfortunately, numerous problems can arise when using complex regression models that involve terms of an order higher than linear (e.g., squares, cubes, and cross products of variables). It has been pointed out (e.g., see McDonald and Schwing, 1973; Marquardt and Snee, 1975) that the estimated coefficients in such models (when obtained by standard least squares procedures) can take values that are far from the true parameter values being estimated (e.g., they can even have the wrong signs), and they can be extremely unstable (i.e., they can change dramatically in value even with small changes in the values of one or two data points). Because of these estimation problems, great care must be exercised in constructing multivariable statistical models for the purpose of quantifying an exposure-disease relationship in the face of confounding and interaction. These issues will be discussed further in Chapters 20–24, which deal with statistical-modeling procedures.

There is a more basic issue concerning the use of regression models to assess interaction. Not enough thought has been given to an understanding of what cross-product terms in such models really mean with regard to measuring interaction. In light of our previous discussions on additive and multiplicative models, we might ask whether a significant interaction term in a regression model is measuring a deviation from an additive or from a multiplicative state of no interaction. As we will now illustrate with a simple example, the answer depends on the form of model being fit.

Let us reconsider, in a regression analysis context, the simple situation described in Section 19.3.1, which involved factors A and B, each at two levels. Let us define the following indicator variables to index the levels of A and B in our regression models:

$$A_i = \begin{cases} 1 \text{ if } i = 1 \\ 0 \text{ if } i = 0 \end{cases} \quad \text{and} \quad B_j = \begin{cases} 1 \text{ if } j = 1 \\ 0 \text{ if } j = 0 \end{cases}$$

The two basic types of regression models typically employed to model risk when analyzing epidemiologic data are the *linear model* and the *logistic model*. If, in the notation of Section 19.3.1, $R_{ij} = \text{pr}(D|A_iB_j)$ for $i = 0, 1$ and $j = 0, 1$, then the linear model is of the general form

$$R_{ij} = \alpha + \beta A_i + \gamma B_j + \delta A_i B_j \tag{19.5}$$

In Model 19.5, α is the intercept, β and γ measure the main effects of A and B, respectively, and δ is the regression coefficient measuring the "interaction" between A and B. The reader may feel more at home with Expression 19.5 by thinking of A as a dichotomous exposure variable and B as a dichotomous extraneous factor with potential confounding and/or effect-modifying characteristics.

From the definitions of A_i and B_j and from 19.5, we have

$$R_{11} = \alpha + \beta A_1 + \gamma B_1 + \delta A_1 B_1$$

$$= \alpha + \beta(1) + \gamma(1) + \delta(1)(1) = \alpha + \beta + \gamma + \delta$$

$$R_{10} = \alpha + \beta, \qquad R_{01} = \alpha + \gamma, \qquad R_{00} = \alpha$$

Clearly, this *linear* model represents effects as being *additive* in nature, so that one might suspect that such a model would quantify interaction as a departure from additivity. This is indeed the case, since the interaction contrast T of Section 19.3.1 takes the value

$$T = R_{11} - R_{10} - R_{01} + R_{00}$$

$$= (\alpha + \beta + \gamma + \delta) - (\alpha + \beta) - (\alpha + \gamma) + \alpha = \delta$$

Thus, T is zero or nonzero when δ is zero or nonzero, and so an assessment of interaction in terms of a deviation from additivity in risk differences (or, equivalently, in excess risk ratios) could be carried out via regression analysis by testing whether the estimated regression coefficient $\hat{\delta}$ for the cross-product (or interaction) variable A_iB_j is significantly different from zero. Thus, a regression analysis based on the linear model in 19.5 would be appropriate for assessing deviations from additivity, which, as we have emphasized, bear directly on public health concerns.

Finally, note that the specific relationship between R_{ij} and A_i and B_j imposed by the linear model, Equation 19.5, is necessarily imposed for RR_{ij} as well, since R_{00} (equal to α) is just a scale factor, and thus also for OR_{ij} when $RR_{ij} \approx OR_{ij}$.

It is possible for the linear model to lead to estimated risks that are negative or greater than one in a given application, although such a result could be due more to the method of estimation of the regression coefficients than to the inappropriateness of the linear model. In contrast, the *logistic model* does not suffer from this drawback, since it specifies the following relationship between R_{ij} and A_i and B_j:

$$R_{ij} = \{1 + \exp[-(\alpha + \beta A_i + \gamma B_j + \delta A_i B_j)]\}^{-1} \qquad (19.6)$$

Thus, the odds $R_{ij}/(1 - R_{ij})$ of developing disease given exposure to level i of factor A and level j of factor B has the form

$$R_{ij}/(1 - R_{ij}) = \exp(\alpha + \beta A_i + \gamma B_j + \delta A_i B_j) \qquad (19.7)$$

In this case, the *log odds*, or *logit*, satisfies the linear law

$$\ln\left(\frac{R_{ij}}{1 - R_{ij}}\right) = \alpha + \beta A_i + \gamma B_j + \delta A_i B_j$$

This is why the logistic function, Equation 19.6, is said to be in the class of *log-linear* models (Bishop et al., 1975).

Since

$$OR_{ij} = \frac{R_{ij}/(1 - R_{ij})}{R_{00}/(1 - R_{00})}$$

it follows from Expression 19.7 that

$$OR_{ij} = \exp(\beta A_i + \gamma B_j + \delta A_i B_j)$$

Then, when $RR_{ij} \approx OR_{ij}$, we have

$$\frac{RR_{11}}{RR_{10}RR_{01}} \approx \frac{OR_{11}}{OR_{10}OR_{01}} = \frac{e^{\beta+\gamma+\delta}}{e^\beta \cdot e^\gamma} = e^\delta$$

Thus, since $OR_{11} = OR_{10} \cdot OR_{01}$ if and only if $\delta = 0$, departures from the multiplicative state of no interaction can be assessed by testing whether the estimated coefficient $\hat{\delta}$ of the product term $A_i B_j$ in the logistic model, Equation 19.6, is significantly different from zero. As we pointed out earlier, such an interaction has been called effect modification by others, including Breslow and Powers (1978).

Although the models we have considered deal with the simplest situation imaginable, a generalization can still be made. *What our findings imply is that linear models like Equation 19.5 are appropriate for detecting deviations from additivity, while logistic models like Equation 19.6 are*

useful for detecting departures from the multiplicative no-interaction state.
For related discussions on this point, see Walker and Rothman (1982).

A further implication is that one could be misled into concluding that
there is no evidence of interaction of any kind on the basis of a logistic
regression analysis when, in fact, there is considerable evidence of a
deviation from additivity (Greenland, 1979). A perfect example of such a
phenomenon would be obtained when analyzing the artificial data in Section 19.3.1 by using the logistic model, 19.6. In this situation, $\hat{\delta}$ in 19.6
would equal zero, which, as we pointed out earlier, necessarily means that
$\hat{\delta}$ in 19.5 would be positive.

More generally, $\hat{\delta} > 0$ based on fitting (19.6) implies $\hat{\delta} > 0$ when
fitting (19.5); i.e., positive interaction in the logistic model means positive
interaction in the linear model. However, a negative $\hat{\delta}$ for (19.6) leads to
no simple connection to the linear model, since it could mean antagonism,
no interaction, or even very weak positive interaction based on (19.5). See
Koopman (1981) for an excellent discussion of additive and multiplicative
models and their use in studying the interaction between discrete causes of
disease.

What does all this mean for the investigator faced with the task of
analyzing a complex epidemiologic data set? If one accepts the argument
that a deviation from additivity is the type of interaction of primary interest
in public health, then a linear model would seem to be more appropriate
than a logistic model for certain analysis purposes. In any case, we emphasize that an investigator must be fully cognizant of the assumptions, both
implicit and explicit, associated with the statistical models he or she uses;
otherwise, the investigator may completely misinterpret the relationships
in the data being analyzed.

As we have demonstrated, the methods for assessing "synergism" that are
encountered in the epidemiologic literature are related to standard statistical procedures for assessing interaction in contingency tables based on
either an additive or multiplicative model for the state of no interaction.
Thus, a statistical test of the null hypothesis of no interaction is really a test
of independence of effects of a certain *specific* type among the factors
under study. As such, interaction can be interpreted only as a departure
from the type of independence that is specified by the particular null
hypothesis or no-interaction model under consideration. If an inappropriate no-interaction state is assumed, then any observed significant
interaction may be nothing more than an indication that the wrong no-
interaction model was used.

19.4 CONCLUDING REMARKS

The following list summarizes the key notation introduced in this chapter.

NOTATION

A, B	Factors.
A_1, A_0	Presence and absence, respectively, of factor A.

B_1, B_0	Presence and absence, respectively, of factor B.
$R_{11} = \text{pr}(D\|A_1B_1)$	Risk when A and B are both present.
$R_{10} = \text{pr}(D\|A_1B_0)$	Risk when A is present and B is absent.
$R_{01} = \text{pr}(D\|A_0B_1)$	Risk when A is absent and B is present.
$R_{00} = \text{pr}(D\|A_0B_0)$	Background risk (A and B are both absent).
$\text{RR}_{11} = R_{11}/R_{00}$	Risk ratio comparing risk when both factors are present to background risk.
$\text{RR}_{10} = R_{10}/R_{00}$	Risk ratio comparing risk when only factor A is present to background risk.
$\text{RR}_{01} = R_{01}/R_{00}$	Risk ratio comparing risk when only factor B is present to background risk.
$T = R_{11} - R_{10} - R_{01} + R_{00}$	Hogan and colleagues' index.
$S = \dfrac{R_{11} - R_{00}}{(R_{10} - R_{00}) + (R_{01} - R_{00})}$	Rothman's index.
RR_{B_1}	Risk ratio measuring A–D association among persons with B present.
RR_{B_0}	Risk ratio measuring A–D association among persons with B absent.
α, β, γ, δ	Coefficients in mathematical models relating R_{ij} to A_i and B_j.

PRACTICE EXERCISES

19.1 This problem concerns a hypothetical study of infectious hepatitis (IH) in the early 1950s. In 1953, an outbreak of IH occurred in rural western Pennsylvania. An emerging theory at that time was that the probable causative agent (a virus) was contained in feces and was transmitted by fecal-oral contact among persons living in close proximity. Public health officials had already observed that IH epidemics were more common in places that had inadequate sanitation, such as crowded institutions, low-cost housing projects, and poor rural areas. Investigating epidemiologists, working for the state health department, decided to study the relationship between disease occurrence during the epidemic and the level of personal hygiene and sanitation. Familial social status (SS) was selected as a proxy indicator for the level of personal hygiene and sanitation; this measure of SS was dichotomized into "high" and "low" for analysis purposes. It was expected that the rate of IH would vary *inversely* with SS; i.e., low-SS children would be more likely to contract the disease than would high-SS children.

Of the 600 children in the outbreak area between the ages of 4 and 18, 56 developed IH during the period of the study. Exercise Table 19.1 gives the numbers of children contracting (IH) and not contracting (IH) the disease, stratified by the age of the child and by the SS of his or her parents.

a. Calculate the estimated crude and internally standardized risk ratios (namely, cR̂R and sR̂R), comparing low-SS children to high-SS children.

Exercise Table 19.1

	AGES 4–9			AGES 10–18	
	Low SS	High SS		Low SS	High SS
IH	20	7		12	17
$\overline{IH}$	80	133		188	143
N_{ij}	100	140		200	160

Test the statistical significance of the observed association, controlling for age. Is the use of the stratified MH test appropriate here?

b. Assess the evidence in the data for a possible interaction effect between age and SS, measured as a deviation from additivity. Test the statistical significance of this interaction effect by using the procedure described by Hogan and colleagues (1978). This procedure utilizes the Z statistic

$$Z = (\hat{T} - 0)/\sqrt{\hat{\text{Var}}(\hat{T})}$$

where

$$\hat{T} = \hat{R}_{11} - \hat{R}_{10} - \hat{R}_{01} + \hat{R}_{00}$$

$$\hat{\text{Var}}(\hat{T}) = \sum_{i=0}^{1} \sum_{j=0}^{1} \frac{\hat{R}_{ij}(1 - \hat{R}_{ij})}{N_{ij}}$$

It is convenient to treat high-SS children under 10 years of age as the referent or $(0, 0)$ group to which the other three groups will be compared, the $(1, 1)$ group being (low SS, 10–18 years).

c. Describe the observed associations among SS, age, and IH. Interpret any important interaction effect in terms of the original theory and the then-current (1953) knowledge of the disease.

d. If the logistic model, Equation 19.6, is fit to these data, would you expect $\hat{\delta}$ to be positive, negative, or zero? Explain.

REFERENCES

ASHFORD, J. R., and COBBY, J. M. 1974. A system of models for the action of drugs applied singly or jointly to biological organisms. *Biometrics* 30: 11–31.

BISHOP, Y. M. M.; FIENBERG, S. E.; and HOLLAND, P. W. 1975. *Discrete multivariate analysis: Theory and practice.* Cambridge, Mass.: MIT Press.

BLOT, W. J., and DAY, N. E. 1979. Synergism and interaction: Are they equivalent? *Am. J. Epidemiol.* 110(1): 99–100.

BRESLOW, N., and POWERS, W. 1978. Are there two logistic regressions for retrospective studies? *Biometrics* 34(1): 100–105.

COLE, P., and MACMAHON, B. 1971. Attributable risk percent in case-control studies. *Br. J. Soc. Prev. Med.* 25: 242–244.

GREENLAND, S. 1979. Limitations of the logistic analysis of epidemiologic data. *Am. J. Epidemiol.* 110(6): 693–698.

HAMILTON, M. A. 1982. Detection of interactive effects in carcinogenesis. *Biomet. J.* To appear in Spring, 1982.

HAMMOND, E. C., and SELIKOFF, I. J. 1973. Relation of cigarette smoking to risk of death of asbestos-associated disease among insulation workers in the United States. In *Biological effects of asbestos,* edited by P. Bogouski, J. C. Gilson, V. Timbrell, and J. C. Wagner, pp. 312–317. Lyon, France: IARC Publications.

HOGAN, M. D.; KUPPER, L. L.; MOST, B. M.; and HASEMAN, J. K. 1978. Alternatives to Rothman's approach for assessing synergism (or antagonism) in cohort studies. *Am. J. Epidemiol.* 108(1): 60–67.

KOOPMAN, J. S. 1981. Interaction between discrete causes. *Am. J. Epidemiol.* 113: 716–724.

KUPPER, L. L., and HOGAN, M. D. 1978. Interaction in epidemiologic studies. *Am. J. Epidemiol.* 108(6): 447–453.

McDONALD, G. C., and SCHWING, R. C. 1973. Instabilities of regression estimates relating air pollution to mortality. *Technometrics* 15(3): 463–481.

MANTEL, N.; BROWN, C.; and BYAR, D. P. 1977. Tests for homogeneity of effect in an epidemiologic investigation. *Am. J. Epidemiol.* 106: 125–129.

MARQUARDT, D. W., and SNEE, R. D. 1975. Ridge regression in practice. *Am. Stat.* 29(1): 3–20.

MIETTINEN, O. S. 1974. Confounding and effect modification. *Am. J. Epidemiol.* 100: 350–353.

PETO, R. 1977. Epidemiology, multistage models, and short-term mutagenicity tests. In *Origins of human cancer,* edited by H. H. Hiatt, J. P. Watson, and J. A. Winsten, pp. 1403–1430. Cold Spring Harbor, N.Y.: Cold Spring Harbor Laboratory.

ROTHMAN, K. J. 1974. Synergy and antagonism in cause-effect relationships. *Am. J. Epidemiol.* 99: 385–388.

———. 1976. The estimation of synergy or antagonism. *Am. J. Epidemiol.* 103: 506–511.

ROTHMAN, K. J.; GREENLAND, S.; and WALKER, A. M. 1980. Concepts of interaction. *Am. J. Epidemiol.* 112(4): 467–470.

SARACCI, R. 1977. Asbestos and lung cancer: An analysis of the epidemiological evidence on the asbestos-smoking interaction. *Int. J. Cancer* 20: 323–331.

———. 1980. Interaction and synergism. *Am. J. Epidemiol.* 112(4): 465–466.

WALKER, A. M., and ROTHMAN, K. J. 1982. Models of varying parametric form in case-referent studies. *Am. J. Epidemiol.* 115(1): 129–137.

WALTER, S. D. 1976. The estimation and interpretation of attributable risk in health research. *Biometrics* 32: 829–849.

WALTER, S. D., and HOLFORD, T. R. 1978. Additive, multiplicative and other models for disease risks. *Am. J. Epidemiol.* 108: 341–346.

WHITTEMORE, A., and KELLER, J. B. 1978. Quantitative theories of carcinogenesis, *Siam Rev.* 20: 1–30.

20

Modeling: Theoretical Considerations

CHAPTER OUTLINE

**20.0
PREVIEW**

In Chapter 16, we pointed out that procedures for the control of extraneous factors in an epidemiologic study may be implemented at both the design stage and the analysis stage. Once the design aspects of the study have been decided (e.g., methods of subject selection, including issues of restriction and matching) and the data have been collected on the basis of the specified study design, the next step is to carry out the statistical analysis to obtain a valid and precise quantification of the exposure-disease relationship. The analysis should involve the use of both stratification methods (see Chapter 17) and mathematical-modeling procedures.

The judicious use of stratified analysis techniques very often leads to a good overall understanding of the key interrelationships among the variables under study. This understanding can then be used to help construct a valid, precise, and parsimonious mathematical model by suggesting some of the important confounding and effect-modifying variables and by identifying uninformative factors. The results obtained from using both stratified analyses and multivariable-modeling techniques should be at least approximately comparable. This analysis plan will be illustrated through several examples in Chapters 22–24.

In this chapter, we provide a technical discussion of the use of mathematical-modeling procedures to control or adjust, at the analysis stage, for the effects of extraneous factors. Major emphasis will be given to *logistic regression analysis*. Our presentation begins with a consideration of the basic mathematical properties of the logistic regression model. Techniques for fitting logistic regression models to data and for subsequently making statistical inferences will then be discussed. This presentation will be followed by a description of unconditional and conditional maximum likelihood procedures, including remarks on the relationship between logistic regression methods for follow-up and case-control study data. Finally, Miettinen's confounder summarization procedure (1976), which involves a combination of model fitting and stratification analysis, will also be described.

This chapter is necessarily somewhat technical, particularly Section 20.3. However, the reader should acquire (even if Section 20.3 is ignored) a general appreciation of the concepts and methods discussed here in order to be able to interpret the results of analyses based on mathematical modeling and to be aware of the assumptions and limitations associated with such analyses. As an aid to understanding, the reader is encouraged to read Chapters 22–24 (which deal with specific numerical applications of the multivariable techniques discussed here) in conjunction with this chapter and Chapter 21 (which concerns analysis strategy). In this way, the reader will better follow the transition from theory to practical application. Exercises covering the material in Chapters 20–24 are presented at the end of Chapter 24.

The *linear logistic regression model* derives from the mathematical function

20.1 LINEAR LOGISTIC REGRESSION MODEL

$$f(y) = 1/(1 + e^{-y}), \qquad -\infty < y < +\infty \tag{20.1}$$

The graph of $f(y)$ is shown in Figure 20.1. Note that $f(y)$ goes from zero to one in a monotonically increasing manner as y increases in value from $-\infty$ to $+\infty$. The word "linear" used above refers to the property that the *logit transformation*

$$\text{logit } f(y) = \ln\left[\frac{f(y)}{1 - f(y)}\right] = y \tag{20.2}$$

is linear in y.

Because $f(y)$ varies between zero and one and has a sigmoid shape, the logistic function is often used by epidemiologists and statisticians to model the risk (or probability) of disease development during some specified time interval as a function of various independent variables known or suspected to be related to disease development. In particular, let D be a dichotomous variable taking the value one or zero, according to whether or not some specific disease develops during the defined study period (from time t_0 to time t, say) in a disease-free individual, with independent variable values $x_1, x_2, \ldots, x_k$ measured at t_0. Then the conditional probability

$$\text{pr}(D = 1 | x_1, x_2, \ldots, x_k) \equiv P(\mathbf{x})$$

where the row vector $\mathbf{x}' = [x_1, x_2, \ldots, x_k]$, is modeled by the *logistic function* in Equation 20.1 as

$$P(\mathbf{x}) = \left\{1 + \exp\left[-\left(\alpha + \sum_{j=1}^{k} \beta_j x_j\right)\right]\right\}^{-1} = \left\{1 + \exp[-(\alpha + \boldsymbol{\beta}'\mathbf{x})]\right\}^{-1} \tag{20.3}$$

where the vector $\boldsymbol{\beta}' = [\beta_1, \beta_2, \ldots, \beta_k]$. Note that Equation 20.3 is exactly of the form of 20.1, with $f(y) = P(\mathbf{x})$ and $y = \alpha + \sum_{j=1}^{k} \beta_j x_j$.

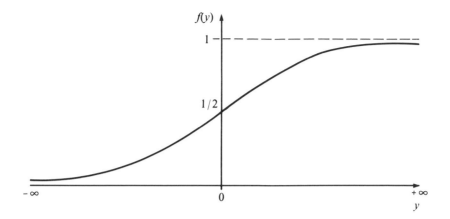

Figure 20.1 Graph of $f(y) = 1/(1 + e^{-y})$

Thus, from Equation 20.2, it follows that

$$\text{logit } P(\mathbf{x}) = \ln\left[\frac{P(\mathbf{x})}{1 - P(\mathbf{x})}\right]$$

$$= \ln\left[\frac{\text{pr}(D = 1 | x_1, x_2, \ldots, x_k)}{\text{pr}(D = 0 | x_1, x_2, \ldots, x_k)}\right] = \alpha + \sum_{j=1}^{k} \beta_j x_j \qquad (20.4)$$

So, α is the log odds of disease development for an individual with a "standard" (i.e., $\mathbf{x} = \mathbf{0}$) set of independent variable values, and β_j measures the change in the log odds for a one-unit change in x_j.

**20.1.1
The Odds
Ratio**

The formula in Equation 20.4 means that the *log risk odds ratio* comparing the risks of disease development for two different sets $\mathbf{x}^*$ and $\mathbf{x}$ of independent variable values is of the form

$$\ln \text{ROR} = \text{logit } P(\mathbf{x}^*) - \text{logit } P(\mathbf{x})$$

$$= \sum_{j=1}^{k} \beta_j (x_j^* - x_j) = \boldsymbol{\beta}'(\mathbf{x}^* - \mathbf{x})$$

so that

$$\text{ROR} = \frac{P(\mathbf{x}^*)/[1 - P(\mathbf{x}^*)]}{P(\mathbf{x})/[1 - P(\mathbf{x})]} = \exp[\boldsymbol{\beta}'(\mathbf{x}^* - \mathbf{x})]$$

$$= \exp\left[\sum_{j=1}^{k} \beta_j (x_j^* - x_j)\right] = \prod_{j=1}^{k} \exp[\beta_j (x_j^* - x_j)] \qquad (20.5)$$

The *multiplicative effect* on the risk odds ratio ROR of a difference in value between x_j^* and x_j is clear from Equation 20.5. For example, if $(x_j^* - x_j) = +1$, then the odds of disease are e^{β_j} times larger when the jth independent variable has the value $(x_j + 1)$ than when it has the value x_j.

Clearly, a large number of possible situations can be modeled by using Equation 20.3. For example, the x_j's can be nominal (e.g., indicator or dummy variables) or interval (i.e., continuous) variables, and they can appear in various forms in the model (e.g., as squares, cross products, and logarithms). Furthermore, the x's can represent exposure variables, confounders, and effect modifiers. The following examples will illustrate the flexibility inherent in Model 20.3.

Consider the familiar 2×2 table for a follow-up study over the period t_0 to t involving just one dichotomous exposure variable, with levels $E = 1$ for exposed and $E = 0$ for unexposed. If $R_1 = pr(D = 1|E = 1)$ and $R_0 = pr(D = 1|E = 0)$ are the risks, then the 2×2 table relating exposure and disease is as follows:

**20.1.2
Logistic Model
for Simple
Analysis**

	$E = 1$	$E = 0$
$D = 1$	R_1	R_0
$D = 0$	$(1 - R_1)$	$(1 - R_0)$
	1	1

For this table, the risk odds ratio is

$$\text{ROR} = \frac{[R_1(1 - R_0)]}{[R_0(1 - R_1)]}$$

Note that $\text{ROR} \approx \text{RR} = R_1/R_0$ when $(t - t_0)$ is small enough and the disease rare enough so that $R_i/(1 - R_i) \approx R_i$, $i = 0, 1$.

In the notation of Model 20.3, if we take $k = 1$, $\beta_1 = \beta$, and $x_1 = E$ (a dummy variable with levels 1 and 0 for exposed and unexposed, respectively), then

$$pr(D = 1|E) = \{1 + \exp[-(\alpha + \beta E)]\}^{-1} \tag{20.6}$$

Thus, by setting $E = 1$ and $E = 0$ in 20.6, we obtain

$$R_1 = \frac{\exp(\alpha + \beta)}{1 + \exp(\alpha + \beta)} \quad \text{and} \quad R_0 = \frac{\exp(\alpha)}{1 + \exp(\alpha)}$$

so that

$$\text{ROR} = \frac{R_1(1 - R_0)}{R_0(1 - R_1)} = e^{\beta}$$

Thus, a test of H_0: ROR = 1 versus H_A: ROR > 1 is equivalent to a test of H_0: $\beta = 0$ versus H_A: $\beta > 0$ on the basis of the logistic model representation in 20.6.

**20.1.3
Logistic Model
for Assessing
Interaction**

As a second example (previously discussed in Chapter 19), consider two exposure factors A and B, each at two levels, with $R_{ij} = \text{pr}(D = 1|A = i, B = j)$, $i = 0, 1$ and $j = 0, 1$. With R_{00} as the baseline disease risk, we define

$$\text{OR}_{ij} = \frac{R_{ij}(1 - R_{00})}{R_{00}(1 - R_{ij})} \qquad i = 0, 1 \text{ and } j = 0, 1$$

The null hypothesis of no interaction on a *multiplicative scale* (see Chapter 19 and also Kupper and Hogan, 1978) is

$$H_0: \text{OR}_{11} = \text{OR}_{10} \cdot \text{OR}_{01} \tag{20.7}$$

which can be easily tested by using logistic regression analysis. In particular, if we consider Equation 20.3 with $k = 3$, $x_1 = A$, $x_2 = B$, and $x_3 = AB$ (with A and B being dichotomous indicator variables, each with levels 1 and 0), then we have

$$\text{pr}(D = 1|A, B, AB)$$
$$= \{1 + \exp[-(\alpha + \beta_1 A + \beta_2 B + \beta_3 AB)]\}^{-1} \tag{20.8}$$

Thus,

$$R_{00} = \frac{\exp(\alpha)}{1 + \exp(\alpha)} \qquad R_{10} = \frac{\exp(\alpha + \beta_1)}{1 + \exp(\alpha + \beta_1)}$$

$$R_{01} = \frac{\exp(\alpha + \beta_2)}{1 + \exp(\alpha + \beta_2)} \qquad R_{11} = \frac{\exp(\alpha + \beta_1 + \beta_2 + \beta_3)}{1 + \exp(\alpha + \beta_1 + \beta_2 + \beta_3)}$$

It then follows that $\alpha = \text{logit } P_{00}$, $\beta_1 = \ln \text{OR}_{10}$, $\beta_2 = \ln \text{OR}_{01}$, and

$$\beta_3 = \ln\left[\frac{\text{OR}_{11}}{\text{OR}_{10} \cdot \text{OR}_{01}}\right]$$

$$= \text{logit } R_{11} - \text{logit } R_{10} - \text{logit } R_{01} + \text{logit } R_{00}$$

So, a test of the null hypothesis 20.7 is equivalent to a test of the null hypothesis H_0: $\beta_3 = 0$ in Model 20.8.

As another illustration, suppose we have attempted to control for confounding in the first example we considered (Section 20.1.2) by forming strata based on the categorization of a single extraneous factor or, more generally, on combinations of levels of several potentially confounding factors; such strata could, in part, be defined by matching carried out before the data were gathered. For the gth of G strata, the 2×2 table is as follows:

20.1.4
Logistic Models
for Stratified
Analysis

	$E = 1$	$E = 0$
$D = 1$	R_{1g}	R_{0g}
$D = 0$	$(1 - R_{1g})$	$(1 - R_{0g})$
	1	1

For this table,

$$\text{OR}_g = \frac{R_{1g}(1 - R_{0g})}{R_{0g}(1 - R_{1g})} \qquad g = 1, 2, \ldots, G$$

Two generalized versions of Model 20.6 can be used to describe such a stratified analysis. The first model is

$$\text{pr}_g(D = 1|E) = \{1 + \exp[-(\alpha_g + \beta E)]\}^{-1}$$

This model allows R_{1g} and R_{0g}, but *not* OR_g, to vary from stratum to stratum. In particular,

$$R_{1g} = \frac{\exp(\alpha_g + \beta)}{1 + \exp(\alpha_g + \beta)} \qquad \text{and} \qquad R_{0g} = \frac{\exp(\alpha_g)}{1 + \exp(\alpha_g)}$$

so that

$$\text{OR}_g = e^\beta$$

Thus, this model assumes uniformity in the odds ratio across strata or no "effect modification" (i.e., no interaction on a multiplicative scale).
    The second model is

$$\text{pr}_g(D = 1|E) = \{1 + \exp[-(\alpha_g + \beta_g E)]\}^{-1}$$

This more general model permits R_{1g}, R_{0g}, and $\text{OR}_g = e^{\beta_g}$ *all* to vary in value across the strata. This model is a "saturated" one in the sense that it involves $2G$ parameters (namely, α_g and β_g, $g = 1, 2, \ldots, G$), which is exactly the number of probabilities to be estimated (namely, R_{0g} and R_{1g}, $g = 1, 2, \ldots, G$). As a result, this model will fit the data perfectly and so will not help with regard to simplification.

In general, when we are representing stratification (or categorization) in the context of logistic regression, it is sometimes convenient to model the gth stratum probability $P_g(\mathbf{x})$ by using a generalized version of 20.3 of the form

$$P_g(\mathbf{x}) = \{1 + \exp[-(\alpha_g + \boldsymbol{\beta}'\mathbf{x})]\}^{-1} \qquad (20.9)$$

Although Model 20.9 implies that the risk odds ratio, given by 20.5, does not vary with g, nonuniformity in ROR across strata can be taken into account by including, as x's, one or more cross-product terms, each involving an exposure variable and an indexing variable depending on g.

A drawback to Model 20.9 is that the confounding effects of the individual variables, whose combinations of categories define the strata, are not explicitly considered separately. Instead, these individual effects are suppressed in favor of the parameters $\{\alpha_g\}$, which simply index the various strata without regard to their structure. Further, Model 20.9 does not take full advantage of confounding and effect-modifying factors that are measured on a continuous scale. Rather than lose information by categorizing such variables, we should incorporate them directly into the logistic model as main effects and as interactions with exposure variables. In this way, specific functional relationships involving such variables can be investigated. Also, the resulting model will involve fewer parameters, leading to better interpretability and increased efficiency. Nevertheless, Model 20.9 does have the advantage of making no assumptions about the form of dose-response effects of extraneous factors.

20.1.5
Logistic Model
with One
Exposure
Variable and
Several
Extraneous
Variables

Now let us discuss an example of a model that quantifies the *separate* effects of several extraneous factors. Consider Model 20.3 when there is a single dichotomous exposure variable $x_1 = E$ and p extraneous variables $C_1, C_2, \ldots, C_p$ to be considered for control. The variables $C_1, C_2, \ldots, C_p$ may be either continuous or categorical. Let $x_2 = V_1$, $x_3 = V_2$, $\ldots$, $x_{p_1+1} = V_{p_1}$ denote a set of functions of the extraneous variables that are thought to account for confounding in the data; e.g., we may have $V_1 = C_1$, $V_2 = C_2^2$, and $V_3 = C_1 C_3$. Further, let $x_{p_1+2} = E \cdot W_1$, $x_{p_1+3} = E \cdot W_2$, $\ldots$, $x_{p_1+p_2+1} = E \cdot W_{p_2}$, where $W_1, W_2, \ldots, W_{p_2}$ denote a set of functions of the extraneous variables that are considered to be potential effect modifiers in the data; e.g., we may have $W_1 = C_1$ and $W_2 = C_1 C_3$. Then, the general logistic model, 20.3, is expressible in the following form (with $k = p_1 + p_2 + 1$):

$$P(\mathbf{x}) = \text{pr}(D = 1|E, V_1, \ldots, V_{p_1}, W_1, \ldots, W_{p_2})$$

$$= \left\{ 1 + \exp\left[-\left(\alpha + \beta E + \sum_{i=1}^{p_1} \gamma_i V_i + E \sum_{j=1}^{p_2} \delta_j W_j \right) \right] \right\}^{-1} \quad (20.10)$$

This particular model form has been considered by Cox (1970), Prentice (1976), and Breslow and Powers (1978).

An alternative representation of this model, using the logit transformation 20.4, is given by the linear function

$$\operatorname{logit} P(\mathbf{x}) = \alpha + \beta E + \sum_{i=1}^{p_1} \gamma_i V_i + E \sum_{j=1}^{p_2} \delta_j W_j \quad (20.11)$$

Also, the risk odds ratio in 20.5 comparing the odds of disease development for exposed ($E = 1$) versus unexposed ($E = 0$) persons, *with the same values for the extraneous factors $C_1, C_2, \ldots, C_p$*, takes the form

$$\operatorname{ROR} = \exp\left[\beta + \sum_{j=1}^{p_2} \delta_j W_j \right] \quad (20.12)$$

which is a function of the modifying variables $W_1, \ldots, W_{p_2}$. If $\delta_j = 0$ for all j (i.e., there is no effect modification), the odds ratio expression (20.12) equals e^β. For such a main effect model in E, deleting one or more of the V_i terms and monitoring any associated changes in the estimate of β is one way to assess whether such factors are really confounders in the data. An application of Model 20.10 to the analysis of follow-up study data will be presented in Chapters 22 and 23.

Before proceeding to discuss the use of the logistic regression model to analyze follow-up and case-control study data, we caution the reader that *there can be situations where the logistic model is not appropriate* (Gordon, 1974). For example, we have already emphasized in Chapter 19 that the linear model

20.1.6 When Is the Logistic Model Inappropriate?

$$P(\mathbf{x}) = \alpha + \sum_{j=1}^{k} \beta_j x_j$$

may be more relevant in situations where the risk difference

$$P(\mathbf{x}^*) - P(\mathbf{x}) = \sum_{j=1}^{k} \beta_j (x_j^* - x_j)$$

is the parameter of interest. [The often-cited argument that this linear model is not useful because it can lead to predicted probabilities lying outside the permissible range (0, 1) may be more an indictment of the method of estimation than of the appropriateness of the linear model. For example, Mason and Webster (1975) have shown that the use of ordinary least squares estimation techniques can lead to estimated coefficients that deviate considerably from the true parameter values, the reason being that the x's are highly correlated in the data so that there is severe "multicollinearity." Also, we have pointed out that deviations from *additivity* in excess risk are directly quantifiable by using a *linear* model with appropriate cross-product terms, while the *logistic* model assumes that a change in the level of a variable x affects the odds ratio in a *multiplicative* manner (see Expression 20.5).

Further, consider the situation where the risk odds ratio itself, rather than the risk, is related to the x_j's through the *linear function*

$$\text{ROR} = \sum_{j=1}^{k} \beta_j (x_j^* - x_j)$$

This relationship could be poorly modeled by erroneously assuming that the logistic model 20.3 and hence the multiplicative structure 20.5 are appropriate. It is sometimes possible to detect such a situation by constructing various graphs relating the sample $\widehat{\text{ROR}}$ values to the x's; the plots may suggest a more appropriate functional form than the one in 20.5.

Although the rest of this chapter will focus on the logistic model, a proper statistical analysis using mathematical modeling always involves the examination of several different model forms, with the final choice of the model being based both on theoretical considerations (e.g., biologic plausibility, disease etiology considerations) and on data-based information (e.g., the signs of the estimated coefficients, the fit of the model to the data, the examination of residual plots, the correlation patterns among the x's, etc.). Thus, despite the fact that the logistic function is very often a reasonable model form to use when dealing with epidemiologic data, we strongly urge the reader to verify as completely as possible its appropriateness in any particular situation.

20.2 MAXIMUM LIKELIHOOD ESTIMATION AND INFERENCE MAKING

The method of maximum likelihood (ML) estimation chooses estimators of the parameters in a likelihood function that maximize the value of that function. The likelihood function represents the probability of observing the data obtained as a function of the unknown parameters. The ML estimators of these parameters, therefore, have the desirable property of being those estimators that agree most closely with the data actually encountered.

20.2.1 ML Estimation of Model Parameters

Suppose that $L \equiv L(\boldsymbol{\theta})$ represents a likelihood function involving an $(r \times 1)$ vector of parameters $\boldsymbol{\theta}$, say. Specific examples of likelihood functions are given in Section 20.3, where we distinguish between two general types: unconditional and conditional.* In these examples, the

---

*Loosely speaking, the term "unconditional likelihood" (or "unconditional likelihood function") refers to the unconditional probability of obtaining the particular set of data under

parameter vector $\boldsymbol{\theta}$ involves the α's and β's in logistic models like Equation 20.3. The ML estimator of $\boldsymbol{\theta}$ is defined mathematically to be that unique vector $\hat{\boldsymbol{\theta}}$ of numerical functions of the observed data for which $L(\hat{\boldsymbol{\theta}})$ is a maximum. Since maximizing $L(\boldsymbol{\theta})$ is equivalent to the computationally easier problem of maximizing $\ln L(\boldsymbol{\theta})$, the elements of $\hat{\boldsymbol{\theta}}$ are usually found as the solutions of the r equations obtained by setting the *partial derivative* of $\ln L(\boldsymbol{\theta})$ with respect to *each* θ_j equal to zero. That is,

$$\partial \ln L(\boldsymbol{\theta})/\partial \theta_j = 0 \qquad j = 1, 2, \ldots, r \qquad (20.13)$$

where $\boldsymbol{\theta}' = [\theta_1, \theta_2, \ldots, \theta_r]$.

Except in certain very special cases, explicit formulas for the ML estimators cannot be obtained. And, in general, Expression 20.13 describes a system of r equations in r unknowns that must be solved in an iterative fashion. However, this condition is no real drawback given the availability of sophisticated computer algorithms designed to perform such complex calculations. Nevertheless, for likelihood methods (like *conditional* ones) which require permutation calculations, there are often time and cost constraints to consider when dealing with data sets of any reasonable size.

The data input to standard ML computer programs consists of each individual's status as diseased or nondiseased (i.e., the dependent variable value) and his or her associated set of independent variable values (i.e., x values). When the data are categorical in nature, meaning that individuals in the same stratum have the same x values, the methods of Bishop and colleagues (1975) can be used to obtain unconditional ML estimates through the iterative proportional fitting of models to the logits of the stratum-specific observed proportions of diseased. Grizzle and colleagues (1969) advocate a weighted least squares estimation approach in this framework, leading to results that are asymptotically equivalent to those of Bishop and co-workers. If these categorical data analysis procedures are to be used with confidence, the stratum-specific sample sizes must be large enough so that the asymptotic theory on which these approaches are based is applicable. As the strata become finer and finer, one must turn, for validity reasons, to the conditional likelihood methods.

---

consideration. More specifically, the unconditional likelihood is the joint probability distribution of the data (e.g., a joint density function when dealing with continuous variables), which depends on the population parameters. The *unconditional maximum likelihood estimates* of these parameters are those data-determined numerical values of the parameters that maximize the value of the unconditional likelihood function.

Conditional maximum likelihood estimators are derived from a likelihood function that gives the conditional probability of obtaining the data configuration *actually observed* given all possible configurations (i.e., permutations) of the data values. An example that we discuss in Section 20.3 considers the conditional probability that the first m_1 out of m subjects are cases given all the possible $(m!/m_1!m_0!)$ ways of dividing m subjects into m_1 cases and m_0 controls.

When the data are such that each individual is best treated separately in the likelihood (e.g., when some of the x's are continuous), then unconditional likelihood methods are appropriate as long as the number of parameters to be estimated is small relative to the number of individuals in the sample. For matched data, however, conditional methods are usually required. Treating continuous variables on an interval scale in the logistic model, rather than forming strata on the basis of a categorization process that is often quite arbitrary, makes the most use of the flexibility of the logistic regression approach. Such modeling allows one to make a quantitative assessment of the joint *functional relationship* of continuous variables to risk. Also, it allows one to consider several variables simultaneously, since the number of parameters to be estimated will generally not be excessive.

Until recently, the most popular method of estimation for logistic regression has been the procedure employed by Cornfield (1962), Truett and colleagues (1967), and others (e.g., Kleinbaum et al., 1971). This method uses estimates derived from linear discriminant analysis, a technique that is equivalent computationally to unweighted least squares regression with a dichotomous dependent variable. The valid use of discriminant function estimates requires the assumption that the distribution of $\mathbf{x}$ is multivariate normal in both the diseased and nondiseased groups. Such an assumption is generally not realistic, in which case the use of such discriminant function–based estimates can lead to considerable bias (see Halperin et al., 1971; Press and Wilson, 1978).

20.2.2 Statistical Inferences

Once the maximum likelihood estimates have been obtained, the next step is to use the $\hat{\beta}$'s to make statistical inferences concerning the exposure-disease relationships under study. This step can be accomplished through the use of two quantities that are part of the output provided by standard ML estimation programs. The first of these is the *maximized likelihood value*, which is simply the numerical value of the likelihood function when the ML estimates are substituted for their corresponding parameter values; this value is $L(\hat{\boldsymbol{\theta}})$ in our earlier notation. The second quantity is the *estimated covariance matrix* of the ML estimators, a matrix that has as its elements their estimated variances (on the diagonal) and covariances (off the diagonal).

To illustrate how these quantities are used, we consider the following three models:

Model 1: $\operatorname{logit} P_1(\mathbf{x}) = \alpha + \beta_1 x_1 + \beta_2 x_2$

Model 2: $\operatorname{logit} P_2(\mathbf{x}) = \alpha + \beta_1 x_1 + \beta_2 x_2 + \beta_3 x_3$

Model 3: $\operatorname{logit} P_3(\mathbf{x}) = \alpha + \beta_1 x_1 + \beta_2 x_2 + \beta_3 x_3$

$$+ \beta_4 x_1 x_2 + \beta_5 x_1 x_3 + \beta_6 x_1 x_2 x_3$$

Let $\hat{L}_1$, $\hat{L}_2$, and $\hat{L}_3$ denote the maximized likelihood values from fitting Models 1, 2, and 3, respectively (either by unconditional or conditional methods). Since the more parameters a model has, the better it fits the data, it is clear that $\hat{L}_1 \le \hat{L}_2 \le \hat{L}_3$. Thus, it follows that

$$-2 \ln \hat{L}_3 \le -2 \ln \hat{L}_2 \le -2 \ln \hat{L}_1$$

where $-2 \ln \hat{L}_1$, e.g., is known as the *log likelihood statistic* for Model 1.

Hypothesis Testing

Although a log likelihood statistic does not in general have any well-defined distribution when considered by itself, the difference between the log likelihood statistics for two models, one of which is a special case of the other (i.e., contains a subset of the parameters in the other), has an approximate chi-square distribution in large samples, with the degrees of freedom being equal to the difference between the numbers of parameters in the two models. Since the degrees of freedom for this χ^2 test are equal to the number of parameters in the larger model that must be set equal to zero to obtain the smaller model, such a χ^2 statistic can be used to test the null hypothesis that all these additional parameters have the value zero (i.e., that the larger model fits the data no better than the smaller one). In fact, this is exactly the null hypothesis being addressed by the difference in log likelihood statistics, and this test is called a *likelihood ratio test* since it is a function of the ratio of maximized likelihoods.

In terms of Models 1, 2, and 3, then,

$$-2 \ln \hat{L}_1 - (-2 \ln \hat{L}_2) = -2 \ln (\hat{L}_1/\hat{L}_2)$$

provides a χ^2 statistic with one degree of freedom for the likelihood ratio test of H_0: $\beta_3 = 0$ versus H_A: $\beta_3 \ne 0$. Also, $-2 \ln (\hat{L}_2/\hat{L}_3)$ is a χ^2 statistic, with three degrees of freedom, that tests H_0: $\beta_4 = \beta_5 = \beta_6 = 0$ (i.e., there is no need to add this particular set of interaction terms to Model 2) versus H_A: *at least one* of β_4, β_5, and β_6 is nonzero.

The above hypotheses can be equivalently tested by comparing the appropriate functions of the estimated coefficients to their standard errors, which are obtained by using combinations of elements from the estimated covariance matrix of the ML estimators. For example, a test of H_0: $\beta_3 = 0$ can be performed by using the statistic $Z = (\hat{\beta}_3 - 0)/\sqrt{\hat{V}ar(\hat{\beta}_3)}$, where $\hat{V}ar(\hat{\beta}_3)$ is the estimated variance of $\hat{\beta}_3$ under Model 2. If Model 1 holds, then $-2 \ln (\hat{L}_1/\hat{L}_2) \approx Z^2 = \chi_1^2$ for large samples. A test of H_0: $\beta_4 = \beta_5 = \beta_6 = 0$ can also be carried out by using the statistic

$$(\hat{\beta}_4, \hat{\beta}_5, \hat{\beta}_6) \, \hat{V}^{-1} \begin{bmatrix} \hat{\beta}_4 \\ \hat{\beta}_5 \\ \hat{\beta}_6 \end{bmatrix}$$

where $\hat{\mathbf{V}}$ is the estimated covariance matrix for $(\hat{\beta}_4, \hat{\beta}_5, \hat{\beta}_6)'$ on the basis of fitting Model 3. (Note that $\hat{\mathbf{V}}$ is a submatrix of the full estimated covariance matrix for Model 3.) For large samples, this statistic will have an approximate χ_3^2 distribution under H_0: $\beta_4 = \beta_5 = \beta_6 = 0$.

Yet another method for testing these hypotheses involves the use of a *score statistic* (see Day and Byar, 1979; Kleinbaum et al., 1982). Since this statistic is not routinely calculated by standard ML programs, and since its use gives about the same numerical χ^2 values as the two techniques just presented, we will not discuss it further.

When one is dealing with grouped data, there are readily available statistics for assessing the goodness of fit of a k-parameter logistic model. With continuous variables, however, the approach is not so straight-forward, though Hosmer and Lemeshow (1980) have suggested several tests. (Also, see Lemeshow and Hosmer, 1982.) Let us assume that the explanatory vector $\mathbf{x}$ defines a small number of strata relative to the number of observations, and that the expected or fitted numbers of cases and controls are not too small. Then, we can assess the fit of a model by using the Pearson χ^2 statistic $\Sigma[(O - E)^2/E]$, where the sum is over all strata defined by $\mathbf{x}$ for cases and controls separately. We may also utilize the likelihood ratio statistic, comparing the saturated model with the model under consideration. Each of these statistics is approximately χ_d^2 under the null hypothesis of interest, where $d = (S - k)$, S being the number of strata determined by $\mathbf{x}$ and k being the total number of model parameters to be estimated.

Interval Estimation

The large-sample $100(1 - \alpha)\%$ confidence interval for β_3 is

$$\hat{\beta}_3 \pm Z_{1-\alpha/2}\sqrt{\hat{\mathrm{Var}}(\hat{\beta}_3)},$$

so that the corresponding interval estimator of the odds ratio e^{β_3} is $\exp[\hat{\beta}_3 \pm Z_{1-\alpha/2}\sqrt{\hat{\mathrm{Var}}(\hat{\beta}_3)}]$.

As another illustration, we consider the case when it is necessary to work with a linear function of estimated β's since, as is the common situation in practice, the odds ratio estimator resulting from a logistic regression analysis is a function of several x's (i.e., there is interaction). For example, with x_1 in Model 3 being a 0–1 exposure variable, the estimated odds ratio comparing exposed ($x_1 = 1$) to unexposed ($x_1 = 0$) individuals, with the same values for the extraneous factors x_2 and x_3, is $\exp(\hat{\beta}_1 + \hat{\beta}_4 x_2 + \hat{\beta}_5 x_3 + \hat{\beta}_6 x_2 x_3)$. The corresponding $100(1 - \alpha)\%$ large-sample confidence interval for the population odds ratio is then

$$\exp[\hat{\ell} \pm Z_{1-\alpha/2}\sqrt{\hat{\mathrm{Var}}(\hat{\ell})}] \tag{20.14}$$

where $\hat{\ell} = \hat{\beta}_1 + \hat{\beta}_4 x_2 + \hat{\beta}_5 x_3 + \hat{\beta}_6 x_2 x_3$. It can be shown that the estimated variance* of the linear function $\hat{\ell}$ is

$$
\begin{aligned}
\hat{\mathrm{Var}}(\hat{\ell}) = {} & \hat{\mathrm{Var}}(\hat{\beta}_1) + x_2^2 \,\hat{\mathrm{Var}}(\hat{\beta}_4) + x_3^2 \,\hat{\mathrm{Var}}(\hat{\beta}_5) + x_2^2 x_3^2 \,\hat{\mathrm{Var}}(\hat{\beta}_6) \\
& + 2x_2 \,\hat{\mathrm{Cov}}(\hat{\beta}_1, \hat{\beta}_4) + 2x_3 \,\hat{\mathrm{Cov}}(\hat{\beta}_1, \hat{\beta}_5) \\
& + 2x_2 x_3 \,\hat{\mathrm{Cov}}(\hat{\beta}_1, \hat{\beta}_6) + 2x_2 x_3 \,\hat{\mathrm{Cov}}(\hat{\beta}_4, \hat{\beta}_5) \\
& + 2x_2^2 x_3 \,\hat{\mathrm{Cov}}(\hat{\beta}_4, \hat{\beta}_6) + 2x_2 x_3^2 \,\hat{\mathrm{Cov}}(\hat{\beta}_5, \hat{\beta}_6)
\end{aligned}
$$

The estimated variances and covariances appearing in the above expression are obtained as the appropriate diagonal and off-diagonal elements of the estimated covariance matrix based on the ML fitting of Model 3. Clearly, the interval estimate 20.14 is a function of the values given to x_2 and x_3. A recommended practice is to use "typical" or "representative" values of x_2 and x_3, such as their mean values in the data, when computing such interval estimates; this practice will be illustrated by example in Chapters 22–24.

In this section, we will discuss logistic regression analysis procedures for both follow-up and case-control studies. The presentation will include unconditional and conditional likelihood methods.

20.3 LOGISTIC REGRESSION ANALYSIS: FOLLOW-UP AND CASE-CONTROL STUDIES

20.3.1 Unconditional Likelihood Procedures

The discussion in Section 20.1 illustrates that the inherent structure of the logistic model 20.3 is ideally suited for a follow-up study situation. This model is suitable because the dependent (or outcome) variable is the occurrence ($D = 1$) or nonoccurrence ($D = 0$) of a particular disease and the independent variables (the x's) are measured on disease-free individuals at the start of the defined study period. [The extension of Model 20.3 to multiple disease outcomes (e.g., $D = 0, 1, 2, \ldots, d$ for $d \geq 2$) has been discussed by Prentice and Pyke (1979) and by Day and Byar (1979), but it will not be pursued here.]

In a case-control study setting, however, the exposure data constitute the outcome or response, this information being gathered *after* samples of

---

*In general, if $\hat{\ell} = \sum\limits_{i=1}^{k} a_i Y_i$, then

$$
\mathrm{Var}(\hat{\ell}) = \sum_{i=1}^{k} a_i^2 \,\mathrm{Var}(Y_i) + 2 \sum\sum_{\text{all } i<j} a_i a_j \,\mathrm{Cov}(Y_i, Y_j)
$$

cases and controls have been selected. This feature has led to the use of logistic analysis with $\text{pr}(E = 1|D)$, rather than $\text{pr}(D = 1|E)$, as the response probability being modeled. This approach, although conceptually sound, has some drawbacks. First, a continuous exposure variable must be categorized to produce a dichotomous (or polychotomous) response measure. Also, it is not obvious how one proceeds when one is considering several exposure variables simultaneously. Fortunately, it is possible to justify* the use of the follow-up study logistic model, 20.3, to analyze case-control data (see Prentice and Pyke, 1979; Breslow and Day, 1981). Essentially, this argument requires a comparison of the (unconditional) likelihood functions for case-control data considered both retrospectively and as if such data had been obtained prospectively.

Follow-up Studies

To describe such likelihoods, we consider that we have m_1 cases, which are associated with the response vectors $x_1, x_2, \ldots, x_{m_1}$, and m_0 controls, which are associated with the response vectors $x_{m_1+1}, x_{m_1+2}, \ldots, x_m$, where $m = (m_0 + m_1)$. Then, the *unconditional likelihood* (UL_F), which is derivable from Model 20.3 and which is based on treating the data prospectively (i.e., as if obtained from a *follow-up* study), is given by the expression

$$\text{UL}_F = \prod_{\ell=1}^{m_1} \text{pr}(D = 1|x_\ell) \prod_{\ell=m_1+1}^{m} \text{pr}(D = 0|x_\ell)$$

$$= \prod_{\ell=1}^{m_1} \exp(\alpha + \boldsymbol{\beta}'x_\ell) \Big/ \prod_{\ell=1}^{m} [1 + \exp(\alpha + \boldsymbol{\beta}'x_\ell)] \quad (20.15)$$

If a parametric model is used to describe the distribution of x in each of the case and control groups, then direct (i.e., noniterative) unconditional maximum likelihood estimation of the parameters in a likelihood function such as 20.15 is sometimes possible. One often-used approach (e.g., see Cornfield, 1962) is to assume that $\text{pr}(x_\ell|D = d)$ refers to a multivariate normal distribution with mean vector $\boldsymbol{\mu}_d$ and covariance matrix $\boldsymbol{\Sigma}$, $d = 0, 1$. In this special situation, the exposure odds ratio takes the specific form $\text{EOR} = \exp[\boldsymbol{\beta}'(x^* - x)]$, where $\boldsymbol{\beta} = \boldsymbol{\Sigma}^{-1}(\boldsymbol{\mu}_1 - \boldsymbol{\mu}_0)$. And, since $\boldsymbol{\Sigma}^{-1}(\boldsymbol{\mu}_1 - \boldsymbol{\mu}_0)$ is exactly the vector of population discriminant function coefficients, ML estimation of $\boldsymbol{\beta}$ follows directly by using normal theory discriminant analysis for two groups. However, this multivariate normality assumption is generally not realistic (e.g., when some of the x_j's are dichotomous), in which case the use of such discriminant function–based estimates can lead to considerable bias (see Halperin et al., 1971; Press and Wilson, 1978).

---

*The specifics of the mathematical theory underlying this justification are complex; the interested reader may consult Breslow and Day (1981) and Prentice and Pyke (1979) for further mathematical details.

Case-Control Studies

In contrast, Prentice and Pyke (1979) have shown that the corresponding *unconditional likelihood* UL_C, which incorporates the retrospective features of the *case-control* study design, is proportional to $UL_1 \cdot UL_2$, where

$$UL_1 = \prod_{\ell=1}^{m_1} \exp(\alpha^* + \boldsymbol{\beta}' \mathbf{x}_\ell) \Big/ \prod_{\ell=1}^{m} [1 + \exp(\alpha^* + \boldsymbol{\beta}' \mathbf{x}_\ell)] \quad (20.16)$$

and

$$UL_2 = \prod_{\ell=1}^{m} \mathrm{pr}(\mathbf{x}_\ell)$$

with $\alpha^* (\neq \alpha)$ a nuisance parameter. They then showed that ML estimation of the parameter $\boldsymbol{\beta}$, using the likelihood $UL_1 \cdot UL_2$, leads to an estimator $\hat{\boldsymbol{\beta}}$ and an estimated asymptotic covariance matrix $\hat{\mathbf{V}}(\hat{\boldsymbol{\beta}})$ that are identical to those obtained by treating the case-control data as though they had been gathered prospectively and by using the likelihood UL_F given by 20.15. This, in essence, is the justification for using the follow-up study model to analyze case-control data. However, the parameter α^* is not interpretable in the case-control study situation. We should not be surprised that α cannot be estimated from a case-control study, since it is the log odds of disease development among the unexposed in a follow-up study setting.

Prentice and Pyke also showed that the ML estimator $\hat{\boldsymbol{\beta}}$ based on 20.15, and its associated covariance matrix estimator $\hat{\mathbf{V}}(\hat{\boldsymbol{\beta}})$, have the usual asymptotic properties, namely, normality for $\hat{\boldsymbol{\beta}}$ and consistency for $\hat{\mathbf{V}}(\hat{\boldsymbol{\beta}})$ as an estimator of $\mathbf{V}(\hat{\boldsymbol{\beta}})$.

More generally, when one is using Model 20.9 for the case-control study situation when there are G strata, with the gth stratum containing m_{1g} cases and m_{0g} controls, then the overall likelihood for all the $m_1 = \sum_{g=1}^{G} m_{1g}$ cases and $m_0 = \sum_{g=1}^{G} m_{0g}$ controls is simply the product of the separate likelihoods for each stratum. This overall likelihood would be of the form

$$\prod_{g=1}^{G} \left\{ \frac{\prod_{\ell=1}^{m_{1g}} \exp(\alpha_g^* + \boldsymbol{\beta}' \mathbf{x}_{\ell g})}{\prod_{\ell=1}^{m_g} [1 + \exp(\alpha_g^* + \boldsymbol{\beta}' \mathbf{x}_{\ell g})]} \cdot \prod_{\ell=1}^{m_g} \mathrm{pr}(\mathbf{x}_{\ell g}) \right\} \quad (20.17)$$

where $m_g = (m_{1g} + m_{0g})$. The corresponding follow-up study likelihood, based on the development of m_{1g} cases from the m_g initially disease-free subjects in the gth stratum, is the left-hand product in Expression 20.17, with α_g replacing α_g^*. We again caution that the estimated values of the

α_g^*'s are usually not interpretable; however, this does *not* mean that the confounding effects that the α_g^*'s represent are not being controlled for but only that the actual numerical values of the $\hat{\alpha}_g^*$'s are not generally meaningful.

Likelihoods for Simple Analysis

By way of illustration, consider the following simple case-control data layout for random samples of m_1 cases and m_0 controls:

	$E = 1$	$E = 0$	
$D = 1$	a	b	$m_1 = (a + b)$
$D = 0$	c	d	$m_0 = (c + d)$

For this simple analysis situation, Model 20.6 is to be used, and the likelihood function 20.16 reduces to the special form

$$\mathrm{UL}_1 = \prod_{\ell=1}^{m_1} \exp(\alpha^* + \beta E) \Big/ \prod_{\ell=1}^{m} [1 + \exp(\alpha^* + \beta E)] \quad (20.18)$$

Now, since a of the m_1 cases and c of the m_0 controls have a history of previous exposure ($E = 1$), while the remaining $b = (m_1 - a)$ cases and $d = (m_0 - c)$ controls do not ($E = 0$), it follows that Expression 20.18 can be written as

$$\mathrm{UL}_1 = \left(\frac{e^{\alpha^*+\beta}}{1 + e^{\alpha^*+\beta}}\right)^a \left(\frac{1}{1 + e^{\alpha^*+\beta}}\right)^c \left(\frac{e^{\alpha^*}}{1 + e^{\alpha^*}}\right)^b \left(\frac{1}{1 + e^{\alpha^*}}\right)^d \quad (20.19)$$

For an analogous table of data from a follow-up study, where a cases develop from $(a + c)$ exposed subjects and b cases develop from $(b + d)$ unexposed subjects, the corresponding follow-up study likelihood (20.15) for Model 20.6 becomes

$$\left(\frac{e^{\alpha+\beta}}{1 + e^{\alpha+\beta}}\right)^a \left(\frac{1}{1 + e^{\alpha+\beta}}\right)^c \left(\frac{e^{\alpha}}{1 + e^{\alpha}}\right)^b \left(\frac{1}{1 + e^{\alpha}}\right)^d \quad (20.20)$$

A comparison of 20.19 and 20.20 clearly shows that these two likelihoods differ only because of α^* and α. It can be shown (see Section 20.2) that the unconditional ML estimator of β under either 20.19 or 20.20 is $\hat{\beta} = \ln(ad/bc)$. Thus, the unconditional ML estimator of either EOR in the case-control study, simple analysis situation or ROR in the follow-up study, simple analysis situation is the well-known sample odds ratio $e^\beta = ad/bc$.

Likelihoods for Stratified Data

Let us consider another example for the dichotomous exposure situation, with the table for the gth stratum as follows:

	$E = 1$	$E = 0$	
$D = 1$	a_g	b_g	$m_{1g} = (a_g + b_g)$
$D = 0$	c_g	d_g	$m_{0g} = (c_g + d_g)$

It follows that the case-control study likelihood, based on 20.17 and the model $\mathrm{pr}_g(D = 1|E) = \{1 + \exp[-(\alpha_g + \beta E)]\}^{-1}$, takes the form

$$\prod_{g=1}^{G} \left(\frac{e^{\alpha_g^* + \beta}}{1 + e^{\alpha_g^* + \beta}}\right)^{a_g} \left(\frac{1}{1 + e^{\alpha_g^* + \beta}}\right)^{c_g} \left(\frac{e^{\alpha_g^*}}{1 + e^{\alpha_g^*}}\right)^{b_g} \left(\frac{1}{1 + e^{\alpha_g^*}}\right)^{d_g} \quad (20.21)$$

The corresponding follow-up study likelihood is 20.21, with α_g replacing α_g^*.

Likelihoods Based on Model 20.10

Note that the use of the likelihood in 20.21 requires the ML estimation (by iteration) of $(G + 1)$ parameters, G of which are nuisance parameters. As we mentioned earlier, it is generally more efficient to control confounding, when possible, with a model like 20.10, involving fewer parameters. In particular, rather than have a separate parameter for each stratum, one might have a model containing main effect terms for just two or three possibly continuous confounders.

If we let $\mathbf{V}' = (V_1, V_2, \ldots, V_{p_1})$, $\boldsymbol{\gamma}' = (\gamma_1, \gamma_2, \ldots, \gamma_{p_1})$, $\mathbf{W}' = (W_1, W_2, \ldots, W_{p_2})$, and $\boldsymbol{\delta}' = (\delta_1, \delta_2, \ldots, \delta_{p_2})$, then Model 20.10 can be written (using matrix notation) as

$$\mathrm{pr}(D = 1|E, \mathbf{V}', \mathbf{W}') = \frac{\exp(\alpha + \beta E + \boldsymbol{\gamma}'\mathbf{V} + E\boldsymbol{\delta}'\mathbf{W})}{1 + \exp(\alpha + \beta E + \boldsymbol{\gamma}'\mathbf{V} + E\boldsymbol{\delta}'\mathbf{W})}$$

It then follows that the corresponding follow-up study likelihood for all m_1 cases and m_0 controls under 20.10 is expressible as the product of the likelihood for the m_1 cases (of which a are exposed), namely,

$$\prod_{\ell=1}^{a} \left[\frac{\exp(\alpha + \beta + \boldsymbol{\gamma}'\mathbf{V}_\ell + \boldsymbol{\delta}'\mathbf{W}_\ell)}{1 + \exp(\alpha + \beta + \boldsymbol{\gamma}'\mathbf{V}_\ell + \boldsymbol{\delta}'\mathbf{W}_\ell)} \right]$$

$$\cdot \prod_{\ell=a+1}^{m_1} \left[\frac{\exp(\alpha + \boldsymbol{\gamma}'\mathbf{V}_\ell)}{1 + \exp(\alpha + \boldsymbol{\gamma}'\mathbf{V}_\ell)} \right] \qquad (20.22)$$

and the likelihood for the m_0 controls (of which c are exposed), namely,

$$\prod_{\ell=m_1+1}^{m_1+c} \left[\frac{1}{1 + \exp(\alpha + \beta + \boldsymbol{\gamma}'\mathbf{V}_\ell + \boldsymbol{\delta}'\mathbf{W}_\ell)} \right]$$

$$\cdot \prod_{\ell=m_1+c+1}^{m_1+m_0} \left[\frac{1}{1 + \exp(\alpha + \boldsymbol{\gamma}'\mathbf{V}_\ell)} \right] \qquad (20.23)$$

The product of 20.22 and 20.23 involves $(p_1 + p_2 + 2)$ parameters to be estimated via ML methods, with α being a nuisance parameter whose numerical estimate based on case-control data (namely, $\hat{\alpha}^*$) is not generally interpretable. Thus, the advantage of Model 20.10 over 20.9 is realized when the control of confounding can be achieved through a model for which p_1 is less than G. In such a situation, ML estimation using the product likelihood based on 20.22 and 20.23 should produce more precise estimates of exposure-related effects than those based on the case-control likelihood (20.17) or its follow-up study counterpart. This claim is based on the principle that the smaller the number of parameters to be estimated relative to the number of data points (i.e., the larger the "degrees of freedom for error"), the better will be the precision.

20.3.2 Conditional Likelihood Procedures

An alternative to the unconditional maximum likelihood estimation of $\boldsymbol{\beta}$ in Model 20.3 is a conditional estimation procedure. We consider again the case-control study format, with $\mathbf{x}_1, \mathbf{x}_2, \ldots, \mathbf{x}_m$ the observed data vectors associated with the $m = (m_1 + m_0)$ cases plus controls. We can then derive the conditional probability that the first m_1 of the vectors $\mathbf{x}_1$, $\mathbf{x}_2, \ldots, \mathbf{x}_m$ actually go with the cases, given that exactly m_1 of the m subjects are cases. Using independence of the $\mathbf{x}$'s, conditional on disease status, and applying Bayes' rule, we can show this conditional probability to be

$$\frac{\displaystyle\prod_{\ell=1}^{m_1} \mathrm{pr}(D = 1|\mathbf{x}_\ell) \cdot \prod_{\ell=m_1+1}^{m} \mathrm{pr}(D = 0|\mathbf{x}_\ell)}{\displaystyle\sum_{\mathbf{u}} \left\{ \prod_{\ell=1}^{m_1} \mathrm{pr}(D = 1|\mathbf{x}_{u_\ell}) \cdot \prod_{\ell=m_1+1}^{m} \mathrm{pr}(D = 0|\mathbf{x}_{u_\ell}) \right\}} \qquad (20.24)$$

where the sum in the denominator is over all partitions of $\{1, 2, \ldots, m\}$ into two subsets, the first of which contains m_1 elements; there are $C_{m_1}^{m} =$

$m! / m_1! m_0!$ such partitions. Now, using the logistic model (20.3) and some simplification, we can write this conditional probability as

$$CL = \prod_{\ell=1}^{m_1} \exp(\boldsymbol{\beta}'\mathbf{x}_\ell) \Bigg/ \sum_{\mathbf{u}} \left[\prod_{\ell=1}^{m_1} \exp(\boldsymbol{\beta}'\mathbf{x}_{u_\ell}) \right] \qquad (20.25)$$

Note that the conditional likelihood 20.25 involves only the $\boldsymbol{\beta}$ vector; the α's (or $\alpha*$'s) have been eliminated through this permutation (or randomization) procedure. Although this conditional likelihood approach thus precludes our having to estimate any nuisance parameters, as is necessary when using the unconditional likelihood (20.15), the evaluation of the denominator in 20.25 quickly becomes laborious as m_1 and m_0 get large. (As these sample sizes are increased, limited numerical work suggests that the estimates of the $\boldsymbol{\beta}$'s and their variances and covariances will be reasonably approximated by the values obtained by using the computationally simpler unconditional likelihood procedures.) As we will see, conditional likelihood procedures work well computationally in precisely those situations when unconditional ML estimation is unreliable, namely, when stratum-specific sample sizes are small (e.g., with pair-matched and R-to-1 matched data).

It can be shown (we omit the details) that the same conditional likelihood of 20.25 is obtained regardless of whether we consider the data to have arisen from a follow-up study or from a case-control study. That these two conditional likelihoods agree perfectly is not surprising, since a similar equivalence is known to hold for the special case of a 2×2 table where the conditional analysis assumes the marginal totals to be fixed; for that simple situation, the permutation argument leads to Fisher's exact test for evaluating the null hypothesis of no exposure-disease association.

Likelihood for Stratified Data

When there are G strata, the full conditional likelihood is the product of G terms of the form of 20.25, where the permutation analysis is carried out separately for the $m_g = (m_{1g} + m_{0g})$ individuals in each stratum. In terms of previous notation, this full conditional likelihood would have the form

$$\prod_{g=1}^{G} \left[\prod_{\ell=1}^{m_{1g}} \exp(\boldsymbol{\beta}'\mathbf{x}_{\ell g}) \Bigg/ \sum_{\mathbf{u}} \left\{ \prod_{\ell=1}^{m_{1g}} \exp(\boldsymbol{\beta}'\mathbf{x}_{u_{\ell g}}) \right\} \right] \qquad (20.26)$$

It is worth noting that Expression 20.26 has precisely the structure of Cox's partial likelihood (1975), based on the proportional hazards model, for analyzing follow-up study data. However, an important distinction is that each stratum-specific set in the denominator of 20.26, instead of involving *all* persons in the study who are disease-free at the time each incident case is identified, consists *only* of the m_{0g} controls specifically associated with (e.g., sampled at the same time as) the m_{1g} cases. For instance, when $m_{1g} = 1$ and $m_{0g} = R$, as in R-to-1 matching, only those R controls matched to a particular case are involved in each stratum-specific permutation calculation.

When m_{1g} and m_{0g} are both large, the calculations required to complete the conditional analysis based on Expression 20.26 are time-consuming. Since the unconditional likelihood approach will give about the same results in such circumstances, it is the method of choice when the stratum-specific sample sizes are large. However, when the number of observations in each stratum is moderate to small, it becomes mandatory to employ conditional likelihood procedures. Such small-sample situations are especially typified by matched case-control studies where each stratum often contains just one case and one or more controls. In fact, Pike and colleagues (1980) have demonstrated numerically that the use of the conditional likelihood approach becomes obligatory in order to avoid bias as the stratification becomes finer and finer, an extreme example being a pair-matched analysis (i.e., one case and one control per stratum).

One reason why unconditional likelihood methods give biased estimators when analyzing finely stratified data is that the number of parameters to be estimated becomes large relative to the amount of data available. This situation results because the use of unconditional likelihoods like Expressions 20.15 and 20.17 requires estimation of nuisance parameters as well as the parameters of interest (the β's), and the number of these nuisance parameters can become quite large. In such situations, unconditional likelihood approaches can result in highly biased parameter estimates (see Cox and Hinkley, 1974). Thus, unconditional ML estimation techniques should be used only when the stratum-specific sample sizes are reasonably large; otherwise, conditional ML procedures are called for.

Likelihood for R-to-1 Matched Data

As an illustration of the conditional likelihood approach, consider a matched case-control study involving G cases, where each case is individually matched to R controls on one or more variables. For the gth of G such matched sets (or strata), $m_{1g} = 1, m_{0g} = R, m_g = (R + 1)$, and the conditional likelihood in 20.26 simplifies to

$$\prod_{g=1}^{G} \left\{ 1 + \sum_{\ell=2}^{R+1} \exp\left[\boldsymbol{\beta}'(\mathbf{x}_{\ell g} - \mathbf{x}_{1g})\right] \right\}^{-1} \tag{20.27}$$

Note that the structure of Expression 20.27 means that any x_j that takes the same value for all $(R + 1)$ subjects in the same matched set will not appear in the likelihood, so that its corresponding β_j cannot be estimated. Of course, by incorporating such matching variables in the model as interaction terms with exposure factors, one can model the variation in the odds ratio across the matched sets (or strata).

An interesting special case of 20.27 obtains when $\mathbf{x}$ is a single dichotomous exposure variable E, taking the value 1 for exposed subjects and 0 for unexposed subjects. In this instance, the conditional ML estimator of the odds ratio reduces exactly to the one proposed by Miettinen (1970). Breslow and colleagues (1978) have illustrated the use of Expression 20.27 in analyzing data from two matched case-control studies of esophageal cancer, the goal being to estimate the odds ratios for persons having different sets of values for several exposure factors of interest.

Likelihood for Pair-matched Data

When $R = 1$ (i.e., the matched pairs situation), the likelihood 20.27 can be written as

$$\prod_{g=1}^{G} \frac{1}{1 + \exp[-\boldsymbol{\beta}'(\mathbf{x}_{1g} - \mathbf{x}_{2g})]} \tag{20.28}$$

This expression has the same form as an unconditional likelihood for logistic regression of a binary response function on the vector of variables $(\mathbf{x}_{1g} - \mathbf{x}_{2g})$, where each pair is treated as a single unit of observation, $\alpha = 0$, and the response is always one. Thus, computer programs written to perform unconditional ML estimation of linear logistic models can be adapted to evaluate this specialized form of conditional likelihood (see Holford et al., 1978).

To appreciate that these generalized, multivariable conditional likelihood methods do, in fact, specialize to give recognizable results in well-known special cases, consider the following 2×2 table, which represents the results of a matched pairs case-control study involving a single dichotomous exposure variable:

		$D = 0$	
		$E = 1$	$E = 0$
$D = 1$	$E = 1$	v_{11}	v_{10}
	$E = 0$	v_{01}	v_{00}

G

Here, v_{11} is the number of matched pairs out of G where both the case and the control were exposed, v_{10} is the number of matched pairs where the case was exposed but the control was not, etc. For this table, the likelihood of 20.28 becomes

$$\left[\frac{1}{1 + e^{-\beta(1-1)}}\right]^{v_{11}} \left[\frac{1}{1 + e^{-\beta(1-0)}}\right]^{v_{10}} \left[\frac{1}{1 + e^{-\beta(0-1)}}\right]^{v_{01}} \left[\frac{1}{1 + e^{-\beta(0-0)}}\right]^{v_{00}}$$

which, since e^β = EOR, equals

$$\left(\frac{1}{2}\right)^{(v_{11}+v_{00})}\left(\frac{\text{EOR}}{1+\text{EOR}}\right)^{v_{10}}\left(\frac{1}{1+\text{EOR}}\right)^{v_{01}}$$

By differentiating the logarithm of the above likelihood with respect to EOR, equating it to zero, and solving, one finds that the ML estimator of EOR is v_{10}/v_{01}, the ratio of the off-diagonal elements. The unconditional ML estimator in this situation can be shown to be $(v_{10}/v_{01})^2$, which dramatically illustrates the potential bias associated with the use of unconditional likelihood methods for finely stratified data (see Breslow and Day, 1981).

20.4 CONFOUNDER SUMMARIZATION

This multivariable procedure, introduced by Miettinen (1976), involves both model fitting and stratified analysis. Confounder summarization is designed to capitalize on the basic principle that confounding hinges ultimately on a univariate dimension, risk (i.e., the probability of developing the disease), and that appropriate stratification on this dimension would be sufficient to control confounding. A model that usually includes a dichotomous exposure variable E plus appropriate terms involving the potential confounders is fit to the data (usually by discriminant analysis). A *confounder summarization score* is then computed for each individual as the value of the fitted model evaluated at the confounder variable values for that particular individual and with the exposure variable E set equal to zero (its value for unexposed subjects). The individuals are then cast into strata according to score—one easy way to accomplish this being to divide the ranked cases into quintiles by score and then to assign the noncases to these defined strata. Miettinen also recommends that, prior to stratification, individuals be deleted if their scores lie outside the range of overlap between comparison groups. Then, one proceeds as in stratified analysis to test null hypotheses of no association with Mantel-Haenszel statistics, to examine stratum-specific effect measures, and to calculate (if appropriate) standardized measures of effect.

According to Miettinen, two advantages result from this approach. One is its simplicity—e.g., stratum-specific effect measures are directly available and the interpretation of a complex multivariable function is avoided. The second advantage is its lack of dependence on the usual assumptions underlying multivariable procedures—e.g., less is demanded of the fitted model since only a proper *relative* ranking of the subjects by score is required, rather than an *absolute* assessment of risk as a complex function of several interrelated factors. In fact, constructing some sort of "best" model through significance tests is not recommended, since "nonsignificance" does not mean "lack of confounding," and deleting "nonsignificant" terms from the model may lead to substantial confounding by the combination of deleted factors.

In using this procedure, one should make an a posteriori comparison of the groups within each stratum with regard to their distributions by the various confounding factors incorporated in the model. The purpose of this comparison is to evaluate the extent to which stratification by the confounder score did actually control confounding and to assess the degree of intrastratum confounding that remains. In practice, there is bound to be some loss in information from stratification, and some residual confounding is usually present.

Very little theoretical statistical work has been done to evaluate the performance of the confounder summarization procedure. One question that remains is whether or not the exposure variable should be included in the model for testing purposes. Miettinen (1976) and Heilbron (1978) have argued that a model that does *not* include the exposure variable will exaggerate the effect of any true nonconfounders in the model and will lead to a less powerful overall test than would have been obtained if the exposure variable had been included. On the other hand, Pike and colleagues (1979) have argued, on the basis of an analogy between confounder summarization and the use of analysis of covariance, that the χ^2 test statistic for overall association is exaggerated in comparison to a standard partial F test statistic for the addition of the exposure variable to a model already containing the variables to be controlled. We find the reasons for including the exposure variable to be more convincing and therefore recommend such inclusion.

Another problem with confounder summarization concerns the procedure by which strata are formed from the scores. In this regard, questions to be considered include how many strata should be used, whether or not individuals should be deleted from the analysis if their scores lie outside the range of overlapping scores, and whether or not strata should be formed by using ranked scores for all subjects, ranked scores on cases (or noncases) alone, or ranked scores on exposed (or unexposed). Unfortunately, the results obtained from a confounder summarization analysis are quite sensitive to such choices (see Chapter 22 for some numerical illustrations). In addition, the interpretation of the strata (once decided on) is still quite difficult, since the stratification is based on the complex multivariable score rather than on combinations of well-defined categories of the confounding factors. Finally, the standard confounder summarization methodology, which involves a model with only a main effect term in E, can be quite misleading when there is effect modification present in the data.

In light of the preceding remarks, we strongly advocate that confounder summarization *never* be used as the sole method of multivariable analysis. It should be employed, when appropriate, only in conjunction with logistic regression analysis techniques.

20.5 CONCLUDING REMARKS

In this chapter, we have provided a theoretical discussion of mathematical-modeling techniques, with particular emphasis being given to logistic regression procedures. Both unconditional ML estimation and conditional ML estimation of the logistic model coefficients have been described. Unconditional ML methods are appropriate for data sets where stratum-specific sample sizes are large. Conditional ML methods should be used when stratum-specific sample sizes are moderate to small, as typified by matched case-control data (e.g., R-to-1 and pair-matched designs); in such situations, unconditional ML estimates will be biased.

We have also described methods for making statistical inferences based on logistic model fitting, methods that are appropriate for both the unconditional and conditional approaches.

The proper use of mathematical-modeling techniques requires a reasonable strategy for model building, which entails deciding which variables should be included in the final model. In particular, in the analysis of epidemiologic data, the goal in model building should be to obtain a *valid* quantification of the exposure-disease relationship, which necessitates making an accurate assessment of interaction and confounding effects in the data. We will describe a model-building strategy in Chapter 21, and we will consider several applications of unconditional and conditional logistic regression analysis methodology in Chapters 22–24.

NOTATION

The following list summarizes the key notation introduced in this chapter.

D, E	0–1 disease and exposure variables, respectively.
$\text{logit}\,(f) = \ln \dfrac{f}{1-f}$	Logit function for some quantity f.
$P(\mathbf{x}) = \text{pr}\,(D = 1 \lvert x_1, x_2, \ldots, x_k)$	Probability of being a case given the values $x_1, x_2, \ldots, x_k$.
$\alpha, \beta_1, \ldots, \beta_k$	Regression coefficients in the logistic model representing $P(\mathbf{x})$.
$C_1, C_2, \ldots, C_p$	Extraneous variables (risk factors) being considered for control; there are p in number.
$V_1, V_2, \ldots, V_{p_1}$	Functions of the extraneous variables C_1, $C_2, \ldots, C_p$ specified as potential confounders in the logistic model; there are p_1 in number.
$W_1, W_2, \ldots, W_{p_2}$	Functions of the extraneous variables C_1, $C_2, \ldots, C_p$ specified as potential effect modifiers in the logistic model; there are p_2 in number.
β	Coefficient of the dichotomous exposure variable E in the logistic model.
$\gamma_1, \gamma_2, \ldots, \gamma_{p_1}$	Coefficients of the potential confounders V_i in the logistic model.
$\delta_1, \delta_2, \ldots, \delta_{p_2}$	Coefficients of product terms of the form $E \cdot W_j$ in the logistic model.
$L(\boldsymbol{\theta}) \equiv L$	Likelihood function involving a vector of parameters $\boldsymbol{\theta}' = [\theta_1, \theta_2, \ldots, \theta_r]$.

$\hat{V} \equiv \hat{V}(\hat{\boldsymbol{\beta}})$	Estimated variance-covariance matrix of ML estimators of logistic model coefficients.
UL_F	Unconditional likelihood function for a follow-up study.
$UL_C = UL_1 \cdot UL_2$	Unconditional likelihood function for a case-control study.
CL	Conditional likelihood function.

REFERENCES

BISHOP, Y. M. M.; FIENBERG, S. E.; and HOLLAND, P. W. 1975. *Discrete multivariate analysis: Theory and practice.* Cambridge, Mass.: MIT Press.

BRESLOW, N. E., and DAY, N. E. 1981. *Statistical methods in cancer research. Vol. I: The analysis of case-control studies.* Lyon, France: IARC Scientific Publications No. 32.

BRESLOW, N. E.; DAY, N. E.; HALVORSEN, K. T.; PRENTICE, R. L.; and SABAI, C. 1978. Estimation of multiple relative risk functions in matched case-control studies. *Am. J. Epidemiol.* 108(4): 299–307.

BRESLOW, N., and POWERS, W. 1978. Are there two logistic regressions for retrospective studies? *Biometrics* 34(1): 100–105.

CORNFIELD, J. 1962. Joint dependence of the risk of coronary heart disease on serum cholesterol and systolic blood pressure: a discriminant function analysis. *Fed. Proc.* 21: 58–61.

COX, D. R. 1970. *The analysis of binary data.* London: Methuen.

———. 1975. Partial likelihood. *Biometrika* 62: 599–607.

COX, D. R., and HINKLEY, D. V. 1974. *Theoretical statistics.* London: Chapman & Hall.

DAY, N. E., and BYAR, D. P. 1979. Testing hypotheses in case-control studies— Equivalence of Mantel-Haenszel statistics and logit score tests. *Biometrics* 35: 623–630.

GORDON, T. 1974. Hazards in the use of the logistic function with special reference to data from prospective cardiovascular studies. *J. Chronic Dis.* 27: 97–102.

GRIZZLE, J. E.; STARMER, C. F.; and KOCH, G. G. 1969. Analysis of categorical data by linear models. *Biometrics* 25(3): 489–504.

HALPERIN, M.; BLACKWELDER, W. C.; and VERTER, J. I. 1971. Estimation of the multivariate logistic risk function: A comparison of the discriminant function and maximum likelihood approaches. *J. Chronic Dis.* 24: 125–158.

HEILBRON, D. C. 1978. Which confounder score? Unpublished manuscript. San Francisco: University of California, Computer Center.

HOLFORD, T. R.; WHITE, C.; and KELSEY, J. L. 1978. Multivariate analysis for matched case-control studies. *Am. J. Epidemiol.* 107: 245–256.

HOSMER, D. W., and LEMESHOW, S. 1980. Goodness of fit tests for the multiple logistic regression model. *Commun. Stat.* A9(10): 1043–1071.

KLEINBAUM, D. G.; KUPPER, L. L.; CASSEL, J. C.; and TYROLER, H. A. 1971. Multivariate analysis of risk of coronary heart disease in Evans County, Georgia. *Arch. Intern. Med.* 128: 943–948.

KLEINBAUM, D. G.; KUPPER, L. L.; and CHAMBLESS, L. E. 1982. Logistic regression analysis of epidemiologic data: Theory and practice. *Commun. Stat.*, to appear in April, 1982.

KUPPER, L. L., and HOGAN, M. D. 1978. Interaction in epidemiologic studies. *Am. J. Epidemiol.* 108(6): 447–453.

LEMESHOW, S., and HOSMER, D. W. 1982. A review of goodness of fit statistics for use in the development of logistic regression models. *Am. J. Epidemiol.* 115: 92–106.

MASON, R. L., and WEBSTER, J. T. 1975. Regression analysis and problems of multicollinearity. *Commun. Stat.* 4: 277–292.

MIETTINEN, O. S. 1970. Estimation of relative risk from individually matched series. *Biometrics* 23: 75–86.

———. 1976. Stratification by a multivariate confounder score. *Am. J. Epidemiol.* 104(6): 609–620.

PIKE, M. C.; ANDERSON, J.; and DAY, N. 1979. Some insights into Miettinen's multivariate confounder score approach to case-control study analysis. *Epidemiol. Community Health* 33: 104–106.

PIKE, M. C.; HILL, A. P.; and SMITH, P. G. 1980. Bias and efficiency in logistic analyses of stratified case-control studies. *Int. J. Epidemiol.* 9(1): 89–95.

PRENTICE, R. 1976. Use of the logistic model in retrospective studies. *Biometrics* 32(3): 599–606.

PRENTICE, R. L., and PYKE, R. 1979. Logistic disease incidence models and case-control studies. *Biometrika* 66: 403–411.

PRESS, S. J., and WILSON, S. 1978. Choosing between logistic regression and discriminant analysis. *J. Am. Stat. Assoc.* 70: 699–705.

TRUETT, J.; CORNFIELD, J.; and KANNEL, W. 1967. A multivariate analysis of the risk of coronary heart disease in Framingham. *J. Chronic Dis.* 20: 511–524.

21

Modeling: Analysis Strategy

21.0
PREVIEW

In this chapter, we propose a general strategy to be employed when analyzing a complex multivariable epidemiologic data set. Our primary focus here will be on the use of logistic regression procedures for the control of extraneous factors at the analysis stage, taking into account, when necessary, pertinent aspects of the design of the study (e.g., matching).

In view of this orientation, we hasten to emphasize that the use of classical algorithms (e.g., stepwise regression) to obtain a "best" regression model can lead to highly misleading interpretations of the data being analyzed, since their use does not *automatically* ensure that confounding and effect modification features will be properly addressed. Such readily available variable selection procedures are designed to include independent variables in a regression model solely on the basis of precision considerations (i.e., according to which factors explain the most variability in the dependent variable, as reflected, for example, by partial correlation coefficient values) and *not* on validity grounds. The control of extraneous factors is primarily a validity issue involving the assessment of factor relationships with the exposure variable(s) as well as with the disease variable, and such validity considerations must take precedence over those concerned with precision.

Furthermore, the implementation of any reasonable analysis strategy is complicated by problems associated with small sample sizes, complex interrelationships among the variables under consideration, and the inherent limitations of the statistical procedures used. Hence, in actual practice, the appropriate application of the general analysis strategy discussed here will involve a great deal of knowledge and expertise. Indeed, the ability to carry out a well-conceived multivariable analysis of a complex epidemiologic data set requires an in-depth theoretical understanding of the statistical procedures involved, an appreciation of the disease etiology as a function of the variables of interest, and considerable experience in working with such data so that one is aware of the analytical pitfalls that often occur. Such analyses are best carried out in an interactive environment that includes both biostatisticians and epidemiologists.

Figure 21.1 provides a flow diagram for a *three-part general analysis strategy*. The first part concerns initial *variable specification*. The remaining two parts, which will be discussed in detail below, involve the assessment of *interaction* and of *confounding*.

21.1
INTER-
ACTION
ASSESSMENT

As the second part of a general analysis strategy, we recommend that the nature of the interaction present in the data, including the identification of specific effect-modifying factors, be assessed before any consideration is given to issues of confounding. This part of the analysis is, in practice, the most difficult to carry out. Even so, it is conceptually the most important, since the failure to detect and quantify the key interaction effects in the data can lead to serious errors in interpreting the exposure-disease relationships under study.

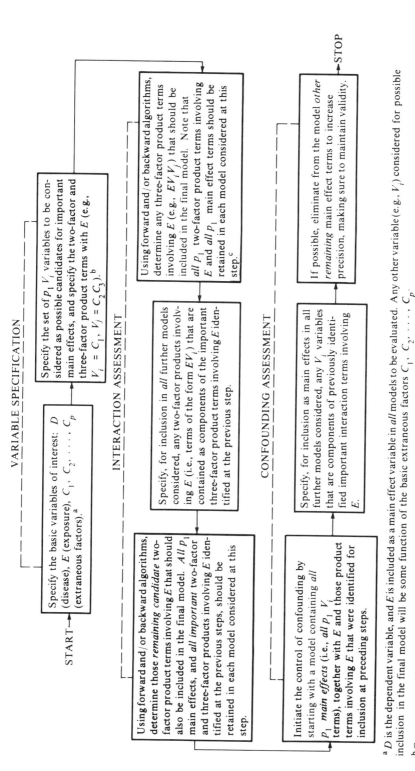

VARIABLE SPECIFICATION

START — Specify the basic variables of interest: D (disease), E (exposure), $C_1, C_2, \ldots, C_p$ (extraneous factors).[a]

Specify the set of p_1 V_i variables to be considered as possible candidates for important main effects, and specify the two-factor and three-factor product terms with E (e.g., $V_i = C_1$, $V_j = C_2 C_3$).[b]

INTERACTION ASSESSMENT

Using forward and/or backward algorithms, determine those *remaining candidate* two-factor product terms involving E that should also be included in the final model. *All* p_1 main effects, and *all important* two-factor and three-factor products involving E identified at the previous steps, should be retained in each model considered at this step.

Specify, for inclusion in *all* further models considered, any two-factor products involving E (i.e., terms of the form EV_i) that are contained as components of the important three-factor product terms involving E identified at the previous step.

Using forward and/or backward algorithms, determine any three-factor product terms involving E (e.g., EV_iV_j) that should be included in the final model. Note that *all* p_1 two-factor product terms involving E and *all* p_1 main effect terms should be retained in each model considered at this step.[c]

CONFOUNDING ASSESSMENT

Initiate the control of confounding by starting with a model containing *all* p_1 *main effects* (i.e., all p_1 V_i terms), together with E and those product terms involving E that were identified for inclusion at preceding steps.

Specify, for inclusion as main effects in all further models considered, any V_i variables that are components of previously identified important interaction terms involving E.

If possible, eliminate from the model *other remaining* main effect terms to increase precision, making sure to maintain validity.

→ STOP

[a] D is the dependent variable, and E is included as a main effect variable in *all* models to be evaluated. Any *other* variable (e.g., V_i) considered for possible inclusion in the final model will be some function of the basic extraneous factors $C_1, C_2, \ldots, C_p$.

[b] Components of interaction terms involving E (e.g., EV_iV_j) have occasionally been denoted as W variables (e.g., $W_i = V_iV_j$); for an example, see model 20.10 in Section 20.1.

[c] When one is evaluating such models, a linear dependency among the columns of the design matrix may be encountered. This dependency requires a redefinition of the model to remove the singularity.

Figure 21.1 Flow Diagram for a Multivariable (Logistic) Analysis Strategy to Control for Extraneous Factors

A popular qualitative approach for obtaining a general impression of the types of interaction present in a data set entails checking for *heterogeneity* among stratum-specific effect measures resulting from various stratified analyses. Such a check might involve appropriate statistical tests for such heterogeneity. The variables so identified by this inspection as potential effect modifiers may then be treated, initially, as such in building a valid regression model. Unfortunately, as we have already seen, when the number of extraneous factors is even moderately large (leading to small stratum-specific samples sizes), the use of stratified analysis procedures *alone* to assess interaction and confounding usually leads to both imprecise and difficult-to-interpret results. In practice, then, although stratification methods are useful for an initial gross examination of the data, the most informative analysis would require that the quantification of key interaction effects be carried out with mathematical-modeling procedures, with the logistic model most often being the regression function of choice.

21.1.1
Baseline
Logistic Model

Although there is no "best" strategy in this regard, a reasonable and often-used approach for assessing interaction starts with a "baseline" logistic model that includes as many main effect terms *as considered appropriate* (i.e., the $\gamma_i V_i$ terms and the βE term in the notation of Model 20.10). One then identifies important effect modifiers by assessing the additional contribution to prediction (relative to this baseline main effects model) of product functions involving E and the V_i's (e.g., functions of the form EV_i, EV_iV_j, etc.).

Note: A product term involving only the V_i's themselves (e.g., a term like $V_iV_jV_k$) can be included in the set of main effect terms by simply defining a new variable (e.g., $V^* = V_iV_jV_k$). Hence, in all that follows, *our discussions on interaction will pertain only to product terms involving the exposure variable E.*

21.1.2
Variable
Selection
Strategies

There are several statistical algorithms that can be used to select those product terms to be included in the final regression model. We will briefly mention a couple of them in this section, and we will illustrate their use in Chapters 22–24. Unfortunately, there is no algorithm that can be called "optimal." And, in fact, there is no guarantee, when using more than one of these variable selection methods on a given data set, that each will lead to the identification of the *same* set of important effect-modifying factors.

When one is using algorithms, in practice, to search for effect modifiers, we strongly advocate considering only functions of the form EV_i (two-factor interactions) and EV_iV_j (three-factor interactions). One reason for restricting the set of potentially important interaction terms is that products involving four or more factors (e.g., functions at least as complex as $EV_iV_jV_k$) are usually not of practical importance. In addition, they are extremely difficult to interpret etiologically (and sometimes even mathematically).

Another compelling argument for such a restriction is that the reliability in the estimation of the coefficients in a regression model becomes worse as the model becomes more complex (e.g., contains several higher-order terms), regardless of whether the method of estimation is ordinary least squares, weighted least squares, standard maximum likelihood, iterative proportional fitting, etc. This unreliability results because independent variables in the model, being mathematical functions of one another when polynomial and interaction terms are used, are highly intercorrelated. This intercorrelation leads to severe multicollinearity (see Mason and Webster, 1975), which is manifested by a "nearly singular" covariance or information matrix. Such ill-conditioning can severely detract from the utility of commonly employed variable selection algorithms.

Even with this restriction on the order of candidate interaction terms, the number of two-factor and three-factor interaction terms expands quickly with only a slight increase in the number of V_i terms considered. Clearly, a judicious specification of the set of V_i variables is crucial to the success of any variable selection algorithm for identifying the key effect modifiers. Moreover, when adding interaction terms to a model, one must take care not to produce a singular design matrix.

Two commonly used variable selection procedures for deciding which interaction terms to include in the final logistic model are the *forward selection procedure* and the *backward elimination procedure*. We recommend that the forward selection procedure *start,* if possible (see footnote c in Figure 21.1), with the model that contains *all* main effects and two-factor interactions involving E. Then one sequentially selects three-factor interactions involving E when the appropriate likelihood ratio statistic is "significant" at some specified α level. The inclusion of such three-factor interaction terms stops when none of the remaining candidates can meet the *appropriately specified* significance level criterion for entry into the model. [See Kupper and colleagues (1976) for a discussion concerning Type I error rates when using forward selection algorithms in a regression setting.] The corresponding backward elimination procedure would start with a model containing all main effects and two-factor interactions. Then one would include as many three-factor interactions as possible without causing a singularity. Finally, one would eliminate statistically insignificant three-factor interactions (e.g., as determined by appropriate likelihood ratio tests), stopping when only statistically significant three-factor interaction terms remain. [Note that a set of main effect or interaction terms pertaining to a single multicategory factor—e.g., when a nominal variable with L levels is represented by $(L - 1)$ dummy variables—must be added or deleted as a group rather than individually.]

As we mentioned earlier, two *different* sets of important three-factor interactions may result from applying both the forward selection and backward elimination procedures to the same data set. If such an undesirable outcome occurs, the final decision regarding which three-factor terms to

21.1.3 Forward and Backward Algorithms

keep in the model should be made after considering all available a priori information about the variables and the disease etiology. Also, the final decision should be made only after examining the fit of the model to the data, the signs of the estimated coefficients (are they realistic?), the evidence regarding the degree of multicollinearity, the behavior of the residuals, etc.

An example when certain backward approaches do not work is given in Chapter 23. In that example, the coefficients in a model containing *all* main effects, two-factor, and three-factor interactions could not be estimated by maximum likelihood, because a singular estimated information matrix was obtained. This *perfect singularity* occurrence (i.e., exact multicollinearity) is not as uncommon as one might think when working with a model involving a large number of terms (including higher-order interactions).

Since the results from any stratified analysis can be exactly duplicated via regression methods by defining the model appropriately, it follows that problems with small stratum-specific sample sizes can only be lessened by reducing the number of terms needed in such regression models. This reduction can often be accomplished by treating some of the extraneous factors (i.e., the C's) as continuous rather than as categorical variables and also by eliminating some of these factors completely from consideration, while at the same time making sure that validity is not compromised by such model simplification. As a final comment, we note that singularity problems are encountered much more often with the backward elimination procedure than with the forward selection procedure, which sometimes necessitates the *sole* use of the latter algorithm (see Chapter 23 for an example).

**21.1.4
Hierarchical
Model
Simplification**

In the use of the above algorithms as described, note that the statistical significance of the three-factor interactions is to be assessed with *all* lower-order terms (i.e., all possible main effect and two-factor interaction terms) present in the model. This statistical hypothesis-testing strategy is based on the philosophy that model simplification should begin with an examination of the highest-order terms and should proceed with an evaluation of the importance of terms of a given order on the basis of likelihood ratio tests involving models that *must* contain all lower-order terms. In other words, *no terms of a given order should be dropped from a model before proper consideration is given to all higher-order terms*. In fact, it has been argued, in a categorical data analysis setting, that retaining an interaction effect of a given order in a model precludes eliminating from that model any lower-order terms involving the variables constituting that effect [e.g., see the hierarchy principle discussed in Bishop and colleagues (1975)]. Under this policy, then, if the three-factor interaction EV_iV_j is retained in the model, then so should be the two-factor products EV_i and EV_j, and also the main effects of V_i, V_j, and, of course, E, regardless of whether they are statistically significant or not. (If the product V_iV_j is originally deemed important as a baseline main effect variable, then it should also be retained.)

A key reason for not automatically dropping statistically insignificant lower-order terms corresponding to an important interaction effect of a given order is that the physical meaning of the coefficients of such lower-order terms depends on how the variables involved are coded. Hence, the interpretations of associated statistical inference-making procedures are likewise affected.

**21.1.5
Effect of
Coding**

To illustrate how such interpretation problems arise, we consider a commonly employed coding scheme thought to help reduce unwanted multi-collinearity [see the paper by Smith and Campbell (1980) and the associated debate in the *Journal of the American Statistical Association*]. This simple procedure, referred to as *centering,* involves subtracting some "typical value" (e.g., a sample mean) from each of the V_i variables *before* fitting a model including these variables to the data. So, we let $V_i^* = (V_i - C_i)$ be the centered variable corresponding to V_i. Then, for example, a model like

$$\text{logit } P(\mathbf{x}) = \alpha + \beta E + \gamma_1 V_1 + \gamma_2 V_2 + \delta_1 EV_1$$
$$+ \delta_2 EV_2 + \delta_3 EV_1 V_2 \tag{21.1}$$

can (after some algebraic manipulations) be equivalently expressed in terms of the centered V_i^* variables as

$$\text{logit } P(\mathbf{x}) = \alpha^* + \beta^* E + \gamma_1^* V_1^* + \gamma_2^* V_2^* + \delta_1^* EV_1^*$$
$$+ \delta_2^* EV_2^* + \delta_3^* EV_1^* V_2^* \tag{21.2}$$

where

$$\alpha^* = \alpha + \gamma_1 C_1 + \gamma_2 C_2$$
$$\beta^* = \beta + \delta_1 C_1 + \delta_2 C_2 + \delta_3 C_1 C_2$$
$$\gamma_1^* = \gamma_1 \qquad \gamma_2^* = \gamma_2$$
$$\delta_1^* = \delta_1 + \delta_3 C_2 \qquad \delta_2^* = \delta_2 + \delta_3 C_1 \qquad \delta_3^* = \delta_3$$

The important thing to note here is that the *only* coefficients in the transformed model, 21.2, that are the same as those in the original model, 21.1, are the ones corresponding to the *highest-order interaction term* (namely, δ_3) and to the main effects of V_1 and V_2. These latter two coefficients (γ_1 and γ_2) remain undisturbed only because the product $V_1 V_2$ does not appear in 21.1.

It follows that the presence of a significant interaction effect of a given order necessarily means that statistical tests about corresponding lower-order terms in that model depend on the coding scheme used for the variables involved. Hence, it would be unwise, from a validity standpoint, to drop such terms from that model solely on the basis of such tests. Note, in particular, that the odds ratio based on Expression 21.1, with E being a 0–1 exposure variable, is

$$\exp(\beta + \delta_1 V_1 + \delta_2 V_2 + \delta_3 V_1 V_2)$$

With some algebraic manipulation, it can be shown that this quantity is exactly equal to

$$\exp(\beta^* + \delta_1^* V_1^* + \delta_2^* V_2^* + \delta_3^* V_1^* V_2^*)$$

the odds ratio under Expression 21.2. Thus, dropping one or more of β^*, δ_1^*, and δ_2^* from 21.2 on the basis of a statistical test when δ_3^* (and hence δ_3) is not zero would introduce a bias in estimating the odds ratio under 21.1.

Of course, the above discussions implicitly considered Model 21.1 to be the correct model in some sense. In this regard, a subtle but very important point is that the V_i variables in 21.1 could themselves be considered as linear transforms of other variables (e.g., as defined by a different, and equally valid, coding scheme), just as the variables in 21.2 are linear transforms of those in 21.1. The true underlying odds ratio will be the same for all such models if no associated lower-order terms involving E are dropped corresponding to any nonzero interaction term of a given order involving E. This result emphasizes the inadvisability, when working with real data, of dropping *any* related lower-order terms in a model corresponding to a statistically significant interaction term of a given order.

A few comments are now in order about the controversy over the usefulness of centering the independent variables. After fitting the centered model (21.2) by any of the standard ML estimation procedures we have discussed, one can easily transform back to Expression 21.1. This linear transformation would produce exactly the same set of estimated coefficients, and also the same estimated information matrix, as would be obtained by fitting Expression 21.1 *directly*. In other words, any apparent reduction in multicollinearity achieved by centering (e.g., as illustrated by Breslow et al., 1978, pp. 303–304) is really only an artifact when using an estimation procedure that is inherently mathematically independent of any linear transformation (e.g., like centering and scaling) of the independent variables. Centering and scaling can make a difference in computational accuracy and in the use of a so-called biased estimation procedure like *ridge regression* (see Marquardt and Snee, 1975). This technique is specifically designed to address real (and *not* artificial) multicollinearity and is not inherently mathematically independent of linear transformations performed on the predictor variables. Although ridge regression is a fairly new procedure, its utility in fitting logistic regression models has been studied in detail by at least one author (see Schaefer, 1979). We will not illustrate ridge regression here, but we encourage its use with highly ill-conditioned data.

A summary of the main points concerning the second part of our general analysis strategy—namely, the assessment of interaction—is provided in the second row of the flow diagram given in Figure 21.1. As an illustration of the strategy to this point, suppose that V_1, V_2, V_3, V_4, and V_5 are five risk factor functions identified for possible control. As we emphasized earlier, the validity of our (or indeed, any) analysis strategy hinges on a proper specification of these factors. Now let us imagine that EV_1V_2 is the only one of the ten possible three-factor interactions deemed significant enough for retention in the final model. According to our strategy, then, EV_1, EV_2, V_1, and V_2 (in addition to E) must also appear in the final model. At the second step, imagine that only EV_3 is found to be significant out of the remaining three candidate two-factor interactions (namely, EV_3, EV_4, and EV_5) not already earmarked for inclusion in the final model. The retention of EV_3 means, according to our system, that V_3 must also be included in the final model. At this penultimate stage in our general analysis strategy, then, the fitted model under consideration is

21.1.6 Summary

$$\text{logit } P(\mathbf{x}) = \hat{\alpha} + \hat{\beta}E + \hat{\gamma}_1 V_1 + \hat{\gamma}_2 V_2 + \hat{\gamma}_3 V_3 + \hat{\gamma}_4 V_4 + \hat{\gamma}_5 V_5$$
$$+ \hat{\delta}_1 EV_1 + \hat{\delta}_2 EV_2 + \hat{\delta}_3 EV_3 + \hat{\delta}_4 EV_1 V_2 \qquad (21.3)$$

Note that the V_4 and V_5 terms are the only remaining ones in the above model for which a decision concerning retention or deletion has not been made.

We have now arrived at the third part of our three-part general analysis strategy, which concerns what to do with those remaining V_i main effect variables not already chosen for retention in the final model. (See the third row of Figure 21.1.) In deciding whether to delete or to retain such terms, one must consider both validity and precision issues, with the former taking precedence (as usual) over the latter.

21.2 CONFOUND- ING ASSESSMENT

If some of these main effect variables are important confounders in the data, then their deletion, even if they are *not* statistically significant, will alter the values of one or more of the estimated exposure-involved coefficients upon fitting the reduced model. This result leads to a potential bias in the estimation of the odds ratio. On the other hand, *if deletion of main effect (V_i) variables does not materially change the exposure-involved coefficients (upon refitting)—and hence the estimated odds ratio—then the use of a reduced model without such terms can sometimes lead to a gain in precision.*

In practice, the deletion of such terms will invariably alter the values of the exposure-involved coefficients somewhat (thus necessitating a difficult, subjective decision about whether such an alteration is "small enough" to ignore). Also, the deletion of such terms (when permissible on validity grounds) will not usually result in any substantial gain in precision. Thus, it is often best just to leave such terms in the final model. In fact, even if such terms, like $\hat{\gamma}_4 V_4$ and $\hat{\gamma}_5 V_5$ in Expression 21.3, are retained in the final model (regardless of their statistical significance), they do not enter into the final odds ratio expression, which, for 21.3 with E being a 0–1 exposure variable, becomes

$$\exp(\hat{\beta} + \hat{\delta}_1 V_1 + \hat{\delta}_2 V_2 + \hat{\delta}_3 V_3 + \hat{\delta}_4 V_1 V_2)$$

Finally, consider the situation when no interaction terms involving E are found to be significant. Then, any simplification of the resulting main effects model (to gain precision) by eliminating one or more of the V_i terms requires a monitoring of the exposure coefficient $\hat{\beta}$.

21.3 CONCLUD- ING REMARKS

This completes our discussion of the general analysis strategy we recommend. The motivation behind this strategy has always been to come up with a *valid* estimate of the odds ratio, even to the point of sacrificing some precision in its estimation. We readily concede that our strategy will not necessarily lead to the most parsimonious (i.e., most simply structured) and most precisely fitting model. Indeed, there are many other model-building algorithms that can be used. However, we feel that this strategy offers a good opportunity for determining the most valid model, with no substantial loss in precision.

REFERENCES

BISHOP, Y. M. M.; FIENBERG, S. E.; and HOLLAND, P. W. 1975. *Discrete multivariate analysis: Theory and practice*. Cambridge, Mass.: MIT Press.

BRESLOW, N. E.; DAY, N. E.; HALVORSEN, K. T.; PRENTICE, R. L.; and SABAI, C. 1978. Estimation of multiple relative risk functions in matched case-control studies. *Am. J. Epidemiol.* 108(4): 299–307.

KUPPER, L. L.; STEWART, J. R.; and WILLIAMS, K. A. 1976. A note on controlling significance levels in stepwise regression. *Am. J. Epidemiol.* 103(1): 13–15.

MARQUARDT, D. W., and SNEE, R. D. 1975. Ridge regression in practice. *Am. Stat.* 29(1): 3–20.

MASON, R. L., and WEBSTER, J. T. 1975. Regression analysis and problems of multicollinearity. *Commun. Stat.* 4: 277–292.

SCHAEFER, R. L. 1979. Multicollinearity and logistic regression. Ph.D. dissertation, University of Michigan. University Microfilms, Ann Arbor, Mich.

SMITH. G., and CAMPBELL, F. 1980. A critique of some ridge regression methods. *J. Am. Stat. Assoc.* 75(369): 74–80.

22

Applications of Modeling with No Interaction

CHAPTER OUTLINE

**22.0
PREVIEW**

In this chapter and in the two chapters to follow, we numerically illustrate the mathematical-modeling procedures discussed in Chapter 20. Moreover, we provide applications of strategies for analysis that we previously outlined in Chapter 21. The examples discussed here and in Chapter 23 use follow-up data on 609 white males from the Evans County heart disease study described in Chapters 1 and 17. These analyses will illustrate the use of unconditional maximum likelihood (ML) estimation of the logistic model, as well as other approaches we have discussed [i.e., log-linear modeling (using weighted least squares estimation) and confounder summarization]. In Chapter 24, we consider the analysis of matched case-control data (using two different data sets) to illustrate the use of conditional ML estimation procedures for the logistic model.

**22.1
EXAMPLES
USING THE
EVANS
COUNTY
DATA**

The reader may recall that the problem addressed via this data set concerned the assessment of the putative association between endogenous catecholamine level (CAT), a dichotomous exposure variable fabricated for illustrative purposes, and the subsequent seven-year incidence of coronary heart disease (CHD). The extraneous variables considered for possible control included AGE, CHL (serum cholesterol), SMK (smoking status), ECG (electrocardiogram abnormality status), and HPT (hypertension status). In the discussions to follow, we illustrate two separate series of analyses. The first of these, which we discuss in this chapter, considers the control of AGE and ECG as if these were the only risk factors of interest. The second set of analyses, described in Chapter 23, considers all five of the above variables to be the risk factors. The reason we first focus only on the two variables AGE and ECG is that we wish to illustrate the various approaches for control in a manageable situation—i.e., one characterized by a minimum number of variables, sufficiently large sample sizes to permit valid stratum-specific analyses, and (as we will demonstrate) no interaction. In contrast, when we later consider all five variables identified above, we will find evidence of interaction, which will allow us to illustrate more complex aspects of analysis. Note that, of the five extraneous variables being considered, two variables (AGE and CHL) inherently have an interval scale, whereas the other three (ECG, SMK, and HPT) are binary. This situation will allow us to compare various modeling approaches when assumptions of multivariate normality are not valid and when interval variables are treated as categorical variables in the analysis.

**22.2
STRATIFIED
ANALYSIS
RESULTS:
CAT VERSUS
CHD, CON-
TROLLING
FOR AGE
AND ECG**

We have previously illustrated the results of stratified analyses carried out on the Evans County data set (see Tables 17.3, 17.4, and 17.7), analyses that involved the variables ECG and/or AGE. As we have mentioned, stratification is a convenient and appealing initial approach commonly taken for the control of extraneous variables. Moreover, since the stratum-specific sample sizes (particularly on the four margins of each relevant two-way table) are relatively large when AGE (treated dichotomously) and ECG abnormality status are the only variables to be controlled, the results from stratification may be viewed with sufficient confidence to provide baseline conclusions that can be compared with conclusions from other more sophisticated analytic approaches. (Of course, misleading interpretations may be made because of a loss in sensitivity from categorizing continuous variables; however, this loss does not occur with this data set.)

Table 22.1 provides a summary of the results of stratification when AGE and ECG are the only control variables considered. It is instructive to review the information in this table in the context of the analytic strategy we have recommended in Chapter 21. Subsequently, we will follow this same strategy when using mathematical-modeling approaches.

Our first concern is with the assessment of interaction. An inspection of the four stratum-specific risk ratios (and risk odds ratios) in Table 22.1, which were obtained by simultaneously stratifying on AGE and ECG, shows that there is little meaningful variation in the estimated CAT–CHD relationship over the four strata. Comparison of the $a\hat{R}R$, $s\hat{R}R$, and $s'\hat{R}R$ values within any row of the table also suggests little interaction. Moreover, the χ_I^2 test for interaction (described in Exercise 17.6 in Chapter 17), which compares observed values to fitted values obtained by using a *common* adjusted odds ratio ($a\hat{O}R = 1.91$) for each of the four strata, is nonsignificant ($P \geqslant .25$).

22.2.1 Interaction Assessment

Assuming, then, that neither AGE nor ECG is an effect modifier, we may now proceed to the assessment of confounding. The baseline statistic for this aspect of the analysis should be some estimated effect measure that simultaneously controls for both AGE and ECG, say, $a\hat{R}R = 1.71$. Monitoring the value of $a\hat{R}R$ when ECG and AGE are treated separately, and when both are ignored, we find the following results. When ECG is the only variable controlled, $a\hat{R}R$ changes from 1.71 to 2.15; when AGE is the only variable controlled, $a\hat{R}R$ becomes 1.91; and when neither variable is controlled, $a\hat{R}R$ (which is equal to $c\hat{R}R$) increases to 2.45. We have argued (Chapter 13) that the presence of confounding depends on the investigator's judgment as to whether any of these $a\hat{R}R$'s is meaningfully different from the baseline value (1.71) obtained when all variables are controlled simultaneously. The data indicate that, when both AGE and ECG are controlled simultaneously, the resulting CAT–CHD effect is clearly weaker ($a\hat{R}R = 1.71$) than it is when both variables are ignored ($c\hat{R}R = 2.45$). Also, of the two control variables, AGE is a stronger candidate for being a confounder, since its control alone yields a result ($a\hat{R}R = 1.91$) closer to the baseline value than that for the control of ECG alone ($a\hat{R}R = 2.15$).

22.2.2 Confounding Assessment

To help solve this dilemma about which, if any, variables should be controlled, we now consider whether a substantial gain in *precision* would be obtained by not controlling for AGE or ECG. Using *reciprocal confidence interval length* as a crude measure of precision, we obtain the results

22.2.3 Precision Considerations

Table 22.1 Summary of Stratified Analyses for CAT–CHD Association, Controlling for AGE and ECG

a. Test Statistics and Estimates Obtained Using Different Sets of Control Variables

Control Variables Involved	Number of Strata	χ^2_{MH} (P-value)	POINT ESTIMATES				95% TAYLOR SERIES INTERVAL ESTIMATES	
			$\widehat{aRR}$	$\widehat{sRR}$	$s'\widehat{RR}$	$\widehat{aOR}$	For aRR	For aOR
None (crude analysis)	1	16.22 (.000)	2.45	2.45	2.45	2.86	(1.58, 3.79)	(1.69, 4.85)
AGE = $\begin{cases} 1 \text{ if} \geq 55 \\ 0 \text{ if} < 55 \end{cases}$	2	6.99 (.004)	1.91	1.88	2.04	2.17	(1.19, 3.07)	(1.22, 3.85)
ECG = $\begin{cases} 1 \text{ if abnormality} \\ 0 \text{ if no abnormality} \end{cases}$	2	9.31 (.001)	2.15	1.98	2.38	2.45	(1.35, 3.42)	(1.39, 4.32)
AGE, ECG[a,b]	4	4.15 (.021)	1.71	1.65	1.83	1.91	(1.03, 2.84)	(1.03, 3.53)

b. Stratum-Specific Information When AGE and ECG Are Controlled Together

Strata	a	b	c	d	n	χ^2_{MH}	$\widehat{RR}_g$	$\widehat{OR}_g$
1 (AGE < 55, ECG = 0)	1	17	7	257	282	.51	2.01	2.16
2 (AGE < 55, ECG = 1)	3	7	14	52	76	.38	1.49	1.59
3 (AGE ≥ 55, ECG = 0)	9	15	30	107	161	2.69	1.88	2.14
4 (AGE ≥ 55, ECG = 1)	14	5	44	27	90	.89	1.54	1.72
Total (crude)	27	44	95	443	487	16.22	2.45	2.86

[a]See the table in part b.

[b]$\chi^2_I = \sum_g (a_g - a'_g)^2 / \hat{V}ar_0(A_g) = .128$, where a'_g is the fitted value for stratum g using the common odds ratio value $a\hat{O}R = 1.91$. (A more detailed explanation of this statistic is given in Practice Exercise 17.6 in Chapter 17.)

Table 22.2   Precision Measured as Reciprocal
Confidence Interval Length

Control Variables	Precision in Estimating aRR
AGE	.53
ECG	.48
AGE, ECG	.55

in Table 22.2, which are based on the interval estimation information in Table 22.1.

These results suggest that the simultaneous control of both AGE and ECG provides the highest precision; in other words, no substantial gain in precision is obtained by dropping AGE or ECG from consideration. We would therefore recommend that both variables be controlled. Thus, on the basis of our stratification analysis, we would conclude that there is a moderate ($P = .021$) CAT–CHD association, as reflected in an adjusted risk ratio value aR̂R of 1.71, with approximate 95% confidence limits of 1.03 and 2.84.

We now turn to an examination of the same data by using the mathematical-modeling approaches discussed in Chapters 20 and 21. Tables 22.3, 22.4, and 22.5 provide modeling results regarding point estimation of overall effect, 95% confidence interval estimation, and hypothesis testing, respectively. The methods illustrated in these tables include logistic modeling, confounder summarization, and log-linear modeling (using weighted least squares estimation). We first describe the results from logistic modeling.

22.3
LOGISTIC
MODELING:
CAT VERSUS
CHD,
CONTROL-
LING FOR
AGE AND
ECG

From Expression 20.10, the particular form of logistic model to be used here (controlling for ECG and AGE) is

22.3.1
The Logistic
Model

$$P(\mathbf{x}) = \mathrm{pr}(\mathrm{CHD} = 1 \,|\, \mathrm{CAT}, V_1, \ldots, V_{p_1}, W_1, \ldots, W_{p_2})$$

$$= \frac{1}{\left\{1 + \exp\left[-\left(\alpha + \beta(\mathrm{CAT}) + \sum_{i=1}^{p_1} \gamma_i V_i + (\mathrm{CAT}) \sum_{j=1}^{p_2} \delta_j W_j\right)\right]\right\}}$$

where the V_i and W_j terms are functions of the control variables ECG and AGE, with the V_i denoting potential confounders and the W_j denoting potential effect modifiers. (Note that, according to the hierarchy principle described in Chapter 21, every W_j must also be included as a V_i.) For this model, the (adjusted) risk odds ratio describing the CAT–CHD association is obtained from Formula 20.12, which reduces to e^β under no interaction (i.e., all $\hat{\delta}_j = 0$).

22.3.2
Variable
Specification

For the above logistic model, the first problem to be addressed concerns the specification of potentially important main effect (V_i) and associated interaction (W_j) terms. In Chapter 21, we recommended, as part of a general analytic strategy, that both the V_i and W_j terms be no more complicated than two-way products of the basic extraneous variables being controlled. Since our example here involves only two extraneous variables, then the only two-factor product eligible to be a V_i or a W_j is the variable AGE $\times$ ECG. Thus, the most complicated (i.e., "saturated") model that we will consider contains the following V_i and W_j terms:

$$V_1 = \text{AGE} = W_1 \qquad V_2 = \text{ECG} = W_2 \qquad V_3 = \text{AGE} \times \text{ECG} = W_3$$

Table 22.3   Point Estimation Results; Evans County Data
(D = CHD, E = CAT, Controlling for AGE and ECG)

Model	V_i Terms in Model	LOGISTIC ($e^{\hat{\beta}}$) MLE$_u$[b]	DISC[b]	LOG–LIN ($e^{\hat{\beta}}$), GSK[b]	STRATIFIED[a] a$\hat{R}R$	a$\hat{O}R$
1	None (crude analysis)	2.86	3.68	2.86	2.45	2.86
2	AGEG[c]	2.17	2.77	2.17	1.91	2.17
3	AGE	2.20	2.98	2.58	—	—
4	ECG	2.45	3.10	2.45	2.15	2.45
5	AGEG, ECG	1.86	2.35	1.86	—	—
6	AGE, ECG	1.92	2.40	1.91	—	—
7	AGEG, ECG, AGEG $\times$ ECG	1.91	2.40	1.91	1.71	1.91
8	AGE, ECG, AGE $\times$ ECG	1.93	2.38	1.95	—	—

[a]Stratified analysis results are provided only for those regression models that lead to theoretically equivalent results. For example, when only age is being controlled, the logistic model incorporating two age strata has the form logit $P(\mathbf{x}) = \alpha + \beta(\text{CAT}) + \gamma(\text{AGEG})$, which contains the binary variable AGEG instead of the interval variable AGE. Correspondingly, when age and electrocardiogram history are being controlled simultaneously, the logistic model incorporating four strata (combinations of categories of the binary variables AGEG and ECG) has the form logit $P(\mathbf{x}) = \alpha + \beta(\text{CAT}) + \gamma_1(\text{AGEG}) + \gamma_2(\text{ECG}) + \gamma_3(\text{AGEG} \times \text{ECG})$.

[b]MLE$_u$, DISC, and GSK denote, respectively, unconditional ML estimation, discriminant function estimation, and Grizzle-Starmer-Koch weighted least squares estimation.

[c]$\text{AGEG} = \begin{cases} 1 \text{ if AGE} \geq 55 \\ 0 \text{ if AGE} < 55 \end{cases}$

Table 22.4 95% Large-Sample Confidence Intervals; Evans County Data (D = CHD, E = CAT, Controlling for AGE and ECG)

Model	V_i Terms	LOGISTIC			STRATIFIED	
		MLE$_u$	DISC	LOG–LIN, GSK	For aRR	For aOR
1	None	(1.69, 4.85)	(1.97, 6.87)	(1.69, 4.85)	(1.58, 3.79)	(1.69, 4.85)
2	AGEG	(1.21, 3.87)	(1.40, 5.49)	(1.22, 3.85)	(1.19, 3.07)	(1.22, 3.85)
3	AGE	(1.23, 3.94)	(1.41, 5.55)	(1.35, 4.96)	—	—
4	ECG	(1.37, 4.38)	(1.57, 6.12)	(1.39, 4.32)	(1.35, 3.42)	(1.39, 4.32)
5	AGEG, ECG	(1.00, 3.48)	(1.13, 4.88)	(1.01, 3.44)	—	—
6	AGE, ECG	(1.03, 3.59)	(1.15, 4.98)	(.93, 3.91)	—	—
7	AGEG, ECG, AGEG × ECG	(1.02, 3.54)	(1.15, 5.02)	(1.03, 3.53)	(1.03, 2.84)	(1.03, 3.53)
8	AGE, ECG, AGE × ECG	(1.04, 3.60)	(1.14, 4.98)	(.95, 3.99)	—	—

Note: All confidence intervals are of the general form

$$\exp\left[\ln\hat{\theta} \pm 1.96\sqrt{\hat{\text{V}}\text{ar}(\ln\hat{\theta})}\right]$$

where $\hat{\theta}$ is the point estimator of the parameter of interest (e.g., aOR) and $\hat{\text{V}}\text{ar}(\ln\hat{\theta})$ is the estimated variance of ln $\hat{\theta}$ (e.g., obtained from the estimated information matrix based on ML model fitting).

Table 22.5   Test Statistics for H_0: No CAT–CHD Association; Evans County Data (D=CHD, E=CAT, Controlling for AGE and ECG)

Model	V_i Terms	$\chi^2_{ML\beta}$	χ^2_{MLR}	F_{DISC}	$\chi^2_{LOG-LIN}$	χ^2_{MHS}
1	None (crude analysis)	15.24	14.13	16.64	15.24	16.22
2	AGEG	6.85	6.66	8.58	6.99	6.99
3	AGE	7.07	6.84	8.67	8.16	—
4	ECG	9.08	8.69	10.67	9.69	9.31
5	AGEG, ECG	3.80	3.73	5.24	3.96	—
6	AGE, ECG	4.16	4.08	5.50	3.14	—
7	AGEG, ECG, AGEG × ECG	4.13	4.04	5.39	4.22	4.15
8	AGE, ECG, AGE × ECG	4.28	4.18	5.36	3.31	—

Note: All test statistics have one degree of freedom. $\chi^2_{ML\beta}$ and χ^2_{MLR} are two alternative test statistics based on unconditional ML logistic model estimation. $\chi^2_{ML\beta}$ is the square of the ML estimate $\hat{\beta}$ divided by its standard error $S_{\hat{\beta}}$. χ^2_{MLR} denotes the chi-square statistic based on a likelihood ratio test. F_{DISC} is obtained from a discriminant function analysis; because the total study size is large ($n = 609$), F_{DISC} has, approximately, a χ^2 distribution under H_0. $\chi^2_{LOG-LIN}$ is derived from a log-linear model estimated by using the Grizzle-Starmer-Koch (GSK) weighted least squares procedure. χ^2_{MHS} denotes the Mantel-Haenszel chi-square for stratified analysis.

Note that each W_j term is incorporated into the logistic model as the product term $W_j \times$ CAT.

We also consider (in Tables 22.3–22.5) models in which AGE is treated as a binary variable, defined as

$$\text{AGEG} = \begin{cases} 1 \text{ if AGE} \geq 55 \\ 0 \text{ if AGE} < 55 \end{cases}$$

**22.3.3
Interaction
Assessment**

On the basis of Formula 20.12, the estimated, adjusted risk odds ratio for the above saturated model takes the form

$$\hat{ROR}(\text{adj.}) = \exp(\hat{\beta} + \hat{\delta}_1 \text{ AGE} + \hat{\delta}_2 \text{ ECG} + \hat{\delta}_3 \text{ AGE} \times \text{ECG})$$

where $\hat{ROR}(\text{adj.})$ denotes an adjusted risk odds ratio obtained from a logistic regression analysis. This estimate is a function of the two control variables AGE and ECG and, thereby, reflects effect modification.

Before using this estimate, however, we must first determine (following our recommended strategy) whether we should even include any W_j terms in the model. Several options for such assessment of interaction are available; we will examine a few of them below (all lead to the same conclusion).

First, using unconditional ML model-fitting procedures, we can perform a likelihood ratio test (see Section 20.2) that compares the following two models:

$$\text{logit } P_1(\mathbf{x}) = \alpha + \beta(\text{CAT}) + \gamma_1(\text{AGE}) + \gamma_2(\text{ECG}) \\ + \gamma_3(\text{AGE} \times \text{ECG})$$

$$\text{logit } P_2(\mathbf{x}) = \alpha + \beta(\text{CAT}) + \gamma_1(\text{AGE}) + \gamma_2(\text{ECG}) \\ + \gamma_3(\text{AGE} \times \text{ECG}) + \delta_1(\text{CAT} \times \text{AGE}) \\ + \delta_2(\text{CAT} \times \text{ECG}) + \delta_3(\text{CAT} \times \text{AGE} \times \text{ECG})$$

The null hypothesis being tested here is H_0: $\delta_1 = \delta_2 = \delta_3 = 0$, and the likelihood ratio statistic is of the form

$$\chi^2_{\text{MLR}} = -2 \ln(\hat{L}_1 / \hat{L}_2)$$

which has a chi-square distribution with three degrees of freedom under H_0; $\hat{L}_j$ denotes the maximized likelihood value based on fitting model $P_j(\mathbf{x})$, $j = 1, 2$. The value obtained for this test statistic is $\chi^2_{\text{MLR}} = .04$, which is clearly nonsignificant.

Two other approaches, which we recommended in Chapter 21, involve forward and backward algorithms (we used $\alpha = .10$), in which the main effect variables CAT, ECG, AGE, and AGE $\times$ ECG are always in the model. The forward algorithm considers, first, whether CAT $\times$ AGE $\times$ ECG should be added to a model already containing CAT $\times$ AGE and CAT $\times$ ECG together with the four main effect variables. If this first test is nonsignificant, then the significance of CAT $\times$ AGE and CAT $\times$ ECG is assessed in a forward manner, again keeping the main effects in the model. The backward algorithm, on the other hand, starts with the saturated model containing E and all V_i and W_j terms specified above and first determines whether or not CAT $\times$ AGE $\times$ ECG should be retained. If not, then the algorithm assesses whether CAT $\times$ AGE and/or CAT $\times$ ECG should be retained. As it turned out, the same results were obtained from each approach: none of the product terms among CAT $\times$ AGE $\times$ ECG, CAT $\times$ AGE, and CAT $\times$ ECG were significant. In fact, no likelihood ratio chi-square among these tests yielded a P-value below .50.

Essentially the same results (i.e., no evidence of interaction) were obtained when AGEG replaced AGE in the models fitted, and/or when discriminant function estimation was used instead of unconditional ML estimation. Thus, as was indicated by the stratified analysis, there is no evidence of interaction when AGE and ECG are the only variables considered for control.

22.3.4 Confounding Assessment

Turning now to the assessment of confounding via mathematical modeling, we consider the adjusted point estimates provided in Table 22.3; these vary as a function of which V_i terms (potential confounders), without any W_j terms (potential modifiers), are in the model. The third column (labeled MLE_u) in this table gives the estimated adjusted odds ratio $e^{\hat{\beta}}$, whose value depends on the particular V_i variables being controlled (second column); $\hat{\beta}$ is the regression coefficient obtained by using unconditional ML estimation methods for the logistic model. Note that the use of unconditional (rather than conditional) ML estimation is appropriate for these data since the stratum-specific sample sizes are large and the number of parameters being estimated is small relative to these sample sizes.

In the use of the MLE_u results to assess confounding, essentially the same interpretation can be made as was previously described for the stratified analysis (see the last two columns in Table 22.3). Controlling for both AGE (treated either as continuous or dichotomous) and ECG gives odds ratios that are somewhat reduced from those obtained when only one or none of these variables is controlled. Note that the differences among the odds ratios when both variables are controlled are very slight, regardless of whether or not a product term involving the control variables is used. Also, AGE appears to contribute more to confounding than does ECG. These results suggest that at least AGE (or AGEG) should be controlled and that, if both variables are controlled, it is not necessary (for validity reasons) to add a product term such as AGE $\times$ ECG.

**22.3.5
Precision
Considerations**

To determine whether a substantial gain in precision would be achieved by dropping one or more of the V_i terms initially considered, we can consider the interval estimates provided in the third column of Table 22.4 (under the MLE_u heading). As occurred in the stratified analyses, these results indicate highest precision when both AGE and ECG are controlled, with little difference in the intervals when adding a product term. We therefore recommend that a logistic model containing just $V_1 = \text{AGE}$ and $V_2 = \text{ECG}$ would be adequate to describe the association. The fitted model in this instance turns out to be

$$\text{logit}[\text{pr}(\text{CHD} = 1 | \text{CAT, AGE, ECG})]$$
$$= -3.911011 + .651607(\text{CAT}) + .028964(\text{AGE})$$
$$+ .342288(\text{ECG})$$

so that the estimated adjusted risk odds ratio is

$$\hat{\text{ROR}}(\text{adj.}) = e^{.651607} = 1.92$$

A printout (using SAS's LOGIST procedure) that provides the necessary information for evaluating this model is as follows:

LOGISTIC REGRESSION PROCEDURE

DEPENDENT VARIABLE: CHD

609 OBSERVATIONS

71 POSITIVES

538   NEGATIVES
  0   OBSERVATIONS DELETED DUE TO MISSING VALUES

VARIABLE	MEAN	MINIMUM	MAXIMUM	RANGE
CAT	.200328	0	1	1
AGE	53.7061	±0	76	36
ECG	.272578	0	1	1

−2 LOG LIKELIHOOD FOR MODEL CONTAINING INTERCEPT ONLY =   438.56

CONVERGENCE OBTAINED IN 6 ITERATIONS.   D = 0.031.
MAX ABSOLUTE DERIVATIVE = 0.2797D-05.   −2 LOG $\hat{L}$ =   419.02.
MODEL CHI-SQUARE =   19.54 WITH   3 D.F.   P = 0.0002.

VARIABLE	BETA	STD. ERROR	CHI-SQUARE	P	D
INTERCEPT	−3.91101143	.80036982	23.88	.0000	
CAT	.65160692	.31929935	4.16	.0413	.007
AGE	.02896361	.01459093	3.94	.0471	.006
ECG	.34228831	.29091165	1.38	.2394	.002

From this printout, a 95% large-sample interval estimate for the adjusted risk odds ratio can be obtained, using the ML estimate of the standard error of the coefficient of the variable CAT, namely,

$$S_{\hat{\beta}} = .31929935$$

Thus, the confidence limits are given by

$$\exp(\hat{\beta} \pm 1.96 S_{\hat{\beta}})$$

or

$$\exp[.65160692 \pm 1.96(.31929935)]$$

or

$$\exp(.65160692 \pm .62582673)$$

To two decimal places the interval is (1.03, 3.59).

Having considered both validity and precision issues in terms of point and interval estimation, we now turn to a discussion of the results of significance testing. In Table 22.5, the statistic $\chi^2_{ML\beta}$ (third column) is obtained from the formula

**22.3.6
Hypothesis-
testing Results**

$$\chi^2_{ML\beta} = (\hat{\beta}/S_{\hat{\beta}})^2$$

The fourth column gives the values of the likelihood ratio statistic

$$\chi^2_{MLR} = -2 \ln(\hat{L}_2/\hat{L}_1)$$

where $\hat{L}_1$ and $\hat{L}_2$ are the maximized likelihood functions based on fitting the models

$$\text{logit } P_1(\mathbf{x}) = \alpha + \beta(\text{CAT}) + \sum_{i=1}^{p_1} \gamma_i V_i$$

and

$$\text{logit } P_2(\mathbf{x}) = \alpha + \sum_{i=1}^{p_1} \gamma_i V_i$$

The printout provided earlier for the control of $V_1 = \text{AGE}$ and $V_2 = \text{ECG}$ gives results for $P_1(\mathbf{x})$ and provides the necessary information for computing $\chi^2_{\text{ML}\beta}$. In particular,

$$\chi^2_{\text{ML}\beta} = \left(\frac{\hat{\beta}}{S_{\hat{\beta}}}\right)^2 = \left(\frac{.6516}{.3193}\right)^2 = 4.16 \qquad \text{(one-sided } P\text{-value} \approx .021)$$

The corresponding likelihood ratio statistic, χ^2_{MLR}, is obtained by fitting model $P_2(\mathbf{x})$ in addition to model $P_1(\mathbf{x})$. This fitting leads to

$$-2 \ln \hat{L}_2 = 423.10 \qquad \text{and} \qquad -2 \ln \hat{L}_1 = 419.02$$

Thus,

$$\chi^2_{\text{MLR}} = -2 \ln(\hat{L}_2/\hat{L}_1) = 423.10 - 419.02 = 4.08 \qquad (P \approx .021)$$

For this particular example, both test statistics yield about the same P-value and provide the same conclusion: The estimated adjusted odds ratio of 1.92 is of borderline significance (i.e., we would reject H_0 at $\alpha = .05$ but not at $\alpha = .01$).

22.4 RESULTS FROM OTHER APPROACHES

We have completed our descriptions of the results based on a stratified analysis and on an unconditional ML fitting of the logistic model. We now return to Tables 22.3–22.5 to see how these results compare with those based on other modeling approaches.

First, with reference to Table 22.3, we see that the MLE_u adjusted odds ratio estimates for models 1, 2, 4, and 7 are identical to the corresponding $a\hat{O}R$'s obtained from comparable stratified analyses. (Remember that $e^{\hat{\beta}}$ is an odds ratio and *not* a risk ratio.) Furthermore, when AGE is treated *continuously* in the logistic model (e.g., models 3, 6, and 8), the results under MLE_u are close (though not identical) to those for the stratified analysis. This result will be the case when important information is not lost upon categorization and when stratum-specific sample sizes are sufficiently large.

The odds ratio estimates obtained when using discriminant (DISC) function analysis are consistently higher than the corresponding MLE_u estimates. Similar discrepancies are found when comparing the interval estimation and testing results in Tables 22.4 and 22.5. These findings demonstrate numerically why the use of discriminant analysis (based on the assumption of multivariate normality) is not recommended for estimating regression coefficients.

**22.4.1
Discriminant
Function
Analysis**

Table 22.3 also allows us to compare the logistic-modeling results with those from log-linear modeling using GSK weighted least squares estimation (Grizzle et al., 1969). The particular form of the log-linear model used has the same general logistic form considered earlier, namely,

**22.4.2
Log-Linear
Modeling**

$$\text{logit}[\text{pr}(D = 1 | \text{CAT}, V_1, \ldots, V_{p_1})] = \alpha + \beta(\text{CAT}) + \sum_{i=1}^{p_1} \gamma_i V_i$$

However, in a fit of this model by using weighted least squares, all independent variables are treated categorically, and the response variable is the logit of the estimated proportion $\hat{p}$ of persons developing CHD. There is an estimated logit for each combination of categories of the independent variables. For example, for the eight categories based on the dichotomous variables CAT, ECG, and AGEG, the values of $\hat{p}$ and $\ln[\hat{p}/(1 - \hat{p})]$ are given in Table 22.6. When AGE is not categorized, the GSK approach treats each distinct age value as a separate category. For these data, there are 30 distinct age values, leading to 120 estimated logits.

**Table 22.6   Data Set for Log-Linear Model Analyses Using
GSK Weighted Least Squares Estimation**

INDEPENDENT VARIABLES				
CAT	AGEG	ECG	Estimated Proportion, $\hat{p}$	Estimated Logit, $\ln[\hat{p}/(1 - \hat{p})]$
0	0	0	17/274	−2.716
0	1	0	15/122	−1.965
0	0	1	7/59	−2.005
0	1	1	5/32	−1.686
1	0	0	1/8	−1.946
1	1	0	9/39	−1.204
1	0	1	3/17	−1.540
1	1	1	14/58	−1.145

From Table 22.3, we see that the log-linear (GSK) odds ratio point estimates $(e^{\hat{\beta}})$ are identical to the corresponding MLE_u estimates whenever the binary variable AGEG is used. In contrast, there are slight discrepancies between MLE_u and GSK estimates when AGE is left ungrouped. This result is to be expected since stratum-specific sample sizes for 120 strata are much smaller than they are for 8 strata (when age is dichotomized) and since both estimation procedures are only "asymptotically" equivalent. Similar comparative results are also found in Tables 22.4 and 22.5.

22.4.3
Confounder
Summarization

To complete this section, we consider results obtained by using confounder summarization (CS). We illustrate this methodology for the case when both AGE and ECG are to be controlled, with AGE being treated as an interval variable. (Note that when all control variables are categorical, the CS method is *identical* to stratified analysis.)

We begin by deriving CS scores based on a logistic model that controls for $V_1 = $ AGE and $V_2 = $ ECG and that has been fitted by unconditional ML estimation. Using the results given previously in the computer printout, we can write the fitted model as

$$\hat{\ell} = \text{lo}\hat{g}\text{it}[\text{pr}(\text{CHD} = 1 | \text{CAT, AGE, ECG})]$$

$$= -3.911011 + .651607(\text{CAT}) + .028964(\text{AGE}) + .342288(\text{ECG})$$

As we pointed out in Section 20.4, the CS scores obtained from such a fitted model simply provide a *relative* (rather than an absolute) *ranking* of risk for all persons in the sample. Thus, for the above fitted model, the same *relative* ranking of scores will be obtained regardless of whether the above logit form of the model is employed or whether the underlying (logistic) probability form of the model, $(1 + e^{-\ell})^{-1}$, is used. Moreover, since the relative ranking of scores is not affected by the value of the intercept, we may focus on the following linear expression:

$$\hat{\ell} + 3.911011 = .651607(\text{CAT}) + .028964(\text{AGE}) + .342288(\text{ECG})$$

Setting CAT = 0 in this expression yields the function

$$\hat{S} = .028964(\text{AGE}) + .342288(\text{ECG})$$

which can then be used to derive a CS score for each of the $n = 609$ individuals in the sample.

As described in Section 20.4, the step following the calculation of the individual scores involves forming strata that lead to a standard stratified analysis. This analysis is designed to control (by stratification) for the newly constructed CS score variable, which is now assumed (on the basis of its structure as a "combination of the potential confounders") to be the only factor requiring control. The strata are constructed so as to be small in number and to represent different "levels of risk." Also, the stratum-specific sample sizes are to be relatively large (particularly on the margins of each table).

In general, several alternative procedures for categorization may be considered—which leaves the CS method open to criticism as being too much of an ad hoc approach. Among the alternative approaches to categorization, we consider the following:

Method 1: Determine the distribution of scores separately by level of the *exposure* variable (CAT), and eliminate those persons whose scores are outside the range of overlap of the two distributions. (This procedure results in the loss of 179 persons from our data set.) Then, form five strata by dividing the total number of *exposed* persons (i.e., CAT = 1) into quintiles.

Method 2: Determine the distribution of scores separately by level of the *disease* variable (CHD), and eliminate those persons whose scores are outside the range of overlap of these two distributions. (This procedure results in the loss of one person from the data set.) Then, form five strata by dividing the total number of *diseased* persons (i.e., CHD = 1) into quintiles.

Miettinen (1976) suggests that either of these methods could be used with follow-up data but that only Method 2 should be used with case-control data. He also recommends that one initially form ten strata and then reduce this number to five or so by pooling strata if no additional confounding is introduced by such pooling.

Tables 22.7 and 22.8 provide stratum-specific and summary information for confounder score strata obtained when using these two methods. From Table 22.8, we see that Method 2 yields results ($a\hat{O}R = 1.99$, $\chi^2_{MH} = 4.16$) that are comparable with the results from ML logistic modeling ($a\hat{O}R = 1.91$, $\chi^2_{ML\beta} = 4.16$), given in Tables 22.3 and 22.5. In contrast, Method 1, which involves the loss of 179 subjects because of nonoverlapping CS scores, yields a point estimate and a test statistic that are smaller than corresponding results from logistic modeling. [It should be noted, for each method, that the use of a summary point estimate may be criticized if the stratum-specific estimates are considered to exhibit meaningful interaction.] Both methods, nevertheless, yield the same general conclusion: evidence of a moderately significant CAT–CHD association, as reflected in an $a\hat{O}R$ value of around 2.

Further research involving other data sets (perhaps simulated) is required to demonstrate more definitively the kinds of discrepancies in results that may arise when using different methods for forming strata. However, this example certainly illustrates the ad hoc nature of the CS method. Other criticisms and related controversies concerning the CS method were documented earlier in Section 20.4.

Table 22.7   Strata Resulting from Categorization of Confounder Summarization Scores, Using Four Methods for Forming Strata; Evans County Data (D = CHD, E = CAT, Controlling for AGE and ECG)

a. Method 1

STRATUM 1

	CAT 1	CAT 0	
CHD 1	4	14	18
CHD 0	20	146	166
	24	160	

STRATUM 2

	CAT 1	CAT 0	
CHD 1	5	8	13
CHD 0	17	77	94
	22	85	

STRATUM 3

	CAT 1	CAT 0	
CHD 1	5	6	11
CHD 0	19	16	35
	24	22	

STRATUM 4

	CAT 1	CAT 0	
CHD 1	4	2	6
CHD 0	18	31	49
	22	33	

STRATUM 5

	CAT 1	CAT 0	
CHD 1	7	4	11
CHD 0	16	11	27
	23	15	

b. Method 2

	CAT		
	1	0	
CHD 1	15	15	
0	193	194	
	208		

	CAT		
	1	0	
CHD 1	4	9	13
0	11	102	113
	15	111	

	CAT		
	1	0	
CHD 1	5	10	15
0	28	93	121
	33	103	

	CAT		
	1	0	
CHD 1	7	6	13
0	30	41	71
	37	47	

	CAT		
	1	0	
CHD 1	11	4	15
0	24	14	38
	35	18	

Table 22.8   Summary Information for Confounder Summarization, Using Methods 1 and 2 for Categorization of CS Score (D = CHD, E = CAT, Controlling for AGE and ECG)

	a. Method 1 ($n = 430$)			b. Method 2 ($n = 608$)		
	CS Boundaries	$\hat{RR}_g$	$\hat{OR}_g$	*CS Boundaries*	$\hat{RR}_g$	$\hat{OR}_g$
Stratum 1	1.4185–1.6515	1.90	2.09	1.1585–1.4485	0	0
Stratum 2	1.6515–1.8545	2.41	2.83	1.4485–1.6225	3.29	4.12
Stratum 3	1.8545–1.9935	.76	.70	1.6225–1.8835	1.56	1.66
Stratum 4	1.9935–2.2015	3.00	3.44	1.8835–2.1675	1.48	1.59
Stratum 5	2.2015–2.4285	1.14	1.20	2.1675–2.5155	1.41	1.60
$\hat{aRR}$	1.53			$1.79^{\dagger}$		
$\hat{aOR}$	1.73			$1.99^{\dagger}$		
χ^2_{MH}	2.95 ($P = .43$)			4.16 ($P = .021$)		
95% CI, aRR	(.94, 2.50)			(1.08, 2.96)		
95% CI, aOR	(.94, 3.20)			(1.07, 3.69)		

Note: The confounder score function is given by the formula

$$\hat{S} = .028964(AGE) + .342288(ECG)$$

which is based on unconditional ML estimation of the model

$$\text{logit } P(\mathbf{x}) = \alpha + \beta(CAT) + \gamma_1(AGE) + \gamma_2(ECG)$$

†Denotes an estimate derived using a stratum containing a zero cell frequency.

22.5 CONCLUDING REMARKS

In this chapter, we have illustrated the use of stratified analysis procedures and various mathematical-modeling approaches to analyze a particular data set involving two extraneous factors, one categorical and one continuous. There was no evidence of interaction between these factors and the dichotomous exposure variable CAT. A comparison of these different analysis methods indicates, for this particular numerical example, that the use of logistic modeling with unconditional ML estimation gives results similar to those based on stratified analysis, log-linear modeling of categorical data, and Miettinen's confounder summarization techniques. Discriminant analysis gives numerical results that are clearly in error, and so its use is not recommended when dealing with categorical variables. Further research, probably involving simulation studies, is needed in order to make definitive statements about the relative merits of these various analytical procedures in situations involving and not involving interaction.

NOTATION

The following list summarizes the key notation introduced in this chapter.

MLE_u Maximum likelihood estimation based on an unconditional likelihood function.

DISC	Two-group discriminant function estimation.
GSK	Grizzle-Starmer-Koch weighted least squares estimation.
$\chi^2_{ML\beta}$	Chi-square statistic calculated as $\hat{\beta}^2/S^2_{\hat{\beta}}$, where $\hat{\beta}$ is a maximum likelihood estimate and $S^2_{\hat{\beta}}$ is its estimated variance.
χ^2_{MLR}	Chi-square statistic based on a likelihood ratio test.
F_{DISC}	F statistic based on a two-group discriminant function analysis.
$\chi^2_{LOG-LIN}$	Chi-square statistic based on fitting a log-linear model by the Grizzle-Starmer-Koch weighted least squares procedure.
$\hat{ROR}$(adj.)	Adjusted risk odds ratio obtained from a logistic regression analysis.

REFERENCES

Grizzle, J. F.; Starmer, C. F., and Koch, G. G. 1969. Analysis of categorical data by linear models. *Biometrics* 25(3): 489–504.

Miettinen, O. S. 1976. Stratification by a multivariate confounder score. *Am. J. Epidemiol.* 104(6): 609–620.

23

Applications of Logistic Regression with Interaction, Using Unconditional ML Estimation

We will now consider a more complicated analysis situation. This situation involves the simultaneous control of five extraneous variables in the Evans County data set, namely, AGE, ECG, SMK, CHL, and HPT. As we mentioned in Chapter 22, we will find evidence of interaction in this analysis, thus making for a somewhat more complicated (and controversial) assessment and interpretation of these data.

    When examining, in Chapter 17, the results of stratified analyses performed on these data, we found considerable variation in the stratum-specific risk ratios when AGE, CHL, and HPT were simultaneously controlled (see Table 17.6). However, specific identification of confounders and effect modifiers was difficult because of small sample sizes within several strata. In spite of this "numbers" problem, inspection of the stratum-specific risk ratios led us to believe that both CHL and HPT suggested themselves as modifiers, with CHL being the more reasonable candidate. This interpretation was also supported by the stratified analyses presented in Table 17.4, which showed, in particular, discrepancies among a$\hat{R}$R, s$\hat{R}$R, and s$'\hat{R}$R values when AGE, CHL, and HPT were controlled simultaneously. (Table 17.4 also contained results, rows 27–29, from stratified analyses carried out within combinations of categories of CHL and HPT.) Nevertheless, the stratified analyses have to be viewed with caution because of the small-numbers problem. In addition, no more than three of the five extraneous variables have been considered together up to this point. The use of mathematical modeling, therefore, is particularly called for here as a feasible way to accurately take into account all five variables at one time. As we discussed in Section 20.2, the advantage in using logistic regression methods is that AGE and CHL can be treated as continuous variables, a feature that may reduce the number of parameters to be estimated (and may enable one to make use of sample information on age trends in risk).

23.0 PREVIEW

The results we will discuss below involve only *unconditional* maximum likelihood (ML) estimation of the logistic model. Although we would certainly advocate the use of conditional ML estimation methods as well for these data because of the small numbers problem, we chose not to illustrate such conditional analyses in order to present clearly the issues attendant with the unconditional ML methods when dealing with interaction and with sparse data. Following the strategy we outlined in Chapter 21, we first concern ourselves with the assessment of interaction. Such an evaluation, however, is more complicated now than when only two extraneous variables were being considered for control. Among the various strategies available for assessing interaction, we have considered the following:

23.1 INTERAC-TION

Strategy 1.   Start with the most saturated model, which involves all main effects and all possible product terms of extraneous variables (with CAT, the exposure variable) up to the highest degree (which, in our case, is the sixth-degree product term CAT × CHL × AGE × ECG × SMK × HPT). Then, work *backward,* in a manner analogous to that described in Chapter 21 (Section 21.1.3), to delete interaction terms that do not make a significant contribution to prediction. Recall that when one is considering the possible deletion of a product term involving k variables, all main effect terms and product terms of lower degree (less than or equal to $k - 1$) need to be included in the model. Not eligible for deletion are product terms of a given degree that contain variables that are also components of higher-degree product terms already found to be significant.

Strategy 2. Start with a model that is saturated only up through third-degree product terms involving CAT (e.g., terms like CAT × CHL × ECG). Then, work *backward,* as in Strategy 1, to delete any nonsignificant interaction terms. This strategy hinges on the viewpoint that product terms involving the exposure variable of degree higher than three are rarely, if ever, either etiologically interpretable or statistically significant. And even if they are apparently significant, the validity of statistical tests about such higher-order terms can be seriously questioned because of multicollinearity considerations. We recommended this backward elimination strategy in Section 21.1.3.

Strategy 3. Start with a model containing all main effect terms and all second-degree product terms with CAT (e.g., like CAT × CHL). Then, work *forward* to add any significant third-degree product terms involving CAT. If no such third-order terms are added, then consider the model just containing all main effect terms and work *forward* to add any significant two-factor product terms involving CAT. If any third-degree products are added, work *backward* to determine whether to delete any second-degree product terms involving variables not contained in the already added third-degree products. However, retain all second-degree terms involving variables contained in the third-degree products already deemed important. (We also recommended this strategy in Chapter 21.)

Strategy 4. Allow for interaction effects in the model only up to second-degree product terms involving CAT. Then, while retaining in the model all main effect terms, work *forward* and/or *backward* to determine if any significant second-degree product terms need to be included in the model. (Although this strategy was not explicitly discussed in Chapter 21, the viewpoint taken here is that product terms higher than second degree are not important.)

A summary of the results obtained by using each strategy above, coupled with unconditional ML estimation of the logistic model, is provided in Table 23.1. These results give a somewhat confused picture regarding the assessment of interaction. First of all, no solution could be obtained when using the backward elimination (saturated model) of Strategies 1 and

Table 23.1 Assessing Interaction in the Evans County Data Set When Controlling for AGE, CHL, SMK, ECG, and HPT, Using Unconditional Maximum Likelihood Estimation of the Logistic Model

Strategy	Description	Results
1	Backward approach ($\alpha = .10$)[a] using saturated model involving all possible higher-degree product terms involving CAT.	No solution—singular information matrix.
2	Backward approach ($\alpha = .10$) using a saturated model up through third-degree product terms involving CAT.	No solution—singular information matrix.
3	Forward approach ($\alpha = .10$), first adding third-degree product terms involving CAT, with all lower-degree terms in model. Repeat forward procedure to determine important second-degree terms only if no third-degree terms are added at the first step. If third-degree terms are added, work backward to delete nonsignificant second-degree terms eligible for removal.	Interaction terms included are CAT × HPT × SMK, CAT × CHL, CAT × SMK, CAT × HPT.
4	Forward and/or backward approaches ($\alpha = .10$) allowing for interaction only in terms of second-degree products, given main effects in the model.	Interaction terms included as significant (both forward and backward approaches) are CAT × CHL (entered first), CAT × HPT (entered second).

[a]The use of this particular (or, indeed, any) *nominal* significance level for entry or deletion of variables is certainly open to criticism (see Kupper et al., 1976).

2. We pointed out in Chapter 21 that such indeterminacies can arise when fitting a model involving higher-degree product terms among categorically treated variables. In such circumstances, some of the coefficients in the logistic model will not be estimable. Translated into matrix terminology, such a condition is manifested by a singular information matrix, which cannot be inverted to provide an ML solution.

Strategies 3 and 4 did not lead to such singularity problems; however, they did yield differing interpretations about the nature of the interaction present in these data. In particular, the model resulting from Strategy 3 identifies CHL, HPT, and SMK as effect modifiers. The results from Strategy 4, however, suggest that CHL (entered first on the basis of forward selection), followed by HPT, are the only two modifiers; this finding corresponds to the interpretation from the stratified analyses performed earlier. It is our opinion that neither of these alternative interpretations can be dismissed outright—which leaves it up to the investigator to choose the model(s) that either seem(s) most meaningful at the substantive (i.e., biological and clinical) level and/or that follow(s) a strategy that is most appealing statistically. In an analysis of a complex epidemiologic data set, it is not an uncommon dilemma to have to choose between two or more statistically plausible models. We will not make such a choice here; instead, we will describe and compare the results obtained from each of the two strategies.

Focusing for now on Strategy 4, we first note that the V_i and W_j variables considered for inclusion in the logistic model are as follows:

$$V_1 = \text{AGE} = W_1 \qquad V_2 = \text{CHL} = W_2 \qquad V_3 = \text{ECG} = W_3$$

$$V_4 = \text{SMK} = W_4 \qquad V_5 = \text{HPT} = W_5$$

In accordance with Strategy 4, we wish to determine whether any of the above W_j variables are important, given that all the V_i variables and CAT are included as main effects in the model. On the basis of either forward or backward algorithms, CAT $\times$ CHL and CAT $\times$ HPT are the only product terms considered significant ($\alpha = .10$). Thus, CHL and HPT are the only W_j variables to be retained as modifiers. Results from *forward selection* ($\alpha = .10$) using unconditional ML estimation are provided in Table 23.2. Note that the product terms competing for entry are CAT $\times$ AGE, CAT $\times$ CHL, CAT $\times$ ECG, CAT $\times$ SMK, and CAT $\times$ HPT.

The chi-square statistic for the addition of the CAT $\times$ CHL term to a model containing all six main effects is

$$\chi^2_{\text{ML}\delta_1}(\text{CAT} \times \text{CHL}|\text{main effects}) = (\hat{\delta}_1/S_{\hat{\delta}_1})^2$$

$$= (.06826746/.01431679)^2 = 22.74$$

where $\hat{\delta}_1$ is the estimated coefficient of the CAT $\times$ CHL variable and $S_{\hat{\delta}_1}$ is its standard error. This statistic is based on the unconditional ML fitting of the logistic model

$$\text{logit } P_1(\mathbf{x}) = \alpha + \beta(\text{CAT}) + \sum_{i=1}^{5} \gamma_i V_i + \delta_1(\text{CAT} \times \text{CHL})$$

The corresponding likelihood ratio chi-square statistic for the addition of CAT $\times$ CHL to the main effects model, which is $\text{logit } P_0(\mathbf{x}) = \alpha + \beta(\text{CAT}) + \sum_{i=1}^{5} \gamma_i V_i$, is

$$\chi^2_{\text{MLR}}(\text{CAT} \times \text{CHL}|\text{main effects}) = -2 \ln (\hat{L}_0/\hat{L}_1)$$

$$= -2 \ln \hat{L}_0 + 2 \ln \hat{L}_1$$

$$= 400.41 - 357.09 = 43.37$$

where $\hat{L}_0$ and $\hat{L}_1$ are the maximized likelihoods corresponding to $P_0(\mathbf{x})$ and $P_1(\mathbf{x})$, respectively. Although $\chi^2_{\text{ML}\delta_1}$ and χ^2_{MLR} are typically quite close in numerical value in the vicinity of the null value, this is not the case here since both statistics are highly significant.

Returning to Table 23.2, we see that CAT $\times$ HPT is the second interaction term to enter, with corresponding $\chi^2_{\text{ML}\delta_2}$ and χ^2_{MLR} statistics of

Table 23.2   Forward Selection ($\alpha = .10$) Using Strategy 4 with Unconditional ML Estimation

Step 0: Main effect variables entered.

$$-2 \ln \hat{L}_0 = 400.41$$

VARIABLE	BETA	STD. ERROR	CHI-SQUARE	P
INTERCEPT	−6.77271400	1.14015940	35.29	.0000
CAT	.59755181	.35197303	2.88	.0896
AGE	.03222424	.01517585	4.51	.0337
CHL	.00873732	.00326262	7.17	.0074
ECG	.36950678	.29363661	1.58	.2083
SMK	.83471545	.30521931	7.48	.0062
HPT	.43932946	.29080920	2.28	.1309

Step 1: CAT × CHL added (this variable has the highest partial chi-square for entry among all product terms not in the model at step 0).

$$-2 \ln \hat{L}_1 = 357.09$$

VARIABLE	BETA	STD. ERROR	CHI-SQUARE	P
INTERCEPT	−3.93111172	1.25020439	9.89	.0017
CAT	−14.07169585	3.12193671	20.32	.0000
AGE	.03225905	.01622780	3.95	.0468
CHL	−.00445368	.00413403	1.16	.2813
ECG	.35728774	.32628149	1.20	.2735
SMK	.80663069	.32641865	6.11	.0135
HPT	.60698251	.30247392	4.03	.0448
CC = CAT × CHL	.06826746	.01431679	22.74	.0000

Step 2: CAT × HPT added (this variable has the highest partial chi-square for entry among all product terms not in the model at step 1).

$$-2 \ln \hat{L}_2 = 347.28$$

VARIABLE	BETA	STD. ERROR	CHI-SQUARE	P
INTERCEPT	−4.04735444	1.25489653	10.40	.0013
CAT	−12.68090667	3.10422354	16.69	.0000
AGE	.03494584	.01613723	4.69	.0303
CHL	−.00546212	.00418385	1.70	.1917
ECG	.36653818	.32780320	1.25	.2635
SMK	.77347950	.32723223	5.59	.0181
HPT	1.04679751	.33163438	9.96	.0016
CH = CAT × HPT	−2.32988654	.74223947	9.85	.0017
CC = CAT × CHL	.06911793	.01435511	23.18	.0000

NO OTHER TWO-FACTOR PRODUCT TERM MET THE $\alpha = .10$ SIGNIFICANCE LEVEL CRITERION FOR ENTRY INTO THE MODEL

$$\chi^2_{\text{ML}\delta_2}(\text{CAT} \times \text{HPT} | \text{main effects and CAT} \times \text{CHL}) = 9.85$$

and

$$\chi^2_{\text{MLR}}(\text{CAT} \times \text{HPT} | \text{main effects and CAT} \times \text{CHL}) = -2 \ln (\hat{L}_1/\hat{L}_2)$$
$$= 357.09 - 347.28$$
$$= 9.81$$

where $\hat{L}_2$ is the maximized likelihood for the model

$$\text{logit } P_2(\mathbf{x}) = \alpha + \beta(\text{CAT}) + \sum_{i=1}^{5} \gamma_i V_i$$
$$+ \delta_1(\text{CAT} \times \text{CHL}) + \delta_2(\text{CAT} \times \text{HPT})$$

Thus, when added sequentially to the main effects model, both CAT × CHL and CAT × HPT contribute significantly to prediction. Also, as we can see from the output (step 2) for the model containing both these product terms, each one is highly significant given that all other variables are in the model. Furthermore, the (two-degrees-of-freedom) χ^2_{MLR} statistic for the simultaneous addition of both CAT × CHL and CAT × HPT to a model already containing the main effect terms is

$$\chi^2_{\text{MLR}} = -2 \ln (\hat{L}_0/\hat{L}_2) = 400.41 - 347.28 = 53.13$$

which is highly significant. (This latter χ^2 test is analogous to a multiple partial F test used in standard least squares multiple linear regression analysis.) Finally, the χ^2_{MLR} or $\chi^2_{\text{ML}\delta}$ statistic for the addition of any other CAT × W_j term to a model already containing all the V_i terms, CAT, CAT × CHL, and CAT × HPT is always clearly nonsignificant (minimum P-value > .24).

In summary, then, the results based on Strategy 4 support the general conclusions drawn from previous stratified analyses, namely, that CHL and HPT are the only two clearly discernible effect modifiers out of the five extraneous variables being considered.

When considering Strategy 3, however, we find a somewhat different interpretation regarding effect modification. In addition to the variables CAT × CHL and CAT × HPT, two other interaction variables, CAT × SMK and CAT × HPT × SMK, are also to be retained in the final model, according to Strategy 3. Table 23.3 summarizes the results from the use of this strategy.

**23.2
POINT
ESTIMATION**

From our assessment of interaction (via Strategies 3 and 4), we have obtained two different impressions of the adjusted CAT–CHD association. On the basis of the general expression (20.12), the following adjusted odds ratio estimates are obtained by using the best models determined from Strategies 3 and 4:

Table 23.3   Best Model Based on Strategy 3; $-2 \ln \hat{L} = 342.32$

VARIABLE	BETA	STD. ERROR	CHI-SQUARE	P
INTERCEPT	−4.28684148	1.32636190	10.45	.0012
CAT	−15.02136655	3.77780014	15.81	.0001
AGE	.03606998	.01694402	4.53	.0333
CHL	−.00541758	.00419511	1.67	.1966
ECG	.35423489	.33620296	1.11	.2921
SMK	.99775692	.40181071	6.17	.0130
HPT	1.05015409	.33272550	9.96	.0016
CC = CAT × CHL	.07480571	.01538951	23.63	.0000
CH = CAT × HPT	−.24270172	1.50039356	.03	.8715
CS = CAT × SMK	1.45981148	1.59421594	.84	.3598
CHS = CAT × HPT × SMK	−3.03940236	1.73110829	3.08	.0791

Strategy 4 (fitted model given in step 2 of Table 23.2):

$$\hat{ROR}(\text{adj.}) = \exp[\hat{\beta} + \hat{\delta}_1(\text{CHL}) + \hat{\delta}_2(\text{HPT})]$$

where $\hat{\beta} = -12.68090667$, $\hat{\delta}_1 = .06911793$, and $\hat{\delta}_2 = -2.32988654$.
Strategy 3 (fitted model given in Table 23.3):

$$\hat{ROR}(\text{adj.}) = \exp[\hat{\beta} + \hat{\delta}_1(\text{CHL}) + \hat{\delta}_2(\text{HPT}) \\ + \hat{\delta}_3(\text{SMK}) + \hat{\delta}_4(\text{HPT} \times \text{SMK})]$$

where $\hat{\beta} = -15.02136655$, $\hat{\delta}_1 = .07480571$, $\hat{\delta}_2 = -.24270172$, $\hat{\delta}_3 = 1.45981148$, and $\hat{\delta}_4 = -3.03940236$.

Each of the above formulas reflects the presence of interaction; in particular, it is necessary to specify numerical values for the modifiers appearing in each adjusted odds ratio expression in order to obtain a corresponding numerical value for the adjusted odds ratio. In other words, each expression describes the odds ratio as varying as a function of the values of the effect modifiers.

To illustrate the complex nature of the CAT–CHD association, we have presented, in Table 23.4 (for each of the two models), several estimated odds ratios based on different combinations of values of the corresponding modifiers. As both the odds ratio expressions and the entries in Table 23.4 indicate, the estimated CAT–CHD association increases exponentially with the level of CHL for each model. Also, for each model, the estimated odds ratio is smaller for persons with a history of hypertension (HPT = 1) than for those without any history (HPT = 0) at each level of CHL. However, the model obtained via Strategy 4 indicates that the estimated odds ratio does not depend on SMK at all, whereas the Strategy 3 model considers SMK to be an effect modifier. In particular, when HPT =

Table 23.4   Estimated Adjusted Odds Ratios for CAT–CHD Association at Various Combinations of Values of Modifiers, Based on Models Determined via Strategies 3 and 4

a. Strategy 4[a]			b. Strategy 3[b]				
	HPT			HPT = 0		HPT = 1	
CHL	0	1	*CHL*	*SMK* = 0	*SMK* = 1	*SMK* = 0	*SMK* = 1
140	.05	.005	140	.01	.05	.01	.002
180	.79	.08	180	.21	.91	.17	.03
200	3.14	.31	200	.94	4.05	.74	.15
220	12.49	1.22	220	4.20	18.10	3.30	.68
240	49.77	4.84	240	18.77	80.79	14.72	3.03
260	198.30	19.30	260	83.77	360.66	65.72	13.54
300	3,147.91	306.31	300	1,669.61	7,187.93	1,309.82	269.90

Note: AGE, CHL, ECG, SMK, and HPT are present as main effect terms in each model considered.

[a]$\hat{ROR}$(adj.) = exp[−12.6809 + .0691(CHL) − 2.3299(HPT)].

[b]$\hat{ROR}$(adj.) = exp[−15.0214 + .0748(CHL) − .2427(HPT) + 1.4598(SMK) − 3.0394(HPT × SMK)].

1, the odds ratio expression involving SMK increases with rising CHL level at a slower rate for smokers than for nonsmokers. On the other hand, when HPT = 0, this odds ratio increases with increasing CHL level at a faster rate for smokers than for nonsmokers. This added complexity in interpretation is due to the presence in the model of the three-factor product CAT × HPT × SMK. (Note: *No* general etiologic interpretations should be made regarding these numerical findings. As we stated earlier, CAT is an *artificially constructed* variable, and the entire example is for illustrative purposes only.)

23.3 INTERVAL ESTIMATION

We have previously described (in Section 20.2) how to construct a large-sample confidence interval for an odds ratio when there are interaction terms in the fitted model. Expression 20.14 provided a general formula for a $100(1 - \alpha)\%$ interval of this type, which we repeat here:

$$\exp[\hat{\ell} \pm Z_{1-\alpha/2}\sqrt{\hat{Var}(\hat{\ell})}]$$

In terms of the notation of this chapter, which corresponds to that for Expression 20.10, the linear function $\hat{\ell}$ has the general form

$$\hat{\ell} = \hat{\beta} + \sum_{j=1}^{p_2} \hat{\delta}_j W_j$$

Actually, we have already used this formula (Section 22.2) in the special situation when there is no evidence of interaction. There, the computation of the confidence interval for the adjusted risk odds ratio e^β was straightforward since there were no terms involving modifiers (i.e., W_j's) to worry about. The computer printout conveniently provided the point estimate $\hat{\beta}$ and its estimated standard error $\sqrt{\hat{V}ar(\hat{\beta})}$, leading to the interval $\exp[\hat{\beta} \pm Z_{1-\alpha/2}\sqrt{\hat{V}ar(\hat{\beta})}]$. With interaction terms in the fitted model, however, the computation of $\hat{V}ar(\hat{\ell})$ is somewhat more complicated.

A general formula for this estimated variance is

$$\hat{V}ar(\hat{\ell}) = \hat{V}ar(\hat{\beta}) + \sum_{j=1}^{p_2} W_j^2\,\hat{V}ar(\hat{\delta}_j) + 2\sum_{j=1}^{p_2} W_j\,\hat{C}ov(\hat{\beta}, \hat{\delta}_j)$$
$$+ 2\sum\sum_{\text{all } j<j'} W_j W_{j'}\,\hat{C}ov(\hat{\delta}_j, \hat{\delta}_{j'})$$

This expression not only contains terms involving the estimated variances of $\hat{\beta}$ and the $\hat{\delta}_j$'s in the model but also contains terms involving the estimated covariances of each $\hat{\delta}_j$ with other $\hat{\delta}_{j'}$ and with $\hat{\beta}$. Fortunately, most available computer packages for ML estimation (e.g., SAS's LOGIST) print out (as an option) the estimated variance-covariance matrix for each fitted model.

As an example, for the Strategy 4 model in which CHL and HPT were identified as the only modifiers, the estimated variance-covariance matrix of estimated coefficients is presented in Table 23.5. We have circled those values in this matrix that will appear in the general odds ratio confidence interval formula based on this Strategy 4 model. More specifically, using the estimated coefficient values given previously (step 2, Table 23.2), we obtain the following general expression for a large-sample 95% interval estimate of the adjusted odds ratio:

$$\exp \{[\hat{\beta} + \hat{\delta}_1(\text{CHL}) + \hat{\delta}_2(\text{HPT})] \pm 1.96\sqrt{\hat{V}ar[\hat{\beta} + \hat{\delta}_1(\text{CHL}) + \hat{\delta}_2(\text{HPT})]}\}$$

where $\hat{\beta} = -12.680907$, $\hat{\delta}_1 = .069118$, $\hat{\delta}_2 = -2.329887$, and

$$\begin{aligned}
\hat{V}ar[\hat{\beta} + \hat{\delta}_1(\text{CHL}) + \hat{\delta}_2(\text{HPT})] &= \hat{V}ar(\hat{\beta}) + (\text{CHL})^2\,\hat{V}ar(\hat{\delta}_1) \\
&\quad + (\text{HPT})^2\,\hat{V}ar(\hat{\delta}_2) \\
&\quad + 2(\text{CHL})\,\hat{C}ov(\hat{\beta}, \hat{\delta}_1) \\
&\quad + 2(\text{HPT})\,\hat{C}ov(\hat{\beta}, \hat{\delta}_2) \\
&\quad + 2(\text{CHL})(\text{HPT})\,\hat{C}ov(\hat{\delta}_1, \hat{\delta}_2) \\
&= 9.636209 + (\text{CHL})^2(.000206) \\
&\quad + (\text{HPT})^2(.550920) \\
&\quad + 2(\text{CHL})(-.043671) \\
&\quad + 2(\text{HPT})(-.005914) \\
&\quad + 2(\text{CHL})(\text{HPT})(-.001604)
\end{aligned}$$

Table 23.5   Estimated Variance-Covariance Matrix of Estimated Coefficients for Strategy 4 Model Containing CHL and HPT as Effect Modifiers

COVARIANCE MATRIX OF ESTIMATES

	INTERCEPT	CAT	AGE	CHL
INTERCEPT	1.574765			
CAT	−.663589	9.636209		
AGE	−.0136081	−.00205291	.0002604102	
CHL	−.00341062	.003591349	−.0000036585	.00001750461
ECG	−.0431337	.02410592	.0001398037	.00004234846
SMK	−.119197	−.0257146	.0005867178	.0000283013
HPT	.001288945	.0013989	−.000031649	−.000247241
CC = CAT × CHL	.003446171	−.0436712	.00000250775	−.0000175592
CH = CAT × HPT	.0550055	−.00591374	−.00103918	.0002580651

	ECG	SMK	HPT	CC	CH
INTERCEPT					
CAT					
AGE					
CHL					
ECG	.1074549				
SMK	.007098607	.1070809			
HPT	−.0135381	−.000391108	.1099814		
CC = CAT × CHL	−.000327954	.00009720329	.0002840077	.0002060692	
CH = CAT × HPT	−.00152621	.002554285	−.107999	−.00160411	.5509195

Note: The fitted model here is

$$\text{logit } \hat{P}_2(\mathbf{x}) = \hat{\alpha} + \hat{\beta}(\text{CAT}) + \hat{\gamma}_1(\text{AGE}) + \hat{\gamma}_2(\text{CHL}) + \hat{\gamma}_3(\text{ECG}) + \hat{\gamma}_4(\text{SMK}) + \hat{\gamma}_5(\text{HPT})$$
$$+ \hat{\delta}_1(\text{CAT} \times \text{CHL}) + \hat{\delta}_2(\text{CAT} \times \text{HPT})$$

where the estimated coefficients are given in Table 23.2 under the "BETA" column at step 2.

To illustrate a typical calculation, suppose we consider computing the interval estimate for the specific values CHL = 220 and HPT = 1. The numerical value of the variance expression above is then

$$
\begin{aligned}
\hat{\text{Var}}[\hat{\beta} + \hat{\delta}_1(220) + \hat{\delta}_2(1)] &= 9.636209 + (220)^2(.000206) \\
&\quad + (1)^2(.550920) + 2(220)(-.043671) \\
&\quad + 2(1)(-.005914) \\
&\quad + 2(220)(1)(-.001604) \\
&= .224701
\end{aligned}
$$

Using this value for the variance in the interval estimate formula given above, we obtain the following result:

$$\exp\{[-12.680907 + (.069118)(220) - (2.329887)(1)] \\ \pm 1.96\sqrt{.224701}\}$$

or

$$\exp(.195166 \pm .929091) \quad \text{or} \quad (1.216)\exp(\pm.929091)$$

or

$$(.48, 3.08)$$

Thus, for hypertensive persons with a cholesterol level of 220, the adjusted CAT–CHD odds ratio, estimated by using the Strategy 4 model, is about 1.22, with a 95% confidence interval of (.48, 3.08). The results from similar computations for other combinations of CHL and HPT values are provided in Table 23.6; on inspection of the table, it becomes evident that most such intervals are quite wide. Therefore, the reliability in the estimation of the regression coefficients and their standard errors can be questioned, with a plausible explanation being a combination of multicollinearity and the use of unconditional ML estimation with insufficient data.

Table 23.6 95% Large-Sample Confidence Intervals for ROR(adj.) Based on Strategy 4 Model

a. HPT = 0

CHL	$\hat{\beta} + \Sigma\hat{\delta}_j W_j$	$\hat{\mathrm{Var}}(\hat{\beta} + \Sigma\hat{\delta}_j W_j)$	$\hat{ROR}$(adj.)	95% Confidence Interval
140	−3.004387	1.445929	.05	(.005, .52)
180	−.239667	.589049	.79	(.17, 3.54)
200	1.142693	.407809	3.14	(.90, 10.96)
220	2.525053	.391369	12.49	(3.67, 42.57)
240	3.907412	.539729	49.77	(11.79, 210.05)
260	5.289773	.852889	198.30	(32.45, 1,211.81)
300	8.054493	1.973609	3,147.91	(200.53, 49,414.68)

b. HPT = 1

CHL	$\hat{\beta} + \Sigma\hat{\delta}_j W_j$	$\hat{\mathrm{Var}}(\hat{\beta} + \Sigma\hat{\delta}_j W_j)$	$\hat{ROR}$(adj.)	95% Confidence Interval
140	−5.334274	1.535901	.005	(.0004, .05)
180	−2.569554	.550701	.08	(.02, .33)
200	−1.187194	.305301	.31	(.10, .90)
220	.195166	.224701	1.22	(.48, 3.08)
240	1.577526	.308901	4.84	(1.63, 14.39)
260	2.959886	.557901	19.30	(4.46, 83.42)
300	5.724606	1.550301	306.31	(26.69, 3,515.80)

**23.4
HYPOTHESIS
TESTING**

To test the null hypothesis that exposure is not related to disease, given specified values of the effect modifiers, one could use confidence intervals as constructed above. If the computed interval does not contain the null value one, reject the null hypothesis of no adjusted effect. Also, one could appeal to the asymptotic normality of $\hat{\beta} + \sum_{j=1}^{p_2} \hat{\delta}_j W_j$ to test such a null hypothesis with the statistic

$$Z = \left(\hat{\beta} + \sum_{j=1}^{p_2} \hat{\delta}_j W_j \right) \Big/ \left[\hat{\mathrm{Var}} \left(\hat{\beta} + \sum_{j=1}^{p_2} \hat{\delta}_j W_j \right) \right]^{1/2}$$

Finally, although its appropriateness is debatable when interaction is present, a test of the global null hypothesis of no overall exposure-disease association (namely, H_0: $\beta = \delta_1 = \delta_2 = \cdots = \delta_{p_2} = 0$ under Model 20.10) can be carried out by using any of the three testing procedures described in Section 20.2. (The reader may recall our comments in previous chapters about the relevance of carrying out tests involving main effects in the presence of interaction.)

To illustrate this global test, let us consider the model resulting from Strategy 4 (Table 23.2, step 2), which includes the two interaction terms CAT × CHL and CAT × HPT in addition to CAT and the five V_i variables AGE, CHL, ECG, SMK, and HPT. The null hypothesis in this particular case is

$$H_0: \beta = \delta_1 = \delta_2 = 0 \qquad \text{(i.e., no overall CAT–CHD association)}$$

for the model

$$\begin{aligned} \mathrm{logit}\, P_2(\mathbf{x}) = {} & \alpha + \beta(\mathrm{CAT}) + \gamma_1(\mathrm{AGE}) + \gamma_2(\mathrm{CHL}) + \gamma_3(\mathrm{ECG}) \\ & + \gamma_4(\mathrm{SMK}) + \gamma_5(\mathrm{HPT}) + \delta_1(\mathrm{CAT} \times \mathrm{CHL}) \\ & + \delta_2(\mathrm{CAT} \times \mathrm{HPT}) \end{aligned}$$

To carry out the appropriate likelihood ratio test, we must compare the likelihood function value based on fitting this model to the corresponding value obtained by fitting the *reduced* (under H_0) model given by

$$\begin{aligned} \mathrm{logit}\, P_0'(\mathbf{x}) = {} & \alpha + \gamma_1(\mathrm{AGE}) + \gamma_2(\mathrm{CHL}) + \gamma_3(\mathrm{ECG}) \\ & + \gamma_4(\mathrm{SMK}) + \gamma_5(\mathrm{HPT}) \end{aligned}$$

The test statistic is given by the formula

$$\chi^2_{\mathrm{MLR}} = -2 \ln (\hat{L}_0' / \hat{L}_2) = -2 \ln \hat{L}_0' + 2 \ln \hat{L}_2$$

which has a chi-square distribution with three degrees of freedom under the null hypothesis, and where $\hat{L}_0'$ and $\hat{L}_2$ are the maximized likelihood values for the fitted models $\hat{P}_0'(\mathbf{x})$ and $\hat{P}_2(\mathbf{x})$, respectively. The degrees of freedom for this test are three, because three linearly independent constraints (namely, $\beta = 0$, $\delta_1 = 0$, $\delta_2 = 0$) are imposed by the null hypothesis.

Using the information provided in Table 23.2 (step 2), we find that

$$-2 \ln \hat{L}_2 = 347.28$$

This table, however, does not provide the other likelihood value we need, since the model $P_0'(\mathbf{x})$ was not considered in the algorithm used to assess interaction. From a separate computer run, however, we find that

$$-2 \ln \hat{L}_0' = 403.27$$

so that

$$\chi^2_{\text{MLR}} = 403.27 - 347.28 = 55.99$$

which is highly significant. The corresponding five-degrees-of-freedom chi-square statistic for assessing the significance of the overall CAT–CHD association under the Strategy 3 model (see Table 23.3) has the value 60.95, which is also highly significant. Both these tests provide strong evidence of an overall CAT–CHD association.

We have pointed out many times (e.g., see Chapter 21) that the precision in an odds ratio estimate may sometimes be improved if nonconfounders can be identified and subsequently eliminated from the fitted model. When illustrating this phenomenon with our previous example (Section 22.3.4), we showed that this elimination of nonconfounders amounted to finding (proper) subsets of the initial set of risk factors (i.e., V_i variables) in the model that gave the same odds ratio value as was obtained when all such risk factors were controlled. With no interaction terms in the model, this procedure entails monitoring only the main effect coefficient of the exposure variable, namely, $\hat{\beta}$. Unfortunately, an analogous approach when significant interaction effects are present is somewhat less manageable, since the interaction coefficients as well as $\hat{\beta}$ would have to be monitored. Nevertheless, if *none* of the estimated coefficients involving the exposure variable change upon refitting, after deletion of one or more V_i variables from the model, a gain in precision may be realized (without loss of validity) by using the more parsimonious model. (We remind the reader that those V_i variables involved in the model as modifiers are not candidates for deletion.)

23.5 DELETING NONCONFOUNDERS

To illustrate this elimination procedure, we will restrict our attention to the model derived from Strategy 4, in which CHL and HPT are the only two variables identified as modifiers. Table 23.7 illustrates how the three estimated coefficients involving CAT (i.e., $\hat{\beta}$, $\hat{\delta}_1$, and $\hat{\delta}_2$) vary in value, depending on which V_i terms are retained in the model. Since there are changes of *varying* amounts in each of the estimated coefficients as variables are deleted, it is difficult to determine precisely how large the "collective" change in all three coefficients has to be in order for the corre-

Table 23.7 Monitoring Coefficients Involving CAT
for Various Subsets of Main Effect (i.e., V_i) Variables,
Based on Strategy 4 Model

Main Effect Variables (V_i) in Model	Main Effect Variables Deleted	$\hat{\beta}$	$\hat{\delta}_1$	$\hat{\delta}_2$
CHL, HPT, AGE, ECG, SMK	—	−12.6809	.0691	−2.3299
CHL, HPT, AGE, ECG	SMK	−12.7187	.0696	−2.3809
CHL, HPT, AGE, SMK	ECG	−12.8367	.0706	−2.3316
CHL, HPT, ECG, SMK	AGE	−12.5611	.0696	−2.2059
CHL, HPT, AGE	ECG, SMK	−12.7787	.0706	−2.3769
CHL, HPT, ECG	AGE, SMK	−12.5767	.0703	−2.2561
CHL, HPT, SMK	AGE, ECG	−12.7131	.0711	−2.2188
CHL, HPT	AGE, ECG, SMK	−12.7324	.0712	−2.2584

Note: The model considered here has the general form

$$\text{logit } \hat{P}(\mathbf{x}) = \hat{\alpha} + \hat{\beta}(\text{CAT}) + \sum \hat{\gamma}_i V_i + \hat{\delta}_1(\text{CAT} \times \text{CHL}) + \hat{\delta}_2(\text{CAT} \times \text{HPT})$$

where the number of V_i terms varies between two and five.

sponding adjusted odds ratio formula to be altered substantially. It is our opinion that any decision to delete such variables is largely subjective, and we urge caution in such deletion for fear of sacrificing validity in exchange for what is typically only a minor gain in precision.

In any case, it is more appropriate to base variable-deletion decisions on comparisons of estimates of the adjusted odds ratio rather than of the individual regression coefficients. In this example, to determine whether AGE, ECG, and SMK can *all* be deleted simultaneously without sacrificing validity, we can compute an odds ratio table (of the type illustrated in Table 23.4) for the corresponding reduced model and compare it with the odds ratio table for the unreduced model. This comparison is provided in Table 23.8 and indicates sufficient discrepancies in corresponding odds ratios to preclude simultaneously dropping AGE, ECG, and SMK from the model.

23.6 CONCLUDING REMARKS

We have attempted to demonstrate, with this second example, the specific kinds of analyses required (point and interval estimation plus hypothesis testing) when interaction is present in one's data. Moreover, we have illustrated the complexity of both the analyses and the strategies involved in the choice of such analyses when interaction effects are important. Regarding our conclusions about this specific data set, it is our opinion that CHL and HPT should be controlled as effect modifiers. However, the specific nature of the CAT–CHD association can only be described in rough terms when

Table 23.8   Comparison of Adjusted Odds Ratios When AGE, ECG, and SMK Are Retained Versus Being Removed from the Strategy 4 Model

a. AGE, ECG, SMK Retained[a]			b. AGE, ECG, SMK Removed[b]		
	HPT			HPT	
CHL	0	1	*CHL*	0	1
140	.05	.005	140	.06	.007
180	.79	.08	180	1.10	.11
200	3.14	.31	200	4.56	.48
220	12.49	1.22	220	18.96	1.98
240	49.77	4.84	240	78.82	8.24
260	198.30	19.30	260	327.69	34.25
300	3,147.91	306.31	300	5,664.64	592.08

[a]$\hat{ROR}(adj.) = \exp[-12.6809 + .0691(CHL) - 2.3299(HPT)]$.
[b]$\hat{ROR}(adj.) = \exp[-12.7324 + .0712(CHL) - 2.2584(HPT)]$.

considering the uncertainty reflected in the interval estimates given in Table 23.6. As mentioned earlier, we would strongly recommend using conditional ML estimation methods to examine these follow-up study data. Chapter 24 discusses two applications of this conditional ML methodology to the analysis of case-control study data.

KUPPER, L. L.; STEWART, J. R.; and WILLIAMS, K. A. 1976. A note on controlling significance levels in stepwise regression. *Am. J. Epidemiol.* 103(1): 13–15.   **REFERENCES**

24

Applications of Modeling: Conditional Likelihood Estimation

CHAPTER OUTLINE

We now turn to examples illustrating the *conditional* method of maximum likelihood (ML) estimation, described in Chapter 20 (Section 20.3.2), for fitting logistic models like 20.10. As we pointed out there, conditional likelihood procedures are appropriate for situations in which unconditional ML estimation is markedly biased, such as when stratum-specific sample sizes are small (e.g., pair-matched and R-to-1 matched data). Consequently, the examples given in this chapter will consider situations in which individual matching has been employed. Discrepancies between the results obtained by using conditional and unconditional methods (the latter giving biased estimates of effect) will also be illustrated.

**24.0
PREVIEW**

In Chapter 18 on matching (Section 18.5), we considered an example of 4-to-1 matching based on a study by Trichopoulos and colleagues (1969). The data for this study are presented in Table 18.10. This study was a case-control study involving 18 women with ectopic (i.e., tubal) pregnancy, each of whom was matched with 4 controls (women with uterine pregnancies) on the basis of order of pregnancy, age, and husband's age. The exposure variable was dichotomous, indicating whether or not there was a history of induced abortion for any previous pregnancy. From a standard stratified analysis that takes the matching into account (i.e., each stratum contains 5 observations corresponding to a case and its 4 matched controls), the following results were obtained regarding the relationship between previous history of induced abortion and the subsequent occurrence of a tubal pregnancy:

**24.1
EXAMPLE:
4-TO-1
MATCHING
WITHOUT
COVARIATES**

$$\text{m}\hat{\text{OR}} = 33.0 \qquad \chi^2_{\text{MHS}} = 16 \qquad (P\text{-value} < 0.001)$$

As an alternative to the m$\hat{\text{OR}}$, a complex iterative method proposed by Miettinen (1970) produces a point estimator of the population exposure odds ratio having the value 22.57, with an associated 90% confidence interval of (3.93, 210.60). Miettinen's point estimator turns out to be mathematically identical to that obtained through the general conditional likelihood estimation procedures to be described here. The Mantel-Haenszel test, although computationally different, is "asymptotically" (i.e., for very large samples) equivalent to the test derived from conditional likelihood methods. (The reader may recall from Chapter 17 that the Mantel-Haenszel chi-square test is a conditional one based on the assumption of fixed margins for each stratum.)

In addition to the above stratified analyses, mathematical-modeling methods were used to analyze these data via the following logistic model:

$$\text{logit } P(\mathbf{x}) = \alpha + \beta E + \sum_{i=1}^{17} \gamma_i V_i$$

where $P(\mathbf{x}) = \mathrm{pr}\,(D = 1 | E, V_1, \ldots, V_{17})$,

$$D = \begin{cases} 1 & \text{if a case} \\ 0 & \text{if a control} \end{cases}$$

$$E = \begin{cases} 1 & \text{if previous history of induced abortion} \\ 0 & \text{if no previous history of induced abortion} \end{cases}$$

$$V_i = \begin{cases} 1 & \text{for a person belonging to the } i\text{th matched set} \\ 0 & \text{otherwise} \end{cases}$$

for $i = 1, 2, \ldots, 17$.

Note that the V_i terms in the model are dummy (i.e., indicator) variables used to index the 18 strata (or matched sets). Also, since the model contains no cross-product terms involving E, we are assuming that there is uniformity in the odds ratio across the strata. The above model is, in fact, equivalent in structure to Model 20.9, which can be written for this example as

$$\mathrm{logit}\,P_g(\mathbf{x}) = \alpha_g + \beta E \qquad g = 1, 2, \ldots, 18$$

where the α_g are nuisance parameters indexing the different strata.

Using the above model, we will now describe two different sets of numerical results (estimated odds ratios, associated confidence intervals, and chi-square statistics), one set generated from unconditional ML estimation and the other by conditional ML estimation. Under unconditional ML estimation, the results are derived from maximizing an appropriate unconditional likelihood function based on the general expression 20.15. When conditional likelihood estimation is used, the results are derived from maximizing an appropriate conditional likelihood of the general form in 20.25. (The reader should be aware that the same underlying logistic model is being used for both likelihoods 20.15 and 20.25. Also, this same general model is appropriate even if the analysis involves only one of the four controls available for each case.)

Table 24.1 provides various statistics obtained from both unconditional and conditional ML estimation of logistic model parameters for the data in Table 18.10. This table also includes results from a pair-matched analysis based on the use of only the first of the four controls in each matched set. For both the 4-to-1 and the 1-to-1 matching situations, we have provided point and interval estimates of the adjusted exposure odds ratio [EOR (adj.)], and chi-square statistics for assessing the strength of the relationship between previous induced abortion and the subsequent occurrence of a tubal pregnancy. [The unconditional ML results were obtained by using SAS's LOGIST program; the conditional ML results were obtained by using a program developed by Smith and colleagues (1981), called "STRAT-Linear Regression Analysis for Stratified Sets."]

Table 24.1   Results from Unconditional and Conditional ML Estimation of the Logistic Model Adjusted Odds Ratio When Analyzing a Matched Case-Control Study Concerning the Relationship Between Previous Induced Abortion and Subsequent Occurrence of a Tubal Pregnancy

	$\exp(\hat{\beta}) = \widehat{EOR}$ (adj.)	90% Confidence Interval	$\chi^2_{ML\beta}$ (One-sided P-Value)
1–1 Matching (n = 36):[a]			
Unconditional	$\exp(2.197222) = 9.00$	(.61, 132.09)	1.81 (P = .089)
Conditional	$\exp(1.098610) = 3.00$	(.45, 20.05)	.91 (P = .171)
4–1 Matching (n = 90):			
Unconditional	$\exp(4.366967) = 78.80$	(8.42, 737.41)	10.32 (P = .001)
Conditional	$\exp(3.116438) = 22.57$	(3.94, 129.37)	8.62 (P = .002)

[a]1–1 matching was achieved by pairing each case with the *first* of its four matched controls listed in Table 18.10.

From Table 24.1, we see that there is considerable discrepancy between the results from the unconditional and conditional estimation methods. As we previously mentioned, the unconditional point estimate of the adjusted odds ratio is misleading whenever the strata being used involve small sample sizes. In particular, for the 1–1 matching situation, the odds ratio based on unconditional ML estimation (namely, 9.00) is the square of the corresponding conditional estimate of 3.00. [Recall (see Section 20.3) that, for a pair-matched design, the unconditional ML estimator is $(v_{10}/v_{01})^2$, whereas the conditional estimator is v_{10}/v_{01}, the ratio of discordant pairs.] When all four controls are used, the odds ratio from unconditional estimation (78.80) is considerably less than the square of the conditional estimator (22.57), although the discrepancy is still quite large. In general, the more controls used, the closer the unconditional and conditional odds ratio estimates will be; the same relationship holds regarding the chi-square values.

Finally, note that the odds ratio from conditional estimation (22.57) is relatively close to the $m\widehat{OR}$ value of 33.0 presented earlier and (as expected) is identical to Miettinen's point estimate. However, Miettinen's interval estimate of (3.93, 210.60), which is based on a complex iterative scheme described in his 1970 paper, has an upper limit considerably larger than 129.37, the conditional likelihood value. The reader can also see from Table 24.1 that there is considerable discrepancy between the conclusions drawn from the pair-matched analysis and those from the analysis of the 4-to-1 matched data. In particular, the 4-to-1 matched analysis reveals a much stronger exposure-disease association. Although one data set is a subset of the other, and involves the same group of cases, such a large discrepancy in results is possible because of the correspondingly large difference in total sample sizes ($n = 90$ for 4-to-1 matching versus $n = 36$ for 1-to-1 matching). For an excellent discussion of sample size considerations in case-control studies, see Chapter 6 of Schlesselman (1982).

24.2 EXAMPLE: 2-TO-1 MATCHING WITH COVARIATES

The previous example involved the use of a model that accounted for extraneous variables only in terms of those actually employed in the matching process. It frequently happens that, in addition to the matching variables, there are other extraneous factors the investigator needs to consider at the analysis state. As we will see, logistic modeling provides a convenient and efficient approach for handling such a situation.

To illustrate, we will consider a (hypothetical) hospital-based data set for a matched case-control study designed to assess the relationship between smoking and myocardial infarction. The cases consist of 39 persons identified over a three-month period as having been treated in a certain hospital for acute nonfatal myocardial infarction (MI). Each of these cases is assumed to be matched on age (± 2 years), race, and gender with *two* controls, each of whom is a noncoronary (NC) patient from the same hospital (i.e., a control has had no signs or history of any cardiovascular disease). Thus, there is 2-to-1 matching, and the data consist of 39 such matched sets. All 117 subjects in the study were asked whether or not they had smoked cigarettes for a total of at least three years, and these subjects were so grouped into smokers (SMK = 1) and nonsmokers (SMK = 0). In addition, two other variables were measured on each individual for possible control at the analysis stage: systolic blood pressure (SBP) and history of electrocardiogram abnormality (ECG = 1 if yes, and ECG = 0 if no). Note that the extraneous factors SBP and ECG were *not* involved in the matching process but may require control at the analysis stage.

Table 24.2 summarizes the study results in terms of the six smoking status configurations possible for each matched set. The entries in the body of Table 24.2 are the numbers of matched sets (out of 39) having the various smoking status configurations. Table 24.3 provides summary statistics for the unmatched variables SMK, SBP, and ECG, broken down by case-control status. Table 24.4 lists the complete (hypothetical) data set, including the values for the variables SBP and ECG.

24.2.1 Preliminary Analysis Considerations

Table 24.2 provides the same kind of information considered in our previous example (Table 18.10). We can assess the relationship between SMK and MI status just from Table 24.2 by using either stratified analysis (involving 39 strata) or conditional logistic modeling, as described in Section 24.1. However, the data in Table 24.2 alone do not allow us to investigate the potential modifying and/or confounding effects of the variables SBP and ECG.

Table 24.3 provides us with some summary data about the three unmatched independent variables: the exposure variable SMK, SBP, and

Table 24.2   Distribution of Matched Sets by Smoking Status for a Hypothetical 2-to-1 Matched Case-Control Study Concerning Smoking and Myocardial Infarction

	NUMBER OF CONTROLS WHO SMOKED		
	2	1	0
Case Smoked	2	4	9
Case Did Not Smoke	2	6	16
			39

Note: Each matched set consists of one case and two controls.

ECG. In particular, we see that the cases are heavier smokers than the controls, have considerably higher blood pressure (on the average) than the controls, and have a higher proportion of persons with ECG abnormality. Nevertheless, this table considers these independent variables only one at a time and, more importantly, completely ignores the matching that has been employed.

What is required for a proper analysis is consideration of the complete data set presented in Table 24.4; this data set will allow us to simultaneously evaluate the effects of all the independent variables while also taking the matching into account. An appropriate method of analysis, which we will now describe, involves conditional ML estimation of a logistic model incorporating the effects of both matched and unmatched independent variables.

Table 24.3   Summary Statistics for SMK, SBP, and ECG for Cases and Controls Based on a Hypothetical 2-to-1 Matched Case-Control Study Concerning Smoking and Myocardial Infarction

Variable	Statistic	Cases ($n = 39$)	Controls ($n = 78$)
SMK	Proportion of smokers	$15/39 = .3846$	$18/78 = .2308$
SBP	Mean blood pressure	145.13	132.05
ECG	Proportion with ECG abnormality	$14/39 = .3590$	$11/78 = .1410$

Table 24.4 Hypothetical Data Set for a 2-to-1 Matched Case-Control Study Concerning Smoking and Myocardial Infarction

Matched Set	Person	Case Status	SMK	SBP	ECG	Matched Set	Person	Case Status	SMK	SBP	ECG
1	1	1	0	160	1	16	48	0	0	160	1
1	2	0	0	140	0	17	49	1	1	160	1
1	3	0	0	120	0	17	50	0	0	140	0
2	4	1	0	160	1	17	51	0	0	120	0
2	5	0	0	140	0	18	52	1	1	160	1
2	6	0	0	120	0	18	53	0	0	140	0
3	7	1	0	160	0	18	54	0	0	120	0
3	8	0	0	140	0	19	55	1	1	160	0
3	9	0	0	120	0	19	56	0	0	140	1
4	10	1	0	160	0	19	57	0	0	120	0
4	11	0	0	140	0	20	58	1	1	160	1
4	12	0	0	120	0	20	59	0	0	140	1
5	13	1	0	160	0	20	60	0	0	120	0
5	14	0	0	140	0	21	61	1	1	160	0
5	15	0	0	120	0	21	62	0	0	140	0
6	16	1	0	160	0	21	63	0	0	120	0
6	17	0	0	140	0	22	64	1	1	120	0
6	18	0	0	120	0	22	65	0	0	120	0
7	19	1	0	160	0	22	66	0	0	120	0
7	20	0	0	140	0	23	67	1	1	140	0
7	21	0	0	120	0	23	68	0	0	140	0
8	22	1	0	160	0	23	69	0	0	140	0
8	23	0	0	140	0	24	70	1	1	120	0
8	24	0	0	120	0	24	71	0	0	140	0
9	25	1	0	160	0	24	72	0	0	160	0
9	26	0	0	140	0	25	73	1	1	120	0
9	27	0	0	120	0	25	74	0	0	160	0
10	28	1	0	160	0	25	75	0	0	140	0
10	29	0	0	140	0	26	76	1	0	160	0
10	30	0	0	120	0	26	77	0	1	140	0
11	31	1	0	120	1	26	78	0	0	120	0
11	32	0	0	120	0	27	79	1	0	120	0
11	33	0	0	120	0	27	80	0	1	120	0
12	34	1	0	120	0	27	81	0	0	120	0
12	35	0	0	120	0	28	82	1	0	160	1
12	36	0	0	120	0	28	83	0	0	140	0
13	37	1	0	120	0	28	84	0	1	120	0
13	38	0	0	120	0	29	85	1	0	160	0
13	39	0	0	120	0	29	86	0	0	140	0
14	40	1	0	140	0	29	87	0	1	120	0
14	41	0	0	140	0	30	88	1	0	120	0
14	42	0	0	140	0	30	89	0	0	140	0
15	43	1	0	120	1	30	90	0	1	160	0
15	44	0	0	140	1	31	91	1	0	140	0
15	45	0	0	160	0	31	92	0	0	140	0
16	46	1	0	120	1	31	93	0	1	140	0
16	47	0	0	140	1	32	94	1	1	160	1

Table 24.4   (*continued*)

Matched Set	Person	Case Status	SMK	SBP	ECG	Matched Set	Person	Case Status	SMK	SBP	ECG
32	95	0	1	140	0	36	106	1	0	160	1
32	96	0	0	120	0	36	107	0	1	140	1
33	97	1	1	160	1	36	108	0	1	120	1
33	98	0	1	140	1	37	109	1	0	120	0
33	99	0	0	120	0	37	110	0	1	140	0
34	100	1	1	120	1	37	111	0	1	160	0
34	101	0	1	120	1	38	112	1	1	160	1
34	102	0	0	120	1	38	113	0	1	140	0
35	103	1	1	160	0	38	114	0	1	120	0
35	104	0	0	140	0	39	115	1	1	120	0
35	105	0	1	120	0	39	116	0	1	120	0
						39	117	0	1	120	0

The traditional alternative to such conditional analyses has involved stratification of the data into subgroups of matched sets with common values for combinations of the unmatched extraneous variables. For example, the data might be divided into six subgroups of matched sets according to combinations of three SBP levels (e.g., low, medium, and high) and the two ECG levels. A severe drawback to this approach, however, concerns discarded data resulting from matched sets that contain subjects with differing values for the unmatched extraneous variables. For example, with these data (see Table 24.4), there are 12 matched sets (involving 36 subjects) for which subjects in the same matched set do not have identical ECG values. This large chunk of data would have to be dropped from any stratified analysis that controls for ECG *and* retains the matching. The logistic-modeling approach, in contrast, does not require any of the data to be dropped in order to evaluate the effects of both matched and unmatched factors.

Since these data involve 39 matched sets (i.e., strata), a logistic model incorporating all the stratum-specific effects would contain 38 indicator variables and an intercept. The model we will consider includes SMK (the exposure variable), the two unmatched extraneous variables (SBP and ECG), and the 38 indicator variables all as main effects, and it allows for interaction of SBP and ECG with SMK (but assumes uniformity in the odds ratio across the matching strata). This "full" model takes the form

24.2.2
The Model

$$\text{logit } P(\mathbf{x}) = \alpha + \beta(\text{SMK}) + \sum_{i=1}^{41} \gamma_i V_i + (\text{SMK}) \sum_{j=1}^{3} \delta_j W_j$$

where

$$V_1 = \text{SBP} = W_1 \qquad V_2 = \text{ECG} = W_2 \qquad V_3 = \text{SBP} \times \text{ECG} = W_3$$

and, for $i = 4, 5, \ldots , 41$,

$$V_i = \begin{cases} 1 \text{ if the subject belongs to matched set number } (i - 3) \\ 0 \text{ otherwise} \end{cases}$$

An equivalent form of this model, using Expression 20.9, is

$$\text{logit } P_g(\mathbf{x}) = \alpha_g + \beta(\text{SMK}) + \sum_{i=1}^{3} \gamma_i V_i + (\text{SMK}) \sum_{j=1}^{3} \delta_j W_j$$

$$g = 1, 2, \ldots , 39$$

where the α_g are nuisance parameters used to index the 39 strata.

Both unconditional and conditional ML estimation methods were used to fit this model, as well as variations of this model involving subsets of the independent variables. As in the previous example, SAS's LOGIST program was used to perform the unconditional ML estimation, and the program STRAT (as developed by Smith et al., 1981) was used to carry out the conditional ML estimation. Only the conditional methods were used to evaluate interaction, so that α and the 38 γ_i effects indexing matched sets did not enter into these conditional ML estimation computations. Not having to estimate these 39 nuisance parameters is a decided advantage of the conditional approach.

24.2.3
Interaction
Assessment

Since the conditional ML estimation program of Smith and colleagues (1981) had not, at the time of this writing, been packaged to include standard forward, backward, and stepwise algorithms, our assessment of interaction entailed fitting only one model at a time. Fortunately, this task was not formidable, since only the *two* extraneous variables SBP and ECG were candidates for modifiers.

The essential question regarding interaction concerns whether or not any product terms among the collection SMK × SBP, SMK × ECG, and SMK × SBP × ECG need to be included in a model already containing the main effects of SMK and the 41 V_i variables. As we described for the follow-up study data in Section 23.1, both forward selection and backward elimination variable-selection approaches are applicable here. For example, the backward type of strategy would begin by determining whether or not the product term SMK × SBP × ECG contributed significantly to a model already containing the variables SMK, all the V_i, SMK × SBP, and SMK × ECG. If SMK × SBP × ECG is deemed significant, then the full model given earlier would be wholly retained, with the variables SBP and ECG being identified as modifiers. If SMK × SBP × ECG is found to be not significant, then the backward elimination algorithm would continue examining various "reduced" models to determine whether SMK × SBP and/or SMK × ECG could be eliminated. In contrast, the forward selection approach would first determine whether any of the two-factor products SMK × SBP and SMK × ECG need to be added to the main effects model, and, if so, whether the triple product SMK × SBP × ECG also needs to be added.

As it turned out, under either the forward or backward strategies, no two-factor or three-factor product term was found to be significant at the 10% level. Table 24.5 provides likelihood ratio chi-square values (χ^2_{MLR}) and chi-square values based on the ML estimates (i.e., $\chi^2_{\text{ML}\delta} = \hat{\delta}^2/S^2_{\hat{\delta}}$) obtained from the backward and forward algorithms just described. We conclude from these values that there is no evidence of interaction, and we will therefore proceed to assess the SMK–MI relationship via a model involving only confounders.

From our conclusion of "no interaction," the full logistic model previously defined can be simplified to the following "reduced" model:

24.2.4 Point Estimation and Tests of Hypotheses: Reduced Model

$$\text{logit } P(\mathbf{x}) = \alpha + \beta(\text{SMK}) + \sum_{i=1}^{41} \gamma_i V_i$$

where the V_i's are defined as before.

Under this reduced model, the estimated odds ratio adjusted for the effects of the V_i variables is given by the familiar expression $\exp(\hat{\beta})$, where $\hat{\beta}$ is the estimated coefficient of the exposure variable SMK. Recalling our discussion on strategy in Chapter 21, we can monitor changes in this adjusted odds ratio estimate (or $\hat{\beta}$ itself) as various subsets of SBP, ECG, and SBP × ECG are dropped in an attempt to increase precision. Furthermore, for any such main effect model (containing SMK and any subset of

Table 24.5 Testing for Interaction Effects in a Logistic Model Using Conditional ML Estimation in the Second Matching Example

Product Terms Already Included[a]	Product Terms Tested[b]	χ^2_{MLR}	$\chi^2_{\text{ML}\delta}$
SMK × SBP, SMK × ECG	SMK × SBP × ECG	2.6962 ($P = .101$)	2.5181 ($P = .113$)
—	SMK × SBP	.2026 ($P = .653$)	.2036 ($P = .652$)
—	SMK × ECG	.0062 ($P = .937$)	.0063 ($P = .937$)

[a]All main effect terms (the intercept, SMK, and all 41 V_i variables) are already included in each model considered, although the stratum-indexing variables do not enter into the conditional likelihood computation.

[b]The null hypothesis being tested in each case is H_0: $\delta = 0$, where δ is the coefficient of a product term in a model containing all main effects and other already included product terms.

V_1, V_2, and V_3), we can assess whether $\hat{\beta}$ is significantly different from zero by using either a likelihood ratio chi-square (χ^2_{MLR}) or the chi-square statistic $\chi^2_{\mathrm{ML}\beta} = (\hat{\beta}/S_{\hat{\beta}})^2$.

The results from point estimation and hypothesis testing, using both conditional and unconditional ML methods for various subsets of V_1, V_2, and V_3, are provided in Table 24.6. From inspection of this table, we see that the unconditional estimation procedure leads to overestimation of the odds ratio (i.e., it is positively biased) and therefore should not be used. Also, despite apparently *large* differences between cases and controls regarding mean SBP and the proportion of individuals with ECG abnormality (see Table 24.3), there is only moderate evidence of confounding due to these variables. In particular, when the model contains SBP, ECG, and SBP × ECG, the adjusted odds ratio from conditional estimation is 2.14, whereas the model containing *no* control variables (other than the matched set indexing variables V_4 to V_{41}) gives only a slightly higher estimate of 2.32. The hypothesis-testing results, however, do indicate a discrepancy in conclusions about evidence regarding the adjusted SMK–MI association; in particular, ignoring SBP and ECG leads to a P-value of .035, as opposed to P-values around .09 otherwise. Consequently, we would recommend the use of a model involving at least one of the two variables SBP and ECG as a main effect.

The reader should not be surprised that there is only moderate evidence of confounding, even though $\widehat{\mathrm{OR}}_{df}$ appears to be much larger than

Table 24.6 Point Estimation and Tests of Significance for the Logistic Model Adjusted Odds Ratio, Controlling for Various Subsets Among SBP and ECG in the Second Matching Example

V_i Variables Included in the Model[a]	ML Estimation Method	$\exp(\hat{\beta}) = \widehat{\mathrm{EOR}}(\mathrm{adj.})$	$\chi^2_{\mathrm{ML}\beta}$ (One-sided P-value)
SBP, ECG, SBP × ECG	Conditional	exp(.759668) = 2.14	1.75 ($P = .093$)
	Unconditional	exp(1.260884) = 3.53	2.97 ($P = .085$)
SBP, ECG	Conditional	exp(.761825) = 2.14	1.80 ($P = .090$)
	Unconditional	exp(1.259975) = 3.53	3.01 ($P = .083$)
SBP	Conditional	exp(.731753) = 2.08	1.83 ($P = .088$)
	Unconditional	exp(1.219944) = 3.39	3.13 ($P = .077$)
ECG	Conditional	exp(.719795) = 2.05	1.91 ($P = .084$)
	Unconditional	exp(1.120436) = 3.07	2.87 ($P = .091$)
—	Conditional	exp(.943344) = 2.32	3.27 ($P = .035$)
	Unconditional	exp(1.311772) = 3.71	4.89 ($P = .027$)

[a]All models considered involve an intercept, the 38 indicator variables for the matching strata, and SMK (the exposure variable with coefficient β); the stratum-indexing variables do not enter into the conditional likelihood computations.

unity (for f = SBP or ECG and d = MI). We have pointed out, in both Chapters 13 and 18, that the appearance of confounding in case-control data requires that both $\hat{OR}_{df|\bar{E}}$ and $\hat{OR}_{ef|\bar{D}}$ be different from unity in the data. In our particular situation, confounding appears to be absent because the second of these two odds ratios is not noticeably different from unity for either variable.

24.3 CONCLUD-ING REMARKS

In this chapter and in Chapters 22 and 23, we have attempted to provide the reader with practical insight regarding the use of mathematical modeling for the control of extraneous variables. We have illustrated the basic steps involved in the formulation of an appropriate logistic model and in the computation of relevant statistics. Moreover, we have demonstrated how to apply various strategies appropriate for different stages of the analysis. We recognize that there is no single strategy that will always provide a clear-cut set of analytical conclusions. On the contrary, several different strategies, types of modeling approaches, and other forms of analyses (e.g., stratified analysis) can and should be applied in any given data analysis situation. The final conclusions to be drawn require a delicate balance of both quantitative and substantive (e.g., clinical) considerations.

One final point is worth emphasizing. In each of our examples, we have restricted our attention to fitting a logistic model involving a single, dichotomous exposure variable. The reader should, nevertheless, be aware that the general form of the logistic model given by Expression 20.3 allows for analyses that incorporate several exposure variables, each of which can be dichotomous, polychotomous, or continuous. In such a situation, the model will contain several exposure variables instead of a single exposure variable, whose joint relationship with the disease variable is to be assessed. The general adjusted odds ratio expression given by 20.5 can be used for this purpose, and multiple partial chi-square statistics involving one or more of the exposure variables can be used to test hypotheses. For brevity's sake, we have not provided in this chapter an example that involves a multiple exposure variable. (The reader can, however, formulate such a situation by using our earlier examples and simply redefining a previously designated extraneous variable as an additional exposure variable.) Examples of logistic modeling with two or more exposure variables are given in Breslow and Day (1980).

PRACTICE EXERCISES

Problems 24.1–24.4 concern the assessment of the relationship between catecholamine level (CAT) and the incidence of coronary heart disease (CHD); they are based on the Evans County study considered throughout the text. In these problems, various subsets of the variables SMK, CHL, ECG, AGE, and HPT (a binary hypertension variable) will be considered for control as potential confounders and effect modifiers of the postulated CAT–CHD association. The first problem considers the application of procedures for the (unconditional) ML fitting of the logistic model involving a single binary exposure variable (E). The second problem considers an extension of logistic modeling to account for two exposure variables. The third and fourth problems require computation and interpretation, using computer printouts that are provided.

24.1 This problem considers the control of SMK, CHL, AGE, and HPT, but not ECG.

a. Give two equivalent expressions for a saturated logistic model that could be used to perform a stratified analysis that simultaneously controls for SMK, CHL, AGE, and HPT and that assumes no interaction. In defining these models, treat each variable in binary fashion, with AGE and CHL categorized as follows:

$$AGEG = \begin{cases} 0 \text{ if less than } 55 \\ 1 \text{ if greater than or equal to } 55 \end{cases}$$

$$CHLG = \begin{cases} 0 \text{ if less than } 220 \\ 1 \text{ if greater than or equal to } 220 \end{cases}$$

Hint: To describe one model, you should use Expression 20.10 to define appropriate V_i and W_j terms in the model. To describe the other model, you should use Expression 20.9 to define an appropriate number of nuisance parameters (i.e., coefficients of indicator variables) that index the different strata.

b. Are there any possible drawbacks to the use of unconditional ML estimation techniques to fit this model?

c. If you were to treat age and cholesterol level as continuous variables, how would you modify the models defined in part a?

d. Would you use discriminant function analysis to obtain estimates and tests for the parameters in these models? Explain.

e. Suppose you allow for the possibility of interaction in controlling for SMK, CHL, AGE, and HPT, treating AGE and CHL as continuous variables. What form of model would you use if you had only these four variables in the model as potential confounders (i.e., as V_i terms) but included up to three-factor interactions (of the form EV_iV_j) to account for effect modification?

f. Of all the three-factor interactions considered in part e, suppose that only the variables $E \times$ CHL $\times$ HPT and $E \times$ SMK $\times$ HPT are deemed significant enough to be retained in the final model. From this result (and using the hierarchy principle described in Chapter 21), what two-factor interactions (EV_i terms) and potential confounder terms (V_i terms) should also appear in the final model?

g. Describe the null hypothesis (H_0), the appropriate likelihood ratio test statistic, and its distribution under H_0 for testing (via unconditional ML estimation) whether or not the variables $E \times$ CHL $\times$ HPT and $E \times$ SMK $\times$ HPT significantly improve model prediction when both are incorporated into the logistic model containing all main effects and all two-factor interactions.

h. At the next step of interaction assessment, suppose that *none* of the remaining candidate interactions (of the form EV_i) not already earmarked for inclusion in the final model are to be found significant. On the basis of this result, give an expression for the final model resulting from this assessment of interaction, making sure to explicitly identify each variable to be included in this final model.

i. Describe what steps you would take to decide whether to eliminate any of the V_i variables not already chosen for retention in the final model. Make sure to state which V_i variables are candidates for such deletion (on the basis of the hierarchy principle).

j. Using the model determined in part h, give an expression for the adjusted odds ratio that describes the CAT–CHD association controlling for the effects of AGE, CHL, SMK, and HPT.

k. Using the model determined in part h for 50-year-old smokers *without* hypertension and with a cholesterol level of 250, give an expression for a 95% large-sample confidence interval for the adjusted population odds ratio describing the CAT–CHD association. Describe how you would obtain the estimate of variance needed to construct such an interval estimate.

l. For 50-year-old smokers *with* hypertension and with a cholesterol value of 250, describe two alternative procedures for testing whether or not there is statistical evidence of a CAT–CHD association.

24.2 In addition to an investigation of the effect of CAT on CHD, suppose it is of interest to consider simultaneously the effect of physical activity level (PAL), again controlling for SMK, CHL, AGE, and HPT. Assume that PAL is a binary variable (PAL = 1 if high, PAL = 0 if low).

a. Treating AGE and CHL as continuous variables and using only primary variables as V_i terms (i.e., no product terms among SMK, CHL, AGE, and HPT should be used as V_i terms), write a logistic model that can be used to describe the combined CAT–PAL effect on CHD, allowing for interaction between CAT and PAL but assuming no effect modification due to the potential confounders SMK, CHL, AGE, and HPT.

b. For 50-year-old nonsmokers with cholesterol values of 250 but no hypertension, write an expression for the adjusted risk odds ratio comparing the risk of disease development for such persons having high CAT and high PAL with the corresponding risk for persons having low CAT and low PAL.

c. Using the model defined in part a, how would you test, via unconditional ML estimation, whether there is significant interaction between CAT and PAL?

24.3 This problem considers five variables for control: AGE, CHL, SMK, HPT, and ECG.

a. Comment on whether the accompanying computer printout could have been obtained from a strategy based on the hierarchy principle. (This printout gives results for unconditional ML estimation of a logistic model.)

b. Using the information in the printout, give an expression for the adjusted risk odds ratio that describes the CAT–CHD association controlling for AGE, CHL, ECG, SMK, and HPT.

c. Using the result in part b, compute the adjusted risk odds ratio for a smoker without hypertension and with a cholesterol value of 220. Compare this result with the computed odds ratio for a smoker with hypertension and with a cholesterol value of 220. What additional information would be helpful in making this comparison?

d. Using the information in the printout, carry out a test of hypothesis to determine whether there is significant interaction based on the variables CAT × CHL, CAT × HPT, and CAT × HPT × SMK. (You will need to use the fact that $-2 \ln \hat{L}_0 = 400.41$ for the logistic model containing only the variables CAT, AGE, CHL, ECG, SMK, and HPT.) In performing this test, be sure to state H_0, the general form of the likelihood ratio test statistic, and its distribution under H_0.

$$-2 \ln \hat{L}_1 = 343.24$$

VARIABLE	BETA	STD. ERROR	CHI-SQUARE	P
INTERCEPT	−4.53815727	1.30008929	12.18	0.0005
CAT	−13.39683469	3.20624063	17.46	0.0000
AGE	0.03925459	0.01647847	5.67	0.0172
CHL	−0.00544935	0.00420535	1.68	0.1950
ECG	0.31825158	0.33472886	0.90	0.3417
SMK	1.11735281	0.39001622	8.21	0.0042
HPT	1.05624334	0.33333646	10.04	0.0015
CC = CAT × CHL	0.07250095	0.01482501	23.92	0.0000
CH = CAT × HPT	−1.28473786	0.89349526	2.07	0.1505
CHS = CAT × HPT × SMK	−1.68841586	0.84731902	3.97	0.0463

24.4 As they were in Problem 24.3, the five variables AGE, CHL, HPT, SMK, and ECG are considered for control here. Answer the following questions by using the computer information provided in Table 23.2.

a. Using the step 1 results, give an expression for the adjusted risk odds ratio that describes the adjusted CAT–CHD relationship and considers CHL to be the only effect modifier among the control variables.

b. Using your result in part a, describe how the CAT–CHD relationship varies according to the level of CHL. (Hint: Form a table of adjusted odds ratios obtained for various values of CHL, and then interpret the tabulated results.)

c. Again using step 1 results for persons with a cholesterol value of 250, give a general expression for a 95% large-sample confidence interval for the adjusted odds ratio. Why can't the variance estimate in this expression be computed by using the estimated variance-covariance matrix given in Table 23.5?

d. Using the step 0 results, give point and 95% interval estimates for the adjusted CAT–CHD odds ratio. Also, test for the significance of this odds ratio, making use of the fact that $-2 \ln \hat{L}_0' = 403.27$ for the logistic model (not shown here) containing all the control variables but not including CAT. Why are these results inappropriate for describing the CAT–CHD association?

24.5 Suppose a case-control study was conducted to assess the effect of (0–1) exposure status E on (0–1) disease status D. Among the six risk factors to be considered for control, the variables C_1, C_2, and C_3 were used as matching variables, with 3 controls matched to each case. The other 3 variables C_4, C_5, and C_6 were left unmatched. The total number of cases identified was 50, so that the study involved a total of 200 subjects.

a. Considering each matched set as a separate stratum and assuming no interaction of any kind, state a "prospective" logistic model that can be used to estimate the odds ratio, controlling only for the variables used in the matching process.

b. How would you modify the model in part a to allow for control of the unmatched variables, including possible effect modification involving these latter variables? In defining this model, use only the primary variables C_1, C_2, and C_3 as V_i terms, and allow for interaction only in terms of two-factor products of the form EV_i for $i = 4, 5, 6$.

c. Which method of ML estimation should be used to fit the model defined in part b, unconditional or conditional? Why?

d. If a follow-up study had been used instead of a case-control study, with C_1, C_2, C_3 again used as matching variables (giving 3 unexposed subjects to each exposed subject), how would the logistic model defined in part b be modified, if at all? (Assume that there were 60 *exposed* subjects in the study.)

e. For the follow-up study described in part d, which method of ML estimation should be used to fit the model? Why?

REFERENCES

BRESLOW, N. E., and DAY, N. E. 1980. *Statistical methods in cancer research. Vol. 1: The analysis of case-control studies.* Lyon, France: IARC Scientific Publications No. 32.

MIETTINEN, O. S. 1970. Estimation of relative risk from individually matched series. *Biometrics* 23: 75–86.

SCHLESSELMAN, J. J. 1982. *Case-control studies: Design, conduct, analysis.* New York: Oxford University Press.

SMITH, P. G.; PIKE, M. C.; HILL, A. P.; BRESLOW, N. E.; and DAY, N. E. 1981. Multivariate conditional logistic analysis of stratum-matched case-control studies. *J. R. Stat. Soc. C* 30(2): 190–197.

TRICHOPOULOS, D.; MIETTINEN, O. S.; and POLYCHRONOPOULOU, A. 1969. Induced abortions and ectopic pregnancy. Unpublished manuscript.

APPENDIX A
Answers to Selected Exercises

CHAPTER 6   **6.1 a.** $\hat{R}_{(0,5)} = .486$ **b.** $\hat{R}_{(0,5)} = .485$

           6.2 a. $\hat{R}_{(55,57)} = .010$ **b.** $\hat{R}_{(55,65)} = .118$ **c.** $\hat{R}_{(55,75)} = .378$

CHAPTER 7   **7.1 a.** period prevalence   **b.** incidence density   **c.** point prevalence (at birth)   **d.** cumulative incidence   **e.** point prevalence   **f.** (prevalence odds)   **g.** incidence density

           7.2 a   **7.3** c

CHAPTER 9   **9.1 a.** $\hat{P}_{1960} = .0476$; $\hat{C}_{1960} = 5000$ **b.** $\hat{RR} = 4.00$; $\hat{RD} = .075$

           c. $\hat{EF} = .545$ **d.** $\hat{EF}_e = .75$

           e. $\hat{T} = 4.42$ years if we assume that there is no loss to follow-up and that new cases occur uniformly over the follow-up period. (Or $\hat{T} = 4.55$ years if we assume that the disease is rare so that CI is $\approx$ ID(Δ).)

           9.2 a. $\hat{POR}_{H/M} = 1.81$; $\hat{POR}_{L/O} = 1.30$

           b. $\hat{P}_{H/M} = .101$; $\hat{P}_{L/O} = .075$; $\hat{P}_{NONE} = .059$

           c. $\hat{EF} = .169$ **d.** $\hat{EF}_e = .446$

           9.3 a. $\hat{IDR} = .530$ **b.** $\hat{IDD} = -.00940/\text{year}$

           c. $\hat{IDR}(\text{corrected}) = .583$ **d.** $\hat{PF} = .085$

           9.4 a. $\hat{ID}_{50-59} = .00040/\text{year}$; $\hat{ID}_{60-69} = .00084/\text{year}$; $\hat{ID}_{70-79} = .00200/\text{year}$

           b. $\hat{IDR}_{50-59} = 2.74$; $\hat{IDR}_{60-69} = 2.37$; $\hat{IDR}_{70-79} = 1.99$

           c. $\hat{EF}_{50-59} = .423$; $\hat{EF}_{60-69} = .289$; $\hat{EF}_{70-79} = .162$

           d. $\hat{ID}_{\bar{s}(50-59)} = .00023/\text{year}$, $\hat{ID}_{\bar{s}(60-69)} = .00060/\text{year}$,

           $\hat{ID}_{\bar{s}(70-79)} = .00168/\text{year}$; $\hat{ID}_{s(50-59)} = .00063/\text{year}$;

           $\hat{ID}_{s(60-69)} = .00142/\text{year}$; $\hat{ID}_{s(70-79)} = .00333/\text{year}$

           e. $\hat{RD}_{(50,80)} = .028$

CHAPTER 10   **10.1** false   **10.3** false   **10.5** false   **10.7** false   **10.9** true

           10.11 true   **10.13** false   **10.15** false

11.1 a. false   **b.** false   **d.** true   **e.** true   **g.** false   **h.** false   **CHAPTER 11**

11.2 b. $OR° = .95$ **c.** $\alpha = .102$, $\beta = .055$, $\gamma = .010$, $\delta = .005$
   d. $BIAS(P\hat{O}R, POR) = -.05$ **e.** $OR° = 1$ **f.** $OR° = .91$
   g. $OR° = .41$; general principle illustrated may be stated as follows: for fixed $pr(H_E)$, $OR° < 1$ if $pr(H_D) > pr(H_{D*})$, whereas $OR° > 1$ if $pr(H_D) < pr(H_{D*})$

11.3 a. $\alpha = \gamma > \beta = \delta$, so that $r_E = 1$, $r_{\bar{E}} = 1$, $\alpha\delta/\beta\gamma = 1$; no selection bias in estimating ROR; no bias in estimating CIR
   b. $\delta > \alpha = \gamma > \beta$, so that $r_E = 1$, $r_{\bar{E}} < 1$; bias in estimating ROR is positive, i.e., away from the null; bias in estimating CIR cannot be clearly determined from given information
   c. no bias in estimating POR or PR
   d. $(1/5)\alpha' = \beta' = \gamma' = \delta'$, where α', β', γ', δ' denote mortality probabilities; bias in estimating ROR using $P\hat{O}R$ is negative, i.e., toward the null
   e. bias in estimating EOR is positive, i.e., away from the null
   f. bias in estimating EOR is negative

12.1 a. true   **b.** false   **c.** true   **d.** true   **e.** true   **f.** false   **CHAPTER 12**

12.2 a. $\phi_E = .65$, $\psi_E = .80$ **b.** $C\hat{I}R(\text{corrected}) = 4.00$
   c. nondifferential assumption must be unreasonable
   e. $C\hat{I}R = 2$ for interview data in part b; $C\hat{I}R° = 1.17$ for data resulting from misclassification of both exposure and disease

13.1 a. $\hat{OR}_{males} = 82.83$, $\hat{OR}_{females} = 82.72$; no evidence of interaction   **CHAPTER 13**
   b. $\hat{OR}_{df} = 1$; no association between gender and disease status
   c. $c\hat{OR} = 10$; evidence of confounding since $c\hat{OR} \neq \hat{OR}_{males} = \hat{OR}_{females}$
   d. $\hat{OR}_{df|E} = .102$, $\hat{OR}_{df|\bar{E}} = .102$; disease and gender associated within each exposure group

13.2 a. $OR_{high} = OR_{low} = cOR = 1$; no population-based confounding due to SES
   b. $\hat{OR}_{high} = \hat{OR}_{low} = 1 \neq c\hat{OR} = 2.01$; evidence of data-based confounding and no evidence of interaction
   c. $a\hat{OR} = 1.0 = aOR \, (= cOR)$
   d. $\alpha = 1$, $\beta = 1$, $\gamma = .00280$, $\delta = .00564$; $\alpha\delta/\beta\gamma = 2.01 \neq 1$
   e. selection bias has led to data-based confounding

13.3 a. $\hat{OR}_M = 2.00$, $\hat{OR}_F = 2.00$, $c\hat{OR} = 2.98$; evidence of confounding by gender
   b. $\mathscr{E}\hat{OR} = 1.49$; gender is a confounder
   c. $s\hat{OR} = 2.00$, which differs from crude estimate of 2.98; moderate association between E and D after controlling for gender

14.1 a. true   **b.** true   **d.** true   **e.** true   **g.** true   **CHAPTER 14**

14.2 a. true   **c.** false   **e.** true   **g.** true

CHAPTER 15   **15.1 a.** $\widehat{\text{EOR}} = 1.91$
  b. $\chi^2 = 2.54$; one-sided P-value $\approx .055$; "borderline" significance
  c. $\widehat{\text{SE}}(\ln \widehat{\text{EOR}}) = .4056$; upper limit $= 4.23$; lower limit $= .86$
  d. $Z/\sqrt{\chi^2} = 1.23$; upper limit $= 4.23$; lower limit $= .86$
15.2 a. $\widehat{\text{IDR}} = .424$
  b. H_0: IDR $= 1$; H_A: IDR < 1; $Z = -1.614$; one-sided P-value $\approx .053$, a borderline situation; exact P-value $\approx .088$
  c. $\chi^2 = Z^2 = 2.605$; lower limit $= .150$; upper limit $= 1.20$
  d. age should be considered as a potential confounding variable

CHAPTER 17   **17.1 a.** $\widehat{\text{cRR}} = 1.88$; moderate association between perception of disease and vaccine acceptance; $\chi^2_{\text{MH}} = 20.5 \ (P \ll .001)$; strong evidence of overall crude association
  b. adjusted estimates not all equal when controlling for gender
  c. ignoring race, gender does not appear to be a confounding variable
  d. ignoring gender, race does not appear to be a confounding variable
  e. controlling simultaneously for both variables, there appears to be no association
  f. simultaneous control of race and gender reveals joint confounding due to these two factors
  g. perception of swine flu does not appear to be a determinant of vaccine acceptance
17.2 a. $\widehat{\text{cOR}} = 2.25$; for one-sided test of H_0: cOR $= 1$, one-sided P-value is .0099
  b. $\widehat{\text{OR}}_{\text{SMK}} = 2.33 \ (P = .077)$; $\widehat{\text{OR}}_{\overline{\text{SMK}}} = 2.00 \ (P = .103)$; no confounding due to smoking status; little evidence of interaction
  c. smoking status does not appear to be a confounding variable
  d. $\chi^2_{\text{MH}} = 3.60 \ (P = .02882)$
  f. 95% Taylor series–based CI for aOR: (.97, 4.74); 95% test-based CI for aOR: (.98, 4.72)
  g. evidence $(P < .001)$ of moderate association between substance E and bladder cancer; 95% Taylor series–based interval: (1.13, 4.46)
17.3 a. no significant evidence of association between education and hypertension
  b. interaction due to race
  c. Whites (controlling for gender): $\widehat{\text{aOR}} = .53$; 95% CI: (.28, .97); $\chi^2_{\text{MH}} = 4.28 \ (P = .19)$; significant protective effect of high education status on prevalence of hypertension. Blacks: $\widehat{\text{aOR}} = 1.93$; 95% CI: (1.15, 3.21); $\chi^2_{\text{MH}} = 6.40 \ (P = .006)$; significant deleterious effect of high education status on prevalence of hypertension.
  d. little evidence that gender is confounding variable in either race-specific data set
17.4 b. $\widehat{\text{aIDR}} = .53$; slight confounding due to age
  c. $\chi^2_{\text{MHD}} = 1.38 \ (P = .121)$; data do not support theory
  d. 95% test-based CI for aIDR: (.18, 1.53); supports result of part c
  e. 95% test-based CI for aPF: $(-.20, .52)$

17.5 a. $\hat{cOR}$(HS vs. NS) = 2.66 (P = .005); $\hat{cOR}$(LS vs. NS) = 1.47 (P = .136); results for separate strata somewhat similar to corresponding crude results
  b. $\hat{mOR}$(HS vs. NS) = 2.39; $\hat{mOR}$(LS vs. NS) = 1.20
  d. χ^2_{MHO} = 5.10 (P = .012, one-sided); significant at α = .05 but not α = .01
  f. $\hat{mEF}$ = .31   **g.** 95% test-based CI for mEF: (.04, .45)
17.6 a. Example 1: χ^2_{Zelen} = 18.09 (P < .001, 1 d.f.); Example 2: χ^2_{Zelen} = .01; use of Zelen's test is inappropriate for testing uniformity in OR estimates
  b. Zelen's procedure actually testing uniformity in standardized differences rather than in odds ratios
  c. Example 1: χ^2_I = 0; Example 2: χ^2_I = 4.01 (P = .045, 1 d.f.); use of χ^2_I appropriate for testing uniformity in odds ratio

18.1 b. yes   **CHAPTER 18**
  d. two estimators are not equal in case of 2-to-1 matching
18.2 a. Population: cOR = 3.00, OR_1 = 3.00, OR_2 = 3.00; no population-based confounding due to maternal age. Study sample: $\hat{cOR}$ = 3.00. Stratified by maternal age: $\hat{OR}_1$ = 3.00, $\hat{OR}_2$ = 3.00, $\hat{sOR}$ = 3.00. Unstratified χ^2 = 17.07, stratified χ^2_{MH} = 15.94; efficiency lost by unnecessary stratification after random sampling in a case-control study. No confounding in data due to maternal age, so crude analysis is preferable.
  b. McNemar χ^2 = 15.00; this χ^2 smaller than unstratified χ^2 in part a, indicating loss in efficiency due to matching on a non–risk factor in a case-control study
18.3 a. χ^2 = 3.33, with one-sided P-value of about .034

19.1 a. $\hat{cRR}$ = 1.34, $\hat{sRR}$ = 1.22; stratified χ^2_{MH} = 1.73 (.05 < P < .10); ex-   **CHAPTER 19** treme nonuniformity of two stratum-specific measures of effect (in particular, being on opposite sides of 1) means stratified χ^2_{MH} test not appropriate
  b. Z = −3.70; strong evidence of deviation from additivity
  d. we would expect $\hat{\delta}$ to be negative

24.1 a. Model 1 using 20.10: logit $P(\mathbf{x}) = \alpha + \sum_{i=1}^{15} \gamma_i V_i + \beta(CAT)$, where   **CHAPTER 24** V_1 = SMK, V_2 = CHLG, V_3 = AGEG, V_4 = HPT, $V_5 = V_1V_2$, $V_6 = V_1V_3$, $V_7 = V_1V_4$, $V_8 = V_2V_3$, $V_9 = V_2V_4$, $V_{10} = V_3V_4$, $V_{11} = V_1V_2V_3$, $V_{12} = V_1V_2V_4$, $V_{13} = V_1V_3V_4$, $V_{14} = V_2V_3V_4$, $V_{15} = V_1V_2V_3V_4$. Model 2 using 20.9: logit $P_g(\mathbf{x}) = \alpha_g + \beta(CAT)$, where α_g is nuisance parameter indexing stratum g, $g = 1, 2, \ldots, 16$.
  e. logit $P(\mathbf{x}) = \alpha + \beta E + \sum_{j=1}^{4} \gamma_i V_i + E \sum_{j=1}^{4} \delta_j V_j + \delta_5 EV_1V_2 + \delta_6 EV_1V_3 + \delta_7 EV_1V_4 + \delta_8 EV_2V_3 + \delta_9 EV_2V_4 + \delta_{10}EV_3V_4$, where V_1 = SMK, V_2 = CHL, V_3 = AGE, V_4 = HPT

    f. $E \times$ CHL, $E \times$ HPT, $E \times$ SMK, CHL, HPT, SMK should be retained in all further models

    h. final model: logit $P_I(\mathbf{x}) = \alpha + \beta E + \sum\limits_{i=1}^{4} \gamma_i V_i + \delta_1 E \times$ CHL $+ \delta_2 E \times$ HPT $+ \delta_3 E \times$ SMK $+ \delta_4 E \times$ CHL $\times$ HPT $+ \delta_5 E \times$ SMK $\times$ HPT

    i. only V_i variable eligible for elimination is $V_3 =$ AGE

    j. $\widehat{\text{ROR}}$(adj.) $= \exp[\hat{\beta} + \hat{\delta}_1$ CHL $+ \hat{\delta}_2$ HPT $+ \hat{\delta}_3$ SMK $+ \hat{\delta}_4$ (CHL $\times$ HPT) $+ \hat{\delta}_5$ (SMK $\times$ HPT)]

    k. $\exp[\hat{\ell} \pm 1.96\sqrt{\widehat{\text{Var}}(\hat{\ell})}]$, where $\hat{\ell} = \hat{\beta} + 250\hat{\delta}_1 + \hat{\delta}_3$ and $\widehat{\text{Var}}(\hat{\ell}) = \widehat{\text{Var}}(\hat{\beta}) + (250)^2 \widehat{\text{Var}}(\hat{\delta}_1) + \widehat{\text{Var}}(\hat{\delta}_3) + 500 \widehat{\text{Cov}}(\hat{\beta}, \hat{\delta}_1) + 2 \widehat{\text{Cov}}(\hat{\beta}, \hat{\delta}_3) + 500 \widehat{\text{Cov}}(\hat{\delta}_1, \hat{\delta}_3)$

24.2 a. logit $P(\mathbf{x}) = \alpha + \sum\limits_{i=1}^{4} \gamma_i V_i + \beta_1(\text{CAT}) + \beta_2(\text{PAL}) + \beta_3(\text{CAT} \times \text{PAL})$, where $V_1 =$ SMK, $V_2 =$ CHL, $V_3 =$ AGE, $V_4 =$ HPT

    b. $\widehat{\text{ROR}}$(adj.) $= \exp(\hat{\beta}_1 + \hat{\beta}_2 + \hat{\beta}_3)$

    c. H_0: $\beta_3 = 0$ for model in part a

24.3 a. printout could not have been obtained from strategy following hierarchy principle

    b. $\widehat{\text{ROR}}$(adj.) $= \exp[\hat{\beta} + \hat{\delta}_1(\text{CHL}) + \hat{\delta}_2(\text{HPT}) + \hat{\delta}_3(\text{HPT} \times \text{SMK})]$

    c. For CHL $= 220$, SMK $= 1$, HPT $= 0$: $\widehat{\text{ROR}}$(adj.) $= 12.85$. For CHL $= 220$, SMK $= 1$, HPT $= 1$: $\widehat{\text{ROR}}$(adj.) $= .66$

    d. $\chi^2_{\text{MLR}} = 57.17$ ($P < .001$, 3 d.f.)

24.4 a. $\widehat{\text{ROR}}$(adj.) $= \exp[-14.07169585 + .06826746(\text{CHL})]$

    b. CAT–CHD association is negative [i.e., $\widehat{\text{ROR}}$(adj.) < 1] when CHL below 206, is positive [i.e., $\widehat{\text{ROR}}$(adj.) > 1] when CHL above 206, and increases with increasing CHL level

    d. For Step 0 results: $\widehat{\text{ROR}}$(adj.) $= 1.82$; 95% interval: $(.91, 3.62)$; for H_0: no CAT–CHD association, $\chi^2_{\text{MLR}} = 2.86$ (one-sided $P = .045$). All results are inappropriate in light of significant CAT $\times$ CHL interaction effect previously identified.

APPENDIX B
Statistical Tables

Table B.1   Standard Normal Cumulative Probabilities

z	0.00	0.01	0.02	0.03	0.04	0.05	0.06	0.07	0.08	0.09
−3.8	0.0001	0.0001	0.0001	0.0001	0.0001	0.0001	0.0001	0.0001	0.0001	0.0001
−3.7	0.0001	0.0001	0.0001	0.0001	0.0001	0.0001	0.0001	0.0001	0.0001	0.0001
−3.6	0.0002	0.0002	0.0001	0.0001	0.0001	0.0001	0.0001	0.0001	0.0001	0.0001
−3.5	0.0002	0.0002	0.0002	0.0002	0.0002	0.0002	0.0002	0.0002	0.0002	0.0002
−3.4	0.0003	0.0003	0.0003	0.0003	0.0003	0.0003	0.0003	0.0003	0.0003	0.0002
−3.3	0.0005	0.0005	0.0005	0.0004	0.0004	0.0004	0.0004	0.0004	0.0004	0.0003
−3.2	0.0007	0.0007	0.0006	0.0006	0.0006	0.0006	0.0006	0.0005	0.0005	0.0005
−3.1	0.0010	0.0009	0.0009	0.0009	0.0008	0.0008	0.0008	0.0008	0.0007	0.0007
−3.0	0.0014	0.0013	0.0013	0.0012	0.0012	0.0011	0.0011	0.0011	0.0010	0.0010
−2.9	0.0019	0.0018	0.0018	0.0017	0.0016	0.0016	0.0015	0.0015	0.0014	0.0014
−2.8	0.0026	0.0025	0.0024	0.0023	0.0023	0.0022	0.0021	0.0021	0.0020	0.0019
−2.7	0.0035	0.0034	0.0033	0.0032	0.0031	0.0030	0.0029	0.0028	0.0027	0.0026
−2.6	0.0047	0.0045	0.0044	0.0043	0.0041	0.0040	0.0039	0.0038	0.0037	0.0036
−2.5	0.0062	0.0060	0.0059	0.0057	0.0055	0.0054	0.0052	0.0051	0.0049	0.0048
−2.4	0.0082	0.0080	0.0078	0.0076	0.0073	0.0071	0.0069	0.0068	0.0068	0.0064
−2.3	0.0107	0.0104	0.0102	0.0099	0.0096	0.0094	0.0091	0.0089	0.0087	0.0084
−2.2	0.0139	0.0136	0.0132	0.0129	0.0125	0.0122	0.0119	0.0116	0.0113	0.0110
−2.1	0.0179	0.0174	0.0170	0.0166	0.0162	0.0158	0.0154	0.0150	0.0146	0.0143
−2.0	0.0228	0.0222	0.0217	0.0212	0.0207	0.0202	0.0197	0.0192	0.0188	0.0183
−1.9	0.0287	0.0281	0.0274	0.0268	0.0262	0.0256	0.0250	0.0244	0.0239	0.0233
−1.8	0.0359	0.0351	0.0344	0.0336	0.0329	0.0322	0.0314	0.0307	0.0301	0.0294
−1.7	0.0446	0.0436	0.0427	0.0418	0.0409	0.0401	0.0392	0.0384	0.0375	0.0367
−1.6	0.0548	0.0537	0.0526	0.0516	0.0505	0.0495	0.0485	0.0475	0.0465	0.0455
−1.5	0.0668	0.0655	0.0643	0.0630	0.0618	0.0606	0.0594	0.0582	0.0571	0.0559

Table B.1 (*continued*)

z	0.00	0.01	0.02	0.03	0.04	0.05	0.06	0.07	0.08	0.09
−1.4	0.0808	0.0793	0.0778	0.0764	0.0749	0.0735	0.0721	0.0708	0.0694	0.0681
−1.3	0.0968	0.0951	0.0934	0.0918	0.0901	0.0885	0.0869	0.0853	0.0838	0.0823
−1.2	0.1151	0.1131	0.1112	0.1093	0.1075	0.1057	0.1038	0.1020	0.1003	0.0985
−1.1	0.1357	0.1335	0.1314	0.1292	0.1271	0.1251	0.1230	0.1210	0.1190	0.1170
−1.0	0.1587	0.1562	0.1539	0.1515	0.1492	0.1469	0.1446	0.1423	0.1401	0.1379
−0.9	0.1841	0.1814	0.1788	0.1762	0.1736	0.1711	0.1685	0.1660	0.1635	0.1611
−0.8	0.2119	0.2090	0.2061	0.2033	0.2005	0.1977	0.1949	0.1922	0.1894	0.1867
−0.7	0.2420	0.2389	0.2358	0.2327	0.2297	0.2266	0.2236	0.2206	0.2177	0.2148
−0.6	0.2743	0.2709	0.2676	0.2643	0.2611	0.2578	0.2546	0.2514	0.2483	0.2451
−0.5	0.3085	0.3050	0.3015	0.2981	0.2946	0.2912	0.2877	0.2843	0.2810	0.2776
−0.4	0.3446	0.3409	0.3372	0.3336	0.3300	0.3264	0.3228	0.3192	0.3156	0.3121
−0.3	0.3821	0.3783	0.3745	0.3707	0.3669	0.3632	0.3594	0.3557	0.3520	0.3483
−0.2	0.4207	0.4168	0.4129	0.4090	0.4052	0.4013	0.3974	0.3936	0.3897	0.3859
−0.1	0.4602	0.4562	0.4522	0.4483	0.4443	0.4404	0.4364	0.4325	0.4286	0.4247
−0.0	0.5000	0.4960	0.4920	0.4880	0.4840	0.4801	0.4761	0.4721	0.4681	0.4641
0.0	0.5000	0.5040	0.5080	0.5120	0.5160	0.5199	0.5239	0.5279	0.5319	0.5359
0.1	0.5398	0.5438	0.5478	0.5517	0.5557	0.5596	0.5636	0.5675	0.5714	0.5753
0.2	0.5793	0.5832	0.5871	0.5910	0.5948	0.5987	0.6026	0.6064	0.6103	0.6141
0.3	0.6179	0.6217	0.6255	0.6293	0.6331	0.6368	0.6406	0.6443	0.6480	0.6517
0.4	0.6554	0.6591	0.6628	0.6664	0.6700	0.6736	0.6772	0.6808	0.6844	0.6879
0.5	0.6915	0.6950	0.6985	0.7019	0.7054	0.7088	0.7123	0.7157	0.7190	0.7224
0.6	0.7257	0.7291	0.7324	0.7357	0.7389	0.7422	0.7454	0.7486	0.7517	0.7549
0.7	0.7580	0.7611	0.7642	0.7673	0.7703	0.7734	0.7764	0.7794	0.7823	0.7852
0.8	0.7881	0.7910	0.7939	0.7967	0.7995	0.8023	0.8051	0.8078	0.8106	0.8133
0.9	0.8159	0.8186	0.8212	0.8238	0.8264	0.8289	0.8315	0.8340	0.8365	0.8389
1.0	0.8413	0.8438	0.8461	0.8485	0.8508	0.8531	0.8554	0.8577	0.8599	0.8621
1.1	0.8643	0.8665	0.8686	0.8708	0.8729	0.8749	0.8770	0.8790	0.8810	0.8830
1.2	0.8849	0.8869	0.8888	0.8907	0.8925	0.8943	0.8962	0.8980	0.8997	0.9015
1.3	0.9032	0.9049	0.9066	0.9082	0.9099	0.9115	0.9131	0.9147	0.9162	0.9177
1.4	0.9192	0.9207	0.9222	0.9236	0.9251	0.9265	0.9279	0.9292	0.9306	0.9319
1.5	0.9332	0.9345	0.9357	0.9370	0.9382	0.9394	0.9406	0.9418	0.9429	0.9441
1.6	0.9452	0.9463	0.9474	0.9484	0.9495	0.9505	0.9515	0.9525	0.9535	0.9545
1.7	0.9554	0.9564	0.9573	0.9582	0.9591	0.9599	0.9608	0.9616	0.9625	0.9633
1.8	0.9641	0.9649	0.9656	0.9664	0.9671	0.9678	0.9686	0.9693	0.9699	0.9706
1.9	0.9713	0.9719	0.9726	0.9732	0.9738	0.9744	0.9750	0.9756	0.9761	0.9767
2.0	0.9772	0.9778	0.9783	0.9788	0.9793	0.9798	0.9803	0.9808	0.9812	0.9817
2.1	0.9821	0.9826	0.9830	0.9834	0.9838	0.9842	0.9846	0.9850	0.9854	0.9857
2.2	0.9861	0.9864	0.9868	0.9871	0.9875	0.9878	0.9881	0.9884	0.9887	0.9890
2.3	0.9893	0.9896	0.9898	0.9901	0.9904	0.9906	0.9909	0.9911	0.9913	0.9916
2.4	0.9918	0.9920	0.9922	0.9924	0.9927	0.9929	0.9931	0.9932	0.9934	0.9936
2.5	0.9938	0.9940	0.9941	0.9943	0.9945	0.9946	0.9948	0.9949	0.9951	0.9952
2.6	0.9953	0.9955	0.9956	0.9957	0.9959	0.9960	0.9961	0.9962	0.9963	0.9964
2.7	0.9965	0.9966	0.9967	0.9968	0.9969	0.9970	0.9971	0.9972	0.9973	0.9974

Table B.1   (*continued*)

z	0.00	0.01	0.02	0.03	0.04	0.05	0.06	0.07	0.08	0.09
2.8	0.9974	0.9975	0.9976	0.9977	0.9977	0.9978	0.9979	0.9979	0.9980	0.9981
2.9	0.9981	0.9982	0.9982	0.9983	0.9984	0.9984	0.9985	0.9985	0.9986	0.9986
3.0	0.9986	0.9987	0.9987	0.9988	0.9988	0.9989	0.9989	0.9989	0.9990	0.9990
3.1	0.9990	0.9991	0.9991	0.9991	0.9992	0.9992	0.9992	0.9992	0.9993	0.9993
3.2	0.9993	0.9993	0.9994	0.9994	0.9994	0.9994	0.9994	0.9995	0.9995	0.9995
3.3	0.9995	0.9995	0.9995	0.9996	0.9996	0.9996	0.9996	0.9996	0.9996	0.9997
3.4	0.9997	0.9997	0.9997	0.9997	0.9997	0.9997	0.9997	0.9997	0.9997	0.9998
3.5	0.9998	0.9998	0.9998	0.9998	0.9998	0.9998	0.9998	0.9998	0.9998	0.9998
3.6	0.9998	0.9998	0.9999	0.9999	0.9999	0.9999	0.9999	0.9999	0.9999	0.9999
3.7	0.9999	0.9999	0.9999	0.9999	0.9999	0.9999	0.9999	0.9999	0.9999	0.9999
3.8	0.9999	0.9999	0.9999	0.9999	0.9999	0.9999	0.9999	0.9999	0.9999	0.9999
3.9	1.0000									

Table B.2   Percentiles of the Chi-Square Distribution

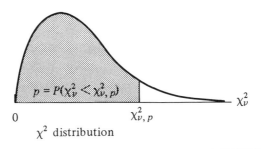

$$p = P(\chi^2_\nu < \chi^2_{\nu,\,p})$$

χ^2 distribution

d.f. \ %	0.5	1	2.5	5	10	20	30	40	50
1	0.0001	0.0002	0.001	0.004	0.016	0.064	0.148	0.275	0.455
2	0.010	0.020	0.051	0.103	0.211	0.446	0.713	1.022	1.386
3	0.072	0.115	0.216	0.352	0.584	1.005	1.424	1.869	2.366
4	0.207	0.297	0.484	0.711	1.064	1.649	2.195	2.753	3.357
5	0.412	0.554	0.831	1.145	1.610	2.343	3.000	3.655	4.351
6	0.676	0.872	1.237	1.635	2.204	3.070	3.828	4.570	5.348
7	0.989	1.239	1.690	2.167	2.833	3.822	4.671	5.493	6.346
8	1.344	1.646	2.180	2.733	3.490	4.594	5.527	6.423	7.344
9	1.735	2.088	2.700	3.325	4.168	5.380	6.393	7.357	8.343
10	2.156	2.558	3.247	3.940	4.865	6.179	7.267	8.295	9.342
11	2.603	3.053	3.816	4.575	5.578	6.989	8.148	9.237	10.341
12	3.074	3.571	4.404	5.226	6.304	7.807	9.034	10.182	11.340
13	3.565	4.107	5.009	5.892	7.042	8.634	9.926	11.129	12.340
14	4.075	4.660	5.629	6.571	7.790	9.467	10.821	12.078	13.339
15	4.601	5.229	6.262	7.261	8.547	10.307	11.721	13.030	14.339
16	5.142	5.812	6.908	7.962	9.312	11.152	12.624	13.983	15.338
17	5.697	6.408	7.564	8.672	10.085	12.002	13.531	14.937	16.338
18	6.265	7.015	8.231	9.390	10.865	12.857	14.440	15.893	17.338
19	6.844	7.633	8.907	10.117	11.651	13.716	15.352	16.850	18.338
20	7.434	8.260	9.591	10.851	12.443	14.578	16.266	17.809	19.337
21	8.034	8.897	10.283	11.591	13.240	15.445	17.182	18.768	20.337
22	8.643	9.542	10.982	12.338	14.041	16.314	18.101	19.729	21.337
23	9.260	10.196	11.689	13.091	14.848	17.187	19.021	20.690	22.337
24	9.886	10.856	12.401	13.848	15.659	18.062	19.943	21.752	23.337
25	10.520	11.524	13.120	14.611	16.473	18.940	20.867	22.616	24.337
26	11.160	12.198	13.844	15.379	17.292	19.820	21.792	23.579	25.336
27	11.808	12.879	14.573	16.151	18.114	20.703	22.719	24.544	26.336
28	12.461	13.565	15.308	16.928	18.939	21.588	23.647	25.509	27.336
29	13.121	14.256	16.047	17.708	19.768	22.475	24.577	26.475	28.336
30	13.787	14.953	16.791	18.493	20.599	23.364	25.508	27.442	29.336
35	17.192	18.509	20.569	22.465	24.797	27.836	30.178	32.282	34.336
40	20.707	22.164	24.433	26.509	29.051	32.345	34.872	37.134	39.335
45	24.311	25.901	28.366	30.612	33.350	36.884	39.585	41.995	44.335
50	27.991	29.707	32.357	34.764	37.689	41.449	44.313	46.864	49.335
60	35.534	37.485	40.482	43.188	46.459	50.641	53.809	56.620	59.335
70	43.275	45.442	48.758	51.739	55.329	59.898	63.346	66.396	69.334
80	51.172	53.540	57.153	60.391	64.278	69.207	72.915	76.188	79.334

Table B.2 (*continued*)

% d.f.	0.5	1	2.5	5	10	20	30	40	50
90	59.196	61.754	65.647	69.126	73.291	78.558	82.511	85.993	89.334
100	67.328	70.065	74.222	77.929	82.358	87.945	92.129	95.808	99.334
120	83.852	86.923	91.573	95.705	100.624	106.806	111.419	115.465	119.334
140	100.655	104.034	109.137	113.659	119.029	125.758	130.766	135.149	139.334
160	117.679	121.346	126.870	131.756	137.546	144.783	150.158	154.856	159.334
180	134.884	138.820	144.741	149.969	156.153	163.868	169.588	174.580	179.334
200	152.241	156.432	162.728	168.279	174.835	183.003	189.049	194.319	199.344

% d.f.	60	70	80	90	95	97.5	99	99.5	99.95
1	0.708	1.074	1.642	2.706	3.841	5.024	6.635	7.879	12.116
2	1.833	2.408	3.219	4.605	5.991	7.378	9.210	10.597	15.202
3	2.946	3.665	4.642	6.251	7.815	9.348	11.345	12.838	17.730
4	4.045	4.878	5.989	7.779	9.488	11.143	13.277	14.860	19.997
5	5.132	6.064	7.289	9.236	11.070	12.833	15.086	16.750	22.105
6	6.211	7.231	8.558	10.645	12.592	14.449	16.812	18.548	24.103
7	7.283	8.383	9.803	12.017	14.067	16.013	18.475	20.278	26.018
8	8.351	9.524	11.030	13.362	15.507	17.535	20.090	21.955	27.868
9	9.414	10.656	12.242	14.684	16.919	19.023	21.666	23.589	29.666
10	10.473	11.781	13.442	15.987	18.307	20.483	23.209	25.188	31.420
11	11.530	12.899	14.631	17.275	19.675	21.920	24.725	26.757	33.137
12	12.584	14.011	15.812	18.549	21.026	23.337	26.217	28.300	34.821
13	13.636	15.119	16.985	19.812	22.362	24.736	27.688	29.819	36.478
14	14.685	16.222	18.151	21.064	23.685	26.119	29.141	31.319	38.109
15	15.733	17.322	19.311	22.307	24.996	27.488	30.578	32.801	39.719
16	16.780	18.418	20.465	23.542	26.296	28.845	32.000	34.267	41.308
17	17.824	19.511	21.615	24.769	27.587	30.191	33.409	35.718	42.879
18	18.868	20.601	22.760	25.989	28.869	31.526	34.805	37.156	44.434
19	19.910	21.689	23.900	27.204	30.144	32.852	36.191	38.582	45.973
20	20.951	22.775	25.038	28.412	31.410	34.170	37.566	39.997	47.498
21	21.991	23.858	26.171	29.615	32.671	35.479	38.932	41.401	49.011
22	23.031	24.939	27.301	30.813	33.924	36.781	40.289	42.796	50.511
23	24.069	26.018	28.429	32.007	35.172	38.076	41.638	44.181	52.000
24	25.106	27.096	29.553	33.196	36.415	39.364	42.980	45.559	53.479
25	26.143	28.172	30.675	34.382	37.652	40.646	44.314	46.928	54.947
26	27.179	29.246	31.795	35.563	38.885	41.923	45.642	48.290	56.407
27	28.214	30.319	32.912	36.741	40.113	43.195	46.963	49.645	57.858
28	29.249	31.391	34.027	37.916	41.337	44.461	48.278	50.993	59.300
29	30.283	32.461	35.139	39.087	42.557	45.722	49.588	52.336	60.735
30	31.316	33.530	36.250	40.256	43.773	46.979	50.892	53.672	62.162
35	36.475	38.859	41.778	46.059	49.802	53.203	57.342	60.275	69.199
40	41.622	44.165	47.269	51.805	56.758	59.342	63.691	66.766	76.095
45	46.761	49.452	52.729	57.505	61.656	65.410	69.957	73.166	82.876
50	51.892	54.723	58.164	63.167	67.505	71.420	76.154	79.490	89.561
60	62.135	65.227	68.972	74.397	79.082	83.298	88.379	91.952	102.695
70	72.358	75.689	79.715	85.527	90.531	95.023	100.425	104.215	115.578

Table B.2   (*continued*)

% d.f.	60	70	80	90	95	97.5	99	99.5	99.95
80	82.566	86.120	90.405	96.578	101.879	106.629	112.329	116.321	128.261
90	92.761	96.524	101.054	107.565	113.145	118.136	124.116	128.299	140.782
100	102.946	106.906	111.667	118.498	124.342	129.561	135.807	140.169	153.167
120	123.289	127.616	132.806	140.233	146.567	152.211	158.950	163.648	177.603
140	143.604	148.269	153.854	161.827	168.613	174.648	181.840	186.847	201.683
160	163.898	168.876	174.828	183.311	190.516	196.915	204.530	209.824	225.481
180	184.173	189.446	195.743	204.704	212.304	219.044	227.056	232.620	249.048
200	204.434	209.985	216.609	226.021	233.994	241.058	249.445	255.264	272.423

Index